ATTACHMENT THEORY APPLIED

Also from Mario Mikulincer and Phillip R. Shaver

Attachment in Adulthood, Second Edition:
Structure, Dynamics, and Change
Mario Mikulincer and Phillip R. Shaver

Attachment Theory Expanded: Security Dynamics
in Individuals, Dyads, Groups, and Societies
Mario Mikulincer and Phillip R. Shaver

Dynamics of Romantic Love:
Attachment, Caregiving, and Sex
Mario Mikulincer and Gail S. Goodman, Editors

Handbook of Attachment, Third Edition:
Theory, Research, and Clinical Applications
Jude Cassidy and Phillip R. Shaver, Editors

Attachment Theory Applied

Fostering Personal Growth through Healthy Relationships

Mario Mikulincer
Phillip R. Shaver

THE GUILFORD PRESS
New York London

A Division of Guilford Publications, Inc.
370 Seventh Avenue, Suite 1200, New York, NY 10001
www.guilford.com

Printed in the United States of America

This book is printed on acid-free paper.

Last digit is print number: 9 8 7 6 5 4 3 2 1

Library of Congress Cataloging-in-Publication Data is available from the publisher.

ISBN 978-1-4625-5233-7 (hardcover)

About the Authors

Mario Mikulincer, PhD, is Professor of Psychology and Founding Dean of the Baruch Ivcher School of Psychology at Reichman University in Israel. His research interests include attachment processes in adulthood, terror management theory, personality processes in interpersonal relationships, evolutionary psychology, human learned helplessness and depression, trauma and posttraumatic processes, and coping with stress. Dr. Mikulincer is a Fellow of the Association for Psychological Science and the Society for Personality and Social Psychology. He is a recipient of Israel's EMET Prize for Art, Science, and Culture and of the Berscheid–Hatfield Award for Distinguished Mid-Career Achievement from the International Association for Relationship Research.

Phillip R. Shaver, PhD, is Distinguished Professor Emeritus of Psychology at the University of California, Davis. He has published numerous books, including *Handbook of Attachment,* and over 400 journal articles and book chapters. Dr. Shaver's research focuses on attachment, human motivation and emotion, close relationships, personality development, and the effects of meditation on behavior and brain. He is a Fellow of the American Psychological Association and the Association for Psychological Science and is past president of the International Association for Relationship Research, from which he received the Distinguished Career Award. He has also received an honorary doctorate from Stockholm University and Distinguished Career Awards from the Society of Experimental Social Psychology and the Society for Personality and Social Psychology. He is an elected member of the American Academy of Arts and Sciences.

Preface

This book began in a conversation with Seymour Weingarten, then Editor-in-Chief of The Guilford Press, at the 2019 convention of the Society for Personality and Social Psychology. We were discussing the number of new books related to attachment theory and research and were considering what might still be missing. We noted that researchers in a variety of fields (e.g., individual and couple psychotherapy, parenting, medicine, education, business management, religion) were beginning to create and evaluate applications and interventions based on attachment theory and the large body of basic research it had inspired. We had been contributors to that research but hadn't been much involved in applications. Seymour invited us to submit a proposal for a book on applications of attachment theory and research. We did, and here, 4 years later, is the result.

We were stunned, and at first somewhat overwhelmed, by the number of applications and interventions already underway. To get a grasp of the large and sprawling literature, indicated by the size of this book's bibliography, we had to do a lot of reading and condensing. We hope the result proves accessible and valuable to several different audiences, including people who might want to adopt one of the interventions we describe, those who want to create and test a novel intervention, or those who merely want to think about attachment issues in their own personal, family, or social lives.

We begin the book with an overview of the basic concepts of attachment theory, a review of research on the "broaden-and-build" cycle of attachment security, and a discussion of the core principles that guide applications of attachment theory aimed at fostering personal growth through healthy relationships. We then show how simple laboratory "security priming" interventions can have beneficial effects on felt security and its psychological and behavioral sequelae. From there, we consider various kinds of existing applications and interventions designed to enhance felt security in parent–child relationships, couple and marital relationships, counseling and psychotherapy relationships, group relationships, and teacher–student relationships, and we propose new applications for medicine, leadership, and organizational development. In each of these domains, we provide the theoretical and research foundation for attachment-based interventions, present their core and distinctive features, and evaluate evidence for their effectiveness.

Along the way we explain what has been missing from some of the evaluation studies and what still needs to be examined. Despite our taking a constructively critical stance toward the studies, we consistently convey our high regard for applied researchers who have had the courage and stamina to undertake complex and time-consuming interventions and evaluations.

We are sincerely grateful to the many people who have contributed their creativity, intelligence, energy, and generosity to this research enterprise. And we are grateful to everyone who helped make this book possible. First, we thank Seymour Weingarten for helping us conceive the book. He and his colleagues at The Guilford Press have been wonderful supporters of attachment theory and the scholars who work within its framework. In creating this book, we had support from Seymour and from Editorial and Contracts Administrator Carolyn Graham, Senior Production Editor Anna Nelson, Art Director Paul Gordon, and copy editor extraordinaire Jacquelyn Coggin. We thank our friend and colleague Professor Jude Cassidy, who encouraged us to write the book and provided useful comments on an early draft. We are also grateful to Professors Chery Marmarosh, Robert Maunder, Angela Rowe, and Sigal Zilcha-Mano, who read the penultimate version of the manuscript and provided insightful comments and helpful suggestions.

Finally, we owe a huge debt of gratitude to our family members, who put up with our frequent absences and moments of distraction while we worked on this book for several years.

Contents

CHAPTER 1

An Overview of Attachment Theory and Research

Attachment theory—a psychological theory concerning the formation, maintenance, and breaking of emotional bonds between people—has had an enormous influence on psychological research in the areas of child–parent relationships and other kinds of close relationships, including friendships and romantic relationships. More recently it has been extended into domains as diverse as education, organizational management, and religion. The measures and basic research methods created in the attachment field are being adapted for practical use in a variety of therapeutic, educational, and management settings.

The purpose of this book is to examine a diverse set of examples of such applications, evaluating them in relation to both the present state of the theory and the goals of the application designers. In each area of application, we also examine evidence (whether existing or still needed) regarding the quality of the applications' results. We begin this chapter with a brief history of attachment theory and research, which should allow the reader to understand how each kind of application is rooted in basic theory and research, and how all of the diverse applications share a core framework, which can be used to create future applications.

Plan of the Book

In his exposition of attachment theory, John Bowlby (1973, 1980, 1969/1982) emphasized the importance of positive interactions with caring, loving relationship partners that, over time, create a persisting sense of attachment security (confidence that one is worthy of love and respect, and that other people will be available and supportive if needed). Bowlby viewed this sense of security as important for physical and mental health, interpersonal relationship quality, and ethical, prosocial behavior. Building on his ideas and on research begun by Mary Ainsworth and her students (Ainsworth, 1967; Ainsworth et al., 1971, 1978), we (Mikulincer & Shaver, 2003) proposed that interactions with caring, loving relationship partners foster a *broaden-and-build* cycle of attachment security, which increases resilience and expands a person's perspectives and capabilities. (The term *broaden-and-build* is borrowed from Barbara Fredrickson's 2001 theory of the evolutionary function of positive emotions.)

By relying on socially sensitive, responsive, and supportive relationship partners, a secure person can remain relatively unperturbed in times of stress, relying on a reservoir of positive beliefs about other people's benevolence and one's own competence and worth. Feeling safe and protected (having a "safe haven," in attachment theory's terms), a secure person can devote mental and physical resources to constructive, useful purposes (e.g., exploration, play, learning) rather than expend them on worry and psychological defenses. Moreover, being confident that support is available when needed (what attachment theorists call a "secure base for exploration"), secure individuals can take calculated risks, experiment with alternative possibilities and make mistakes, and engage in challenging activities that broaden their skills and perspectives.

During the past 30 years, attachment researchers have provided extensive cross-sectional, prospective-longitudinal, and laboratory-experimental evidence concerning the psychological benefits of possessing a sense of attachment security and of experiencing the broaden-and-build effects of actual and imagined interactions with caring, loving others. (We include "imagining" such interactions because people often think about, reminisce about, and dream about interactions with security providers, including ones who are no longer around or who "exist" in a spiritual realm or dimension; Mikulincer & Shaver, 2007.) Studies conducted around the world have largely supported the universality of the broaden-and-build effects of attachment security (see Erdman et al., 2010, for review chapters), but much of the research, beginning with Bowlby, has been based on White European and North American samples (Dawson, 2018), so we still need more research involving non-White nations and minorities, especially African Americans, in the United States (Stern et al., 2022). (It's worth mentioning that Ainsworth's first book, published in 1967, was based on an observational study in Uganda, so her understanding of attachment, elaborated in studies of White American mother–infant dyads, was informed by research in Africa.)

The large body of subsequent research on attachment, especially in its adolescent and adult forms, was reviewed and integrated in our 2016 book *Attachment in Adulthood* (Mikulincer & Shaver, 2016; see also Cassidy & Shaver, 2016). This body of research and its contribution to the further elaboration of attachment theory has encouraged researchers and practitioners in various fields to apply the theory in the development of interventions to foster people's well-being and successful relationships across the lifespan.

The proposed interventions are intended to enhance people's sense of attachment security and support the resulting broaden-and-build effects. These interventions expose people to positive interactions with a responsive and caring relationship partner either by priming thoughts and memories of such interactions or by training an actual relationship partner to become more responsive, compassionate, and caring in times of need (i.e., to serve as a "safe haven") and to provide a "secure base" for exploration. Evidence is accumulating that such interventions can produce positive changes in mental health, relationship quality, prosocial behavior, and the pursuit of personal goals.

Attachment theory and research have been successfully applied in diverse interventions in the domains of parent–child relationships, friendships, couple and family relationships, teacher–student relationships, and therapist–client relationships. Numerous studies indicate, or at least suggest, that the same principles and methods can be applied in other life domains such as health and medicine, management and organizational behavior, and intra- and intergroup relations. The time has arrived, therefore, for a book that integrates the growing body of knowledge concerning applications of attachment theory, organizes this knowledge for a diverse audience, and provides a foundation for new investigators and professionals in various fields who wish to apply what has been learned so far. In this book, we systematically survey and evaluate existing attachment-based interventions and provide a theoretical and empirical foundation for applying what has been learned to the many life domains that can benefit from security-enhancing interventions.

After briefly reviewing attachment theory's core concepts in the present chapter, and then summarizing evidence for the broaden-and-build cycle of attachment security in the next chapter, we devote the remaining chapters to analyzing and evaluating existing attachment-based interventions and proposals for new applications, including ones relevant to higher levels of social organization (e.g., businesses, governments).

Specifically, in Chapter 3, we review laboratory interventions, labeled "security priming" interventions, which momentarily enhance a person's sense of attachment security and thereby improve emotion regulation, personal well-being, goal pursuit, and prosocial behavior. In Chapters 4–10, we consider interventions designed to enhance attachment security in parent–child relationships, couple and marital relationships, counseling and psychotherapy relationships, group relationships, and teacher–student relationships. In all of these domains, the goal is to encourage a key relationship partner (e.g., parent, spouse, psychotherapist, teacher) or a group to be more effective at providing security. With respect to each of these domains, we explain the theoretical and research foundation for the interventions, review existing intervention programs, evaluate the evidence for their effectiveness, and propose new avenues for research and application. In Chapters 11 and 12, we turn to additional life domains in which applications of attachment theory may be useful, such as medicine and health care, and business management and organizational behavior.

Our goals are to showcase what has been accomplished so far in applying attachment theory and research, and to encourage experts and practitioners in the fields of counseling, psychotherapy, education, medicine, social work, public health, leadership, and business administration to develop additional or improved attachment-based interventions.

But before examining the many promising applications of attachment theory, we need to provide, in the remainder of this chapter, a brief overview of attachment theory and research so readers can understand the theory that is being put into application. We begin with an account of the origins of attachment theory during the 1960s and 1970s in the work of John Bowlby and Mary Ainsworth. We then explain how we became involved with extensions of the theory in the 1980s. Next, we describe the theory itself, placing special emphasis on both (1) its normative (species-general) components (e.g., the attachment behavioral system, the interplay of this system with other behavioral systems) and (2) its individual-differences components (e.g., working models of self and others, attachment orientations or styles). Finally, we consider the development of a person's attachment orientation or style from infancy to adulthood, and its stability and change across the lifespan.

The Origins of Attachment Theory

Attachment theory was created by John Bowlby, a British psychoanalyst, and then greatly strengthened by the theoretical and empirical contributions of Mary Ainsworth, an American child-developmental psychologist. As we explain later in this chapter, Bowlby's theory and Ainsworth's theoretical contributions and research findings were extended into adult personality and social psychology by Hazan and Shaver (1987). Their work has generated an enormous and sprawling research and intervention literature over the last 35 years.

John Bowlby

Bowlby was born in England, in 1907, to economically comfortable and well-educated parents. His father was a physician, and John eventually became one as well—a psychiatrist. While studying to become a child psychiatrist, Bowlby undertook psychoanalytic training with a famous mentor, Melanie Klein, and was psychoanalyzed for several years by Joan Riviere, a close associate of Klein. From these mentors, Bowlby learned about the importance of early infants' interactions with their primary caregivers; the tendency of troubled children to deal with traumatic separations and losses from caregivers by defensively excluding these painful experiences from conscious memory; and the arousal of anxiety, anger, and sadness during frustrating parent–child interactions. Despite absorbing many of Klein's and Riviere's ideas, however, Bowlby rejected their exclusive emphasis on children's fantasies at the expense of ignoring children's actual experiences, and on sexual drives rather than other social motives.

Attachment theory grew out of Bowlby's experiences as a family therapist at the Tavistock Clinic in London, where social and family relationships were considered alongside individual psychodynamics as causes of psychological and social disorders. Bowlby was also influenced by preparing a report for the World Health Organization on children who were orphans following World War II.

As Bowlby's clinical observations and insights accumulated, he became increasingly interested in explaining what, in his first major statement of attachment theory, he called "the child's tie to his mother" (Bowlby, 1958). In formulating the theory, he was influenced by Konrad Lorenz's (1952) ideas about "imprinting" in precocial birds and the writings of other ethologists and primatologists, including the primatologist Robert Hinde (1966). These authors, along with the American psychologist Harry Harlow (1959), had begun to show that immature animals' ties to their mothers were not due simply to classical conditioning based on feeding, as learning theorists (and, using different language, psychoanalysts) had thought. Instead, Bowlby viewed the human infant's reliance on, and emotional bond with, its mother to be the result of a fundamental instinctual behavioral system that, unlike Freud's sexual libido concept, was viewed as social-relational rather than sexual.

Bowlby expanded his preliminary articles and lectures about core aspects of attachment into three substantial books, *Attachment and Loss*, Volumes 1, 2, and 3, which are now recognized as landmarks of modern psychology, psychiatry, and social science. The first volume, *Attachment*, was published in 1969 and revised in 1982; the second, *Separation: Anxiety and Anger*, was published in 1973; and the third, *Loss: Sadness and Depression*, was published in 1980. These comprehensive volumes were accompanied in 1979 by a published collection of Bowlby's lectures, *The Making and Breaking of Affectional Bonds*, and were supplemented in 1988 by *A Secure Base*, a book devoted to applying attachment theory and research to psychotherapy. Bowlby died in 1990, having won many professional awards.

Mary Ainsworth

Bowlby's major collaborator, Mary Salter Ainsworth, was born in Ohio in 1913, and received her PhD in developmental psychology from the University of Toronto in 1939, after completing a dissertation on security and dependency that was inspired by her advisor William Blatz's security theory. In her dissertation, *An Evaluation of Adjustment Based on the Concept of Security* (1940), Ainsworth mentioned for the first time what eventually became a central part of attachment theory, the secure-base construct, which emphasized the importance of parents' provision of what Ainsworth called a "secure base" from which children can explore the world with the confidence that parents' support and protection will be available when needed.

When she moved to London with her husband, Ainsworth answered a newspaper ad for a research position with Bowlby, without having known about him or his work beforehand. Part of her job was to analyze films of children's separations from mother. These films convinced her of the value of behavioral observations, which were the centerpiece of her contributions to attachment research. When her husband decided in 1953 to advance his career by undertaking cultural research in Uganda, Ainsworth moved there as well and began an observational study of mothers and infants, whom she visited every 2 weeks for 2 hours of observation over a period of several months. Eventually, after returning to North America and becoming a faculty member at Johns Hopkins University, in 1967 Ainsworth published a book entitled *Infancy in Uganda: Infant Care and the Growth of Love.*

One of the intellectually and historically significant features of Ainsworth's 1967 book was an appendix that sketched different patterns of infant attachment. Although these patterns were not precisely the same as the three attachment types for which Ainsworth later became famous (called *secure, anxious,* and *avoidant* in our work; see Ainsworth et al., 1978, for the original descriptions and labels), some definite similarities are evident. The three main patterns of attachment delineated in the 1978 book were based on its 1967 predecessor, but they were greatly refined by intensive studies of White middle-class American infants in Baltimore, Maryland. In these American studies, Ainsworth and her students recorded detailed home observations during infants' first year of life and supplemented them with a new laboratory assessment procedure, the Strange Situation.

Ainsworth et al.'s 1978 book explains how to code an infant's behavior with mother in the Strange Situation, and also shows how the three major forms of infant attachment are associated with particular patterns of maternal behavior at home. The measures and ideas advanced in the 1978 book, taken in conjunction with Bowlby's theoretical books on attachment, separation, and loss, form the backbone of all subsequent discussions of normative attachment processes and individual differences in attachment behavior. Having published numerous pathbreaking papers, won many awards, and mentored several central figures in the attachment field, Mary Ainsworth died in 1999.

Our Extension of Attachment Theory into Social Psychology

By the time we began to use attachment theory, in the late 1980s, it had been extensively tested in studies of infant and child development, and Ainsworth's infant attachment categories were well known. For various reasons, including (we believe) the increasing number of women entering the field of social psychology (Elaine Hatfield and Ellen Berscheid being two prominent and highly influential examples), the increasing divorce rate in the United States, and a concern with growing prevalence of loneliness in industrialized societies (e.g., Peplau & Perlman, 1982), social psychologists were beginning to concern themselves with the formation, maintenance, and dissolution of close relationships. This concern was manifested in the creation of new professional organizations focused on the study of romantic and marital relationships and in a landmark 1983 book, *Close Relationships,* edited by Harold Kelley, one of the most prominent social psychologists of his (or any other) generation, along with Ellen Berscheid and seven others. Suddenly the study of love was not merely professionally acceptable, it was highly visible, even in such top-tier journals as *Psychological Review* (e.g., Sternberg, 1986).

A problem during that period, at least in our estimation, was the prominence in social psychology of the *attitude* construct, which had concerned the field for decades. Its familiarity caused researchers, at first, to consider love to be just another attitude (e.g., Hendrick & Hendrick, 1986). Little consideration was given to the fact that romantic and parental love had existed for millennia, and that the inherent importance of love, separation, and loss could be seen in the lives of both humans and nonhuman primates (Bowlby, 1980; Harlow, 1959). These were the days before evolutionary perspectives became popular in social psychology. Moreover, social psychologists were generally unaware that psychoanalysts from Freud to Bowlby had written a great deal about the psychodynamics of filial and romantic love, and about the relation of romantic love to sexuality. We were unusual among social psychologists in having been deeply interested in psychoanalysis since first encountering it during our undergraduate years.

In our view, anyone who pays close attention to what goes on in people's lives, or who reads romantic novels or poems or studies art or film, realizes that the issues raised by psychoanalysts, beginning with Freud, are crucial: sexual attraction and desire; romantic love and longing; the development of personality in the crucible of family relationships; painful, corrosive emotions such as anger, fear, jealousy, grief, hatred, shame, and remorse, which contribute to intrapsychic conflicts, defenses, and psychopathology and to intergroup hostility and war. Given our personal interests, social psychology at first seemed superficial compared with psychoanalysis. Nevertheless, social psychology's strong point—which was the fatally weak point of psychoanalysis—was the use of experimental methods and creative experimental manipulations and interventions to test theory-based hypotheses. Psychoanalytic theorists seemed capable of endlessly inventing hypothetical constructs and invisible mental processes without being constrained by operational definitions, sound psychometrics, or replicable empirical methods. Fortunately, social psychology was capable of rendering certain aspects of psychodynamic theories testable.

Both of us began our careers as experimental researchers pursuing then-popular topics in social and personality psychology (stress and learned helplessness in Mikulincer's case, self-awareness and fear of success in the case of Shaver), but our interest in psychoanalytic theory never waned. When we encountered Bowlby's books, we realized that a psychoanalytic theorist could incorporate and integrate the full range of scientific perspectives on human behavior, seek empirical evidence for psychoanalytic propositions, and amend or reformulate psychoanalytic theory based on empirical research. Ainsworth's development of the laboratory Strange Situation assessment procedure, which allowed her to systematically classify infants' attachment behavior into clear patterns and relate them to reliable observations of parent–child interactions at home, added to our confidence that extending attachment theory and its research methods into the realm of adolescent and adult love relationships might be possible and fruitful.

In the mid-1980s, Shaver was studying adolescent and adult loneliness (e.g., Rubenstein & Shaver, 1982; Shaver & Hazan, 1984) and noticing both that attachment theory was useful in conceptualizing loneliness (e.g., Weiss, 1973) and that patterns of chronic loneliness were similar in certain respects to the insecure infant attachment patterns identified by Ainsworth and her colleagues in the Strange Situation (1978). Building on this insight, one of Shaver's doctoral students, Cindy Hazan (now a faculty member at Cornell University), wrote a seminar paper suggesting that attachment theory could be used as a framework for studying romantic love—or "romantic attachment," as she and Shaver called it in their initial article on the topic (Hazan & Shaver, 1987).

This article caught the eye of Mikulincer, who had become interested in attachment theory while studying learned helplessness, depression, combat stress reactions, and posttraumatic stress disorder in Israel. He noticed similarities between (1) certain forms of helplessness in adulthood and the effects of parental unavailability in infancy; (2) intrusive images and emotions in the case of posttraumatic stress disorder and the anxious attachment pattern described by Ainsworth et al. (1978) and Hazan and Shaver (1987); and (3) avoidant strategies for coping with stress and the avoidant attachment pattern described by these same authors. In 1990, Mikulincer, Florian, and Tolmacz published a seminal study of attachment patterns and conscious and unconscious death anxiety, one of the first studies to use the preliminary self-report measure of adult attachment patterns devised by Hazan and Shaver (1987), and the first to show its ability to illuminate unconscious mental processes.

From then on, both of us continued to pursue the application of attachment theory in studies of adults' emotions, emotion-regulation strategies, and close relationships, noticing that we were both interested in the experimental study of what might be called attachment-related psychodynamics: the kinds of mental processes, including intense needs, powerful emotions and conflicts, and defensive strategies, that had captivated the attention of both Freud and Bowlby. We decided to pool our efforts to craft a more rigorous formulation of adult attachment theory (e.g., Mikulincer & Shaver, 2003; Shaver & Mikulincer, 2002), test the model in many different ways, including the use of priming techniques developed by cognitive psychologists, and incorporate within our theory some of positive psychology's emphasis on personal growth and social virtues (e.g., Seligman, 2002). Today, adult attachment theory, as summarized in our 2016 book, is one of the leading approaches to research on social relationships, personality processes, and the psychodynamic nature of the human mind.

Normative Aspects of Attachment Theory

Having considered the biographical backgrounds of Bowlby and Ainsworth, as well as our own histories, we can turn to attachment theory itself, placing special emphasis on Bowlby's notion of the "attachment behavioral system." There are two crucial parts of attachment theory, one of which is called "normative" because it deals with normal, universal features of the attachment behavioral system, and the other of which concerns individual differences in attachment-related mental representations and behavioral orientations. We begin our account of the theory by focusing first on its normative component.

The Attachment Behavioral System: Goals, Activation, and Functioning

One of the core tenets of attachment theory (Bowlby, 1973, 1980, 1969/1982) is that human beings are innately equipped with a psychobiological system (the *attachment behavioral system*) that motivates them to seek proximity to caring and protective others (whom Bowlby [1982] called *attachment figures*) in times of danger, threats, and challenges. The main function of this species-universal, biologically evolved neural system, or "program," is to protect people from danger and sustain their healthy development (especially during infancy and early childhood) by motivating them to maintain proximity to another person who is "stronger and wiser," and who can effectively provide them with safety, comfort, assistance, and encouragement. In Bowlby's view, the innate propensity to seek proximity and support from attachment figures in times of need evolved in relation to the prolonged helplessness and dependence on caregivers of human infants who cannot defend themselves from predators and other dangers. According to Bowlby's evolutionary reasoning, infants who maintained proximity to a supportive caregiver were more likely to survive and eventually to reproduce, causing genes that fostered seeking proximity and support from attachment figures to be selected for and passed on to subsequent generations.

In Bowlby's (1969/1982) view, assuring or maintaining proximity to an attachment figure (*attachment behaviors*) in times of need is not a goal in itself but only a means for sustaining or restoring a sense of safety and security—the "set goal" of the attachment system. This inner sense is rooted in beliefs that the world is generally safe, that one is loved and cared for, and that one can explore the world and move away from attachment figures with the confidence that they will be available if needed.

Elaborating the theory, Ainsworth (1991) proposed that people turn to attachment figures for two main security-related provisions: a physical and emotional *safe haven* (i.e., protection, distress alleviation, comfort, and reassurance) and a *secure base* from which to explore, learn, and thrive in a confident and relaxed manner. In her view, the set goal of the attachment system is twofold: (1) to feel protected and comforted by an attachment figure when threatened and (2) to feel that one's strivings for competence and autonomy are encouraged and supported by this figure. In other words, when working properly, attachment behavior can restore emotional equanimity following threats and dangers, and can sustain safe exploration when one is presented with novel opportunities and challenges. Attachment behavior can move a person from distress to relief (its safe-haven function) but then, of special importance in this book, also move him or her beyond safety to exploration and further development (attachment's secure-base function).

Bowlby discussed several kinds of stimuli and situations that trigger proximity and support seeking: environmental threats that endanger a person's survival; "natural clues of danger" (stimuli that are not inherently dangerous but increase the likelihood of danger; e.g., darkness and loud or strange noises); physical illness, fatigue, and pain; anticipated or actual loss of personal resources (e.g., status, money, self-esteem); daily hassles, life stressors, and traumatic events; and reminders of mortality. After a particular person or group becomes an actual or potential safe haven and secure base, any sign of this figure's disapproval, criticism, or rejection can trigger efforts to restore proximity and support. These proximity-seeking efforts can also be triggered by impending or actual separation from, or loss of, an attachment figure (Bowlby, 1973, 1980). In other words, the possible unavailability of an actual or potential attachment figure can, like other dangers, activate the attachment system (Bowlby, 1973, 1982).

Besides being activated by threats and dangers, proximity seeking can also be activated when a person encounters new opportunities for exploration, learning, and personal development but feels afraid, uncertain, or ambivalent about them (Ainsworth, 1991). In such cases, a person can use an attachment figure for support, and as a reference point, or a *secure base*, for courageously moving forward. Serving as a secure base, an attachment figure can provide both encouragement to tackle new challenges and a safe place to which to retreat if a challenge becomes too difficult, threatening, or demoralizing (Ainsworth, 1991). People of all ages seem to seek a secure base whenever they need help in taking advantage of challenging opportunities or wish to be validated for their efforts and accomplishments (Feeney & Collins, 2019).

According to Bowlby (1969/1982), seeking proximity to a stronger and wiser person (a caregiver, an attachment figure) is the attachment system's natural and primary strategy when the need arises for protection, comfort, or reassurance in times of threat (*safe-haven support*) or support, encouragement, and validation when confronting novel or demanding challenges (*secure-base support*). Support- seeking includes signals (interaction bids) that tell a relationship partner one is interested in restoring or maintaining proximity; overt displays of negative emotion (e.g., anger, anxiety, sadness) that call upon a partner to provide support and comfort; active approach behaviors that result in greater physical or psychological contact, including what Harlow (1959) called "contact comfort"; and explicit requests for emotional or instrumental support. According to Bowlby, not all of these behaviors are likely to be manifested in every threatening or challenging situation; that is, they are not controlled by rigid reflexes. Rather, they are part of a repertoire of behaviors from which an individual can choose (consciously or unconsciously) the most appropriate or available means of attaining a safe haven or secure base in a given situation. These bids for support persist until security is attained, and the comforted and empowered individual can move on to other activities.

This latter step is worth emphasizing, because attachment theory does not view continual clinging or perpetual dependency as the evolutionary function of attachment behavior. The function is to provide safety and protection (safe-haven support), while at the same time encouraging the supported individual to move on to greater autonomy (secure-base support). The ultimate payoff, viewed from an evolutionary perspective, is the ability to grow up, find a mate (or mates), reproduce, and foster viable offspring (where viability depends on parental care, at least early on, as well as cooperation with other family and community members and groups).

Cognitive Aspects of the Attachment Behavioral System

Bowlby (1969/1982) claimed that the attachment system operates in a complex goal-corrected manner. A person evaluates the progress he or she is making toward achieving a safe haven or secure base and then, if necessary, corrects his or her behavior to produce the most effective action sequence. Viewed somewhat abstractly, this flexible, goal-directed and goal-corrected adjustment of attachment behavior requires at least three cognitive operations: (1) monitoring and appraising changes in the environment and one's own internal state (e.g., distress, security); (2) monitoring and appraising the attachment figure's responses to one's bids for safe-haven or secure-base support; and (3) monitoring and appraising the utility of the chosen behaviors in a given context, so that an effective adjustment of these behaviors can be made in accordance with contextual opportunities and constraints. These same cognitive mechanisms are included in every cybernetic, control-system model of self-regulation (e.g., Carver & Scheier, 2012), some of which influenced Bowlby's theorizing.

Bowlby (1973, 1969/1982) stressed that the goal-corrected nature of attachment behavior requires the storage of relevant information in the form of mental representations of one's interactions with attachment figures. Based on the theoretical writings of Craik (1943) and Young (1964), he called these representations *working models* and seemed to intend the word *working* to carry two senses: (1) The models allow for mental simulation and prediction of likely outcomes of attachment behaviors (i.e., they provide context-sensitive representations of complex social situations); and (2) the models are provisional (in the sense of "working" drafts or changeable plans); they can be altered if conditions warrant revisions.

Bowlby (1969/1982) distinguished between two kinds of working models: "If an individual is to draw up a plan to achieve a set-goal not only does he have some sort of working model of his environment, but he must have also some working knowledge of his own behavioral skills and potentialities" (p. 112). That is, everyone, after repeatedly seeking proximity and support from attachment figures in times of need, holds mental representations of the attachment figures' responses (*working models of others*) as well as representations of their own self-efficacy and value, or the lack thereof, during interactions with attachment figures (*working models of self*). These working models organize a person's memories of attachment figures and oneself during attempts to gain protection in times of need. These organized models include expectations about the kinds of behavior that will likely to lead to a sense of security (and those that will lead to rejection or punishment).

In his writings, Bowlby (1969/1982) also discussed the interplay between the attachment system and other behavioral systems. Because coping with threats and dangers must have high priority for biological survival, engagement in proximity- and support-seeking behavior usually inhibits or interferes with engagement in other activities. Under conditions of threat, people turn to others as providers of support and comfort rather than as partners for exploratory, affiliative, or sexual activities. Moreover, at such times, they are likely to be so focused on their own needs for protection and support that they lack the mental resources needed to explore and learn new things or to attend empathically and altruistically to others' needs. Only when relief is attained and a sense of attachment security is restored can the individual deploy ample attention and energy to other goal pursuits and engage fully and effectively in nonattachment activities.

Attachment-System Activation over the Course of the Lifespan

Bowlby (1969/1982, 1988) believed that the attachment system, which is critical for survival during infancy and early childhood, continues to operate throughout life, as indicated by adults' needs for positive regard, affection, comfort, and support (Zeifman & Hazan, 2016). Although Bowlby (1988) acknowledged that age and psychological development result in an increased ability to gain comfort and security from one's own inner resources (self-efficacy, memories of past support, self-soothing, and other emotion-regulation techniques), he also claimed that no one of any age is completely free of reliance on external protective figures when confronting illness, injury, death of loved others, aging, and other threats and traumas.

Of course, the attachment system may operate somewhat differently at different ages, despite needs for support and protection being similar across the lifespan. For example, the identity and type of targeted attachment figures tend to change with development. During infancy, primary caregivers (usually parents or other family members) occupy the role of attachment figures. During adolescence and adulthood, other relationship partners become additional potential targets for proximity and support seeking, including close friends and romantic and marital partners (see Zeifman & Hazan, 2016, for a review).

Beyond these relationship partners, people seek protection and support from people who are experts in particular domains, such as teachers, coaches, and mentors in educational settings, managers in work settings, therapists in clinical settings, health workers in medical settings, and leaders in organizational settings (Mikulincer & Shaver, 2020). Any of these people, depending on circumstances, can be perceived as potential sources, in context, of a safe haven and secure base and therefore become a target for support and proximity seeking in times of need. Moreover, other social or symbolic entities can be recruited as potential attachment figures: small groups (e.g., a work team, a group of friends); religious and community groups; larger social institutions (e.g., the workplace); pets; and God and other supernatural figures (e.g., Granqvist, 2020; Smith et al., 1999; Zilcha-Mano et al., 2012). These actual and symbolic sources of security provide the rationale for applying attachment theory and attachment-based interventions to different kinds of relationships and across different levels of social organization.

The tactics people use for attaining attachment security also tend to be different at different ages. In infancy, the tactics are largely innate (e.g., crying when frightened, reaching out to be picked up and held). As a child develops and enters more complex social relationships, the search for sources of protection becomes increasingly flexible, context-sensitive, and skillful (i.e., communicating needs and feelings verbally, regulating need expression in line with the preferences and role demands of an attachment figure). In adolescence and adulthood, the tactics are expanded to include many other methods of establishing contact and seeking support (e.g., phoning or FaceTiming an attachment figure, sending an email or text message). Moreover, the search for comfort and protection does not necessarily require actual contact with another person; it can include calling upon soothing, comforting mental representations (e.g., memories, visual and auditory images) of loving attachment figures. These mental representations can be activated not only intentionally (e.g., through memory/imagination exercises, Buddhist love and kindness meditation, prayer, nostalgic reveries), but also activated automatically, without conscious deliberation, when a threat arises (Mikulincer & Shaver, 2007).

Bowlby's ideas about the predisposition to seek proximity to others as a means of obtaining care and protection have received extensive empirical support. In times of need, infants show a clear preference for their familiar caregiver(s), engage in intense proximity seeking, and are soothed by a caregiver's presence and support (e.g., Ainsworth, 1991). During adolescence and adulthood, research has shown that people are likely to turn to close relationship partners for support when threatened or distressed (e.g., Kammrath et al., 2020). Using laboratory cognitive techniques, we (e.g., Mikulincer et al., 2002) found that adults react to even minimal threat cues with activation of mental representations of attachment figures. In these studies, fast (implicit) exposure to a threat-related word (e.g., illness, failure) measurably increased the cognitive accessibility of attachment-figure representations, as indicated by faster lexical-decision times for the names of figures identified earlier in a questionnaire to be sources of safety and care (e.g., the name of a parent, spouse, or friend). Interestingly, these effects were not found for the names of people other than attachment figures, including family members who were not nominated as special security providers. Similar findings have been obtained in subsequent studies, where threats have been found to increase mental access to representations of symbolic sources of attachment security, such as a person's pet or God (Granqvist et al., 2012; Zilcha-Mano et al., 2012). These and many other research findings support Bowlby's claim that the human mind/brain turns automatically to attachment figures in times of threat.

There is also extensive evidence that separation from and loss of attachment figures is a powerful source of distress. Ethological observation of infants separated from their mothers (e.g., Robertson & Bowlby, 1952) revealed early in the history of attachment research that absence of an attachment figure causes intense distress, anxiety, anger, protest, and yearning. In adulthood, bereavement research has found that the death of a close relationship partner is one of the most painful experiences a person can endure, one that typically elicits extreme sorrow, despair, and painful longing for the deceased partner that can last for months or years (see Fraley & Shaver, 2016, for a review). Similar emotional reactions have been observed following the breakup of romantic relationships and divorce (for reviews, see Feeney & Monin, 2016; Sbarra et al., 2019).

Attachment-Related Individual Differences

As explained earlier, Bowlby (1969/1982) postulated an innate predisposition to seek proximity to supportive others in times of need in order to obtain a safe haven and secure base. But his ideas might not have captured the attention of developmental, personality, social, and clinical researchers if he had done only that. What captured research psychologists' attention were the patterns or styles of attachment emphasized in Bowlby's (1973, 1980) theory and operationalized in Ainsworth's research on mother–infant dyads (Ainsworth et al., 1978). Most of the research inspired by the theory focuses on those individual differences.

Although all human beings are born with the desire and capacity to seek proximity and comfort from attachment figures in times of need, important individual differences arise in the context of relationships from birth on. According to Bowlby (1973), a person's innate inclination for support-seeking and actual proximity-seeking behavior toward an attachment figure can be affected or shaped by the figure's responses. Over time, social encounters with an attachment figure adjust the parameters of a person's proximity-seeking bids in ways that produce fairly stable individual differences in cognition, emotion, and behavior. A person's neural and behavioral capacities become "programmed" to fit with the responses of major attachment figures. Bowlby assumed that the residues of such social encounters are stored in internal (i.e., mental) working models of self and other, and that these mental representations shape the way a person reacts to threats and searches for protection from an attachment figure.

Bowlby (1973) placed great emphasis on the individual differences in attachment behavior that develop as a result of the availability, responsiveness, and supportiveness of key attachment figures, especially in times of threat or need. When attachment figures are reliably available when needed, sensitive to one's attachment needs, and willing and able to respond warmly to bids for proximity and support, a person of any age feels more secure, valued, and understood and is more able to explore the physical and social environment curiously and competently. These experiences increase a person's confidence in proximity and support seeking as protective measures and build positive working models of self and others, which are important for maintaining emotional stability and for forming mature, mutually satisfying close interpersonal relationships.

However, when attachment figures are not reliably available and supportive, this sense of security is not attained, doubts about one's lovability and worries about others' motives and intentions are formed, and a person loses confidence in the efficacy of his or her proximity-seeking bids as means to achieve protection and security. As a result, *secondary strategies* of affect regulation come into play. According to Cassidy and Kobak (1988), there are two kinds of secondary strategies: *hyperactivation* and *deactivation* of the attachment system.

Hyperactivation (which Bowlby, 1969/1982, called "protest") is characterized by energetic, insistent attempts to induce a relationship partner, viewed as insufficiently available or responsive, to pay more attention and provide better care and support. Hyperactivating strategies are exaggerations of the primary attachment strategy—intense, anxious monitoring of attachment figures and strong efforts to gain and maintain proximity. They include clinging, controlling, and coercive responses; cognitive and behavioral efforts to establish physical contact and experiences a sense of oneness; and overdependence on relationship partners as a source of protection (Shaver & Mikulincer, 2002). Hyperactivation keeps the attachment system chronically activated and constantly on the alert for threats, separations, and betrayals; it therefore unintentionally exacerbates relational conflict, heightens distress associated with attachment-figure unavailability, and reinforces doubts about one's ability ever to attain a sense of security (Mikulincer & Shaver, 2003).

Deactivation refers to inhibition or down-regulation of proximity-seeking inclinations and actions, suppression or discounting of threats that might activate these inclinations, and determination to handle threats and distress alone (a stance that Bowlby [1969/1982] called "compulsive self-reliance"). These strategies involve maintaining physical and emotional distance from others, being uncomfortable with intimacy and interdependence, ignoring or downplaying threat- and attachment-related cues, and suppressing threat- and attachment-related thoughts (Cassidy & Kobak, 1988). These tendencies are bolstered by an attitude of self-reliance that reduces dependence on others and discourages acknowledgment of personal faults.

It is important to note that both anxious hyperactivation and avoidant deactivation of the attachment system are well-organized, adaptive responses to interactions with a cold, frustrating, unstable, unreliable, or rejecting relationship partner. When developed in infancy, they can be viewed as reasonable, perhaps necessary forms of adaptation to a non-optimal caregiving environment. When continued into adolescence and adulthood, however, hyperactivation and deactivation strategies tend to be problematic for both oneself and one's relationship partners (for a review of relevant research, see Mikulincer & Shaver, 2016).

Assessing Attachment-Related Individual Differences in Early Childhood

In examining these individual differences in attachment-system functioning, researchers have focused mainly on a person's *attachment style*—the pattern of relational needs, cognitions, emotions, and behaviors that results from satisfying or frustrating interactions with attachment figures (Fraley & Shaver, 2000). These styles were first described by Ainsworth (1967; Ainsworth et al., 1978) based on observations of infants' responses to separations from and reunions with mother in the laboratory Strange Situation, mentioned earlier, which was designed to activate an infant's attachment behaviors. Ainsworth classified infants into one of three categories, which we label *secure, anxious,* or *avoidant.* Main and Solomon (1990) later added a fourth category, *disorganized,* characterized by odd, disoriented behavior and unusual alternations or mixtures of anxiety and avoidance.

Infants classified as secure seem to possess easily accessible working models of successful proximity-seeking attempts and security attainment. In the Strange Situation, they tend to exhibit distress during separations from mother but then recover quickly following reunions and continue to explore the environment with interest. When reunited with the mother, they greet her with joy and affection, initiate contact with her, and respond positively to being held, after which they quickly reestablish interest in the toys provided in the experimental setting (i.e., they explore). During home observations, mothers of these infants are emotionally available in times of need and responsive to their child's proximity-seeking behavior (Ainsworth et al., 1978). It seems reasonable to characterize these mothers as sources of attachment security and as reinforcing reliance on what attachment theorists consider to be the primary attachment strategy (seeking proximity and comfort when needed).

Avoidant infants seem to possess working models conducive to attachment-system deactivation. In the Strange Situation, they show little distress when separated from their mother and tend to avoid her when she returns. In home observations, the avoidant infants' mothers tend to be emotionally rigid, as well as angry at and rejecting of their infants' proximity-seeking efforts (Ainsworth et al., 1978).

Anxious infants seem to possess working models related to attachment-system hyperactivation. In the Strange Situation, they are extremely distressed during separations and exhibit conflicted, angry, or ambivalent responses to their mother during reunions (e.g., they may cling one moment and angrily resist comforting the next, which was Ainsworth's reason for sometimes calling them "anxious/ambivalent" or "anxious/resistant"). During home observations, interactions between anxious infants and their mothers are characterized by lack of harmony and lack of caregivers' consistent responsiveness (Ainsworth et al., 1978).

Mothers of both avoidant and anxious infants seem to thwart security attainment, thereby fostering their children's adoption of secondary attachment strategies. However, whereas avoidant infants deactivate their attachment system in response to attachment-figure unavailability, anxious infants tend to hyperactivate the system in an attempt to gain more reliable support from their attachment figure.

Disorganized/disoriented infants, the fourth style or type of attachment, seem to suffer from a breakdown of organized attachment strategies (primary/secure, hyperactivating, or deactivating). They either randomly oscillate between strategies or do something bizarre like lying face down on the floor without moving when their mother appears following a separation or sitting passively under a table, evincing no clear proximity-seeking strategy (Main & Solomon, 1990). These odd behaviors seem to be a response to disorganized, unpredictable, and discomfiting behavior on the part of an attachment figure who, research shows, is likely to be suffering from unresolved losses or unresolved attachment-related traumas (e.g., Lyons-Ruth & Jacobvitz, 2016). When her child approaches her for comfort and reassurance, she sometimes looks frightened, looks away, or "spaces out" in a dissociative way, causing the child to stop abruptly, express confusion, and adopt whatever momentary strategy seems to reduce discomfort, such as turning away, diverting attention, or behaving self-protectively (e.g., hiding under a table). Longitudinal studies have linked attachment disorganization in the Strange Situation to severe emotional and personality disorders and poor relationship quality in adolescence and adulthood (Sroufe, 2020).

As we show in Chapters 2 and 4, several longitudinal studies and meta-analyses have found support for Ainsworth's original hypotheses and observations (e.g., Sroufe et al., 2005; Verhage et al., 2016; Zeegers et al., 2017). However, despite several cross-cultural studies of infant attachment around the world (e.g., Mesman, 2021; Mesman et al., 2016, 2018), most of this research has been conducted with predominantly White samples. Only a handful of attachment studies have been conducted in the United States with African American families (see Malda & Mesman, 2017, for a review). In these studies, African American families tend to be characterized by lower rates of both maternal sensitivity (as traditionally measured in White samples) and infant attachment security in the Strange Situation. These tendencies seem to reflect the action of broader ecological factors, such as inadequate financial resources, which interferes with consistent, effective caregiving (e.g., Bakermans-Kranenburg et al., 2004). This kind of interference is likely exacerbated by systemic racism, which contributes to parent–child separations, caregiver loss, and family trauma via disproportionate rates of incarceration, exclusionary school discipline, maternal and infant mortality, stress-related illnesses, police brutality, and child welfare removals (e.g., Barbarin, 2021). Although Bowlby's (1944) initial observations concerned delinquent boys from poor families, he did not consider these specific contextual factors. However, these kinds of factors are critical for understanding caregiving patterns, attachment, and socioemotional development within Black families.

Assessing Attachment-Related Individual Differences in Adolescence and Adulthood

In the 1980s, researchers from different psychological subdisciplines (developmental, clinical, personality, and social) created new attachment measures to extend attachment theory into adolescence and adulthood. Based on a developmental and clinical approach, Main and her colleagues (George et al., 1985; Main et al., 1985; see Hesse, 2016, for a review) devised the Adult Attachment Interview (AAI) to study adolescents' and adults' mental representations of attachment to their parents during childhood. One of the major findings of this approach to studying adult attachment is that an adult's AAI classification (secure, dismissing, preoccupied, or unresolved) predicts his or her infant's attachment pattern in the Strange Situation (see van IJzendoorn, 1995, for a review), even if the interview is conducted before the infant is born. In other words, there is good evidence for the intergenerational transmission of attachment patterns, which seems not to be primarily attributable to shared genes (Vaughn & Bost, 2016) but rather is a result of social experience.

In the AAI, interviewees answer open-ended questions about their childhood relationships with parents and are classified into three major categories paralleling Ainsworth's infant typology (George et al., 1985). A person is classified as *secure* (or free and autonomous with respect to attachment) if he or she describes parents as available and responsive, and verbalizes memories of relationships with parents that are clear, convincing, and coherent. Avoidant individuals (those who are *dismissing* of attachment) play down the importance of attachment relationships and tend to be unable or unwilling to recall specific episodes of emotional interactions with parents. Anxious individuals (those *preoccupied* with attachment) are entangled in worries and angry feelings about parents; are hypersensitive to rejection, separation, and loss; and can easily retrieve negative memories but have trouble discussing them coherently without becoming anxious, angry, or lost in long, emotional monologues. Both dismissing and preoccupied individuals are, in effect, inattentive to and uncooperative with the interviewer's needs, just as they tend to be out of tune with the needs of their infants.

Main et al. (1985) called their measurement strategy a "move to the level of representation," because, unlike the Strange Situation, which emphasizes an infant's behavior, the AAI assesses current adult mental representations of childhood attachment relationships as these are articulated in "coherent" or "incoherent" discourse with an interviewer. Despite the richness of AAI narratives, which are particularly useful in clinical settings, the interview is costly to administer and to score, and deals largely with memories of child–parent relationships. It does not directly measure attachment orientations in current close relationships or in other interpersonal and social contexts.

Working from a personality and social-psychological perspective, Hazan and Shaver (1987, 1990) developed a self-report measure of adult attachment style suitable for use in experiments and surveys. In its original form, the measure comprised three brief descriptions of feelings and behaviors in close relationships that were intended to characterize adult romantic analogues of the three infant attachment styles identified by Ainsworth et al. (1978), not including disorganized (which was discovered and named years after publication of Ainsworth et al.'s 1978 book). Participants were asked to read the descriptions and place themselves into one of the three attachment categories according to their predominant feelings and behavior in romantic relationships. The three descriptions were as follows:

- *Secure:* "I find it relatively easy to get close to others and am comfortable depending on them and having them depend on me. I don't worry about being abandoned or about someone getting too close to me."
- *Avoidant:* "I am somewhat uncomfortable being close to others; I find it difficult to trust them completely, difficult to allow myself to depend on them. I am nervous when anyone gets too close and often, others want me to be more intimate than I feel comfortable being."
- *Anxious:* "I find that others are reluctant to get as close as I would like. I often worry that my partner doesn't really love me or won't want to stay with me. I want to get very close to my partner and this sometimes scares people away."

In subsequent years, numerous researchers developed similar self-report measures, in some cases to improve the precision of the simple forced-choice measure and in other cases to tap attachment orientations beyond the romantic domain (see Crowell et al., 2016, for a review). With cumulative evidence, attachment researchers in the personality and social fields reached the conclusion that attachment styles are best conceptualized as regions in a two-dimensional (anxiety-by-avoidance) space. These two dimensions appear consistently in factor analyses of attachment measures (e.g., Brennan et al., 1998). (They were also obtained from a statistical discriminant-functions analysis of Ainsworth's Strange Situation data on mothers and infants; see Ainsworth et al., 1978. But few readers seemed to pay attention to the dimensional results.)

Researchers have found that dimensional representations of adolescent and adult attachment styles are more precise and accurate than categorical representations (e.g., Fraley et al., 2015). The first dimension, *attachment-related avoidance,* is concerned with discomfort with closeness and dependence on relationship partners, preference for emotional distance, and reliance on deactivating strategies. The second dimension, *attachment-related anxiety,* is concerned with a strong desire for closeness and protection, intense worries about others' responsiveness and one's own value and lovability, and reliance on hyperactivating strategies. People who score low on both dimensions are said to be secure or to have a secure attachment style. People who score high on both dimensions are sometimes called "fearful avoidant" (Bartholomew, 1990) and are perhaps adult versions of "disorganized" attachment in infants.

The two attachment-style dimensions can be measured with the 36-item Experiences in Close Relationships inventory (ECR; Brennan et al., 1998), which has high reliability, as well as construct, predictive, and discriminant validity (Crowell et al., 2016). (See Lafontaine et al., 2015, for a reliable and well-validated short form of the ECR.) This scale can be used to assess a person's global attachment orientation across relational domains, as well as his or her attachment orientation in a particular relational domain, or toward a specific attachment figure, or on a particular occasion (Fraley, Heffernan, et al., 2011; Gillath et al., 2009).

Studies using self-report measures of adult attachment style have found them to be predictably and coherently related to relationship quality, mental health, social adjustment, ways of coping, emotion regulation, self-esteem, interpersonal behavior, and social cognitions (see Chapter 2 for a review of these findings). Importantly, these individual differences in attachment style are not well explained by less specific, more global personality traits such as extraversion, neuroticism, or self-esteem, although there are predictable and meaningful associations between attachment measures and such personality traits (Mikulincer & Shaver, 2016).

Attachment-Related Mental Structures

Bowlby (1973, 1988) believed that individual differences in attachment style can be explained in terms of stored experiences of significant interactions or relationships with attachment figures, organized within an associative memory network. This stored knowledge allows a person to predict future interactions with attachment figures and adjust proximity-seeking efforts in times of need without having to rethink each one from the ground up. As reviewed earlier, Bowlby (1969/1982) called these cognitive structures *working models* of self and others. These mental models presumably operate at least partially at a conscious level and in a relatively reflective and intentional manner. But with repeated use, they can become automatic and may often operate outside of awareness either by habit or because of defensive maneuvers (e.g., repression, suppression, or deliberate inattention; Bowlby, 1980). These working models lie at the core of relatively stable attachment-style differences (Shaver et al., 1996).

During infancy, working models are based on particular interactions, or kinds of interactions, with an attachment figure. As a result, a child can hold multiple situation-specific working models that differ according to the outcome of the interaction (success or failure to attain security) and the strategy used to deal with insecurity during the interaction (hyperactivating or deactivating). With experience, and in the context of cognitive development, these working models form excitatory and inhibitory associations with each other. For example, experiencing or thinking about a security-enhancing interaction activates memories of similar security-enhancing episodes and renders memories of attachment insecurities and worries less accessible. These associations favor the formation of a more abstract and generalized working model of a specific attachment figure. Gradually, through excitatory and inhibitory links with models of other attachment figures, even more generic working models are formed that summarize attachment relationships in general.

This process of continual model construction and integration results, over time, in the creation of a hierarchical associative network that includes a wide variety of secure and insecure episodic memories, relationship-specific models, and generic working models of self and others. As a result, a person can sometimes think about an attachment figure in more secure terms and at other times in less secure terms (Mikulincer & Shaver, 2007). Moreover, the person can think about some attachment figures in more secure terms and about other attachment figures in less secure terms (Baldwin et al., 1996).

In a pioneering study, Overall et al. (2003) provided evidence for this hierarchical cognitive network of attachment working models. They asked people to complete attachment measures for three specific relationships within each of three domains—family, friendship, and romantic—and then examined the structure of these nine relationship descriptions. They found that a hierarchical arrangement of specific and global working models fit the data best, indicating that models of specific relationships (e.g., with a particular family member) are nested within relationship-domain representations (e.g., family members), which in turn are nested within a more global model.

The cognitive/neural network of attachment-related models has all of the usual properties of any such network—for example, differentiation, integration, and coherence among various models and model components (Collins & Read, 1994). In addition, each working model within the network differs in cognitive accessibility (the ease with which it can be activated and used to guide the functioning of the attachment system in a given social situation). As with other mental representations, the strength or accessibility of each model is determined by the amount of experience on which it is based, the number of times it has been applied in the past, and the density of its connections with other working models (Collins & Read, 1994). At a relationship-specific level, the model representing the typical interaction with an attachment figure has the highest accessibility in subsequent interactions with that person. At a more generic level, the model that represents typical interactions with major attachment figures (e.g., parents, romantic partners) becomes the most chronically accessible representation across situations and over time.

Consolidation of a chronically accessible working model is the most important psychological process accounting for the enduring effects on personality functioning of attachment interactions during infancy, childhood, and adolescence (Bowlby, 1973). Given a fairly consistent pattern of interaction with primary caregivers during infancy and childhood, the most representative or prototypical working models of these interactions become part of a person's implicit procedural knowledge, tend to operate automatically and unconsciously, and are resistant to change. Thus, what began as representations of specific interactions with primary caregivers during childhood become core personality characteristics, tend to be applied in new situations and relationships, and shape a person's overall attachment style in adulthood.

In the following passage, Bowlby (1979) described how these chronically accessible models shape a person's experience:

> [One] tends to assimilate any new person with whom he may form a bond, such as a spouse, or child, or employer, or therapist, to an existing model (either of one or other parent or of self), and often to continue to do so despite repeated evidence that the model is inappropriate. Similarly he expects to be perceived and treated by them in ways that would be appropriate to his self-model, and to continue with such expectations despite contrary evidence. (pp. 141–142)

Although the dominance of a particular working model depends on the history of attachment-related interactions, attachment theory also emphasizes the importance of contextual factors that contribute to model activation (Collins & Read, 1994). An individual can possess multiple, even conflicting, attachment inclinations, beyond the attachment orientation that was formed in childhood experiences with parents, and these models or inclinations can become dominant in particular relational, social, or laboratory contexts. As reviewed throughout this book, there is substantial evidence that a current interaction with a sensitive and responsive attachment figure, or even just thinking about this security-enhancing figure, has beneficial effects on attachment security, emotion regulation, social cognition, and relational behavior, even among people who are chronically insecure with respect to attachment (see Gillath & Karantzas, 2019; Gillath et al., 2022; Rowe et al., 2020, for reviews).

Developmental Aspects of the Theory: Stability and Change in Attachment Orientations

One of the pillars of attachment theory is the claim that childhood experiences play an important role in forming what will become a person's adult personality (Bowlby, 1973). This does not mean, however, that attachment theory can simply be equated with Freudian or object relations approaches to psychoanalysis. In fact, attachment theory offers a unique perspective on the development of working models and their interplay with contemporary interpersonal contexts as determinants of adult feelings, behaviors, and relationship outcomes. Specifically, Bowlby (1973) believed that the developmental trajectory of working models is not linear or simple, and that these mental representations in adulthood are not exclusively based on early experiences. Rather, they can be updated throughout life and affected by a broad array of contextual factors, such as current interactions with a relationship partner, the partner's attachment style and dynamics, and a person's current life situation, which can moderate or even override the effects of mental residues of past experiences. In fact, Bowlby (1973) preferred to use the term *working models* rather than *mental representations* or *schemas* in order to emphasize the changing, flexible nature of these cognitions.

Thus, attachment theory does not assert that a person's current attachment orientation must mirror or match his or her attachment orientations with parents during childhood. Rather, the current orientation is a complex amalgam of historical and contemporary factors, and it can be changed by updating and reworking mental representations of self and attachment figures. This assertion is worth emphasizing, because it allows for the development of interventions aimed at reworking a person's attachment-related working models and thereby heightening his or her sense of security.

Borrowing from Waddington's (1957) epigenetic landscape model, Bowlby (1973) proposed that the development of adult attachment orientations is constrained by two kinds of forces: (1) "homeothetic forces" that buffer changes in attachment orientations from infancy to adulthood, making it less likely that they will deviate from early working models, and (2) "destabilizing forces" that cause deviation from early working models given powerful experiences that demand revision and updating of attachment representations. Attachment research has provided evidence for both homeothetic and destabilizing forces. With regard to homeothetic forces, numerous studies have shown that attachment styles tend to remain stable over time (see Booth-LaForce & Roisman, 2021, for a review). Pinquart et al. (2013), for example, meta-analyzed results from 127 samples (N = 21,072 individuals) in studies that examined the stability of attachment security at 225 different time intervals, ranging from 2 weeks to 29 years. The overall stability coefficient for attachment security was .39 regardless of time interval. However, lower stability coefficients were found in intervals larger than 15 years. In short, attachment scores (assessed with self-report scales or the AAI) during adolescence and young adulthood do relate in theoretically meaningful ways to attachment patterns in early childhood (assessed with Ainsworth's laboratory Strange Situation procedure), but these associations are relatively small in magnitude (Fraley, 2019).

Some of the longitudinal studies that have assessed attachment patterns at different ages have also provided evidence of the action of destabilizing forces. In these studies, researchers gathered data concerning stressful attachment-unrelated events (e.g., natural disasters, financial crises, systemic racism) and stressful attachment-relevant events (e.g., death of a parent, parental divorce, physical or sexual abuse by a family member) and found that occurrence of these events during childhood or adolescence destabilized the trajectory of attachment patterns (e.g., Aikins et al., 2009; Booth-LaForce et al., 2014; Van Ryzin et al., 2011). Specifically, they increased the likelihood that what were once securely attached infants would later be classified as insecure. For example, Becker-Stoll et al. (2008) found that adolescents classified as securely attached at both age 1 and age 16 experienced significantly fewer stressful events than adolescents with unstable attachment patterns. Pinquart et al. (2013) reached a similar conclusion in their meta-analysis of studies of attachment stability. Specifically, they found that secure infants with a history of stressful events were less likely to maintain security during adolescence than secure infants who grew up in less stressful environments.

There is also evidence that changes in maternal sensitivity over time are associated with changes in an offspring's attachment security (e.g., Booth-LaForce et al., 2014). These changes may result from a mother's experience of stressful events that may impair her sensitive responsiveness or from more positive events that may improve her caregiving. In any case, this finding highlights the crucial role of caregiving quality, because "the most proximal variable of interest—the ongoing quality of the mother–child relationship—may serve as a significant modifier of early mother–child attachment security" (Booth-LaForce et al., 2014, p. 82).

Along the same lines, Van Ryzin et al. (2011) found a wide variety of attachment pathways across time that were closely associated with stressful events occurring during childhood or adolescence. They concluded that early attachment security does not imply invulnerability to later insecurity, and that continuity in attachment security over time is not just a function of the power of early parental caregiving in shaping the developing child's working models. In fact, the presence of stressful events seems to disrupt family stability and thereby increase vulnerability to insecurity, even in those with early security.

Influenced by findings of lawful discontinuities in attachment styles, Carlson et al. (2004) reanalyzed longitudinal data from the Minnesota Longitudinal Study of Risk and Adaptation, and examined the joint contribution of Strange Situation classifications at 12 months and attachment representations and socioemotional functioning during early childhood (4.5 years of age), middle childhood (8 years), and early adolescence (12 years) to AAI classifications at age 19. Interestingly, although Strange Situation classifications were not directly associated with AAI classifications 19 years later, infant attachment was found to be indirectly related to adult attachment via its effects on attachment representations and socioemotional functioning throughout childhood and adolescence. Specifically, infant attachment in the Strange Situation had significant influences on attachment representations and socioemotional functioning during early childhood, which in turn contributed to later representations and functioning during middle childhood and adolescence. And adolescents' mental representations and socioemotional functioning contributed to AAI classifications at age 19.

According to Simpson et al. (2014), these findings suggest that continuity of attachment patterns from infancy to adulthood is a dynamic process resulting from successive transactions between the person and the environment across the lifespan. Infant attachment patterns are carried from one time point to another by an infant's working models of self and others, but these are also responsive to relational experiences in a wide variety of settings (peer relationships, romantic relationships). Thus, later attachment patterns are always a reflection of the early working models and accumulated subsequent experiences.

This conclusion fits with a railway system metaphor used by Bowlby (1973). People may get on a particular train leading out of London, but they will not all end up in the same place, because some will take different branch lines along the way. In life, people take different routes through socioemotional development, including attachment patterns, depending on their different histories of social relationships. According to Bowlby, people experience different "branch points" in their route through childhood, adolescence, and adulthood, and these branch points place them on different trajectories and cause them to arrive at different adult destinations. Constructively changing a person's attachment pattern is like creating a new trajectory that leads to a more favorable destination.

This dynamic conception of socioemotional development has been supported in longitudinal studies of attachment, beginning with infants in the Strange Situation and following them all the way through adolescence and young adulthood (e.g., Englund et al., 2011), including the study of their romantic and marital relationships and their performance as young parents (e.g., Oriña et al., 2011; Raby, Roisman, Simpson, et al., 2015; Simpson, Collins, et al., 2007). For example, Raby, Roisman, Simpson, et al. (2015) found that receipt of sensitive caregiving in infancy and early childhood predicted children's social competence during childhood and adolescence, which in turn predicted romantic relationship functioning during young adulthood, which in turn predicted supportive parenting in adulthood.

Concluding Remarks

Beginning with Bowlby's insights into the nature of a child's tie to his or her parents, supplemented by the watershed contribution of Ainsworth's home-observational and laboratory research, the focus of attachment researchers has expanded to include not only child–caregiver relationships of various kinds but also couple relationships in adolescence and adulthood, and—as we explain in subsequent chapters—relationships of clients with therapists, students with teachers, workers with managers and work teams, and people with physical illness with health care providers. Bowlby's clinical observations and his exploration of ethological and cognitive research has now been expanded, tested, and operationalized in several ways.

The body of research inspired by attachment theory is ripe for clinical, educational, and organizational applications. In each domain in which applications are developed, the basic concepts of attachment, attachment figures, threats and distress, working models, attachment security, and individual differences in attachment anxiety and avoidance continue to be relevant and important. Moving a person toward greater security in a particular relationship or fostering a more secure attachment style across relationships requires understanding people's internal working models, characteristic expectations and worries, and behavior in relationships with key figures in their lives. Creating successful interventions often requires developing new therapeutic techniques and context-relevant measures, which we discuss throughout this book.

CHAPTER 2

The Broaden-and-Build Cycle of Attachment Security

As explained in Chapter 1, Bowlby and Ainsworth's attachment theory has been tested in thousands of studies of infants, children, adolescents, and adults, all illustrating the importance of attachment security for mental health, social adjustment, and general well-being. This research has encouraged further study of the psychological processes that underlie the adaptive benefits of security and has motivated the creation and evaluation of security-enhancing interventions.

Before discussing actual and potential interventions, we need to examine in a bit more detail what is known about the positive effects of attachment security on a person's motives, cognitions, feelings, and behaviors. For this purpose, we (Mikulincer & Shaver, 2003) have proposed that actual, recalled, and imagined interactions with loving and caring attachment figures activate what, following Fredrickson (2001), can be called a *broaden-and-build cycle of attachment security*. This cycle builds a person's capacity for dealing with threats and challenges, contributes to emotion regulation and relationship quality, fosters the acquisition of knowledge and skills, and moves a person from an egocentric defensiveness to a successful pursuit of prosocial and growth-oriented goals.

In this chapter, we present our theoretical ideas concerning the broaden-and-build cycle of attachment security and review related research. We also describe the characteristics of attachment figures that enhance the broaden-and-build process, and we formulate the core principles that guide the applications of attachment theory to be reviewed in subsequent chapters. Throughout this discussion, we establish contact with other important social-developmental and relational theorists whose concepts and research bases mesh with those guided by attachment theory.

Attachment Security and the Broaden-and-Build Cycle of Attachment Security

When kind and loving attachment figures provide people with safe havens and secure bases in times of need, they instill a sense of attachment security—or what Sroufe and Waters (1977) called "felt security." This subjective sense of safety has many positive emotional and motivational implications. Feeling secure, people can devote attention to pursuing goals other than self-protection. Being well cared for, they can appreciate the feeling of being loved and valued, and can be more loving and kinder to their generous relationship partners and to other people. In this way, felt security not only helps with distress management but it also encourages confident engagement in activities that satisfy what self-determination theorists (SDTs; Ryan & Deci, 2017) call *basic psychological needs*—for competence, autonomy, and relatedness. There is research evidence linking attachment security with satisfaction of these three basic needs (e.g., La Guardia et al., 2000).

In our opinion, the sense of attachment security is not limited to people who have what in Chapter 1 we called a secure attachment orientation or style. When the sense of security is, at a particular moment, the most accessible and dominant psychological state within a person's network of attachment-related memories and working models, whether this condition is characteristic or uncharacteristic of the person, it can engender some of the psychological and behavioral patterns characteristic of a chronically secure person. In other words, secure thoughts (e.g., "I am worthy and other people are generous"), feelings (e.g., "Expressing sadness is acceptable and will elicit care from others"), and behaviors (e.g., "I can ask for help when I need it") are available to almost everyone, but in chronically insecure people these states are less readily accessible and less often dominant.

At particular times, the sense of security can be associated with the actual presence of a loving and caring relationship partner; at other times, it can arise from particular episodic memories or imagined social interactions (e.g., remembering a partner's hug when one was sad; imagining reunion with a loving partner when one's flight lands). For the chronically insecure person, although states of security are neither easily nor frequently engaged, they can become more accessible when an actual, recalled, or imaginary partner successfully provides a safe haven and secure base. In our view, even in the minds of some of the least secure individuals, there are "islands of security" that can be located and highlighted either experimentally or naturally, depending on the context. For example, a person who is generally insecure with respect to attachment can exhibit mistrust and defensiveness with others, based on past trauma, but soften when recalling a positive memory of being cared for by a loving grandmother.

The sense of attachment security includes both declarative knowledge (knowledge of facts and concepts) and procedural knowledge (knowing how to do something) organized around a relational prototype or a "secure-base script" (Mikulincer et al., 2009; Waters & Waters, 2006). This script is acquired during interactions in which loving and caring attachment figures sensitively and effectively meet one's needs for protection and comfort (safe-haven support) or one's needs for support and encouragement when confronting challenges or pursuing desired goals (secure-base support). Knowing that coping with threats and challenges can be accomplished in part by assistance from attachment figures gives a person a model, or script, for regulating distress, sustaining valuable relationships, and moving toward autonomous growth.

The secure-base script contains something like the following if–then propositions: "If I encounter an obstacle, threat, or challenge and/or become distressed, I can approach an attachment figure for safe-haven or secure-base support; he or she is likely to be emotionally available, sensitive, responsive, and capable of providing a safe haven and a secure base; I will feel calm, comforted, and empowered as a result of approaching this figure; I can then confidently return to other activities" (see Figure 2.1). The construction of this script within a particular relationship or across different relational contexts increases confidence that support will be available if one's autonomous coping efforts fail. As a result, a person can remain emotionally stable when confronting threats and challenges, calmly analyze situations, and determine the best ways to cope with them.

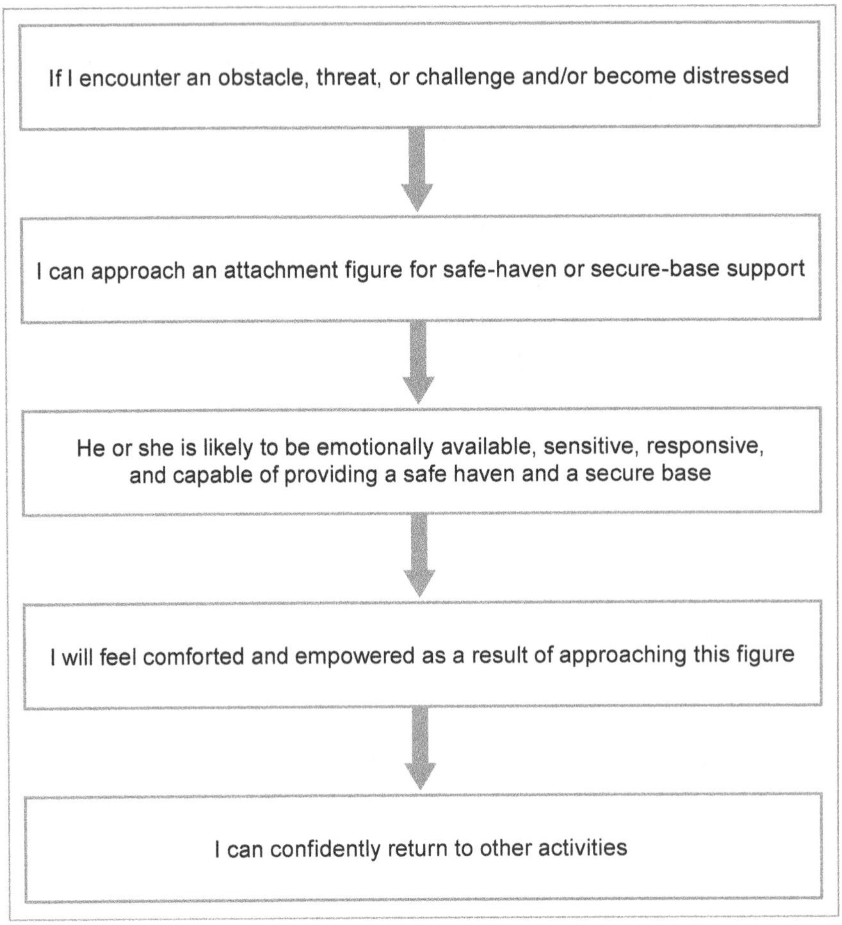

FIGURE 2.1. The secure-base script.

Importantly, this script indicates that interpersonal closeness and support for autonomous functioning are mutually sustainable. When one is distressed or worried, it is useful to seek support from others; when distress is alleviated, it is possible to engage autonomously in other activities and entertain other priorities. Thus, when attachment relationships function well, a person learns that autonomy is compatible with reliance on others.

In our model of attachment-system functioning (Mikulincer & Shaver, 2003), we proposed that interactions with responsive attachment figures and the resulting activation of the secure-base script have proliferating effects on a person's motives, cognitions, feelings, and behaviors—what (as explained earlier) we call, following Fredrickson (2001), a broaden-and-build cycle of attachment security (see Figure 2.2). The secure-base script includes positive beliefs about threats and challenges, one's own value and efficacy, others' benevolence, and the benefits of relational interdependence and closeness. It also includes procedural knowledge about constructive ways of managing distress. All of these security-related cognitions have beneficial emotional effects and contribute to a two-pronged transformation in a person's motives. Instead of being focused exclusively on self-protection and threat prevention, people can also focus on other people's needs and interests and adopt a cooperative

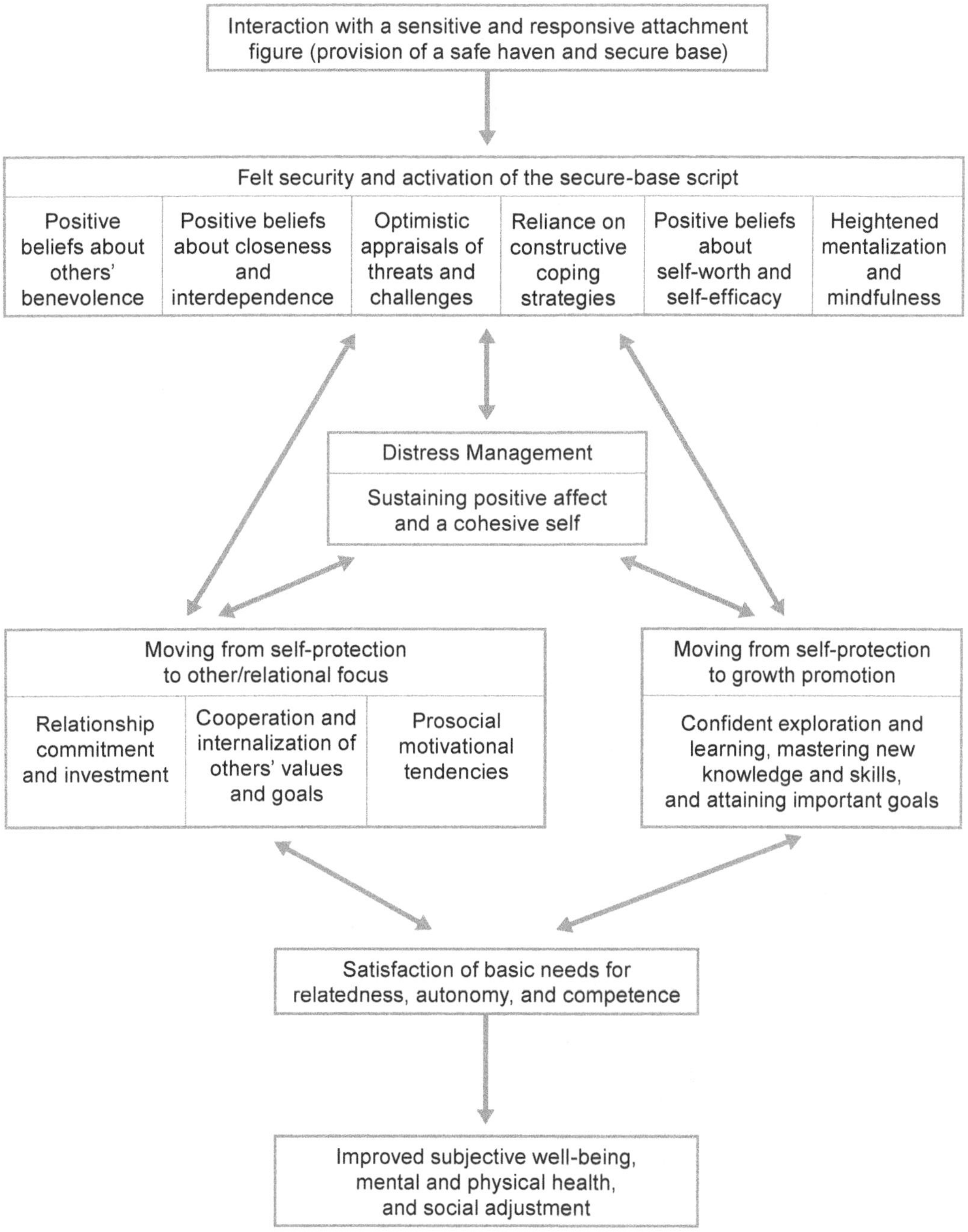

FIGURE 2.2. A schematic representation of the broaden-and-build cycle of attachment security.

stance toward others (which Bowlby, 1973, called a *goal-corrected partnership*). They can also confidently engage in exploration, learning, and pursuit of personal goals that expand their perspectives and competences, and promote their autonomy and self-reliance.

In the long run, repeated activation of the secure-base script during interactions with responsive attachment figures has enduring effects on intrapsychic organization and interpersonal functioning. At the intrapsychic level, such experiences can be called upon as resilience resources that sustain emotional stability, without relying on reality-distorting defenses, such as narcissistic self-inflation (an avoidant defense) or attempts to merge symbiotically with powerful others (an anxious defense), and autonomous growth. At the interpersonal level, repeated experiences of attachment-figure responsiveness allow a person to develop the skills and attitudes associated with a secure attachment style, which facilitates the maintenance of mutually satisfying and stable, persisting relationships.

The broaden-and-build cycle of attachment security emanates from the set of positive beliefs embedded in the secure-base script. First, adhering to the script makes it easy to believe that most of life's threats and challenges are manageable, because the script implies that approaching an attachment figure in times of need will result in comfort, support, and distress management. Hence, a well-supported person can maintain a hopeful and optimistic outlook. Second, the secure-base script includes positive beliefs about other people's benevolence, kindness, and goodwill, because others have usually been responsive to one's support-seeking bids. Third, the secure-base script implies that relational dependence and closeness are rewarding (approaching others and relying on them in times of needs results in comfort and support) and that it is not generally necessary to worry about being disapproved of, rejected, or betrayed by others. As a result, holding such a script makes it easy for a person to maintain a positive outlook on personal and social relationships.

In a complementary way, interactions with responsive attachment figures lead people to perceive themselves as valuable, lovable, and special—thanks to being valued, loved, and viewed as special by caring others (Mikulincer & Shaver, 2004). Moreover, they learn to view themselves as active, strong, and competent, because they can effectively mobilize an attachment figure's support and restore emotional stability, while turning their attention to exploration, learning, and autonomous goal pursuit (thanks to the "secure base" provided by responsive attachment figures). People with a secure attachment orientation, or style, habitually hold positive beliefs about themselves and others across different relational contexts, whereas people with a less secure style maintain these positive beliefs only in contexts in which actual, recalled, or imagined interactions with a responsive relationship partner arouse temporary feelings of being cared for and loved. (As we explain in Chapter 3, this possibility makes it possible for us to experimentally enhance insecure people's sense of security in laboratory experiments.)

The procedural knowledge included in the secure-base script also contributes to the broaden-and-build cycle of attachment security. People who possess such a script expect that support seeking will result in protection and support. They then have confidence that turning to others will be an effective way to cope with threats and challenges. Moreover, the secure-base script implies that self-disclosure of one's needs, feelings, and thoughts will result in beneficial responses from others. In fact, for individuals whose attachment figures have been responsive, expression of negative emotions has usually led to distress-alleviating support and guidance. According to Cassidy (1994), "the experience of security is based not on the denial of negative affect but on the ability to tolerate negative affects temporarily in order to achieve mastery over threatening or frustrating situations" (p. 233).

A related kind of procedural knowledge embedded in the secure-base script concerns attitudes toward mental states. During interactions with a responsive attachment figure, people learn to expect that awareness of, reflection on, and expression of feelings, desires, and thoughts will result in positive outcomes. These positive expectations encourage openness to mental states and what Fonagy et al. (1991) call self-reflective or *mentalizing* capacity—the ability to notice, think about, and accurately understand mental states (e.g., desires, feelings, beliefs, intentions), including one's own and those of other people. These security-based expectations about the benefits of openness to mental states can also foster *mindfulness*—the moment-by-moment awareness of one's thoughts, feelings, and bodily sensations without fear, self-criticism, and defensive biases (Kabat-Zinn, 1994). These aspects of security—mentalizing and mindfulness—are parts of what qualifies a person for a secure classification in the AAI (Hesse, 2016).

Interactions with responsive attachment figures also facilitate problem solving. Part of effective problem solving is recognizing that one's previous course of action was unsuccessful and must be changed if the problem is to be solved. Experiencing, or having experienced, an attachment figure as loving and accepting facilitates revision of erroneous beliefs and strategies, because people feel that this steadfast individual will continue to love and value them even after they make mistakes or misbehave. In addition, believing that support will be available if needed (the core component of the secure-base script) allows people to open their minds to new information and revise their plans to deal realistically with whatever is happening at the moment.

The most immediate psychological effect of activating the secure-base script is distress management. The optimistic appraisals and constructive ways of regulating emotion embedded in the script can assuage distress, elicit positive emotions (anticipatory relief and comfort), and thereby maintain emotional stability. People who adhere to a secure-base script can remain relatively unperturbed in times of stress and enjoy longer runs of positive affect. Over time, relying on the script and experiencing felt security contributes to sustained emotional well-being and mental health.

Besides contributing to emotional stability, the secure-base script allows people to attend not only to their own needs but also to others' needs and to confidently engage in pro-relational and prosocial behavior. At the relational level, a positive assessment of close relationships along with positive beliefs about others' benevolence makes it easier to get emotionally close to relationship partners; feel comfortable with intimacy, commitment, and interdependence in a relationship; and increasingly invest efforts in maintaining and strengthening relationship quality and stability. In this way, adherence to the secure-base script can promote what Wieselquist et al. (1999), whose work is rooted in interdependence theory (Thibault & Kelley, 1959), call "mutual growth cycles" in relationships. In these cycles, a person's felt security increases his or her dependence on the relationship, as well as his or her relational investment and responsiveness to a partner's needs. This, in turn, increases the partner's felt security, interdependence, investment, and responsiveness, thereby heightening the trust and commitment of the two partners. This means that people who feel safe and protected are likely to enjoy mutually satisfying relationships while experiencing opportunities for exploration and personal growth.

With regard to the move from an egoistic to a more prosocial orientation, Bowlby (1969/1982) noticed that when facing threats and challenges, people focus mainly on their own safety and need for protection and care. They are less able or willing than usual to attend empathically and respond compassionately to other people's needs or suffering. At such times, people are likely to be so focused on their own vulnerability that they lack the mental resources required to attend sensitively to others' needs. Only when a sense of attachment security is restored can a person perceive others not only as potential sources of support but also as worthy and benevolent people who also need and deserve sympathy and care. Moreover, possessing a secure-base script implies that one has witnessed, experienced, and benefited from generous attachment figures' effective care, which provides models to follow when another person is in need. In other words, one's orientation toward others' suffering is based partly on a supported sense of security and partly on modeling the behavior of one's caring attachment figures. This is a point of compatibility between attachment theory and various forms of social learning theory (e.g., Bandura, 1986).

Feeling safe and protected, people can also devote attention and effort to their own growth-promoting activities (e.g., exploration, learning, goal pursuit) and intrinsically motivated behaviors (doing an activity because it is interesting and enjoyable). By reducing the need for self-protection, felt security makes it less necessary to be constantly focused on preventing threats and injuries. Instead, people are able to open themselves to experiences and activities that can broaden their perspectives and competences, such as exploration of new objects, places, or ideas and mastering new knowledge and skills. They can also intentionally deploy mental resources in the service of other activities that advance their personal interests and talents, such as effortful pursuit of personal goals and successful completion of personal tasks and plans. Moreover, being confident that attachment figures are available, responsive, and generous, people can accept important challenges that may contribute to personal growth and flourishing.

Empirical Evidence for the Broaden-and-Build Consequences of Security

In the following sections we review some of the evidence for the hypothesized cascade of mental and behavioral processes associated with felt security (see Figure 2.2). In particular, we focus on the psychological correlates of felt security, as manifested in self-report scales or clinical interviews concerned with attachment orientations or states of mind. Specifically, we consider attachment-related individual differences in (1) the psychological reality of the secure base script, (2) mental representations of the self and others, (3) emotion regulation and well-being, (4) mentalization and mindfulness, (5) pro-relational beliefs and behaviors and relationship quality, (6) compassion and prosocial behavior, and (7) exploration and autonomous growth. In subsequent chapters, we review laboratory experiments (Chapter 3) and randomized clinical trials (Chapters 4–10) examining whether and how interventions aimed at contextually heightening felt security contribute to the activation of the broaden-and-build cycle and move a person toward a more vibrant and fulfilling life.

The Psychological Reality of the Secure-Base Script

There is good evidence for the psychological reality of the secure-base script in the minds of adults. For example, Mikulincer et al. (2009) found that people who score lower on self-report scales measuring attachment anxiety or avoidance (i.e., the more secure participants) were more likely to include elements of the secure-base script (support seeking, support provision, and distress relief) when writing about projective-test pictures of a troubled person or when narrating their own dreams about distressing events. Moreover, the two main kinds of insecurity, anxiety and avoidance, were associated with different gaps in the secure-base script (Mikulincer et al., 2009). People who scored relatively high on attachment anxiety tended to omit or deemphasize the final step in the script (relief and return to other activities): They more often wrote about an injured person who was seeking support without achieving relief. People who scored relatively high on avoidance tended to omit the part about benefiting from social support: They more often wrote about a person achieving relief without seeking or receiving others' support.

Other studies have shown that the secure-base script is highly accessible in the minds of secure individuals. For example, self-reports of attachment security are positively associated with the degree to which the secure-base script is evident in dreams about romantic partners (Selterman et al., 2012) and in narratives concerning current relationships (McLean et al., 2014). Similarly, greater security exhibited in the AAI (Main et al., 1985) has been linked with higher scores on the Attachment Script Assessment (ASA; Waters & Waters, 2006), a measure of the propensity to create stories from word prompts that follow the structure of the secure-base script (e.g., Dykas et al., 2006; Steele et al., 2014).

There is also longitudinal evidence linking parental sensitivity and responsiveness during infancy and childhood to the propensity of individuals to create secure-base stories in the ASA during adolescence and young adulthood (e.g., Waters et al., 2017). Recent findings also link higher ASA scores with more sensitive and responsive parenting, higher emotional engagement during interactions with romantic partners, and higher levels of satisfaction in couple relationships (e.g., Groh & Haydon, 2018; Huth-Bocks et al., 2014; Waters et al., 2018). Overall, it seems that possessing a well-developed, coherent secure-base script is a marker of felt security, which promotes a pro-relational and prosocial orientation.

Security-Based Representations of Self

Dozens of studies have indicated that lower scores on attachment anxiety scales (indicating greater security) are associated with more positive beliefs about one's self-worth and self-efficacy (see Tables 6.1 and 6.2 in Mikulincer & Shaver, 2016, for a summary of these studies). For example, Schmitt and Allik (2005) conducted a study in 53 nations and found a strong negative association between attachment anxiety and self-reports of self-esteem in 49 countries. In another key study, Dewitte et al. (2008) asked participants to perform a self-related variant of the Implicit Association Test (IAT), and found that participants who scored lower on attachment anxiety had more positive implicit (i.e., nonconscious) self-views as measured by the IAT.

Interestingly, avoidant people's self-views tend to be positive and resemble those of secure people (Shaver & Mikulincer, 2011). However, whereas avoidant people's self-views seem to result from defensive self-enhancement, secure people's self-views seem to reflect an authentic sense of self-worth. Indeed, avoidant attachment has been associated with higher scores on measures of defensive self-enhancement (Gjerde et al., 2004), overt/grandiose forms of pathological narcissism and unrealistic self-praise (e.g., Miller et al., 2013; Rohmann et al., 2012), and "splitting" defenses—that is, attempts to protect desirable self-aspects by detaching them from undesirable self-aspects (e.g., Lopez, 2001). In contrast, attachment security is associated with higher scores on measures of self-authenticity (e.g., Gillath et al., 2010), self-clarity (e.g., Davila & Cobb, 2003), and coherent integration of self-representations (e.g., Mikulincer, 1995).

Felt security seems also to facilitate maintenance of a stable positive self-view, presumably because this appraisal is derived from attachment figures' love, understanding, and acceptance (Cheng & Kwan, 2008). Hepper and Carnelley (2012) conducted a 14-day diary study and found that the daily self-esteem of more secure participants (those with lower attachment anxiety scores) fluctuated less with daily interpersonal feedback conveying rejection or acceptance coming from a romantic partner. In two experimental studies, Carvallo and Gabriel (2006) found that whereas more avoidant people reported higher state self-esteem after receiving positive feedback (compared with no feedback), the relatively high self-esteem of more secure participants was not much affected by the experimental feedback. In addition, Mikulincer (1998a) and Hart et al. (2005) found that avoidant individuals viewed themselves in a more positive light following an experimentally induced threat than a neutral condition (indicating defensive self-inflation). Secure individuals' self-views did not differ substantially across threat and neutral conditions: They made relatively stable and unbiased self-appraisals even when coping with threats.

Attachment security has also been associated with self-acceptance and self-compassion (e.g,, Thompson & Zuroff; 2004; Pepping, Davis, O'Donovan, & Pal, 2015). It seems that secure individuals incorporate their attachment figures' love and kindness into their own self-representations, evaluating and treating themselves in the same accepting and compassionate manner in which they have been treated by these responsive figures. Indeed, Dunkley et al. (2012) conducted a 7-day diary study and found that participants who reported higher daily felt security during the study period (lower fears of closeness, dependency, and loss) tended to score lower on a trait-like measure of self-criticism. Another way of saying this, which is supported by research, is that secure individuals experience greater self-compassion (Neff & McGehee, 2010).

Security-Based Representations of Others

People with a chronic sense of attachment security tend to have a positive view of humanity in general and of relationship partners in particular (Collins & Read, 1990). For example, lower scores on attachment anxiety or avoidance scales have been associated with higher esteem for others (e.g., Luke et al., 2004) and fewer doubts about others' trustworthiness (e.g., Hofstra et al., 2005). And attachment security is associated with higher ratings of relationship partners' responsiveness, dependability, authenticity, and faithfulness (e.g., Beck et al., 2014; Feeney, 2002; Wickham et al., 2015) and faster access to memories of a romantic partner's trustworthy behavior (Mikulincer, 1998b). This association between felt security and positive views of others has also been observed in a 31-year longitudinal study: 52-year-old women with a self-reported secure attachment style had rated others as more trustworthy and dependable at ages 27 and 43, and still did so at age 52, compared with insecure women (Klohnen & Bera, 1998).

Attachment security is associated with more positive expectations concerning a partner's behavior. For example, as compared with insecure people, secure ones have been found to react with shorter lexical-decision times (reflecting greater cognitive accessibility) to words naming positive partner behaviors (e.g., acceptance, love) than to words naming negative behaviors (e.g., rejection, criticism) (Baldwin et al., 1993). Similarly, self-reports of attachment security are related to stronger automatic associations (indicated by faster associative responses in the IAT between either current romantic partner or mother and positive personal attributes (Zayas & Shoda, 2005). For secure people, exposure to the name of a romantic partner or the name of their mother seems to automatically activate associations with positive traits, implying the existence of implicit positive representations of partners in their associative memory network.

Secure people's positive working models of others are also manifested in the provision of more positive, empathic, forgiving explanations of partners' hurtful behavior. Findings indicate that people scoring lower on attachment anxiety or avoidance (i.e., those who are more secure) are more likely to offer forgiving and constructive explanations of hypothetical vignettes about a romantic partner's disappointing behavior (e.g., "Your partner didn't comfort you when you were feeling down"). Moreover, they are less likely to believe that their partner's negative behavior was caused by lack of love and are more likely to attribute it to unstable, situational causes unrelated to the partner's traits or intentions (Collins, 1996; Collins et al., 2006).

A host of adult attachment studies has also consistently found that attachment security is associated with greater confidence in others' supportiveness and more satisfaction with support received (see Table 6.4 in Mikulincer & Shaver, 2016, for a summary of these studies). Several of these studies were based on prospective designs, showing that attachment security assessed at a particular time point predicted subsequent increases in perceiving others' supportiveness across periods ranging from 1 month to 6 years (e.g., Brock & Lawrence, 2014). This kind of positive perception has also been noted in the interpretations of a partner's everyday helpful behavior: Across two weeks of a daily diary study, attachment security was associated with more daily positive appraisals of partner support (Campbell et al., 2005). Taken together, the findings indicate that secure individuals are predisposed to perceive and remember a partner's behavior in times of need as more supportive and helpful.

Felt Security, Emotion Regulation, and Psychological Well-Being

A large body of evidence supports the hypothesized link between attachment security and effective emotion regulation. This link has been examined in a wide variety of stressful situations not specifically related to attachment, such as combat training, war captivity, terrorism, transition to college, abortion, infertility, financial problems, and job loss, and also with regard to specifically attachment-related stressors, such as a partner's hurtful behavior, a relationship breakup, or the death of a relationship partner (see Tables 7.2 and 7.3 in Mikulincer & Shaver, 2016, for a summary of these studies). With regard to the cognitive appraisal of stressful events, more secure people (with lower scores on attachment anxiety or avoidance scales) have been found to appraise stressful events in less threatening and more optimistic ways and to appraise themselves as better able to cope effectively with threats (e.g., Berant et al., 2001). This pattern of findings has been replicated using a wide variety of scales measuring optimism, hope, ego-resilience, perceived coping resources, and positive expectations about regulation of negative emotions (e.g., Caldwell & Shaver, 2012; Tosone et al., 2010).

With regard to ways of coping with stressful events, people with a strong sense of attachment security tend to rely on the guidelines implied by the secure-base script, showing greater openness to negative emotions, fuller disclosure of feelings, and more active support seeking. For example, secure people are more willing and able to access painful memories and reexperience the accompanying negative affect (e.g., Dykas et al., 2014; Edelstein et al., 2005). Using either self-report or behavioral measures of self-disclosure, researchers have found that secure people are more likely to appropriately disclose personal feelings to others and express their emotions more openly than insecure people (e.g., Collins et al., 2002; Garrison et al., 2012). Observational studies of actual support seeking during distressing situations have revealed that attachment security is associated with more frequent direct requests for support, understanding, and validation from partners (e.g., Collins & Feeney, 2000).

Several studies have shown that dispositional measures of attachment security are associated with self-reports of diminished distress and heightened well-being during and following stressful events (see Mikulincer & Shaver, 2016, for a review). Moreover, some of the studies have compared the emotional reactions of secure and insecure people undergoing stressful experiences with those of controls, revealing that stressful events arouse distress mainly among those who are less secure. For secure people, there is often no notable difference in emotional reactions between neutral and stressful situations (e.g., Berant et al., 2001); that is, secure people seem to be relatively calm under stressful conditions. This conclusion is further reinforced by experimental studies finding that attachment security is associated with lower levels of cardiovascular reactivity, cortisol release, and amygdala activity during and following laboratory stressors (e.g., Diamond et al., 2006; Kidd et al., 2011; Lemche et al., 2006).

Secure people also tend to react less intensely than insecure people—cognitively, emotionally, and behaviorally—to partner criticism, rejection, or betrayal (e.g., Carnelley et al., 2007; Dewitte et al., 2010). In particular, attachment security seems to buffer the intensity and duration of distress following wartime separations from marital partners (Borelli et al., 2014), temporary separations from a romantic partner (e.g., Diamond et al., 2008), romantic relationship breakup (e.g., Fagundes et al., 2012), divorce (Halford & Sweeper, 2013), or spouse's death (e.g., Field et al., 2014). For example, Sbarra (2006) collected daily emotion data for 4 weeks from a sample of young adults who had recently experienced a romantic relationship breakup and found that attachment security was associated with faster recovery from sadness and anger. A similar pattern of findings has been observed in longitudinal studies assessing the trajectory of grief reactions following the death of a loved one: Attachment security (assessed at early stages after the loss) was associated with lower levels of psychological distress and depression 4, 10, 15, and 50 months later (e.g., Field & Sundin, 2001; Fraley & Bonanno, 2004).

Overall, existing evidence supports the hypothesis that a sense of attachment security is associated with a reduction in biopsychological markers of distress. Evidence also indicates that attachment insecurities interfere with effective distress down-regulation (at both psychological and physiological levels) and increase the risk of developing emotional and physical disorders.

Felt Security, Mentalization, and Mindfulness

Comforting interactions with responsive attachment figures who understand, accept, and validate a person's needs and feelings may strengthen the person's ability to reflect on and understand these mental states via two related pathways. The first pathway is provided by a secure base for exploration, which empowers secure individuals to explore not only their external surroundings but also their own needs, feelings, thoughts, and memories. They can pursue this internal exploration with confidence that support will be available if they come upon difficult, conflictual, or confounding material, as almost every complex human being is bound to do. The second pathway is made possible by the mentalizing stance of responsive attachment figures. Loving parents and caregivers are genuinely interested in understanding what the child in their care needs and how he or she feels, so that they can draw correct inferences from the child's behavior, make accurate decisions about the child's needs, and provide empathic and effective care. This kind of caregiver serves as not only a safe haven and secure base but also a role model who encourages the child to reflect on mental states and gain a clearer understanding of them. Both pathways converge in sustaining secure individuals' mentalizing capacity.

Attachment researchers have linked the sense of attachment security with positive and open attitudes toward mental states and the ability to mentalize (see Luyten & Fonagy, 2014, for a review). In both cross-sectional and prospective longitudinal studies, children with a more secure attachment to their mother have been found more capable of making sense of their own behavior in terms of desires, feelings, and intentions (e.g., Raikes & Thompson, 2006). Also, more secure children are better able to understand how the behavior of story characters is influenced by mental states (Humfress et al., 2002) and to identify the mental states of their own mothers (Repacholi & Trapolini, 2004).

Conceptually similar findings have been reported in studies conducted with samples of adolescents and adults. Venta and Sharp (2015) used the Movie for the Assessment of Social Cognition task (MASC; Dziobek et al., 2006) and found that secure adolescents (assessed with the AAI) made more accurate inferences about story characters' mental states (based on characters' social behavior in a video clip) than attachment-insecure adolescents. Felt security (assessed with self-report scales) has also been associated with higher mentalization scores on the Reading the Mind in the Eyes Test and the Parental Reflective Functioning Questionnaire (Burkhart et al., 2017; Fossati et al., 2014).

Secure people's positive and open attitudes toward their own and others' mental states can also be seen in their adoption of a mindful attitude toward the flow of subjective experience. According to Shaver et al. (2007), mindfulness is negatively associated with insecure patterns of attachment. Whereas mindfulness is a calm and accepting approach to sensations, feelings, and thoughts, attachment-anxious people tend to be overwhelmed by self-doubts and worries and are unable to disengage from negative automatic thoughts and compulsive behavior patterns. Attachment-related avoidance is also incompatible with mindfulness, because avoidance involves diverting attention away from threatening thoughts and information, repressing painful memories, and suppressing the experience and expression of distress-related feelings and thoughts. In contrast, with the actual and perceived support and encouragement of responsive attachment figures, secure individuals can remain mindful with respect to the full range of subjective experiences.

This theorizing has received empirical support in correlational studies that yield positive associations between self-reports of attachment security and measures of dispositional mindfulness. In 2017, Stevenson et al. meta-analyzed findings from 33 studies and concluded that both dimensions of attachment insecurity (anxiety and avoidance) are associated with lower levels of mindfulness (with averaged correlations of –.36 for anxiety and –.28 for avoidance). In one of these studies, Shaver et al. (2007) measured mindfulness using Baer et al.'s (2006) five-factor mindfulness scale in a sample of adults who volunteered to participate in a 3-month full-time meditation retreat (the Shamatha Project) and found that lower avoidance scores (on the ECR measure of attachment style; Brennan et al., 1998) were associated with higher scores on all five assessed facets of mindfulness: nonreactivity to inner experience, acting with awareness, observing/noticing/attending to sensations/perceptions/feelings, describing/labeling with words one's experience, and nonjudging of experience.

The link between attachment security and mindfulness was also evident in Mikulincer et al.'s (2020) 15-day diary study of the quality of dream experience. Participants completed the ECR scale, measuring attachment anxiety and avoidance, before the study; then each evening they rated their daily sense of attachment security. Each morning they described in writing any dreams they recalled and rated the extent to which they (1) were aware of their sensations and mental states while dreaming and (2) reflected on their subjective experience during the dream. Two judges made similar ratings for each dream. Findings indicated that lower scores on ECR attachment anxiety and avoidance scales (indicating greater security) were associated with higher levels of within-dream awareness and reflection across the 15-day period. In addition, attachment security on a given day was associated with greater within-dream awareness and reflection that night. These findings suggest that dispositional attachment insecurities can interfere with mindfulness, and that even momentary feelings of security on a given day can enhance and sustain mindfulness.

Felt Security, Pro-Relational Beliefs and Behaviors, and Relationship Quality

In the original studies of adult attachment style, Hazan and Shaver (1987) provided evidence for an association between a person's sense of attachment security (as measured with the three-category measure described in Chapter 1) and the way he or she construes experiences of romantic love. Specifically, they found that participants who endorsed a secure attachment style were more likely to report that these relationships were friendly, warm, trusting, and supportive than were those who endorsed either an anxious or avoidant style. In addition, they were more likely to emphasize intimacy as the core feature of these relationships and to believe in the existence of romantic love and the possibility of maintaining intense love over a long period of time. Subsequent studies using continuous (rather than categorical) measures of adult attachment style have replicated and extended these findings, indicating that people with stronger felt security are more likely to experience and emphasize the beneficial aspects of being in a relationship (e.g., Spielmann et al., 2013).

A large body of evidence shows that people who are secure with respect to attachment not only hold positive beliefs about close relationships but also tend to be more committed to their partner and to invest more effort in a relationship than their insecure counterparts (reviewed by Mikulincer & Shaver, 2016, Table 10.3). This tendency is manifested in secure people's willingness to sacrifice to improve relationship quality and their partner's well-being (e.g., Impett & Gordon, 2010). In a behavioral test of relational investment, Vicary and Fraley (2007) asked people to choose between two options in several "Choose Your Own Adventure" dating story tasks. One option was always a relationship-enhancing option; the other option was detrimental to the relationship. They found that felt security was associated with choosing relationship-enhancing options.

Hundreds of studies, summarized in Tables 10.5 and 10.6 of our book (Mikulincer & Shaver, 2016), confirm that secure individuals tend to maintain more stable romantic relationships than their insecure counterparts (whether anxious, avoidant, or both) and report higher levels of relationship satisfaction. This pattern has been consistently obtained in cross-sectional and prospective longitudinal studies of both dating and married couples and cannot be explained by other personality factors, such as the "Big Five" personality traits or self-esteem. For example, Davila et al. (1999) reported that attachment security within the first 6 months of marriage predicted greater marital satisfaction over the next 3 years, and Hirschberger et al. (2009) found that attachment security predicted greater marital satisfaction over a period of 15 years after the birth of a first child. Several diary studies have found that dispositional measures of attachment security are associated with higher daily reports of relationship satisfaction across study periods ranging from 1 to 3 weeks (e.g., Gosnell & Gable, 2013).

Attachment security seems to be involved in three interpersonal processes that facilitate the maintenance of a satisfying relationship. First, attachment security is associated with more constructive, mutually sensitive patterns of dyadic communication (e.g., Wegner et al., 2018). Secure partners maintain more positive patterns of nonverbal communication (expressiveness, pleasantness, attentiveness) than do less secure partners and are more accurate in interpreting their partner's nonverbal messages (e.g., Guerrero, 1996; Overall et al., 2015). Second, attachment security is related to reliance on effective strategies of conflict resolution—compromising and integrating own and partner's positions (e.g., Creasey, 2014). In contrast, insecure people tend to rely on less effective conflict resolution strategies that leave conflicts unresolved and may lead to conflict escalation (e.g., Rholes et al., 2014; Tran & Simpson, 2009). Third, attachment security is associated with more pro-relational, accommodative responses to a partner's hurtful behavior—"voice" (active attempts to talk with the hurtful partner) and "loyalty" (understanding the temporary nature of a partner's behavior and waiting for improvement) (e.g., Pizzano et al., 2013).

Using the Rochester Interaction Record (Wheeler & Reis, 1991), several studies have found that dispositional measures of attachment security are associated with higher levels of satisfaction, intimacy, self-disclosure, supportive behaviors, and positive emotions during daily interpersonal interactions over the course of 1 to 2 weeks (e.g., Kafetsios & Nezlek, 2002; Sibley et al., 2005). There is also evidence linking attachment security with more constructive expressions of anger (nonhostile protests) and a more forgiving stance toward others' offenses and hurtful behaviors (e.g., Kachadourian et al., 2004; Mikulincer, 1998c). Moreover, attachment security is associated with a stronger inclination to feel and express gratitude to generous others (e.g., Algoe et al., 2010) and more respect for romantic partners (Frei & Shaver, 2002).

Felt Security, Compassion, and Prosocial Behavior

The predicted link between felt security and a prosocial orientation has received support in studies assessing caregiving and support provision within parent–child relationships and within romantic and marital relationships (see Chapters 4–6 for reviews of these studies). Observational studies of actual parent–child interactions reveal that more secure parents are rated by independent observers as warmer and more supportive, more attentive to their child's needs and feelings, and less intrusive when responding to their child's distress (e.g., Bernier & Matte-Gagné, 2011; Crowell et al., 2010; Shlafer et al., 2015). In addition, using the Caregiving Questionnaire (Kunce & Shaver, 1994) with dating and marital couples, several studies have found that secure people, compared with their insecure counterparts, score higher on scales measuring sensitivity and responsiveness to a relationship partner's needs (e.g., Péloquin et al., 2014). Similar findings have been reported in laboratory studies of the actual provision of support to a romantic partner (e.g., Collins & Feeney, 2000). Feeney and Collins (2003) reported that, as compared with insecure adults, secure adults tended to endorse more altruistic reasons for helping a relationship partner, such as to reduce the partner's suffering. Attachment-avoidant people tended to report more egoistic reasons (e.g., to receive something explicit in return), and attachment-anxious people tended to report reasons reflecting unmet needs for security (e.g., to gain a partner's love and approval).

Attachment security is also a foundation for prosocial tendencies outside the domain of close relationships, in the wider social world. Several studies of preschoolers and school-age children have shown that attachment security in the Strange Situation at 12 months is associated with greater empathic concern for an adult stranger's or another child's distress years later, as indicated by teachers' ratings and researchers' observations of children's behavior (e.g., Bohlin et al., 2000; Kestenbaum et al., 1989; van der Mark et al., 2002). Similarly, studies of attachment in adolescence and adulthood have consistently found that reports of attachment security are associated with higher scores on scales measuring compassion, generosity, gratitude, kindness, and a sense of communion with others (see Shaver et al., 2016, for a review). In addition, young adults who are more secure are more likely to endorse personal values reflecting concern for others' welfare (Mikulincer et al., 2003) and engage in altruistic volunteering such as caring for the elderly and donating blood (Gillath, Shaver, et al., 2005).

In an observational laboratory study, Westmaas and Silver (2001) videotaped people while they interacted with a confederate of the experimenter whom they thought had recently been diagnosed with cancer. Findings indicated that secure people tend to provide more effective support than insecure people. Whereas attachment-avoidant participants were rated by observers as less supportive, attachment-anxious participants reported greater discomfort while interacting with the confederate. In another observational laboratory study, B. Feeney et al. (2008) found that higher attachment security (based on the AAI) was associated with providing more responsive support to an unfamiliar peer who was disclosing a personal problem and with less self-focus during the discussion (as coded by external observers).

Felt Security, Exploration, and Autonomous Growth

According to Bowlby (1988), soothing and empowering interactions with responsive caregivers and the resulting sense of felt security allow children to confidently venture out from their secure base and explore the world on their own (reinforced by confidence that they can return to this safe haven and secure base when needed). These exploratory and learning activities might, in turn, provide secure children with more opportunities to practice and improve their evolving executive functions (working memory, response inhibition, cognitive flexibility) and organizational skills (e.g., setting goals and priorities, means–end planning). Because of this developmental process, attachment-secure children and adults are more likely than their insecure counterparts to possess the needed self-regulatory skills to effectively pursue important personal goals throughout life (Mikulincer & Shaver, 2016).

Attachment studies conducted with adolescents and adults support Bowlby's (1988) hypothesis that attachment security provides support for exploration and learning of new skills and perspectives. More attachment-secure people (assessed with either the AAI or self-report scales) tend to score higher on self-report measures of novelty seeking, curiosity, exploratory interest, and cognitive openness (e.g., Lattifian & Delavarpour, 2012; Mikulincer, 1997). Moreover, whereas people who report a secure attachment style are likely to report intrinsic motives for engaging in exploration (e.g., curiosity, joy), attachment-anxious people are likely to report extrinsic reasons, such as distracting oneself from a negative mood (e.g., Martin et al., 2010). Self-reports of attachment security are also associated with lower scores on measures of close-mindedness, dogmatic thinking, intolerance of ambiguity, and rejection of information that challenges the validity of one's beliefs (e.g., Green-Hennessy & Reis, 1998; Mikulincer, 1997; Weber & Federico, 2007). For example, Mikulincer (1997) found that secure people are less likely than insecure ones to rate a target person based on the first information received and to ignore subsequent information (showing a stronger *primacy effect*). In addition, Mikulincer and Arad (1999) found that more secure participants are more likely to adjust their perception of a romantic partner after receiving expectation-incongruent information about his or her behavior.

Attachment studies of both children and adults have found that felt security is positively associated with self-regulation capacities—a prerequisite for effective autonomous goal pursuit. Specifically, children who were more securely attached to their mothers during infancy showed better performance on self-regulation tasks (e.g., inhibition of automatic or distracting responses) and were rated by their teachers as having fewer self-regulation problems at school (e.g., Bernier et al., 2015, 2020; Matte-Gagné et al., 2018). Using data from the National Institute of Child Health and Human Development (NICHD) Study of Early Child Care, Drake et al. (2014) found that attachment security measured at 15 and 36 months of age predicted better self-regulation (as rated by teachers and external observers) and heightened engagement in learning during elementary school. In adolescence and adulthood, measures of attachment security have been associated with higher scores on self-control scales (Tangney et al., 2004) and improved response inhibition in the Stroop color–word task (C. Li et al., 2016).

Secure attachment also facilitates the successful completion of adolescents and adults' major life tasks, such as identity formation, career development, school and academic performance, and performance on the job. Indeed, cross-sectional and prospective studies have shown that measures of attachment security contribute to predicting higher levels of identity achievement—exploring among alternatives and autonomously committing to a unique identity (e.g., Ávila et al., 2012; see Årseth et al., 2009, for a meta-analysis). Self-reports of attachment security have also been associated with career exploration and commitment (e.g., Keller & Brown, 2014), and with better academic and socioemotional adjustment to college (e.g., Marmarosh & Markin, 2007). For example, Larose et al. (2005) found that attachment security measured at the end of high school predicted better academic achievement during the first three semesters in college. These findings indicate that felt security is an important antecedent of favorable career development and academic functioning.

In their pioneering study of "love and work" viewed from an attachment-theoretical perspective, Hazan and Shaver (1990) found that people who were securely attached had more positive attitudes toward work and suffered from fewer work-related problems; they were more satisfied with their work activities and less likely than their insecure peers to allow work to interfere with relationships. Subsequent studies have also found that attachment security is associated with higher levels of job engagement and job satisfaction, and lower levels of work-related distress, burnout, and turnover intentions (e.g., Gama et al., 2014; Krpalek et al., 2014). These associations have been corroborated in longitudinal studies. For example, Burge et al. (1997) found that attachment security predicted increases in adolescents' performance at work 2 years later, and Bartley et al. (2007) reported that a secure attachment style at ages 30–35 years was associated with higher salaries and ranks in the British civil service at midlife. In summary, various desirable aspects of work life are positively affected by felt security.

Enhancing the Broaden-and-Build Cycle of Attachment Security

The broaden-and-build cycle of attachment security is renewed and strengthened every time a person experiences actual, recalled, or imagined interactions with a loving and responsive attachment figure: one who provides a safe haven and secure base. Therefore, from a clinical or interventionist perspective, if we want to enhance a person's felt security and the associated broaden-and-build cycle, we should increase the frequency and personal significance of such interactions. For example, we can ask a person to remember, think, imagine, or interact with loving and responsive attachment figures. Alternatively, we can encourage, guide, and help a person's attachment figure to become a more reliable provider of a safe haven and secure base. These alternative approaches can both increase the cognitive accessibility of the secure-base script and make it easier for a person to feel valued and loved, and to engage in more effective exploration and growth-oriented activities.

This attachment-based interventionist reasoning raises two main questions. First, what are the key characteristics of an attachment figure that we want to instill or strengthen? Second, to what extent can the physical or mental presence of a security-enhancing figure launch a broaden-and-build cycle for a person with a history of insecure relationships? In other words, can interactions with a loving and responsive attachment figure in the present counteract the detrimental psychological effects of dispositional insecure attachment and move a person toward greater security? We tackle these two questions in the following sections.

Key Characteristics of Security-Enhancing Attachment Figures

In the earliest studies of infant attachment, Ainsworth et al. (1978) identified several maternal behaviors, based on home observations of mother–child interactions, that were associated with attachment security exhibited by an infant in the Strange Situation. These behaviors included, for example, soothing a distressed infant, being sensitive to the infant's signals and needs, being emotionally accessible when the infant was distressed or sought support, not intruding when the infant engaged with interest in other activities, and accepting the infant's needs and actions. On this basis, Ainsworth et al. developed rating scales to assess maternal sensitivity versus insensitivity, acceptance versus rejection, cooperation versus interference, and psychological accessibility versus ignoring, finding that these scales significantly differentiated between secure and insecure infants in the Strange Situation.

These findings led Ainsworth to conclude that sensitivity and responsiveness are the key characteristics of a caregiver that contribute to an infant's felt security. Ainsworth et al. (1974) stated that security-enhancing maternal behaviors included four components: "(a) her awareness of the signals; (b) an accurate interpretation of them; (c) an appropriate response to them; and (d) a prompt response to them" (pp. 127–128). Therefore, infants might feel more secure when their caregiver is sensitive to their signals (able to perceive and accurately interpret infant cues) and responsive to their needs (able to respond promptly in an appropriate way). (Notice that these characteristics are closely related to the later concept of mentalization, discussed below.) In conceptualizing sensitivity, Ainsworth also highlighted the importance of mutual delight during parent–infant interactions and the ongoing attunement (moment-by-moment matching) of caregiving to the infant's state.

In her book *Infancy in Uganda* (1967), Ainsworth wrote: "Sensitivity to signals tends to ensure that the care the mother gives the baby, including her playful interaction with him, is attuned to the baby's state and mood at the baby's own timing, not the mother's timing "(p. 397). As we will see in Chapter 4, there is now extensive evidence that Ainsworth et al.'s (1978) rating scales of caregiver sensitivity and responsiveness are predictive of attachment security in infancy and childhood.

Searching for other aspects of early caregiving that might contribute to an infant's attachment security, Fonagy et al. (2002) focused on a caregiver's "mentalizing" ability—being able to take a child's perspective and hold in mind his or her needs, feelings, and thoughts. According to Fonagy and Target (1997), a child of a highly mentalizing parent feels that his or her needs and feelings are accurately recognized, allowing the child to feel secure about the parent's sensitive responsiveness when needed. This parental characteristic has been empirically associated with children's attachment security over and above the contribution of parental sensitive responsiveness (see Chapter 4 for a review of the evidence). From the parental side, mentalization is closely associated with sensitivity, because taking into consideration the mental states and perspective of one's child allows a parent to respond sensitively and appropriately to the child's needs (Meins et al., 2012). However, it is not enough simply to mentalize correctly; a caregiver can make accurate inferences about a child's needs yet not be willing or able to provide the needed care, and that care is crucial to the child's felt security.

Recently, Woodhouse et al. (2020) emphasized that effective responsiveness to both attachment and exploration needs, and not mere sensitivity (or its cognitive underpinnings), is critical for enhancing an infant's sense of felt security. In their own words, a security-enhancing caregiver is able "to meet an infant's needs on both sides of the attachment–exploration continuum (e.g., fully soothing a crying infant chest-to-chest and allowing the exploring infant to experience calm, regulated states), even in the presence of high levels of insensitive behavior" (p. 250). This kind of caregiver is characterized by prompt and effective responsiveness (1) when the child is afraid or distressed and wants to be held, protected, soothed, and reassured (safe-haven support), and (2) when the child is curiously exploring the environment and wants the attachment figure to support, applaud, and celebrate his or her growing autonomy and capacities, and to soothe and reassure him or her when exploration becomes too difficult or threatening (secure-base support). Therefore, a child's felt security can be thwarted not only by caregivers who are rejecting or insensitive to proximity-seeking bids when threatened, but also by caregivers who are sensitive to these bids but do not support bids for exploration and autonomy. This is the case of overprotective, overcontrolling, intrusive caregivers who might prefer their children to remain needy, vulnerable, and dependent rather than becoming more mature and independent.

In analyzing the characteristics of a security-enhancing attachment figure in the context of adult relationships, attachment researchers (e.g., Collins et al., 2010) have built upon Ainsworth's work on parental caregiving, focusing on what Batson (1991) called "empathic concern" for others' well-being. This empathic stance involves sensitive responsiveness to others' needs and feelings and the provision of prompt and appropriate support aimed at reducing distress and facilitating autonomous growth (Feeney & Collins, 2015). According to Reis and Shaver (1988), sensitive responsiveness to a needy person's support-seeking bids (as perceived by the support seeker) is defined by three qualities. The first is *understanding*—support seekers believe that the partner accurately perceives and understands what is important to them and has appropriately "gotten the facts right" about them (a quality that corresponds to Fonagy et al.'s [2002] construct of mentalization). The second quality is *validation*—support seekers feel that the partner values and appreciates their traits and abilities, and likes and accepts them. The third quality is *caring*—support seekers sense that the partner is concerned for their welfare and is doing the best he or she can to meet their needs.

During the last decade, several self-report scales have been developed to assess perceived partner responsiveness by asking support seekers to rate the extent to which they feel understood, validated, and cared for by their partner in times of need (e.g., Crasta et al., 2021). People scoring low on these scales often dismiss or misinterpret their partner's needs and feelings, and either avoid adopting the attachment-figure role or insert themselves awkwardly or intrusively into the needy person's affairs. As a result, they thwart their partner's sense of felt security and undermine his or her ability to confidently rely on them in times of need.

As in parent–child relationships, an understanding, validating, and caring adult attachment figure is capable of enhancing support seekers' felt security only if he or she also effectively meets their needs for a safe haven and secure base. As described in Chapter 1, threats and dangers elicit the search for safe-haven provisions (e.g., protection, reassurance, comfort, relief), and new opportunities and challenges for exploration and goal pursuit elicit the search for secure-base provisions (e.g., encouragement, empowerment, autonomy support). Without such provisions, a person may fail to quell distress and cope with life difficulties or fail to pursue opportunities for exploration and growth. Moreover, he or she may not feel confident that the attachment figure will provide effective support when needed. In other words, he or she may not feel secure with respect to the attachment figure's benevolence and competence.

In their model of thriving with the benefit of healthy relationships, Feeney and Collins (2015) supplied a detailed description of the specific components of safe-haven support and secure-base support that a responsive attachment figure can provide as ways of launching what we are calling a *broaden-and-build process*. When people facing threats or dangers seek a safe haven, a security-enhancing attachment figure provides safety and protection, emotional or physical comfort, reassurance, guidance, or tangible aids that can alleviate distress and ease the care-seeker's burdens. This figure also provides what Feeney and Collins called *fortification*—"assisting in the development of a close other's strengths and abilities relevant to coping with the adversity either by pointing out strengths and abilities that the person already has but may not recognize (helping them learn about the self through adversity) or by recognizing a strength or ability that is needed for successful coping and assisting them in attaining it" (p. 117). A security-enhancing attachment figure also encourages and helps support seekers to solve the problem on their own, to take a more positive outlook on the threat (as surmountable and controllable), and to renew or rebuild their sense of self-efficacy and mastery. According to Feeney and Collins, these safe-haven and secure-base provisions not only help people to restore emotional equanimity but they also allow them to learn and grow from life adversities.

When people facing new opportunities and challenges call for a secure base for exploration, a security-enhancing attachment figure assists them in recognizing and articulating the opportunities, fosters an optimistic outlook on the challenge, and encourages them to take the challenge and stretch beyond their comfort zone. This figure also validates their goals and aspirations, expresses enthusiasm for their opportunities, celebrates their achievements, and responds sensitively and nonjudgmentally to failures and setbacks. He or she also assists the secure-base seeker in setting attainable goals and developing suitable goal-related plans and strategies, provides guidance or tangible aids that support exploration and goal pursuit, and provides safe-haven support when the seeker encounters unexpected difficulties during exploration or goal pursuit. All of these behaviors and inclinations are part of what Feeney (2004) called *secure-base support*, and Feeney and Collins (2015) called *relational catalyst support*, which can bolster support seekers' felt security.

The provision of secure-base support involves not only assistance and encouragement but also noninterference with the support seeker's exploration and goal pursuit (Feeney, 2004). A security-enhancing attachment figure respects the support seeker's choices and decisions, and refrains from providing support that is not needed or wanted, from becoming intrusive and emotionally overinvolved, and from impeding the seeker's autonomy (by fostering overdependence and helplessness). This component of secure-base support resembles Ryan and Deci's (2017) construct of *autonomy support*—supporting and assisting another person while acknowledging his or her feelings and unique perspective, encouraging choices and options, and refraining from excessive control, pressure, or conditional forms of regard ("I like you if you will behave in the way I told you to"). In our view, autonomy support is an integral component of secure-base support that contributes greatly to favorable broaden-and-build processes.

In line with Woodhouse et al. (2020) and Feeney and Collins (2015), we believe that a security-enhancing attachment figure is supportive at both ends of the attachment–exploration continuum. In other words, he or she is willing and able not only to meet a seeker's needs for proximity and protection in times of threat but also to support the seeker's autonomous growth. Overcontrolling and intrusive attachment figures who offer protection and comfort to a person in times of need but disrespect or reject the person's bids for autonomy fail to provide a secure base for exploration and therefore cannot be viewed as security-enhancing attachment figures.

On the whole, from a clinical or interventionist perspective, if we want to enhance a person's sense of felt security, we need to heighten the sensitivity and responsiveness of his or her attachment figures with respect to the full attachment–exploration continuum. This goal can be met by cultivating the attachment figure's mentalization and by fostering his or her provision of more empathic and effective forms of safe-haven and secure-base support. We can also direct a person's attention, reflection, memory, and imagination toward interactions with sensitive and responsive attachment figures who respect and meet needs for both secure attachment and exploration. Although each attachment-based intervention we review in subsequent chapters emphasizes specific, unique components of the path to greater security, they share the assumption that the physical or mental presence of a sensitive and responsive provider of both a safe haven and a secure base is the heart of any successful psychological transformation.

Moving Insecure People toward Greater Felt Security

During infancy, interactions with sensitive and responsive parents contribute to the mental construction of the secure-base script and promotion of the broaden-and-build cycle of attachment security. In later stages of development, interactions with other sensitive and responsive attachment figures can reinforce and elaborate the existing broaden-and-build cycle in those who grew up in a secure familial environment. But can these interactions really instill felt security and promote positive psychological outcomes on the part of less secure individuals?

Fortunately, the answer appears to be yes, although the path to security can be long, arduous, and sometimes frustrating. As we mentioned in Chapter 1, insecure people, despite their predominantly negative working models, usually possess nondominant representations of security in their associative memory networks (Baldwin et al., 1996). Interactions with sensitive and responsive partners, as well as reflecting upon their positive experiences, can strengthen and increase the mental accessibility of the secure-base script. When positive, script-enhancing interactions are personally relevant and repeated across time and situations, they can expand a person's psychological islands of security, compensate for attachment-related vulnerabilities, and allow insecure people to feel cared for, loved, appreciated. Indeed, as we explain in subsequent chapters, research confirms that interacting with responsive attachment figures in different kinds of relationships (e.g., romantic, teacher–student, therapist–client, manager–worker) has long-term positive effects on a person's felt security, relationship quality, and mental health (e.g., Arriaga et al., 2014; Davidovitz et al., 2007; Håvås et al., 2015).

Despite this optimistic conclusion, there is also reason to doubt that security-enhancing experiences in adulthood, either naturally produced or deliberately provided (e.g., experimentally or clinically), can completely overcome strongly dominant and deeply rooted insecure working models and the conscious and unconscious memories on which they are based. Rather, these later experiences can only increase the relative accessibility of the secure-base script, while leaving in place insecurities that originated in prior attachment relationships.

This possibility fits with a "prototype" approach to attachment working models (e.g., Fraley, 2002), which suggests that two different kinds of mental representations jointly determine a person's state of mind with respect to attachment at any given moment: (1) early "prototype" models and (2) currently accessible working models. The prototype working models formed during the first few years of life do not change, and they contribute a stable core to later models, increasing the likelihood that attachment patterns later in life will reflect early childhood patterns. However, attachment patterns at a given developmental stage are also a function of currently accessible working models that result from past and current experiences with a wide variety of nonparental attachment figures. These experiences can be compatible with model stability if they converge with the prototype models, but they can induce changes in attachment orientation if they deviate significantly from these models (e.g., interacting in the present with sensitive and responsive partners who refute insecure working models formed during early childhood).

This approach has been supported in longitudinal studies examining the stability of attachment patterns across various time spans in childhood, adolescence, and adulthood (for meta-analyses, see Fraley, 2002; Fraley & Brumbaugh, 2004; for an updated review, see Fraley & Roisman, 2019). For example, Fraley, Vicary, et al. (2011) examined data from two longitudinal samples. Attachment orientations to the mother, the father, and a romantic partner were assessed daily over a 30-day period (Sample 1) or weekly over a year (Sample 2). In both samples, the observed patterns of stability in attachment scores were consistent with the idea that there is a stable foundation underlying temporary variations in attachment orientation. Moreover, structural statistical models indicated that the data were easier to explain with the assumption that there is a latent, enduring factor (e.g., a prototype) underlying the attachment dimensions at each assessment wave. However, at the same time, the fact that this latent, enduring factor explained only a moderate portion of the variance in attachment scores over time leaves considerable room for change and suggests that adult attachment patterns are also sensitive to changing life circumstances. This finding has been conceptually replicated in a 5-year study on the trajectory of attachment patterns during adolescence (Jones et al., 2018) and in a 2-year study examining stability and change in first-time mothers' attachment style (Stern et al., 2018).

The prototype approach implies that although new security-enhancing experiences can lead insecure people to feel more secure, traces of early experiences of insecurity might still negatively bias their perceptions, thoughts, and emotions, and might reemerge when there are indications that a current attachment figure is failing to be sensitive and responsive. As a result, as clinicians or interveners, we need to encourage insecure people to be aware of, reflect on, and work through their prototypical models and memories in order to allow the broaden-and-build cycle to emerge and function properly. Some of the interventions we review in subsequent chapters put strong emphasis on this working-through process as a necessary step for consolidating long-term positive changes and cultivating a solid sense of felt security.

In our opinion, any attachment-based intervention that aims to foster security-based broaden-and-build processes should consider the following four principles that we draw from Bowlby's (1988) clinical writings:

1. When interacting with others who fulfill the role of attachment figure in a particular relational or social context, a person's dominant working models and dispositional attachment orientation will shape and bias his or her motives, feelings, cognitions, and behaviors in that context (via prototype-driven processing).
2. A person's motives, feelings, cognitions, and behaviors in a given relational or social context are also affected by the quality of actual, recalled, or imagined interactions with others who fulfill the role of attachment figure in that context (via experience-driven processing).
3. Actual, recalled, or imagined interactions with an attachment figure who is sensitive and responsive to both ends of the attachment–exploration continuum in a given relational or social context set in motion broaden-and-build processes and move an insecure person along the path to greater security.
4. Recurrent and personally significant interactions with this beneficial kind of attachment figure will increase the likelihood of long-term changes in felt security. This gradual consolidation of a stable sense of felt security over time and across contexts can be further solidified by exploring, reflecting, and working through early insecure and painful experiences, memories, and working models with the guidance and assistance of a reliable secure-base provider.

With these principles in mind, attachment theory can be applied to any relational or social context in which others are perceived as providing a safe haven and secure base when a person feels a need for this. These contexts include relationships with close partners (e.g., family members, close friends, dating partners, spouses), as well as social contexts in which the potential security provider is a domain expert and occupies the role of a "stronger and wiser" (Bowlby's terms) caregiver in a formal hierarchy or organization (e.g., teacher, coach, priest, therapist, manager, physician). Groups, organizations, and social institutions (e.g., the judicial system, government) as well as nonhuman figures (e.g., God, deceased loved ones, pets) that are perceived to be sensitive and responsive to one's support-seeking bids, can also infuse a sense of felt security and improve psychological well-being, social adjustment, and quality of life.

At the beginning of a relationship, people's prototypical working models (either secure or insecure), especially their early implicit models of others, tend to be automatically projected onto the potential security provider (Brumbaugh & Fraley, 2007), thereby interfering with a change in working models. Andersen and Chen (2002), following Freud, explained this projection of working models in terms of the transference of mental representations. When a representation of a significant other is activated by resemblance cues in a new relationship partner, this representation will affect the way the perceiver responds to the new partner (e.g., Berk & Andersen, 2000). Moreover, since representations of significant others are linked to self-representations (e.g., Bowlby, 1973), the transference of a significant-other representation onto the new partner will bias self-appraisals within the new relationship (e.g., Kraus & Chen, 2009). This makes it likely that prototypical working models can be transferred to new attachment figures throughout life, shaping a person's appraisals of self and others in new relationships.

However, repeated meaningful interactions with a sensitive and responsive attachment figure when one hopes for a safe haven or secure base may counteract the projection of old insecure models onto new relationship partners and allow for an increase in attachment security. Moreover, attending, recalling, reflecting on, and imagining instances of an attachment figure's love, kindness, and sensitive responsiveness can foster the creation and activation of the secure-base script, thereby increasing well-being and adjustment. Thus, attachment-based interventions aimed at positive psychological change should (1) target a person's attachment figure as an agent of change, (2) attempt to heighten this figure's empathic concern and capacity to provide effective care in times of threat and support engagement in challenging and growth-oriented activities when threats abate, and (3) encourage the person to attend to, recall, and reflect upon this and other attachment figures' love and care while working through and gaining new perspective on early or previous painful experiences and insecure working models.

Concluding Remarks

A large body of research, which despite the length of this chapter we have merely touched upon, indicates, once again (Lieberman, 2013) that the human mind/brain is a highly social entity that heavily relies on others for its successful development and functioning. At the heart of each person's psychology is a need for reliable social support and its satisfaction in relationships with loving and accurately empathic attachment figures. This need is obviously critical during infancy, but is not unimportant in any other phase of the lifespan. A fundamental sense of security rooted in personal and social relationships makes it easier for a person to respond effectively to all kinds of threats and challenges; to be calm, happy, and satisfied; to achieve personal goals; and to behave more compassionately toward other people. In other words, a history of security-enhancing experiences is the bedrock of a fully functioning, self-actualized person (Maslow, 1971; Rogers, 1961), one whose sense of security, far from being selfish or self-focused, supports concern for and generosity toward others. In Chapter 3, we review and evaluate laboratory-experimental interventions that increase the short-term mental accessibility of the secure-base script, with measurable beneficial effects on the broaden-and-build cycle of security.

CHAPTER 3

Boosting Felt Security in the Laboratory

The Broaden-and-Build Effects of Security Priming

Before describing attachment-related interventions involving parents, spouses, therapists, and teachers, we examine a range of laboratory-experimental interventions designed to increase felt security and its broaden-and-build sequelae. In the laboratory, it is easier than in the outside world to try out simple interventions, rigorously assess their causal influence on outcomes of interest, and study possible mediators. The laboratory can be an incubator for interventions that might be extended into the more complex "real world." As will be seen, the results from scores of laboratory intervention studies are fascinating in their own right and a source of optimism regarding real-world applications.

The interventions reviewed in this chapter were designed to increase the accessibility of mental representations of attachment security and thereby alter a person's momentary or short-term attachment-related emotions, thoughts, and behavior. These kinds of applications rely on priming procedures that, before being used by social psychologists, had been well-established in cognitive psychology. Typically, a person is exposed to a stimulus (the *prime*) that can activate related mental representations and, in turn, alter a person's responses in the given context. In applying this technique in studies of attachment dynamics, we (e.g., Mikulincer & Shaver, 2007) have called it *security priming*, because the prime is intended to induce a feeling of security and thus activate a broaden-and-build cycle, with all of its psychological benefits (see Chapter 2). (It is also possible to use insecurity primes, but we have not often done that, for obvious ethical reasons.)

We begin by reviewing various methods of security priming. Next, we evaluate their effectiveness in fostering positive thoughts, sustaining emotional stability and well-being, heightening pro-relational and prosocial orientations, and increasing exploration and learning. These are the basic components of the broaden-and-build cycle of attachment security.

Principles and Methods of Security Priming

In cognitive and social psychology, the term *priming* refers to the activation of a conscious or unconscious mental representation by an environmental stimulus (the *prime*), as well as the effects of this activation on a person's goals, thoughts, feelings, and behavior (e.g., Bargh &

Chartrand, 2014). Typically, priming interventions involve exposing participants to a prime (e.g., word, picture, phrase, or sentence) and measuring some of the psychological effects. For example, we might expose a person to the word *cow* in a lexical decision task (where the person must quickly decide whether a string of letters appearing on a computer screen is or is not a word) and determine whether this makes it easier to quickly perceive that m-i-l-k is a word (Stanovich & West, 1983). (And in fact it does make it easier—i.e., faster.) Or we could expose people to pictures of libraries and examine whether this increases their tendency to be quiet (Aarts & Dijksterhuis, 2003).

Explanations of these priming effects focus on the *accessibility* of mental representations in a person's associative memory network—that is, their readiness to guide information processing and behavior (Molden, 2014). A prime can heighten the accessibility of related mental content (e.g., the mental construct "cow" or "library" in the examples), which in turn can affect a person's subsequent cognitive, affective, and behavioral responses.

Priming effects can be observed even when people are unaware of the prime (e.g., Bargh & Chartrand, 2014). In fact, primes can be presented in either an explicit manner, involving a person's awareness (e.g., asking him or her to look at a picture and remember its details), or in more subtle, implicit ways (e.g., placing a picture in the top-right corner of a computer screen while people are responding to other stimuli presented in the center of the screen). Primes can be either generic—in which case all study participants are exposed to the same stimulus—or idiosyncratic, with each participant being exposed to a stimulus that is especially tailored to him or her (e.g., priming the word *mother* versus priming the first name of a person's actual mother). Moreover, primes can be presented in well-controlled laboratory settings or outside the laboratory (e.g., when encountering an experimental confederate walking in a park and wearing a T-shirt with a picture of a cemetery on it, which is an implicit reminder of mortality).

In many cases, exposure to a prime immediately activates a related mental representation and has immediate effects, and those effects then evaporate over time because of naturally occurring interference from other stimuli or trains of thought (Dijksterhuis & van Knippenberg, 1998). However, there is evidence that repeatedly exposing a person to a prime on several different occasions can produce psychological effects that are more sustained over time (e.g., Lowery et al., 2007).

A primed mental representation can affect behavior in many ways (Wheeler & DeMarree, 2009). First, the primed mental representation can directly alter behavior. For example, exposure to the face of an elderly person may increase the accessibility of the stereotyped slow movements of an aged person, influencing the primed individual to walk more slowly (e.g., Bargh et al., 1996). Second, the primed mental representation may activate specific goals, which then direct behavior. For example, the presence of business-related objects in a room can increase the accessibility of the concept or feeling of competitiveness, which may increase a person's motivation to excel at a task (Kay et al., 2004). Third, the primed mental representation may bias perceptions of other people, oneself, or a current situation, which can activate relevant goals and behaviors. For example, priming the concept of hostility can cause a person to perceive others as hostile, which may activate self-protection goals and defensive behaviors (e.g., Srull & Wyer, 1979).

In searching for ways to contextually, experimentally enhance a person's felt security and its beneficial consequences, attachment researchers have used priming procedures to heighten the accessibility of security-related mental representations (the process that we, as mentioned, call *security priming*). Security priming involves either explicit or implicit exposure to generic attachment-related stimuli (the word *loving* or a picture of an infant holding an adult's hand) or idiosyncratic attachment-related stimuli (the name or photo of a person's main security provider), which can momentarily increase felt security and renew a person's confidence in the availability of support when needed. We hypothesize that this primed felt security is similar to that induced by the actual presence of a supportive and loving attachment figure in times of need, which has the effect of causing a person to feel, think, and react more like a secure person. In other words, security priming can elicit, at least in the short term, the broaden-and-build cycle of attachment security and put a person on a better path of personal development.

As with other primes, the psychological effects of security primes seem to involve a cascade of changes in a person's cognitions, emotions, and goals. Priming mental representations of security seems to cause people to think about themselves, others, and their current situation through the lens of the secure-base script, facilitating healthy emotion regulation and moving them beyond egoistic neediness and self-protection goals. Figure 3.1 is a schematic representation of the hypothesized cascade of mental processes involved in security priming.

The immediate effect of security priming is to activate security-related mental representations that may be either abstract (e.g., the construct of being loved) or relationship-specific (e.g., the representation of a specific secure relationship), depending on the type of prime used (generic or relationship-specific). Once these security-related mental representations are activated, related neural networks of social-relational memories, self-representations, and procedural knowledge may be triggered by a process of *spreading activation* (e.g., Collins & Loftus, 1975), heightening access to the core components of the secure-base script. As a result, a person may think positively about self, others, and close relationships; adopt an

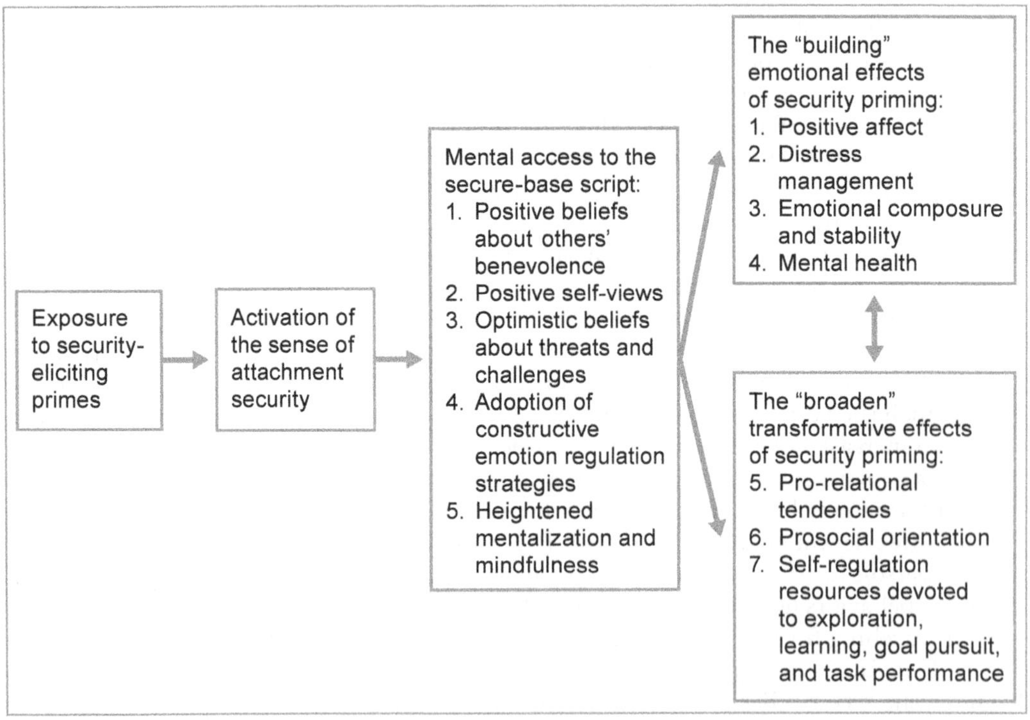

FIGURE 3.1. A schematic representation of the cascade of mental processes involved in security priming.

optimistic outlook on the ability to deal with threats and challenges; and endorse constructive emotion-regulation strategies, including mentalization and mindfulness. This heightened access to the secure-base script creates a relatively calm and confident state of mind, which contributes to distress management, emotional composure, and mental health (the "building" emotional effects of security priming). It also facilitates the endorsement of a pro-relational, prosocial orientation, energizes exploration and learning, improves goal pursuit and task performance, and sustains the cultivation of autonomous action and the further development of personal talents (the "broaden" transformative effects of security priming).

In the last 20 years, the effectiveness of security priming at fostering positive psychological outcomes has been examined in more than 100 published studies (for reviews and meta-analyses, see Gillath & Karantzas, 2019; Gillath et al., 2022; Rowe et al., 2020). In all of them, participants are first exposed to a security-inducing or neutral prime, and the effects of this exposure are examined in a subsequent activity or task. However, the studies differ in the stimuli and techniques used to prime attachment security (see Figure 3.2 for a summary). In the following section we review different kinds of security primes and priming techniques.

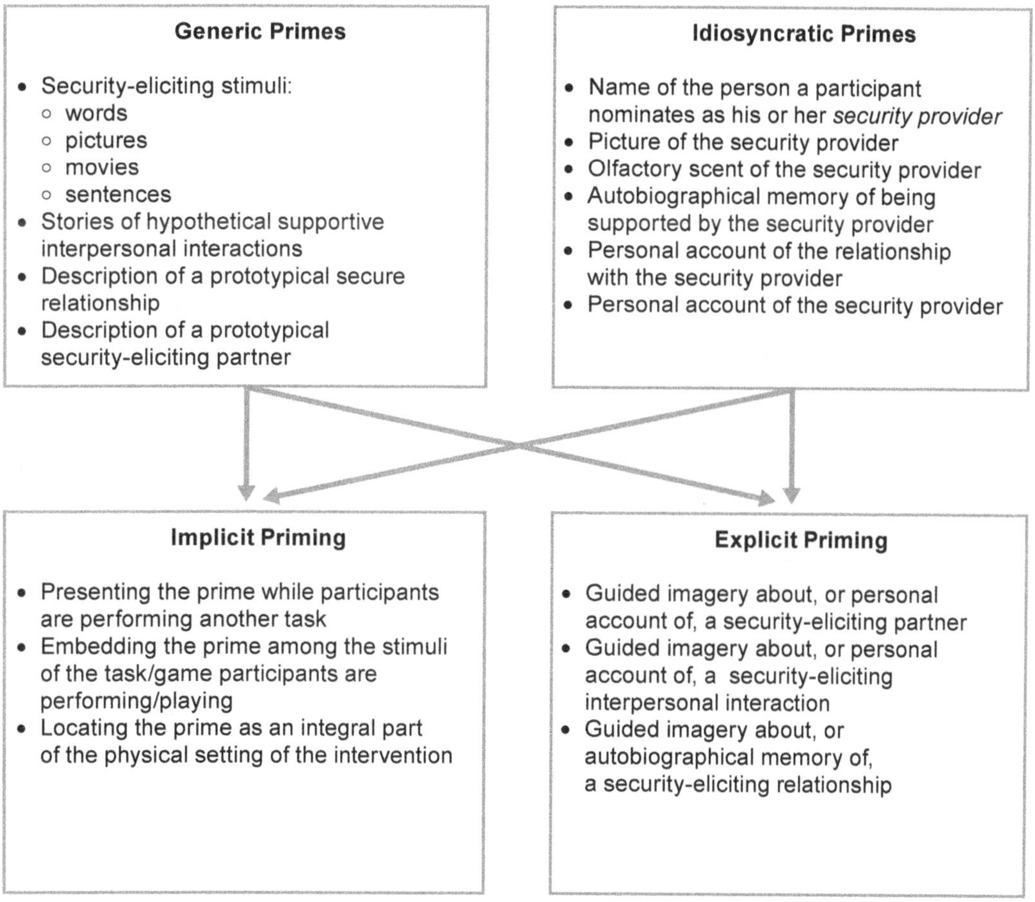

FIGURE 3.2. A schematic representation of different types of security primes and priming techniques.

Types of Security Primes

Security primes include both generic and personally tailored, idiosyncratic stimuli. In studies using generic primes, researchers select a stimulus that is typically suggestive of attachment security, and the same prime is given to all participants in a particular experimental condition. (There are also one or more control, or comparison, priming conditions.) In such studies, it is important to ensure that the selected prime is strong enough to boost security in most of the participants, which is based on conducting systematic pretests and having separate large groups of participants rate the degree to which the potential prime is conceptually related to felt security. In studies using idiosyncratic (person-specific) primes, researchers must identify a stimulus that is suggestive of attachment security for a given participant (usually a relationship partner with whom he or she feels secure), then expose the person to the selected prime. In such studies, it is important to ensure that the prime is the most, or one of the most, prototypical examples of a security provider, which is done by asking each participant to nominate his or her most important source of felt security (see below for a review of nomination techniques).

Although a generic prime is easier than an idiosyncratic prime to create and manipulate (because a standard stimulus is used for all participants), it might fail to increase felt security among chronically insecure people because of negative or ambivalent thoughts and feelings associated with the prime (e.g., the word *love*). In contrast, an idiosyncratic prime might be associated with security-related mental representations in both secure and insecure people, because it represents the most important source of security for each participant. (Still, we cannot rule out the possibility that even these best examples of support might arouse less than completely positive mental representations for some insecure individuals.)

Generic Primes

Studies relying on generic primes have used words, pictures, film clips, sentences, and narratives of hypothetical interpersonal interactions or relationships. Verbal primes include words that connote some of the core features of felt security, such as *loved, hug, comforted, embraced, caring, accepted, wanted,* and *cherished* (e.g., Charles-Sire et al., 2012; Canterberry & Gillath, 2013; Gabriel et al., 2010). Pictorial primes include pictures that connote loving and comforting interactions, such as a mother and her baby gazing lovingly at each other (Bowles & Meyer, 2008), a distressed person being physically comforted by a partner (Mikulincer, Gillath, et al., 2001), or a young boy saying to his father, "Even if there is an ocean between us, I know you will be there for me" (Taubman-Ben-Ari & Mikulincer, 2007). Oehler and Psouni (2019) used pictures depicting a peaceful moment surrounded by family members, time spent with a group of close friends, or the empowering feeling of belonging to a team; and Dandeneau et al. (2007) used photos of accepting faces (expressing genuine Duchenne smiles).

Some studies have used security-related sentences (e.g., Green & Campbell, 2000; McGuire et al., 2018), such as "I feel close to and secure with other people," "I feel relaxed knowing that close others are there for me right now," and "I am comfortable depending on other people." These sentences are usually taken from Hazan and Shaver's (1987) or Bartholomew and Horowitz's (1991) prototypical descriptions of secure attachment or from the security subscale of the State Adult Attachment Measure (SAAM; Gillath et al., 2009). In another study (Taubman-Ben-Ari & Mikulincer, 2007), the security prime was a short video portraying a young boy and his father talking about their good relationship and recalling past situations in which the father was sensitive and responsive to his son's needs. Finally, other researchers have asked participants to read short accounts of hypothetical security-eliciting interpersonal interactions or relationships. For example, Gillath and Shaver (2007, p. 971) provided the following description:

> Imagine a relationship in which your partner, for a fairly long time, has consistently been available to you, sensitive to your needs, and highly reliable, having your interests at heart and supporting you in every way he/she can. That is, imagine that this person is about as reliable as any other human being could be.

Idiosyncratic Primes

Studies relying on idiosyncratic primes include exposure to the name or picture of an actual person a participant nominates as a security provider, visualization of this person's face, or guided imagery focused on the relationship with this person or a security-eliciting interaction with him or her. In some studies, participants are directly asked to nominate the person with whom they feel secure and they trust will be available and responsive when needed. For example, Bartz and Lydon (2004) provided Hazan and Shaver's (1987) prototypical description of a secure relationship (see Chapter 1) and asked participants to nominate a relationship partner who fits this description. Alternatively, Cassidy et al. (2018, p. 578) asked participants to nominate "the person you can most depend on to be there to comfort you in times of trouble."

In other studies, the nomination process is more complex. For example, Baldwin et al. (1996) asked participants to list the names of 10 close relationship partners and to indicate whether the relationship with each partner fits Hazan and Shaver's (1987) prototypical description of secure attachment. Then, from those partners who fit the secure description, participants selected the partner with whom they felt most secure. In Mikulincer et al.'s (2005) study, participants completed the six-item WHOTO scale (Fraley & Davis, 1997) and provided the name of a person who fit the role of a security provider in the situation mentioned in an item. The WHOTO items tap proximity-seeking tendencies (e.g., "Who is the person you most like to spend time with?"), safe-haven provision (e.g., "Who is the person you turn to when you are feeling down?"), and secure-base provision (e.g., "Who is the person you want to share your successes with?"). The primed figure is the partner named most frequently across the six items.

Methods of Security Priming

Both generic and idiosyncratic stimuli can be primed in an implicit or explicit manner. *Implicit priming* refers to incidental exposure to a prime without participants being either fully aware of the manipulation or having been instructed not to attend to or think about the prime (Bargh & Chartrand, 2014). *Explicit priming* refers to conscious exposure to a prime, with participants being explicitly asked to think about and reflect on the prime and sometimes to write about associated feelings and memories. Because of its transparent nature, explicit priming may raise suspicion, discomfort, or self-presentation concerns, especially among insecure people, that could interfere with the smooth activation of security-related mental representations. However, due to its elaborative nature, explicit priming might contribute to a deeper level of cognitive processing than implicit priming, and thus to a broader spread of activation from the primed representation. The details of this complex process have yet to be fully studied.

Implicit Priming

A common implicit priming technique involves presenting a security prime while participants are performing another task on which they are fully concentrating. For example, Gillath et al. (2010) asked participants to rate the similarities between two pieces of furniture (e.g., lamp–rug) presented as words on a computer screen for 25 trials, and before each trial participants were exposed to a generic security-related word for 22 milliseconds in the middle of the screen. In Selcuk et al.'s (2012) study, participants were exposed to a picture of their security provider (presented at the center of a monitor screen) for 30 trials while they were asked to indicate the position of a triangle that was presented at one of six possible locations (i.e., upper left, middle left, lower left, upper right, middle right, and lower right side of the screen).

Another implicit priming technique involves presenting a security prime within the set of stimuli of the task or game that participants are performing or playing. For example, McGuire et al. (2018) used a word search puzzle in which some of the words were security-related, and Norman et al. (2015) presented security-related pictures on the left or right side of a screen and asked participants to indicate the position of the picture. Dandeneau et al. (2007) asked participants to engage in a picture-detection task and quickly detect an accepting target face in a 4 × 4 matrix of otherwise rejecting faces.

Alternatively, the security prime can be presented as an integral part of the physical setting of the intervention (e.g., locating a security-inducing picture on one of the room's walls or as a logo on a computer monitor). For example, Charles-Sire et al. (2012, 2016) printed the word *loving* on the T-shirt an experimental confederate wore during the session, and Karremans et al. (2011) inserted the name of the nominated security provider in the lower right-hand corner of the computer screen that participants were using to complete the experimental tasks. Mikulincer, Gillath, et al. (2001) placed a security-related picture on the inside cover of a folder that included the self-report scales participants were asked to complete, and Dimri (2018) printed such a picture on the mouse pad participants were using during the experimental session.

Explicit Priming

One of the most frequently used explicit priming techniques involves visualization of the person a participant nominates as his or her main security provider. For example, Baldwin et al. (1996) asked participants to "picture this person's face" and "try to imagine being with this person" for 2 minutes. In Carnelley's studies (e.g., Carnelley et al., 2016, 2018), participants received instructions to visualize the face of the nominated relationship partner and to think about a time when this person made them feel safe, secure, and comforted. Bartz and Lydon (2004, p. 1393) added instructions to this visualization task aimed at eliciting feelings and memories associated with the nominated partner. Their instructions were as follows:

> "Now, take a moment and try to get a visual image in your mind of this person. What does this person look like? What is it like being with this person? You may want to remember a time you were actually with this person. What would he or she say to you? What would you say in return? How do you feel when you are with this person? How would you feel if they were here with you now?"

Another explicit priming technique involves guided imagery connected with a prototypical secure relationship. Sutin and Gillath (2009), for example, provided Hazan and

Shaver's (1987) prototypical description of secure attachment (see Chapter 1) and asked participants to describe how being in that relationship would make them feel. In other studies (e.g., Dewitte & De Houwer, 2011), participants were asked to recall, reflect on, and describe a close relationship of theirs, either ongoing or past, that fit Hazan and Shaver's (1987) prototypical description.

In some security priming studies, participants are instructed to imagine and reflect on a hypothetical security-enhancing interpersonal interaction. Mallinckrodt et al. (2013), for example, asked participants to read a story depicting such an interaction, to visualize the situation and the faces of the persons involved as vividly as possible, and to describe the feelings and thoughts this visualization elicited. In other studies, participants have been asked to remember and describe a particular time or situation in which they felt secure or cared for by a relationship partner (e.g., Julal & Carnelley, 2012; Schoemann et al., 2012).

Effects of Security Priming on the Secure-Base Script

Are security-priming interventions capable of heightening a person's sense of attachment security? Can these interventions activate the various components of the secure-base script (positive views of self and others, optimistic appraisals of threats and challenges, constructive emotion-regulation strategies, mentalization, and mindfulness)? In this section, we review security-priming studies that have directly addressed these questions.

The Sense of Attachment Security

Thirty-four studies have examined the effects of security primes (vs. neutral, positive-affect, self-esteem, or attachment-insecure primes) on the sense of attachment security. (Thirty-three of them were conducted among adolescents and young adults, and only one was conducted with children.) Some researchers have used brief self-report scales that tap participants' current feelings of being cared for, esteemed, loved, and protected. For example, Luke et al. (2012) constructed a "Felt Security Measure" to assess the extent to which participants were feeling comforted, supported, looked after, cared for, secure, safe, protected, unthreatened, valued, better about themselves, loved, cherished, treasured, and adored. Other studies have assessed emotions and cognitions associated with attachment security using the Security subscale of the SAAM (e.g., Millings et al., 2019). Still others have examined whether security priming reduces attachment insecurities, as evidenced by participants' scores on the ECR Anxiety and Avoidance scales (e.g., Hudson & Fraley, 2018). Table 3.1 summarizes the methods used in the 34 studies.

The vast majority of the studies included in Table 3.1 (32 of 34) found that, as compared to control primes, security primes increased children's and adults' sense of attachment security and led to lower scores on the ECR anxiety or avoidance scales. Interestingly, similar effects have been found when participants freely wrote about their current feelings without being explicitly asked about their sense of security. Specifically, Carnelley and Rowe (2010) analyzed the texts produced by participants in different priming conditions using the Linguistic Inquiry and Word Count program (Pennebaker et al., 2007) to examine the frequency with which specific themes emerged in the text. They found that visualization of a security provider yielded more themes related to felt security, positive care, and a sense of togetherness than visualization of a mere acquaintance or a funny TV or film character.

Regarding the possibility of creating long-term priming effects, eight studies have used repeated-priming methods, producing strong evidence for the sustainability of

TABLE 3.1. Summary of Studies Examining Security Priming Effects on Felt Security

Author	Type of prime	Prime modality	Priming technique	Control conditions	Number of priming sessions	Felt security assessment	Delay between priming and assessment
Mikulincer, Gillath, et al. (2001, Study 1)	Generic	Hypothetical supportive story	Explicit	Neutral and positive-affect primes	Single session	Four-item scale	No delay
Mikulincer, Gillath, et al. (2001, Study 2)	Generic	Security-eliciting picture	Implicit	Neutral and positive-affect primes	Single session	Four-item scale	No delay
Carnelley & Rowe (2007)	Generic and Idiosyncratic	Hypothetical supportive story; recall of a secure relationship	Explicit	Neutral prime	Every day for 3 consecutive days	Two-item scale and ECR scales	2 days later
Gillath et al. (2009, Study 5)	Idiosyncratic	Recall of a secure relationship	Explicit	Neutral prime	Single session	SS-SAAM	No delay
Gillath et al. (2009, Study 6)	Generic	Hypothetical secure relationship	Explicit	Neutral, positive-affect, and self-esteem primes	Single session	SS-SAAM	No delay
Carnelley & Rowe (2010)	Idiosyncratic	Visualization of security provider	Explicit	Neutral and positive-affect primes	Single session	Open-ended probes	No delay
Luke et al. (2012, Study 1)	Idiosyncratic	Visualization of security provider	Explicit	Attachment-anxious and avoidant primes	Single session	FSS	No delay
Luke et al. (2012, Study 2)	Idiosyncratic	Visualization of security provider	Explicit	Neutral prime	Single session	FSS	No delay
Luke et al. (2012, Study 3)	Idiosyncratic	Visualization of security provider	Explicit	Positive-affect prime	Single session	FSS	No delay
Rowe et al. (2012)	Idiosyncratic	Visualization of security provider)	Explicit	Neutral and attachment-insecurity primes	Single session	FSS	No delay
Bosmans et al. (2014)	Idiosyncratic	Recall of security-eliciting episodes	Explicit	Neutral and attachment-insecurity primes	Single session	SAAM	No delay
Pepping, Davis, & O'Donovan (2015a, Study 2)	Idiosyncratic	Recall of a secure relationship	Explicit	Neutral prime	Single session	SS-SAAM	No delay

Pepping, Davis, O'Donovan, & Pal (2015b, Study 2)	Idiosyncratic	Visualization of security provider	Explicit	Neutral prime	Single session	SS-SAAM	No delay
Deng et al. (2016)	Generic	Hypothetical supportive story	Explicit	No prime	Single session	Four-item scale	No delay
Li, Bunke, et al. (2016, Study 2)	Idiosyncratic	Visualization of security provider	Explicit	Neutral prime	Single session	Seven-item scale	No delay
Otway et al. (2014)	Idiosyncratic	Recall of security-eliciting episodes (texting)	Explicit	Neutral prime	Every day for 3 consecutive days	FSS	2 days later
Norman et al. (2015)	Generic	Security-eliciting pictures	Implicit	Neutral prime	Single session	SAAM	No delay
Boag & Carnelley (2016, Study 1)	Idiosyncratic	Visualization of security provider	Explicit	Neutral prime	Single session	FSS	No delay
Carnelley et al. (2016, Study 1)	Idiosyncratic	Visualization of security provider	Explicit	Neutral, attachment-anxious, and avoidant primes	Single session	FSS	No delay
Carnelley et al. (2016, Study 2)	Idiosyncratic	Recall of security-eliciting episodes (texting)	Explicit	Neutral prime	Every day for 4 consecutive days	FSS	1 day later
Carnelley et al. (2018)	Idiosyncratic	Recall of security-eliciting episodes (texting)	Explicit	Neutral prime	Every day for 4 consecutive days	Four-item scale	1 day later
Hudson & Fraley (2018)	Idiosyncratic	Recall of security-eliciting episodes	Explicit	Neutral prime	Every week for 16 consecutive weeks	ECR	Every 2 weeks
McGuire et al. (2018, Study 2)	Generic and idiosyncratic	Recall of security-eliciting episodes; exposure to security-eliciting pictures, words, and sentences	Explicit and implicit	Neutral prime	Every other day for five sessions over 14 days	SAAM-short version (9 items)	Immediately after the last priming session
Oehler & Psouni (2019)	Idiosyncratic	Recall of security-eliciting episodes (texting)	Explicit	No prime	Every day for 7 consecutive days	SS-SAAM	1 week later

(continued)

TABLE 3.1. *(continued)*

Author	Type of prime	Prime modality	Priming technique	Control conditions	Number of priming sessions	Felt security assessment	Delay between priming and assessment
Millings et al. (2019, Study 1)	Idiosyncratic	Recall of a secure relationship	Explicit	Neutral prime	Single session	SS-SAAM	No delay
Sood & Newman-Taylor (2020)	Idiosyncratic	Recall of security-eliciting episodes	Explicit	Threat-eliciting prime	Single session	FSS	No delay
Sun et al. (2020)	Idiosyncratic	Visualization of security provider	Explicit	Neutral prime	Single session	Five-item scale	No delay
Karl et al. (2021)	Idiosyncratic	Recall of security-eliciting episodes	Explicit	Neutral prime	Single session	FSS	No delay
Ma et al. (2021)	Generic and Idiosyncratic	Recall of security-eliciting episodes; exposure to security-eliciting pictures and films; keeping a diary of security-related interactions	Explicit	Neutral prime	Every day for 30 consecutive days (15 laboratory sessions; 15 days of diary entries)	SS-SAAM	Immediately after the last priming session
Newman-Taylor et al. (2021)	Idiosyncratic	Recall of security-eliciting episodes	Explicit	Attachment-avoidant prime	Every day for 4 consecutive days	FSS	No delay
Sood et al. (2021)	Idiosyncratic	Recall of security-eliciting episodes	Explicit	Attachment-anxious and avoidant primes	Single session	FSS	No delay
Stevenson et al. (2021, Study 2)	Idiosyncratic	Visualization of loving relationship partner	Explicit	Neutral prime and mindfulness exercise	Single session	SAAM	No delay
Sood et al. (2022)	Idiosyncratic	Recall of security-eliciting episodes	Explicit	Attachment-anxious and avoidant primes	Single session	FSS	No delay
Cuyvers et al. (2023)*	Idiosyncratic	Recall of security-eliciting episodes with mother	Explicit	Neutral and attachment-avoidant primes	Single session	SAAM (brief version)	No delay

Note. ECR, Experiences in Close Relationships; FSS, Felt Security Scale, SAAM, State Adult Attachment Measure; SS-SAAM, Security subscale of the State Adult Attachment Measure. An asterisk (*) indicates that the sample comprised school-age children (ages 9–13 years).

security-priming effects on felt security. In these studies, participants were exposed to security or neutral primes every day for 3, 4, 5, 7, or 30 consecutive days or every other day for a total of five sessions over a 2-week period (see Table 3.1). Data on felt security were collected after each priming session, only at the last session, or 1, 2, or 7 days later (see Table 3.1). In all of these studies, with the exception of McGuire et al. (2018), a secure prime led to stronger felt security than a neutral prime at all of the assessed time points, even 1 week after the last priming session.

Hudson and Fraley (2018) assessed attachment anxiety and avoidance (using the ECR) every 2 weeks for 4 months and found that exposing participants to a security prime (vs. a neutral prime) every week during this 4-month period led to a significant and steady decrease in attachment anxiety. However, attachment-related avoidance was unaffected over time by the security prime. Overall, findings obtained to date indicate that repeated security priming is effective in producing long-term (rather than just momentary) changes in the sense of attachment security or insecurity (perhaps mainly along the attachment anxiety dimension).

Positive Beliefs about Relationship Partners

Security priming can also increase positive beliefs about relationship partners. Asking participants to write about a past relationship in which they felt secure leads to more positive evaluations of a current romantic partner and more positive expectations about his or her behavior than writing about an insecure relationship (Dewitte & DeHouwer, 2011; Rowe & Carnelley, 2003). Extending these findings, Carnelley and Rowe (2007) repeatedly asked participants to recall or imagine security-enhancing interpersonal interactions or neutral events across 3 consecutive days. Two days later, they assessed the participants' expectations about a current relationship partner's behavior (not preceded by any prime). Findings indicated more positive expectations following the security prime than the neutral prime. Similar effects were found when text messages were sent to participants' mobile phones instructing them to visualize a security-enhancing or neutral experience (Otway et al., 2014).

Positive Self-Views

Security-priming interventions also have beneficial effects on another component of the secure-base script: positive beliefs about one's social value and lovability. Research indicates that exposure to cues of another's acceptance (e.g., a picture of a smiling, accepting face paired with the participant's own name) results in higher state self-esteem than exposure to neutral cues (Baccus et al., 2004). Directing participants' attention to these kinds of security-enhancing cues also appears to increase state self-esteem (Dandeneau et al., 2007). For 5 days, participants in the security priming condition were asked to quickly detect a smiling, accepting target face in a 4 × 4 matrix of otherwise negative faces. In the control condition, participants had to find a five-petaled flower in a 4 × 4 array of seven-petaled flowers. By the end of the study, the self-esteem of the participants in the security-priming group had increased significantly. No such change occurred in the control condition (Dandeneau et al., 2007). Similar positive effects of security priming have been found in reports of self-compassion (e.g., Oehler & Psouni, 2019; Pepping, Davis, O'Donovan, et al., 2015), indicating that this intervention not only heightens self-esteem but also encourages more accepting and compassionate attitudes toward oneself (attitudes modeled on those of the primed security providers).

Three other studies show that security priming can instill a sense of self-worth that is sufficient to render defensive self-enhancement unnecessary (Arndt et al., 2002; Reis et al., 2018; Schimel et al., 2001). This security-priming effect can be seen in the reduction of five kinds of self-enhancement maneuvers: (1) defensive social comparison (searching for information that suggests that one performs better than others), (2) defensive self-handicapping (emphasizing factors that impair performance in an effort to avoid attribution of negative outcomes to lack of ability), (3) the "better than average effect" (rating oneself as better than an average peer), (4) the "I-knew-it-all-along" effect (believing that one knew the answer to a question or problem all along), and (5) overclaiming personal responsibility for household activities shared with a romantic partner. Along these lines, Kumashiro and Sedikides (2005) found that visualization of a responsive friend (as compared to a control condition) increased willingness to learn about potential personal weaknesses. It seems that security priming bolsters a person's self-concept to the point that it is possible to seek accurate information about personal weaknesses and liabilities despite its self-threatening nature.

Optimistic Beliefs about Threats and Challenges

Several studies have shown that security-priming interventions strengthen optimistic beliefs about threats and challenges. For example, participants who were asked to recall security-enhancing relational experiences on a daily basis (through mobile phone instructions) for a 7-day period reported less perceived stress and viewed themselves as more able to recover from hardships 1 week later than those who received no prime (Oehler & Psouni, 2019). Similar effects of security priming were observed on an implicit measure of threat appraisal—the extent to which participants categorized stimuli as threatening (Wu et al., 2020). Specifically, participants who were asked to recall a security-enhancing relational experience were less likely to categorize ambiguous pictures as threatening than those who recalled a neutral, affect-irrelevant situation (buying some daily necessities). There is also evidence that, as compared to a neutral prime, visualization of a secure relationship results in a higher threshold for and greater tolerance of physical pain in the cold pressor task (Meredith et al., 2021; Rowe et al., 2012).

Using an immersive virtual environment, Kane et al. (2012) asked young adults to complete a threatening cliff-walking task while the avatar of their romantic partner was either absent, present and responsive (waving, clapping at successes, nodding his or her head, and actively orienting toward the participant), or present but inattentive (looking away from the participant). Participants in the responsive-partner condition experienced the task as less stressful than those who were alone; they also reported feeling more secure during the task and were less vigilant of their partner's behavior compared to those in the inattentive-partner condition. Security priming can also make challenges in the physical world appear less daunting (Schnall et al., 2008). While wearing a heavy backpack, participants judged a hill to be less steep when thinking about a loving and caring friend than when thinking about an acquaintance.

There is preliminary evidence that security priming leads not to illusory, unrealistic patterns of optimistic beliefs but to more adaptive, reality-tuned appraisals (Deng et al., 2016). As compared to neutral priming, reflecting on a hypothetical security-enhancing story increased optimistic causal attributions concerning positive and negative events among participants who held an extremely pessimistic explanatory style (fully attributing successes to external factors and failures to themselves). However, the same security-priming intervention reduced optimistic causal attributions among participants who held an extremely optimistic explanatory style (fully attributing successes to themselves and failures to external factors). In this way, security priming resulted in a more balanced outlook on life events in both groups of participants.

Constructive Strategies of Emotion Regulation

As described in Chapter 2, the secure-base script includes useful procedural knowledge concerning emotion regulation and coping with stress: disclosing one's vulnerabilities, needs, and feelings to others; seeking others' support and comfort; and engaging in problem solving without succumbing to catastrophizing worries and self-defeating thoughts. Findings indicate that security priming encourages or allows greater reliance on these useful strategies. Pierce and Lydon (1998), for example, exposed young women to security-related words (e.g., *caring, supportive*), insecurity-related words (e.g., *rejecting, hurtful*), or no words, and asked them to describe how they would cope with an unexpected pregnancy. Women in the security-priming condition were more likely than those in the control conditions to say they would seek more support, comfort, and reassurance from loved others in coping with this troubling event. In addition, as compared to neutral priming, security priming (exposure to the name of a security provider, visualization of a secure relationship) increases participants' willingness to share personal information and inner feelings with others, and to seek their support in times of need (Dawson et al., 2015; Gillath et al., 2006).

Security priming has also been found to reduce maladaptive responses, such as anxious rumination on self-related worries and suppression of negative emotions. Troyer and Greitmeyer (2018) asked participants to think of either a trustworthy person they rely on or a person toward whom they have no strong feelings. These researchers found that security priming (vs. neutral priming) lowered reliance on anxious rumination and emotional suppression.

These beneficial effects of security priming on maladaptive emotion-regulation strategies were also evident in Cassidy et al.'s (2009) study of cognitive and emotional reactions to hurtful experiences in close relationships. Participants wrote a description of an incident in which a close relationship partner hurt them and were primed with either security-related words (*love, secure, affection*) or neutral words (*lamp, staple, building*). They were then asked to think again about the hurtful event they had recalled and to describe how they would react to such an event if it happened in the future. In the neutral priming condition, attachment-related avoidance was associated with more defensive/hostile reactions, and attachment anxiety was associated with more crying and more negative emotions. These correlations were dramatically reduced in size after security priming. In other words, security priming reduced the tendency of avoidant people to react with cool hostility or denial, and reduced the tendency of anxious people to react histrionically to hurtful episodes. Overall, security priming seems to reduce the maladaptive, defensive tendencies of insecure people.

Mentalization and Mindfulness

Security priming also improves performance on tasks that involve mentalization of inner states (e.g., wishes, feelings, beliefs). Fuchs and Taubner (2019) asked participants to complete a mentalization task (the MASC), assessing their ability to accurately recognize others' mental states during social interactions. After performing half of the task, they were exposed to either a security prime (recall of secure attachment experiences from the past

2 years) or a neutral prime (description of every meal participants ate the day before). After that, they completed the second half of the mentalization task. Findings indicated that security priming (rather than neutral priming) led to better mentalization performance mainly among participants who often have difficulties in mentalizing and reaching accurate self-understanding (those who scored relatively high on the ECR Anxiety scale).

Further support for the effects of security priming on people's attitudes toward mental states can be found in Rowe et al.'s (2016) study on the willingness to engage in mindfulness meditation training. The researchers primed meditation trainees with either a security prime (visualization of a responsive relationship partner) or a neutral prime (visualization of a recent shopping trip) prior to an introductory mindfulness exercise and measured their postsession willingness to engage in further training. Findings indicated that participants in the security-priming condition were more willing to engage in further mindfulness training than participants in the control condition. This suggests that even a simple induction of felt security can increase engagement in mindfulness meditation.

Two other studies confirmed that contextual activation of attachment security or insecurities can alter reports of state-like mindfulness (Melen et al., 2017; Stevenson et al., 2021). In one study, participants assigned to write about a relationship characterized by attachment anxiety or avoidance reported lower levels of mindfulness after the intervention than those assigned to write about a neutral issue (Melen et al., 2017). In another study, security priming (visualization of a secure relationship) led to greater increases in state-like mindfulness than a brief mindfulness meditation exercise or a control condition (Stevenson et al., 2021). We should note, however, that Pepping, Davis, and O'Donovan (2015) found no significant effect of security priming on reports of mindfulness. Still, overall, the research findings obtained to date suggest that security priming can sometimes enhance and sustain mindfulness.

The "Building" Emotional Effects of Security Priming

By inducing feelings of being loved and valued, thereby activating the secure-base script, security priming can increase positive affect, reduce negative affect, and facilitate distress management and emotional stability. In the following sections, we review research documenting the effects of security priming on emotion regulation and aspects of mental health.

Emotion Regulation

There is substantial evidence that security priming facilitates constructive emotion regulation (see Rowe et al.'s [2020] meta-analysis of 30 security-priming studies). Specifically, it increases positive affect, reduces negative emotions in response to threats, inhibits the learning of fear responses, and interferes with activation of distressing memories.

Security Priming Infuses Positive Affect

Several studies have shown that people exposed to security primes report stronger positive emotions than those exposed to either neutral primes or attachment-irrelevant positive primes (e.g., Gillath & Karantzas, 2015; Guerra et al., 2012; Liao et al., 2017). Moreover, as compared to neutral primes, security-related pictures or words, or the name of a security provider lead to greater liking of previously unfamiliar Chinese ideographs (Canterberry & Gillath, 2013; Mikulincer, Hirschberger, et al., 2001)—an implicit indicator of positive affect

(Zajonc, 1984). It seems that security priming increases positive affect, which then "spills over" onto other stimuli.

Research also provides evidence concerning the neural and cognitive underpinnings of the emotional effects of security primes. As compared with neutral words, exposure to security-related words increases neural activation in the striatum (e.g., putamen, globus pallidus, caudate), insula, and anterior cingulate cortex (Canterberry & Gillath, 2013)—areas that have previously been associated with positive affect and approach motivation. Moreover, security priming facilitates attention to positive stimuli (i.e., faster reaction times for detecting positive facial expressions) and activity in left-hemisphere regions involved in the spread of activation of positive mood (Tang et al., 2017).

Security Priming Reduces Negative Emotional Reactions to Threats

There is strong support for the soothing effects of security priming. For example, as compared to control conditions, viewing a photo of a loving partner or visualizing his or her face after recalling an upsetting personal event leads to faster emotional recovery and less negative thoughts in a stream-of-consciousness task (Selcuk et al., 2012). Security priming also attenuates self-reported negative emotions (e.g., anger, anxiety) following failure on a cognitive task (Karreman et al., 2019) or exposure to negative self-relevant feedback or an audio recording of interpersonal conflict (Dutton et al., 2016; Park, 2007). Interestingly, Hofer et al. (2018) found that women exposed to the olfactory scent of their romantic partner (from his T-shirt) reported less negative emotion during the Trier Social Stress Test (in which they were asked to deliver a speech to an audience of experts) than women exposed to the scent of a stranger or a neutral scent.

The soothing effects of security priming have also been measured in terms of neural responses to threats. Exposure to a picture of a self-designated security provider (vs. pictures of strangers or objects) led to lowered activity in neural regions associated with pain responses (dorsal anterior cingulate cortex, anterior insula) during a cold pressor task (Eisenberger et al., 2011). Security priming also appears to attenuate another typical brain response to threats—amygdala reactivity (Norman et al., 2015). Specifically, participants who were primed with security-enhancing pictures exhibited lower amygdala activation in response to threat-related words and faces than those primed with neutral pictures.

In a related line of research, Karremans et al. (2011) examined whether security priming could reduce affectively negative brain responses to social exclusion. They replicated Eisenberger et al.'s (2003) functional magnetic resonance imaging (fMRI) study, in which participants experienced social exclusion during a computerized ball-tossing game (Cyberball) played with two other alleged participants (actually digital avatars). While being socially excluded, participants were primed with either the name of their security provider or a neutral name. In the neutral name condition, Karremans et al. (2011) replicated Eisenberger et al.'s (2003) findings: heightened activation in brain areas related to the experience of pain and distress (e.g., ventrolateral prefrontal cortex, hypothalamus) during episodes of social exclusion. More important, they found that security priming attenuated hypothalamus activation during these episodes, thereby supporting the hypothesized soothing effects of security priming at the neural level.

Additional support for the soothing effects of security priming can be found in studies that assess physiological responses to threats. In these studies, security priming, as compared to neutral priming, reduces the release of stress hormones (e.g., cortisol) and weakens autonomic arousal responses (skin conductance level and heart rate) during a cold pressor task or while watching emotionally upsetting film clips or reflecting on a painful relationship breakup (Ai et al., 2020; Bryant & Chan, 2015; Karl et al., 2021). Beyond this inhibition of sympathetic arousal, security priming seems to potentiate parasympathetic regulatory responses: It heightens heart rate variability (a physiological sign of emotional composure) during exposure to various stressors, such as ice water, social exclusion, and threatening pictures (Bryant & Hutanamon, 2018; Liddell & Courtney, 2018; Stupica et al., 2019).

The soothing effects of security priming are also evident at a cognitive level. In a study of autobiographical memories, Bryant and Bali (2018) found that security priming buffered the effects of negative mood on the specificity of these memories. Following a negative mood induction that has been found to elicit categorical, nonspecific personal memories, participants went through a priming process (visualization of either a security provider or an acquaintance) and were asked to retrieve autobiographical memories in response to neutral and negative cue words. Participants who visualized a security provider reported less distress and retrieved more specific memories than those who visualized an acquaintance.

Security Priming Interferes with Fear Conditioning

Security primes act as what learning researchers call "safety cues" (Jacobs & Lolardo, 1977), which reduce the strength of fear conditioning to a threatening stimulus. (In everyday terms, there is less fear available to condition.) In two experiments, Hornstein et al. (2016, Studies 1 and 2) found that pairing an electric shock with a picture of a security provider did not lead to a heightened fear-potentiated skin conductance response (SCR) to this picture, although pairing the shock with images of strangers or neutral objects lead to heightened SCR to these images.

In an additional experiment, Hornstein et al. (2016, Study 3) found that pairing the picture of a security provider (vs. the picture of stranger) with a previously conditioned stimulus (that was paired with an electric shock during a learning phase) during the test phase reduced fear-related SCR to this stimulus. Hornstein and Eisenberger (2017) extended this line of research and found that pairing a picture of a security provider (vs. the picture of a stranger) with the conditioned stimulus during the fear-acquisition phase of the procedure subsequently reduced SCR to this stimulus in the test phase. These findings imply that security priming not only inhibits or reduces fear responses that otherwise are elicited by a previously conditioned stimulus but also prevents the formation of new fear responses, thereby reducing the number of learned fears people acquire as they explore the environment.

These fear-reducing effects of security priming are also evident during fear extinction, implying that mental representations of responsive attachment figures can protect people against relapse of fear after a frightening situation ends. Hornstein et al. (2018) exposed participants to a picture of either a security-inducing attachment figure or a stranger during each trial of the extinction phase of fear conditioning (the conditioned stimulus was presented in the absence of the aversive outcome). Findings indicated that when the conditioned fear stimulus was paired with a picture of a security provider during extinction, return of the fear (heightened fear-potentiated SCR) was weaker both immediately after extinction and during a fear reinstatement test 24 hours later, although return of the fear occurred when the conditioned stimulus was paired with a picture of a stranger. Importantly, all of the observed inhibitory effects of security primes were not just a matter of increasing generic positive affect, because attachment-irrelevant positive primes failed to reduce fear-potentiated responses to conditioned stimuli (Toumbelekis et al., 2018, 2021a, 2021b).

Security Priming Reduces Activation of Distressing Memories

In a series of studies, Bryant and colleagues (Bryant & Chan, 2017; Bryant & Datta, 2019; Bryant & Foord, 2016) reported that security priming can inhibit consolidation and intrusive eruption of distressing memories. Bryant and Foord (2016), for example, exposed participants to distressing pictures, which were preceded by a brief presentation of either security-enhancing or neutral images. Two days later, participants were asked to recall the pictures and report the number of times these pictures had intruded into consciousness during the previous 2 days. Participants in the security-priming condition recalled fewer distress-eliciting pictures and reported fewer intrusive thoughts of these pictures than participants in the control condition. Similar effects have been found when the priming intervention was conducted during the recall session (Bryant & Chan, 2017) and when this session was conducted 1 week after the training session (Bryant & Datta, 2019).

Mental Health

Security priming has beneficial effects on participants' mental health. In two studies, exposure to security primes (vs. neutral primes) via text messages, conducted for 4 consecutive days, improved depressed and anxious moods (measured with the Profile of Mood States scale) among both college undergraduates (Carnelley et al., 2016) and outpatients diagnosed with primary depressive disorder (Carnelley et al., 2018). Similarly, McGuire et al. (2018, Study 1) found that implicit exposure to security-related words (vs. neutral words) reduced reports of depressive symptoms (using the Beck Depression Inventory) 1 week later in a nonclinical sample of undergraduates. In a second study, McGuire et al. (2018, Study 2) exposed adolescents to security or neutral primes every other day for a total of five sessions over a 2-week period and assessed changes in depressive symptoms (using the Hopkins Symptom Checklist). Adolescents who were repeatedly exposed to security primes reported fewer symptoms of depression than those exposed to neutral primes.

In a study conducted during Palestinian terrorist attacks on Israeli cities, Mikulincer et al. (2006) examined whether security priming could reduce cognitive responses to trauma. Israeli undergraduates were asked to complete a measure of posttraumatic symptoms (PTS) related to the terror attacks and to perform a Stroop color-naming task that included words connoting terror (e.g., *Hamas, car bomb*), as well as negatively valenced words not related to terror and some emotionally neutral words. On each trial, participants were primed with either a security word (the Hebrew word for "being loved"), a positively valenced but attachment-unrelated word (*success*), or a neutral word (*hat*). Following positive or neutral primes, participants who scored high on the PTS scale took longer, on average, to name the colors in which terror-related words were presented (indicating greater mental availability of the words) than participants who scored low on this scale. However, security priming lowered the color-naming latencies for terror-related words of participants who suffered from PTS and nullified differences between the PTS and non-PTS groups. Similar buffering effects of security priming were found in a sample of Israeli ex-prisoners of war 35 years after the war (Mikulincer, Solomon, et al., 2014). Overall, it seems that traumatized individuals respond favorably to the activation of security-related mental representations, at least at the preconscious or unconscious level.

Additional studies have found that security priming reduces (1) obsessive hand-washing tendencies among attachment-anxious young adults (Doron et al., 2012), (2) preoccupation with food and body-image distortions among psychiatric impatient women diagnosed with eating disorders (Admoni, 2006), and (3) craving for a cigarette among heavy smokers (Le et al., 2020). In a recent series of studies, Newman-Taylor and colleagues (2021; Sood et al., 2021; Sood & Newman-Taylor, 2020) found that visualization of a secure relationship lowered paranoid thinking among people with high levels of nonclinical paranoia (but see Hutton et al., 2017, for null results). There is also evidence that exposure to the olfactory scent of a loved partner before going to sleep results in better sleep (as assessed by actigraphy) than exposure to the scent of a stranger (Hofer & Chen, 2020).

The "Broadening" Transformative Effects of Security Priming

As described in Chapter 2, the sense of attachment security not only has beneficial effects on emotions but also contributes to a dual transformation in a person's motives. Instead of being exclusively focused on self-protection, secure people can also focus on (1) improving the quality of their close relationships and responding to others' suffering, and (2) exploring, learning, and promoting their own autonomy, skills, and talents. In the following sections, we review studies examining whether security priming facilitates these motivational transformations.

Pro-Relational Tendencies

Security priming has indeed been found to increase pro-relational tendencies that contribute to relationship quality and stability. For example, participants who were implicitly exposed to the name of their security provider were more inclined to forgive others who committed relational offenses (e.g., lying, cheating, insulting) than participants exposed to the name of an acquaintance or a neutral name (Karremans & Aarts, 2007). Moreover, asking participants to recall security-enhancing interactions with a close relationship partner (vs. neutral interactions with an acquaintance) increases participants' reported efforts to initiate and maintain relationships, while reducing tendencies to dissolve relationships (Gillath et al., 2017). These effects were observed mainly among attachment-insecure participants (those scoring high on the ECR Avoidance and/or Anxiety scales).

The pro-relational effects of security priming are evident in Bartz and Lydon's (2004) study of communal, relational traits (e.g., warmth in relations with others, being able to devote oneself to others). Participants who visualized a secure relationship were more likely to rate these pro-relational traits as self-descriptive than were those who visualized an insecure relationship. Security priming has also been found to increase the tendency to modify internal aspects of the self to make them congruent with a relationship partner's preferences, even when those accommodations have negative implications for the self (Gabriel et al., 2010). In addition, security priming seems to benefit relationship quality by increasing trust in others, as is evident in participants' cooperative choices in trust-related games (Ma et al., 2021; McClure et al., 2013).

Security priming softens destructive relational tendencies that compromise relationship sustainability (Selterman & Maier, 2013). As compared to visualization of attachment-irrelevant positive or neutral situations, visualization of a security-enhancing situation reduced jealousy and feelings of hurt and anger toward a romantic partner who was described as behaving flirtatiously with a potential rival. In addition, security-priming interventions reduce dishonesty (lying and cheating) toward a romantic partner (Gillath et al., 2010), as well as attachment-anxious people's tendency to feel regret and ambivalence in close relationships (Bartz & Lydon, 2004; Schoemann et al., 2012).

These beneficial relational effects of security priming have been found even during relationship dissolution. Specifically, recall of a secure relationship (vs. a neutral memory) reduced avoidant people's tendency to use indirect withdrawal breakup strategies in ending a relationship (e.g., "I ceased doing favors for my partner") and attachment-anxious people's tendency to keep open the option of getting back together (Collins & Gillath, 2012). More generally, security priming increased the use of more constructive breakup strategies.

Prosocial Orientation

Security Priming Promotes Prosocial Virtues

Studies show that security-priming interventions enhance the prosocial virtues of kindness and compassion. In a pioneering study, Mikulincer, Gillath, et al. (2001, Study 1) asked participants to read a security-enhancing story or an attachment-irrelevant positive or neutral story and then provided them with a brief story about a student whose parents had been killed in an automobile accident. Participants rated how much they experienced compassion and personal distress when thinking about the distressed student. As compared to positive and neutral priming, security priming strengthened compassion and reduced personal distress in reaction to others' distress. These findings were replicated in subsequent studies (Kogut & Kogut, 2013; Mallinckrodt et al., 2013).

The prosocial effect of security priming is also evident in studies that assess a person's value system and endorsement of generous, other-oriented behavior. For example, as compared to positive or neutral priming, security priming strengthens the endorsement of two self-transcendent values, *benevolence* (concern for close others) and *universalism* (concern for all humanity) and reduces the endorsement of materialistic values and the importance people assign to material objects (Clark et al., 2011; Mikulincer et al., 2003; Sun et al., 2020). This prosocial orientation has also been found in heightened willingness to donate money to health-promoting organizations, give blood, or share monetary resources or food with others following security priming (Charles-Sire et al., 2012; Gillath et al., 2020; Gregersen & Gillath, 2020; Guéguen et al., 2011). In addition, asking participants to think about a security provider (vs. an acquaintance) increases willingness to care for a homeless woman and reduces caregiving-related worries and anxieties (e.g., "I would get anxious if I thought this woman or someone like her didn't want my help"), which can compromise effective helping (Cassidy et al., 2018).

Mikulincer et al. (2005) examined the effects of security priming on the actual decision to help or not to help a stranger in distress. In the first two experiments, participants watched a confederate while she performed a series of increasingly aversive tasks. As the study progressed, the confederate became increasingly upset about the aversive tasks, and the actual participant was given an opportunity to take the distressed person's place, in effect sacrificing self for the welfare of another. Shortly before the scenario just described, participants were exposed to security or neutral priming either implicitly (rapid subliminal presentation of the name of a security provider or an acquaintance) or explicitly (asking participants to recall an interaction with a security provider or an acquaintance). In both studies, participants exposed to security primes (either implicitly or explicitly) reported more compassion toward the distressed woman than those exposed to neutral primes and were more willing to take her place in the subsequent aversive tasks. This finding was conceptually replicated by Charles-Sire et al. (2016), who found that, as compared to neutral priming, participants who were implicitly exposed to the word *loving* printed on a woman's

T-shirt (a confederate of the experimenter) were more likely to spontaneously help her to load a large, heavy carton into her car in a supermarket parking lot.

In two additional studies, Mikulincer et al. (2005, Studies 3 and 4) examined the hypothesis that security priming overrides egoistic motives for helping, such as mood enhancement and empathic joy, and results in genuinely altruistic helping. Indeed, findings indicated that expecting to improve one's mood by means other than helping or expecting not to be able to share a needy person's joy when helped reduced compassion and willingness to help in the neutral priming condition, but it failed to affect these emotional and behavioral reactions in the security-priming condition. It seems that contextual activation of the sense of attachment security heightens compassion and willingness to help even when there was no egoistic reason for helping. These findings fit well with the theoretical view that the sense of attachment security reduces selfishness (defensive self-protection) and moves a person to adopt an empathic and compassionate attitude toward others' distress.

The prosocial effects of felt security can be extended to pro-environmental behaviors (Nisa et al., 2021). In three studies, as compared to neutral priming, security priming (asking participants to recall a supportive interaction or exposing them to security-enhancing pictures or a video clip) increased acceptance of, and perceived responsibility for, human-generated climate change, as well as monetary donations to a proenvironmental group. In a subsequent field study conducted in a university cafeteria, students' actual daily food waste was smaller in quantity during periods in which a security-enhancing banner (a picture of a pregnant woman with an Earth-shaped belly and the phrase "love your mother earth") was located at the entry of the cafeteria than during periods in which a banner linking food waste to carbon emissions was located in the same position (Nisa et al., 2021). It seems that contextual activation of felt security promotes a proenvironmental orientation that can help to mitigate climate change.

Security Priming Increases Positive Parenting-Related Responses

A recent experimental study conducted by Jones et al. (2022) provided initial evidence that security priming can increase parents' positive attitudes toward their offspring. Mothers and childless undergraduates were randomly assigned to a neutral or a secure prime condition (visualization of the face of an acquaintance or a security-enhancing relationship partner), then completed measures of implicit attitudes (a child-focused version of the Go/No-Go Association Task) and explicit attitudes (self-reported) toward children. Following the priming manipulation, mothers in the secure prime condition had more positive implicit attitudes toward their children compared to mothers in the neutral prime condition. Security priming also increased mothers' positive explicit attitudes toward their children, but only among mothers who scored high on self-reported attachment-related avoidance. Importantly, security priming failed to affect nonparents' attitudes toward children, suggesting that these effects may be specific to people who have lived (rather than simply imagined) experiences of parenthood.

Security Priming Increases Empathic Concern for a Relationship Partner's Needs

In a direct examination of the prosocial effects of security priming in close relationships, Mikulincer et al. (2013) conducted a study, in both the United States and Israel, to see whether experimentally augmented security would improve responsiveness to a romantic partner who was asked to discuss a personal problem. A second goal of the study was to examine the extent to which security priming could overcome barriers to responsive caregiving induced by mental depletion or fatigue. Dating couples came to the laboratory and were informed that they would be video-recorded during an interaction in which one of them (whom we regarded as the "care-seeker") disclosed a personal problem to the other (the "caregiver"). Care seekers chose and wrote about any personal problem they were willing to discuss (except ones that involved conflict with the partner). And at the same time, caregivers performed a Stroop color-naming task in which they were or were not mentally depleted. During this task, participants were also implicitly exposed to either the names of security providers (other than the current dating partner) or names of unfamiliar people. Then, couple members were videotaped while they talked about the problem that the care seeker wished to discuss, and independent judges, viewing the video recordings, coded participants' responsiveness to their disclosing partner.

Security priming led to greater responsiveness to the disclosing partner (as coded by judges) than did neutral priming. Moreover, security priming overrode the detrimental effects of mental depletion and of dispositional attachment-related avoidance on responsiveness, and it counteracted the tendency of attachment-anxious participants to be less responsive following experimentally induced mental depletion. These findings were replicated by Mikulincer, Shaver, et al. (2014) in their assessment of secure-base support provision: Security priming increased responsiveness (as coded by judges) to a romantic partner who was exploring personal goals. Overall, the findings emphasize that security priming facilitates effective provision of safe-haven and secure-base support to a romantic partner and can counteract dispositional (insecure attachment orientations) and situational (mental depletion) barriers to responsive caregiving.

Security Priming Increases Tolerance of Out-Groups

The prosocial effects of security priming are also evident in increased tolerance of out-group members—people who are different from oneself and do not belong to one's own social groups. In five studies, Mikulincer and Shaver (2001) found that, as compared to neutral priming, security priming (by implicitly presenting security-related words, e.g., *love* and *closeness,* or by asking participants to read a security-enhancing story or visualize the face of a supportive relationship partner) promoted more tolerant and accepting attitudes to a variety of out-groups (as perceived by heterosexual, secular Israeli Jewish students): Israeli Arabs, ultra-Orthodox Jews, Russian immigrants, and homosexuals. In subsequent studies, security priming has also increased White American participants' empathy for racially different others and reduced British undergraduates' prejudice and discriminatory behavior toward immigrants and Muslims (Boag & Carnelley, 2012, 2016; Mallinckrodt et al., 2013).

Building on these studies, Mikulincer and Shaver (2007) found that security priming can reduce actual aggression between contending or warring social groups. Specifically, Israeli Jewish undergraduates participated in a study together with another Israeli Jew or an Israeli Arab (in each case, the same confederate of the experimenter given different names). They were then implicitly exposed to the name of their security provider, the name of a familiar person who was not viewed as an attachment figure, or the name of a mere acquaintance. Following the priming procedure, the experimenter informed participants that they would evaluate a food sample and that they had been randomly selected to give the confederate hot sauce to evaluate. They also learned indirectly that the confederate disliked spicy foods. (This procedure has been used in other studies of interpersonal aggression; e.g., McGregor et al., 1998.) The dependent variable was the amount of hot sauce allotted to the confederate.

When participants had been primed with the name of someone who was not a security provider, they delivered more hot sauce to the Arab confederate than to the Jewish confederate, a sign of intergroup aggression. But security priming eliminated this difference: Participants whose sense of security had been enhanced allotted equal (relatively low) amounts of hot sauce to both the Arab and the Jewish confederate. This finding fits Saleem et al.'s (2015) discovery that security priming reduces American undergraduates' negative emotions and aggressive behavior toward Arabs. Thus, it seems that people who are contextually induced to feel more secure are better able to tolerate intergroup differences and to refrain from intergroup aggression.

Broadening Capacities and Perspectives

As explained in Chapter 2, the sense of attachment security contributes to the broadening of a person's knowledge and skills; opens his or her mind to new possibilities, experiences, and perspectives; and helps him or her effectively pursue personal goals. One reason for these beneficial effects is that felt security reduces anxiety, vigilance, and preoccupation with attachment-related worries, allowing a person to devote more attention and effort to exploration, learning, goal pursuit, and task performance.

This line of reasoning implies that security priming might enhance a person's curiosity and encourage relaxed exploration of new, unusual information despite the uncertainty and perplexities that this cognitive activity can elicit. In support of this idea, several researchers have found that security priming increases both willingness to explore and cognitive openness to novel information (e.g., Jarvinen & Paulus, 2017; Luke et al., 2012; Millings et al., 2019). Green and Campbell (2000), for example, asked people to read sentences describing secure or insecure close relationships and found that security priming led to greater endorsement of exploration-related behavior and greater liking for novel pictures than did insecurity priming. And Mikulincer and Arad (1999) reported that participants who were asked to visualize a responsive relationship partner (as compared to those who visualized a rejecting partner) showed increased cognitive openness and were more likely to revise knowledge about a relationship partner following behavior on the part of the partner that seemed inconsistent with prior actions.

Following this line of research, Mikulincer et al. (2011, Study 1) implicitly exposed participants to the name of either a security provider or an acquaintance and assessed their performance in a creative problem-solving task (the Remote Associations Test [RAT]). Findings indicated that security priming led to better RAT performance than neutral priming, regardless of variations in dispositional attachment insecurities. However, the positive effects of explicit security priming (recalling experiences of being well cared for) on RAT performance were found mainly among participants scoring low on attachment anxiety (Mikulincer et al., 2011, Study 2).

The calm, relaxed, and confident mental state that security priming creates can facilitate cognitive functioning and task performance. Indeed, using a wide variety of tasks assessing executive functions (*n*-back task, working memory updating task, Stroop color-naming task, rule-switch task), three studies have found that security priming, as compared to neutral priming, improves working memory, response inhibition, and cognitive flexibility (Bai et al., 2019; Benistri, 2019; Li, Bunke, et al., 2016). Research also indicates that contextual activation of the sense of attachment security improves behavioral self-control, task persistence, signal-detection accuracy, and hearing acuity (lowered auditory thresholds) in a standardized audiometric test (Milyavskaya et al., 2012; Nagar et al., 2022; Sakman & Sümer, 2018; Wilkinson et al., 2013).

Critical Overview of Security-Priming Interventions

The Effectiveness of Security-Priming Interventions

Overall, security-priming interventions can clearly have positive psychological consequences. They have been found effective in infusing a state-like sense of attachment security and producing positive changes in a person's cognitions about self, others, and life threats and hardships. Moreover, they have positive effects on emotions: They increase a person's positive emotions, reduce distress during threatening events, encourage reliance on constructive ways of emotion regulation and coping with stress, and support mental health. Security-priming interventions can also strengthen pro-relational and prosocial attitudes and behaviors; foster curiosity, exploration, mentalization, and cognitive openness; and improve performance on sensory, perceptual, and cognitive tasks. From an attachment perspective, these interventions can be viewed as activating the secure-base script, launching a broaden-and-build cycle, and ushering people onto and along a path to greater security, well-being, and thriving.

The observed psychological and physiological effects of security-priming interventions are robust, replicable, and distinct from positive mood inductions. The vast majority of studies examining the effectiveness of these interventions have been conducted in well-controlled settings and have compared a security-priming condition with an active control condition (i.e., participants go through identical procedures in the two conditions, differing only in the prime they receive) rather than an empty control condition (in which participants receive no intervention). Moreover, in most of these priming studies, participants were randomly assigned to the various experimental conditions; the conditions were matched in instructions, materials, and procedures; and researchers relied on well-validated priming techniques and on reliable and valid self-report and behavioral outcome measures. These methodological strengths increase our confidence in the internal validity of the observed effects of security priming.

Our confidence is further reinforced by Gillath et al.'s (2022) meta-analysis of 119 published and unpublished security-priming studies, which found that the overall effect size for security priming (as compared to neutral, positive-affect, or insecurity-related primes) was large (d = 0.51). In Gillath et al.'s words, "priming people with attachment security yielded a large positive effect size, and the effectiveness of security priming extended across affective, cognitive, and behavioral domains. Concerning these broad outcome domains, the largest effect was found for affect-related outcomes, followed by cognitive and behavioral outcomes, which had similar overall effect sizes" (p. 232).

Importantly, the positive effects of security priming are replicable across different priming techniques (explicit, implicit), types of prime (idiosyncratic, generic), and prime modalities (pictorial, verbal). However, Gillath et al.'s (2022) meta-analysis revealed that the size of these effects was larger for implicit than explicit priming techniques (d = 0.61 vs. d = 0.47). Moreover, implicit exposure to security-enhancing pictures yielded the largest effect size (d = 0.64). Rowe et al. (2020) reached an identical conclusion in their meta-analysis of 30 studies examining affective outcomes of security priming. It is possible that pictures are better than words in eliciting affective, somatosensory, and motor responses, perhaps because they have privileged access to the associative memory network and a broader spread of activation over this network (Winkielman & Gogolushko, 2018), which results in larger psychological effects.

In their meta-analysis, Gillath et al. (2022) also evaluated the size of the effects of security priming when compared to different kinds of control primes (neutral, insecurity-eliciting, positive-affect, self-esteem) and found that the positive effects of security priming hold up against all of these kinds of control primes. Importantly, Gillath et al. also found that, as compared to neutral primes, security primes yield larger effects than positive-affect or self-esteem primes, indicating, as mentioned earlier, that security priming is not just a matter of increasing positive affect or self-esteem. In addition, studies that have involved repeatedly exposing participants to security primes over multiple occasions, often separated by one or more days, reveal that such interventions can have lasting effects, at least up to a month after the last prime. The time course and persistence of the effects, however, still needs more research.

In the vast majority of the studies we have reviewed here, the positive effects of security priming occurred in both secure and insecure research participants. In fact, there are few reported statistical interactions between the manipulations and individual differences on measures of secure versus anxious or avoidant attachment. Based on their exhaustive meta-analysis, Gillath et al. (2022) concluded that "the overall findings . . . suggest a moderate effect size regardless of a person's attachment style" (p. 233). As explained in Chapter 2, insecure people, despite their predominantly negative working models, harbor nondominant representations of security in their associative memory networks, and security-priming interventions can apparently strengthen the accessibility of these nondominant representations and temporarily move an insecure person toward greater security.

It is worth noting, however, that the psychological effects of explicit security-priming techniques tend to be more dependent on a participant's attachment orientation than the effects of implicit techniques (e.g., Bryant & Chan, 2017; Mallinckrodt et al., 2013; Mikulincer et al., 2011), perhaps because explicit (conscious) primes activate certain kinds of defenses and motivational biases not activated by implicit primes. Unfortunately, the current state of knowledge does not allow us to specify the precise primes and techniques that would be most effective for enhancing security in attachment-avoidant and attachment-anxious people.

Limitations of the Current Security-Priming Interventions and Future Challenges

Along with the methodological strengths of the reviewed studies and their promising findings, they represent only a first step in using priming techniques for moving a person toward attachment security. And, as always, in a complex and still relatively new research area, there are limitations worth mentioning.

Most of the security-priming studies have been conducted in well-controlled laboratory settings, so their effects are difficult to generalize to real-life situations. In addition, most of the experimental interventions are based on a single priming session, and their effects probably disappear soon after the experimental session. Fortunately, however, security priming does not need to be restricted to sterile laboratory conditions; it could include multiple priming sessions in different real-life contexts and for extended time periods. In fact, Charles-Sire and colleagues have shown that security priming can be conducted in real-life settings (supermarket parking lots; university lawns), for example, by exposing participants to security-associated words printed on confederates' T-shirts (Charles-Sire et al., 2012, 2016; Guéguen et al., 2011). Moreover, a few studies that have involved multiple sessions of security priming across periods spanning from 3 days to 4 months have shown that the positive effects of the intervention can endure over days and weeks after the last priming session (e.g., Carnelley et al., 2016, 2018; McGuire et al., 2018). These findings are certainly encouraging in relation to future long-term interventions, but we need more repeated security-priming studies conducted outside the laboratory in order to determine the number of priming sessions and the optimal time lag between these sessions required to produce lasting effects on people's attachment orientations.

One step in this direction would be to embed security-enhancing images, words, sentences, or brief stories in a person's environment, and repeatedly expose him or her to these primes in an implicit manner for extended time periods (as Nisa et al., 2021, did in one of their studies). For example, we could print these primes on signs and posters, locate them along roads and streets, and in parks and neighborhoods, then examine their long-term psychological effects on people who were inadvertently exposed to them on a daily basis. Security primes could also be located in schools to increase teachers' and students' sense of security, thereby facilitating both teaching and learning processes. They could also be located in medical centers and hospitals as a means of reducing clients' distress and facilitating healing. They could be placed on the walls of therapy rooms in order to strengthen client–therapist relationships and improve therapeutic work.

Another step in increasing the generalizability and sustainability of security-priming effects would be to design electronic applications (apps) that deliver security primes (e.g., photos, voice, or videos of a primary security provider) or ask people to engage in a brief security-enhancing exercise (e.g., speaking or writing about a security provider or a specific supportive interaction with him or her) each time the app is activated. Carnelley and colleagues have made initial steps in this direction by using simple text messages asking people to engage in security-enhancing exercises (Carnelley et al., 2016, 2018; Otway et al., 2014).

A more advanced step would be to construct a sophisticated machine-learning app that could prime security in the ways described earlier immediately upon detection of elevations in a person's physiological or behavioral signs of arousal and distress. (This kind of detection is already possible with some sophisticated wrist watches.) In this way, the app could boost security in the same way that security primes have been proven to do in the laboratory, or in the way a supportive attachment figure does in normal social life. Researchers could then determine whether using these devices over an extended time period has lasting effects on subjective feelings, social functioning, and health.

One could also use mobile platforms for repeatedly challenging insecure attachment working models and training people to be more attentive and receptive to security primes. One example of this kind of mobile platform is GGtude (e.g., Giraldo-O'Meara & Doron, 2021), which has been designed to reduce negative thoughts and maladaptive beliefs related to specific psychological disorders (e.g., obsessive–compulsive disorders, eating disorders). In each session, users are exposed on their mobile screen to statements or images that are consistent or inconsistent with maladaptive beliefs. They are then instructed to accept statements/images that challenge maladaptive beliefs by pulling them toward the bottom of the screen (moving the statements/images toward themselves) and to reject statements/images consistent with maladaptive beliefs by throwing them upwards in the screen, away from themselves.

One can easily adapt GGtude as a security-priming device by using insecurity-eliciting and security-eliciting words, sentences, or images and train people to reject the insecurity-eliciting stimuli and accept the security-enhancing stimuli. This kind of easy-to-use app, which involves the pleasure of gaming and requires only a short attention span, may be an effective intervention for repeatedly priming mental representations of security.

Of course, these kinds of interventions are not likely to be sufficient to move an insecure person all the way to stable security, especially a person who has suffered from severe attachment injuries. As reviewed in Chapter 2, because of the persistence of early frustrating and painful memories and working models, effective attachment-based interventions with insecure people will probably require them to become aware of, reflect upon, and work through their negative models and memories. In other words, even if it is possible to increase an insecure person's moments of feeling more secure, it will probably take additional work to revise and renovate the cognitive and emotional structures established early on and rehearsed and defended against for years. As a result, security-priming interventions probably need to be integrated with other interventions (discussed in the following chapters) that assist insecure people in the working-through process.

This doesn't mean that security priming has no important benefits for insecure people. Although security priming does not include a working-through component, it might temporarily encourage insecure people to explore experiences, memories, models, and habits. In fact, as consistently documented in the studies just reviewed, this kind of intervention can increase trust in others' good intentions, soothe distress, and allow more confident and mindful exploration of painful memories and dysfunctional working models. We can therefore use security priming to improve the effectiveness of other attachment-based interventions that assist insecure people in gaining new perspective on previous painful experiences. For example, incorporating security priming within individual psychotherapy (see Chapter 7) might help insecure clients to be more attentive and receptive to their therapist's care and attention, more tolerant of the therapist's occasional empathic failures, and more open to explore painful attachment memories and revise maladaptive working models with the therapist's assistance and support.

Concluding Remarks

In summary, security priming studies provide strong and encouraging evidence that security enhancement is possible and has many measurable benefits. This knowledge gives us insights, courage, and optimism to explore creative, diverse, and potentially powerful attachment interventions in the world beyond the laboratory. This is the purpose of the remaining chapters.

CHAPTER 4

Enhancing Attachment Security in Relationships between Parents and Young Children

Having reviewed, in Chapter 3, evidence that adults' felt security can be experimentally enhanced, at least in the short run, and have predictable beneficial effects on a person's broaden-and-build cycle, we now turn to attachment interventions in various kinds of real-world relationships. In a major overview volume on this topic, Steele and Steele (2018) called such applications *attachment-based interventions*.

We begin with the type of relationship that most concerned Bowlby and Ainsworth, and that has been the focus of most attachment-based interventions created so far: the one between young children and their adult attachment figures. Interventions in this domain are designed to improve adult caregivers' sensitivity and responsiveness, with a resulting improvement in the sense of security of their young offspring. A key premise of these interventions is that in order to promote children's secure attachment to parents or other caregivers and support a successful broaden-and-build cycle of healthy development, it is useful to cultivate parents' sensitive responsiveness, mentalization, and effective provision of a safe haven and secure base for the children who are attached to them.

We start by describing the research bases for this kind of intervention, reviewing a host of cross-sectional and prospective-longitudinal studies showing that caregivers' (usually the parents') attitudes and behaviors are key to the formation and maintenance of their children's felt security. We then review intervention programs designed to improve caregivers' security-enhancing attitudes and behaviors, evaluating each program with respect to its efficacy in promoting children's felt security and healthy development. Finally, we offer an integrative perspective on the interventions and suggest further avenues for research and application.

Parental Attitudes and Behavior Contribute to Children's Attachment Security

In this section, we review some of the research on which parenting interventions are based. Fortunately, there are hundreds of studies showing that three parental characteristics are key to enhancing a child's felt security: (1) sensitive responsiveness to the child's signals and needs (which Ainsworth et al. [1978] simply called *parental sensitivity*); (2) mentalization (understanding and considering the child's perspective and treating the child as a mental agent); and (3) effective provision of a safe haven and secure base (Cassidy et al.'s, 2005, construct of *secure base provision*). In addition, there is a large body of research showing that parents' own attachment security is important for fostering their children's felt security, because secure parents are more likely than insecure parents to exhibit the three positive parenting characteristics just mentioned (see Jones et al., 2015a, 2015b, for reviews). From a clinical and educational perspective, this issue is critical, because parents' attachment insecurities can reduce the effectiveness of attachment-based parenting interventions.

The Contribution of Parental Sensitivity

Over the past 40 years, dozens of studies and several major meta-analytic reviews have been published concerning the link between observers' ratings of parental sensitivity and different forms of insensitivity (rejection, ignoring, interfering; see Chapter 2) within parent–infant interactions and infant attachment security (assessed with Ainsworth's laboratory Strange Situation procedure). Of the four meta-analyses focused on maternal sensitivity, the one by Goldsmith and Alansky (1987) included 13 studies (based on 691 mother–child dyads); that by de Wolff and van IJzendoorn (1997) included 66 studies (4,176 dyads); that by Atkinson et al. (2000) included 41 studies (2,243 dyads); and the one by Verhage et al. (2016) included 21 studies (1,211 dyads). Two meta-analyses were conducted on fathers' sensitivity: van IJzendoorn and de Wolff (1997) meta-analyzed eight studies (including 546 dyads) and Lucassen et al. (2011) meta-analyzed 16 studies (1,355 dyads). An additional meta-analysis was conducted by Zeegers et al. (2017) on data from 50 studies involving 5,871 mother–infant dyads and 793 father–infant dyads.

In general, these several meta-analyses revealed statistically significant mild-to-moderate associations between parental sensitivity during infancy and infant attachment security, with effect sizes varying from 0.12 (Lucassen et al., 2011) to 0.35 (Verhage et al., 2016). Although these effect sizes are not large, de Wolff and van IJzendoorn (1997) explained that the 0.24 effect size they obtained implies that mothers who are sensitive and responsive increase the likelihood of their infant being securely attached from 38 to 62%. Of considerable importance, all of the meta-analyses revealed substantial effect size variability across studies due to different methods of assessing parental sensitivity and different time spans separating the assessments of parental caregiving and infant attachment. Studies conducted after the Zeegers et al. (2017) meta-analysis have continued to find that parental sensitivity is significantly associated with infant security (e.g., Bailey et al., 2017; Leerkes & Zhou, 2018; Sirois & Bernier, 2018).

As expected theoretically, parental sensitivity also contributes to the broaden-and-build cycle of healthy development. Sensitive parental caregiving during infancy fosters effective regulation of negative emotions, sustains psychological well-being and mental health, and supports prorelational and prosocial orientations during childhood and adolescence (e.g., Bernier et al., 2016; Kochanska et al., 2019; Sirois & Bernier, 2018; Somers & Luecken, 2021). Moreover, it supports the development of self-regulation skills and facilitates cognitive functioning by the time children reach preschool and elementary school (e.g., Bernier et al., 2012; Bindman et al., 2015; Vrijhof et al., 2020). In addition, young adults who have experienced more sensitive parenting during childhood are more likely to form high-quality romantic relationships, to maintain emotional composure during distressing interpersonal interactions, and to provide empathic care to their own children (Raby,

Lawler, et al., 2015; Raby, Roisman, et al., 2015; Waters et al., 2018). Early parental sensitivity even predicts better academic performance and reduced risk for cardiovascular diseases at midlife (Farrell et al., 2019; Raby, Roisman, et al., 2015).

There is also prospective evidence that parental sensitivity during infancy and early childhood has a formative influence on adolescents' and adults' later sense of attachment security. Relying on data from the Minnesota Longitudinal Study (Sroufe et al., 2005), Haydon et al. (2012) and Roisman et al. (2001) found that sensitive parenting during infancy and childhood increased the likelihood of receiving a secure AAI classification when the participants were 19 and 26 years old. Behavioral observations of maternal sensitivity during early childhood in the NICHD study of early child care and youth development also predicted more secure attachment states of mind in the AAI at age 18 (Booth-LaForce et al., 2014; Waters et al., 2021). Similar long-term security-enhancing effects of early maternal sensitivity have been documented in studies that rely on self-report scales for assessing attachment security during adolescence and young adulthood (e.g., Chopik et al., 2014; Fraley et al., 2013; Zayas et al., 2011).

Overall, the large body of evidence from cross-sectional and longitudinal studies consistently supports Ainsworth et al.'s (1978) hypothesis linking parental sensitivity during infancy and early childhood with children's concurrent and later attachment security. However, the observed associations are generally only moderate in size, suggesting that additional factors are involved. As a result, attachment researchers have undertaken a search for other parental characteristics that contribute to children's development of felt security.

The Contribution of Parental Mentalization

One such parental characteristic is *parental mentalization,* the ability to take a child's perspective and to hold in mind his or her needs, feelings, and thoughts (see Chapter 2). Research on parental mentalization is based on three different but related operationalizations of the construct: parental mind-mindedness (Meins, 1997), parental insightfulness (Oppenheim & Koren-Karie, 2002), and parental reflective functioning (Slade, Grienenberger, et al., 2005). *Parental mind-mindedness* is defined as a tendency to treat one's child as a mental agent. It is assessed by analyzing how frequently and appropriately a parent attributes mental states to his or her child during parent–child interactions or in an interview about the child (Meins & Fernyhough, 2015). *Parental insightfulness* refers to a parent's capacity to consider the motives underlying the child's emotions and behaviors in an elaborated, positive, and child-focused manner. It is assessed by analyzing parental mind-related speech during an interview about the thoughts and feelings that underlie children's behavior exhibited in short videotaped vignettes of parent–child interactions (Koren-Karie & Oppenheim, 2001). *Parental reflective functioning* refers to a parent's capacity to hold the child's mental states in mind. This capacity is assessed with the Parent Development Interview (PDI; Slade et al., 2003) or the Parental Reflective Functioning Questionnaire (Fonagy et al., 2016).

Although the three constructs are operationalized and assessed in somewhat different ways, all focus on the degree to which parents demonstrate frequent, coherent, and appropriate mentalizing in relation to their infant. Moreover, all of them view low parental mentalization as resulting from either lack of awareness or disregard of the mental world of the child or inaccuracy in interpreting the child's needs, thoughts, or feelings.

Most of the studies examining the contribution of parental mentalization to children's felt security have assessed parents' mind-mindedness. These studies have consistently found that infants whose parents made more frequent and appropriate mind-related comments were more likely to be classified as secure in the Strange Situation procedure (e.g., Tarabeh et al., 2019). Also, researchers have found that parents' nonattuned mind-related comments at infant age 6 or 8 months predicted less secure attachment at 12 or 15 months (e.g., Arnott & Meins, 2007; Meins et al., 2002, 2012). Finally, parents' tendency to make frequent and appropriate mind-related comments during their child's infancy is predictive of the child's greater attachment security during toddlerhood and middle childhood (Meins et al., 2018; Miller et al., 2019).

The parental insightfulness construct has also been related to children's greater attachment security in community samples, a sample of mothers suffering from clinical depression, and a sample of children with autism spectrum disorder (Koren-Karie et al., 2002; Oppenheim et al., 2012; Ramsauer et al., 2014). Studies using the PDI have shown that parental reflective functioning is both cross-sectionally and prospective longitudinally associated with children's attachment security (Slade, Grienenberger, et al., 2005; Stacks et al., 2014). These findings have been replicated in recent studies using the Parental Reflective Functioning Questionnaire (Fonagy et al., 2016). In a meta-analysis of 13 studies ($N = 974$), Zeegers et al. (2017) found a significant moderate association between parental mentalization (assessed by one of the three constructs) and child attachment security.

Regarding our interest in not just attachment security but also the associated broaden-and-build cycle, there is evidence that parental mentalization is associated with favorable child-developmental outcomes (see Katznelson, 2014, for a review). For example, children of parents who scored relatively high on mind-mindedness or reflective functioning were less likely to exhibit emotional and behavioral problems (e.g., Colonnesi et al., 2019). Moreover, parental mentalization is positively associated with children's capacities for distress regulation and self-control (e.g., Borelli, Lai, et al., 2021; Zeegers et al., 2018); their ability to reflect on their own and others' mental states (e.g., Rosso & Airaldi, 2016); and their prosocial orientation (e.g., Goffin et al., 2020). Recent studies have found positive associations between mothers' mind-mindedness during infancy and children's school readiness in kindergarten and academic achievements during childhood and adolescence (Bernier et al., 2017; Meins et al., 2019).

Several studies have included assessments of both parental mentalization and parental sensitivity, consistently finding a positive association between them (e.g., Planalp et al., 2019). Zeegers et al. (2017) meta-analyzed 14 of these studies (2,029 parents) and found a significant moderate association between the two parental characteristics. Some of these studies have found that parental sensitivity mediates the link between parental mentalization and child felt security (e.g., Dollberg, 2022): Parents who are more able to hold in mind their child's needs score higher on parental sensitivity, which in turn contributes to the child's felt security. Other studies found that parental mentalization contributes to child felt security over and above the contribution of parental sensitivity (e.g., Meins et al., 2012). It seems that although closely related, these two parental characteristics offer two somewhat distinct routes to children's development of security. This indicates that optimal interventions should address both parental characteristics.

The Contribution of Parental Secure-Base Provision

Noting the moderate (rather than strong) association between parental sensitivity and child attachment security, Cassidy et al. (2005) conducted an in-depth, qualitative analysis of parental caregiving and concluded that one of the major problems in assessing parental sensitivity is the lack of specificity and consensus regarding the parental behaviors that get coded. There are large differences among studies of parental sensitivity in the contexts in which it is assessed, including feeding, putting to sleep, dressing, playing, and responding to child distress. Moreover, there are large discrepancies in the specific components of sensitivity assessed, such as positive attitude, stimulation, and mutuality.

According to Cassidy et al. (2005), a solution to this problem is to narrow the focus to parents' ability to effectively resolve episodes of child distress and dysregulation that can interfere with nonattachment activities (e.g., exploration, play, learning) and forestall healthy psychological development. These authors recommend focusing on what they call *secure-base provision*—the degree to which a caregiver is able to ensure emotion regulation and safety (safe-haven support) and provide a secure base from which the child can calmly explore and navigate the world (secure-base support). Cassidy et al. noted that some children may tolerate a degree of parental insensitivity and still develop a secure attachment as long as parents are effective in soothing the child when he or she is distressed and helping the child transition to calm and joyful exploration.

Both constructs, parental sensitivity and secure-base provision, emphasize the extent to which parents appropriately perceive, interpret, and respond to their child's needs. However, secure-base provision spotlights a narrower and more focused range of parental responses than parental sensitivity; that is, parental responses during episodes in which a child asks for safe-haven or secure-base forms of support. In addition, unlike parental sensitivity, promptness and attunement to the child's feelings in a moment-by-moment manner are not core aspects of the construct of secure-base provision. In coding secure-base provision, parents' capacities for resolving episodes of infant crying and for sustaining calm exploration are more important than how quickly and with what degree of attunement they react (Woodhouse et al., 2020).

Only one study has empirically examined Cassidy et al.'s (2005) construct of secure-base provision and its contribution to child attachment security (Woodhouse et al., 2020). In this study, a sample of mother–infant dyads completed laboratory tasks at infant's age 4.5 months and were observed at home three times between 7 and 9 months of age. Coders rated the level of maternal sensitivity (according to guidelines set forth by the NICHD Early Child Care Research Network, 1999) and secure-base provision (using a coding manual developed by the authors). The child's attachment security was assessed at 12 months using the Strange Situation procedure. Findings indicated that mothers' secure-base provision significantly contributed to child attachment security over and above the contribution of mothers' sensitivity.

Although Woodhouse et al.'s (2020) findings are promising, more studies are needed to examine the unique contribution of parents' secure-base provision to children's security coded independently of global parental sensitivity. Nevertheless, we want to keep Cassidy et al.'s (2005) conceptualization of secure-base provision in mind when analyzing and evaluating the attachment-based interventions reviewed later in this chapter.

The Interfering Effects of Parents' Attachment Insecurities

There is an impressive body of research showing that parents' own attachment insecurities interfere with their parental sensitivity, which in turn can prevent the formation of a secure attachment on the part of a their child (for reviews, see Fearon & Belsky, 2016; Jones et al., 2015a, 2015b). In one of the first studies of attachment-related predictors of maternal sensitivity, Haft and Slade (1989) videotaped interactions between mothers and their infants, later coding the tapes with respect to the mother's noticing of and attunement to the child's positive and negative emotions. As compared with secure mothers (assessed with the AAI), insecure mothers were less consistent in reacting to their baby's emotions. Anxious mothers attuned inconsistently to both positive and negative emotions, whereas avoidant mothers seemed to ignore negative emotions.

Following up this pioneering research, dozens of studies have found that insecure mothers are less sensitive than secure mothers to their infant's needs, and are more distressed and intrusive when interacting with their infant (e.g., Bernier & Matte-Gagné, 2011; Biringen et al., 2000; Shlafer et al., 2015; Tarabulsy et al., 2005). Similar parental-attachment-related individual differences have been found in studies assessing the quality of support mothers provide to their preschool children during challenging cognitive tasks: Insecure mothers were rated by independent judges as colder and less supportive than secure mothers (e.g., Bosquet & Egeland, 2001; Crowell & Feldman, 1989; Whipple et al., 2011). In addition, whereas avoidant mothers were less sensitive and more controlling and task-focused, anxious mothers gave confusing instructions, were distressed and intrusive when trying to help their children, and failed to provide secure-base support.

Insecure mothers also seem to have difficulty providing a safe haven and secure base. Crowell and Feldman (1991) videotaped mothers' behavior during separation and reunion episodes with their infant in the Strange Situation. Insecure mothers were less affectionate with their child than secure mothers and had greater difficulty calming the child upon reunion. These difficulties have also been noted when insecure mothers attempt to soothe their infants' distress during the reunion episode of the still-face procedure (e.g., Haltigan et al., 2014) or when trying to calm their child during a threatening medical procedure (e.g., Edelstein et al., 2004).

There is also evidence concerning the association between parents' attachment insecurities and mentalization. For example, Kim et al. (2014) found that, as compared to secure mothers, insecure mothers (based on an AAI administered during pregnancy) were less likely to provide empathic verbalizations about the mental state of their 7-month-old infant during the still-face procedure (e.g., "Oh, you are so upset. This is so upsetting"). Accordingly, Dollberg (2022) found that mothers' reports of attachment anxiety during pregnancy were associated with less appropriate mind-mindedness utterances during a free-play interaction with their 3-month-old baby. However, three studies found no association between mothers' attachment patterns and their mind-mindedness (Arnott & Meins, 2007; Bernier & Dozier, 2003; Milligan et al., 2015).

Overall, there is solid evidence that parents' attachment insecurities interfere with their sensitivity and responsiveness. This interfering effect is likely to compromise the effectiveness of attachment-based interventions and hinder the enhancement of children's felt security. Indeed, there is compelling evidence for the intergenerational association between parental and child attachment patterns. In a meta-analysis of 18 studies (based on 854 mother–child dyads), van IJzendoorn (1995) reported a strong association ($r = .47$) between mothers' AAI classification and their infant's attachment security in the Strange Situation. In a meta-analytic replication of 58 studies conducted 23 years later (4,396 dyads), Verhage et al. (2018) found a significant moderate intergenerational association between parental and child attachment patterns ($r = .29$). These two meta-analyses have also shown that this intergenerational association is partially mediated by parental sensitivity; that is, parental attachment insecurities seem to interfere with parents' sensitivity, which in turn puts children at risk for insecure attachment.

Summary

Based on 40 years of ambitious and systematic research, we can confidently conclude that early positive experiences of parental caregiving increase children's chances of attaching securely and moving along a path of healthy psychological development, and that parents' attachment insecurities can interfere with effective parental caregiving and place children at risk for emotional problems. Based on attachment theory and this large body of research, attachment-based interventions have been designed to strengthen one or more of the three key parental security-enhancing characteristics that can benefit children's security (sensitivity, mentalization, secure-base provision). Some of the interventions are focused mainly on changing parents' behavior, while others also attempt to reduce the parents' own attachment insecurities.

Attachment-Based Interventions Focused on Early Childhood

Several researchers have conducted experimental intervention studies aimed at improving parental caregiving and examining postintervention effects on children's attachment security. These experiments are important because random assignment of parents to intervention and control groups allows us to determine whether experimentally induced changes in parenting have a causal effect on children's security. In 2003, Bakermans-Kranenburg et al. meta-analyzed 70 studies (7,636 parent–child dyads) that had assessed postintervention changes in parental sensitivity, as well as 23 studies (1,255 dyads) that also measured children's attachment security. The analyses revealed moderate and statistically significant effects of the interventions on enhanced parental sensitivity and enhanced children's attachment security. Importantly, there was a fairly strong correlation (r = .45) between experimentally induced changes in parental sensitivity and infant security; that is, interventions that were more successful in improving parental sensitivity were also more effective in enhancing children's security. In a subsequent meta-analysis of 15 studies (842 dyads), Bakermans-Kranenburg et al. (2005) detected a significant moderate association between interventions aimed at improving parental sensitivity and a lower rate of disorganized infant attachment—the most insecure form of attachment.

In the past two decades, partly based on these meta-analyses, there has been a proliferation of attachment-based interventions focused on early childhood. Some are fairly brief (6–20 weeks), mostly relying on parents' psychoeducation and video feedback concerning their behavior during parent–child interactions. Others are more extended in time (1–2 years) and include therapeutic techniques that deal with parents' attachment insecurities. Although Steele and Steele (2018) included 12 interventions in their book about attachment-based interventions with young children, we focus here on only five interventions (1) whose rationale and techniques are coherently based on attachment theory and research; (2) which involve carefully developed standardized protocols, manuals, and methods of training and supervising interveners; and (3) whose effectiveness has been examined in randomized controlled trials (RCTs). Despite this focus, we recommend the book by Steele and Steele (2018) for anyone contemplating an intervention effort.

Video-Feedback Intervention to Promote Positive Parenting and Sensitive Discipline

The Video-Feedback Intervention to Promote Positive Parenting and Sensitive Discipline (VIPP-SD; Juffer et al., 2008, 2018) is a short-term behavioral intervention targeting Ainsworth's construct of parental sensitivity. The intervention is constructed around provision of positive, empowering video feedback to parents concerning their sensitive responses during recorded interactions with their child. According to Juffer and Steele (2014), this feedback provides a "useful 'looking glass' through which parents can see their child and their own behavior with 'new' eyes and relive shared positive moments" (p. 313). In VIPP-SD, the intervener functions as a supportive attachment figure to parents and provides them with a secure base (through empowering feedback) for exploring and reflecting on their attitudes and reactions to their child and learning more sensitive parental responses.

VIPP-SD is currently being implemented with children from birth to age 6 years in the context of their homes or child care centers. It includes a standardized protocol of six biweekly, 90-minute sessions with the child and one of his or her caregivers (usually the mother). However, as can be seen in Table 4.1, the intervention can be extended to 13 sessions (with mothers diagnosed with depression or eating disorders) and tailored to specific characteristics of the parents (e.g., parents with intellectual or visual disabilities) or the children (e.g., twins, adopted children, children with behavioral problems). The intervention can be implemented with or without the Sensitive Discipline (SD) module, depending on the age of the child. (Usually, this module is included when children are older than 1 year.) The VIPP portion follows the same protocol in the two variants of the intervention.

During the first part of each session, the intervener videotapes brief episodes of common daily parent–child interactions (e.g., playing together, having a meal) to be discussed with the parent in the next session. During the second part of the session, the intervener and the parent together watch recorded fragments of the previous visit, and the intervener pauses whenever he or she wants to show the parent a positive interaction moment, verbalize the child's signals and behavior ("speaking for the child"), or reinforce a sensitive parental behavior. Feedback is focused on positive interaction moments and sensitive parental responses, so the parent can feel empowered by the feedback and become more receptive to the intervener's tips and suggestions. In the case of insensitive responses, parents are encouraged to use the more sensitive kinds of behaviors they displayed at other moments in the video, using themselves as a model of sensitive parenting. Interveners prepare the feedback in advance by reviewing the recorded interactions in accordance with the VIPP-SD manual. They then write a script for the video-feedback session, specifying the moments they want to focus on, the messages they want to convey, and the questions they want to ask the parent concerning his or her own and the child's behavior.

VIPP-SD comprises four thematic sessions and two booster sessions (Sessions 5 and 6), in which all four themes are reviewed and integrated for parents. The four themes of the intervention are constructed around the two components of Ainsworth's parental sensitivity construct: (1) accurate perception and interpretation of the child's signals and (2) prompt and adequate reactions to these signals. Beyond these sensitivity-related themes, the variant of the intervention that includes the SD module is focused on encouraging parents to explain to the child the reason for their commands, to give compliments for compliant child behavior, and to use distraction and time-out as ways of dealing with difficult child behavior.

During the first two sessions, the intervener attempts to consolidate a trusting relationship with parents while encouraging them to accurately observe and interpret their child's behavior in the video clip. In the first session, the video feedback focuses on the child's attachment and exploration bids, allowing parents to learn when the child needs them as a safe haven for comfort, and when the child needs them as a secure base for exploration. In the second session, parents are invited to verbalize their child's behavior ("speaking for the child"), and the intervener helps parents notice their child's feelings and needs, and interpret them accurately.

During the third and fourth sessions, video feedback deals mainly with parental responsiveness; the parents are encouraged to respond to their child's feelings and needs in a prompt and appropriate way. In the third session, the video feedback focuses on chains of positive interactions (a child's signal followed by an adequate parental response and the child's consequent expression of positive affect) and the importance of these chains for children's well-being and healthy development. In the fourth session, video feedback focuses on moments of shared emotions (e.g., comforting a sad child, sharing joy) and the importance of these moments for children's openness to their own emotions and development of effective emotion regulation.

The effectiveness of VIPP-SD has been examined in 27 published RCTs (see Table 4.1 for a summary of these studies' methods). As can be seen in Table 4.1, samples have included same-sex twins, adopted children, children in foster care, children at risk for externalizing problem behavior, children with autism, and infants at risk for autism. They have also included children living with insecure or insensitive mothers, depressed mothers, mothers with eating disorders, mothers with intellectual or visual disabilities, maltreating mothers, and women of low socioeconomic status (SES). In addition, the effectiveness of VIPP-SD has been assessed in community samples of Turkish mother–child dyads and among caregiver–child dyads in home-based or center-based child care settings. VIPP-SD has been compared to a control group that received either a brochure with information about child development, telephone calls in which parents talk about their child's development, treatment as usual, or supportive counseling (see Table 4.1).

Observational measures of parental sensitivity during parent–child interactions before and after the intervention have been collected in 24 of the 27 studies, and parents' caregiving attitudes have been assessed in 10 studies. Researchers have also assessed postintervention changes in children's attachment security (11 studies) and externalizing behavioral problems (10 studies, see Table 4.1).

In two-thirds of the RCTs that have included observations of parental sensitivity during parent–child interactions (16/24), VIPP-SD led to higher postintervention increases in these measures than a control condition. However, VIPP-SD was found to result in more positive attitudes toward parental sensitivity in only half of the studies that included a relevant measure (5/10). In addition, whereas more than 70% of the studies that assessed postintervention changes in children's attachment security (8/11) found that VIPP-SD led to greater security than a control condition, only three of the 10 studies that assessed children's behavioral problems found a significant intervention effect. Beyond these core intervention effects, VIPP-SD has been found to increase children's relational engagement and autonomy (e.g., Barone et al., 2019; Poslawsky et al., 2015; Stein et al., 2006). The positive effects of VIPP-SD on parental sensitivity and children's outcomes have been found both immediately after the intervention, and at follow-ups varying from 3 months to 7 years.

Meta-analyses conducted by Juffer et al. (2018) on 12 RCTs (N = 1,116) and by van IJzendoorn et al. (2022) on 25 RCTs (N = 2,201) revealed that VIPP-SD (vs. control groups) resulted in significant moderate-to-large postintervention increases in both parental sensitivity and children's attachment security. van IJzendoorn et al. also analyzed a subset of 11 studies that assessed postintervention changes in both parental sensitivity and child's attachment security and found that larger increases in parental sensitivity following VIPP-SD tended to be accompanied by larger increases in child's attachment security (r = .50). This finding implies that VIPP-SD seems to improve parents' sensitive responsiveness, which in turn sustains a child's secure attachment.

Overall, the findings are encouraging and attest to the effectiveness of VIPP-SD for enhancing both parental sensitivity and children's attachment security. However, it is important to note that, thus far, no study has examined the effectiveness of VIPP-SD with parents suffering from serious attachment injuries or severe mental health disorders. In such samples, a short video-feedback intervention might not be sufficient to enhance parental sensitivity, and VIPP-SD might have to be combined with other therapeutic techniques

TABLE 4.1. Summary of RCTs on Effectiveness of VIPP-SD

			Pre- and postintervention assessments	
Authors	Sample	Conditions	Parent	Child
Juffer et al. (2005) Follow-up: Stams et al. (2001) (7 years later)	130 adoptive mothers and their 6-month-old adopted infants	Three-session VIPP vs. a book-only group (mothers received a booklet on parenting)	• Behavioral observations of parental sensitivity	• Attachment security • Internalizing and externalizing behavioral problems • School adjustment
Bakermans-Kranenburg, Breddels-van Baardewijk, et al. (2008) Follow-up: Klein Velderman et al. (2006) (40 months later)	81 insecure mothers and their 7-month-old infants	Four-session VIPP vs. a book-only group (mothers received a booklet on parenting)	• Behavioral observations of parental sensitivity	• Attachment security • Internalizing and externalizing behavioral problems
Stein et al. (2006)	77 mothers with eating disorders and their 4- to 6-month-old infants	13-session VIPP vs. 13 sessions of supportive counseling	• Behavioral observations of parental sensitivity during mealtime	• Infant autonomy at 13 months
Van Zeijl et al. (2006) Follow-up: Bakermans-Kranenburg et al. (2008) (1 year later)	237 mothers and their 1- to 3-year-old children at risk for externalizing behavioral problems	Six-session VIPP-SD vs. six phone talks about child development	• Behavioral observations of parental sensitivity and sensitive discipline • Self-reported attitudes toward sensitivity and sensitive discipline	• Externalizing behavioral problems • Daily cortisol production
Woolley et al. (2008)	80 mothers with eating disorder and their 4- to 6-month-old infants	13-session VIPP vs. 13 session of supportive counseling	• Behavioral observations of parental sensitivity during mealtime	• Behavioral observations of autonomy during mealtime
Kalinauskiene et al. (2009)	54 insensitive mothers and their 7-month-old infants	Five-session VIPP vs. five phone talks about child development	• Behavioral observations of parental sensitivity • Self-reported attitudes toward sensitivity and sensitive discipline	• Attachment security

Groeneveld et al. (2011)	48 caregivers in home-based child care and children under the age of 4 years	Six-session VIPP-SD vs. six phone talks about child development	• Behavioral observations of parental sensitivity • Self-reported attitudes toward sensitivity and sensitive discipline	—
Moss et al. (2011)	67 maltreating mothers and their 1- to 5-year-old children	Eight-session VIPP-SD vs. eight monthly visits by a counselor	• Behavioral observations of parental sensitivity	• Attachment security • Externalizing behavioral problems
Negrão et al. (2014)	43 highly deprived, high-risk mothers and their 1- to 4-year-old children	Six-session VIPP-SD vs. six phone talks about child development	• Behavioral observations of parental sensitivity • Self-reports of quality of family relations	• Attachment security • Behavioral observations of involvement and positive affect
Poslawsky et al. (2014, 2015)	76 mothers and their 16- to 61-month-old children with autism spectrum disorder	Five-session VIPP-SD vs. care as usual	• Behavioral observations of parental sensitivity • Self-reported attitudes toward sensitivity and sensitive discipline	• Attachment security • Behavioral observations of involvement and positive affect
Yagmur et al. (2014)	76 Turkish minority mothers and their 20- to 47-month-old children	Six-session VIPP-SD vs. six phone talks about child development	• Behavioral observations of parental sensitivity and sensitive discipline	—
Cassibba et al. (2015)	32 Italian mothers with their 7-month-old infants	Seven-session VIPP vs. two "dummy" visits at home	• Behavioral observations of parental sensitivity	• Attachment security
Green et al. (2015) Follow-up: Green et al. (2017) (24 months later)	54 mothers and their 9- to 14-month-old infants with high risk for autism	Six-session VIPP (and six booster sessions) vs. no intervention	• Behavioral observation of parental sensitivity	• Attachment security • Externalizing behavioral problems
Hodes et al. (2017, 2018)	85 mothers with mild intellectual disabilities and their 1- to 5-year-old children	Six-session VIPP-SD (adapted for learning disabilities) vs. care as usual	• Behavioral observation of parental sensitivity and sensitive discipline • Self-reported attitudes toward sensitivity and sensitive discipline	—

(continued)

TABLE 4.1. *(continued)*

			Pre- and postintervention assessments	
Authors	Sample	Conditions	Parent	Child
Barone et al. (2018, 2019)	77 adoptive mothers with their 0- to 5-year-old adopted children	Six-session VIPP-SD vs. six phone talks about child development	• Behavioral observations of parental sensitivity	• Attachment security • Externalizing behavioral problems • Relational engagement and autonomy
Platje et al. (2018)	77 mothers with visual disabilities and their 1- to 5-year-old children	Seven-session VIPP-SD (adapted for visual disabilities) vs. care as usual	• Behavioral observations of parental sensitivity • Self-reported attitudes toward sensitivity and sensitive discipline	—
Stein et al. (2018)	131 clinically depressed women with their 4- to 9-month-old infants	13-session VIPP vs. 13 sessions of muscle relaxation	• Behavioral observations of parental sensitivity	• Attachment security • Externalizing behavioral problems
Werner et al. (2018)	64 caregivers in center-based child care and children under age of 4 years	Six-session VIPP-SD vs. six phone talks about child development	• Behavioral observations of parental sensitivity • Self-reported attitudes toward sensitivity and sensitive discipline	—
Alsancak-Akbulut et al. (2021)	68 Turkish low-SES mothers with their 1- to 2-year-old children	Four-session VIPP-SD vs. four phone talks about child development	• Behavioral observations of parental sensitivity	—
Schoemaker et al. (2020)	55 foster mothers with their 1- to 6-year-old children	Six-session VIPP-SD vs. six phone talks about child development	• Behavioral observations of parental sensitivity and sensitive discipline • Self-reported attitudes toward sensitivity and sensitive discipline	—

van der Asdonk et al. (2020)	56 maltreating mothers with their 1- to 6-year-old children	Six-session VIPP-SD vs. regular assessment procedure	• Evaluation of parents' capacity to care	• Externalizing behavioral problems
Barone, Carone, Salazar-Jimenez, & Ortíz Muñoz (2021)	25 Colombian low-SES mothers and their 1- to 3-year-old children	Six-session VIPP-SD vs. six phone talks about child development	• Behavioral observations of parental sensitivity	—
Euser et al. (2021)	202 mothers of same-sex twins with their 4- to 7-year-old children	Five-session VIPP-SD vs. five phone talks about child development	• Behavioral observations of parental sensitivity and sensitive discipline	—
Kolijn et al. (2021)	66 mothers of same-sex twins with their 4- to 7-year-old children	Six-session VIPP-SD vs. six phone talks about child development	• Behavioral observations of sensitive discipline	—
O'Farrelly et al. (2021)	300 mothers and their 1- to 3-year-old children with behavioral problems	Six-session VIPP-SD vs. treatment as usual	• Self-reported attitudes toward sensitivity and sensitive discipline	• Externalizing behavioral problems
Cyr et al. (2022)	69 maltreating mothers with their 0- to 6-year-old children	Six-session VIPP-SD vs. psychoeducation activities	• Evaluation of parents' capacity to care • Behavioral observations of parental sensitivity	• Attachment security • Externalizing behavioral problems
Runze et al. (2022)	243 mothers of twins with their 7- to 8-year-old children	Five-session VIPP-SD vs. five phone talks about child development	• Behavioral observations of parental sensitivity and sensitive discipline • Self-reported attitudes toward sensitivity and sensitive discipline	—

Note. SES, socioeconomic status.

that address parents' insecurities or psychopathology. In addition, since VIPP-SD includes a component of sensitive discipline that is not derived from attachment theory, we can't tell whether its effects on children's attachment security are mainly driven by the parental sensitivity training. However, the fact that similar effects were obtained in studies that included the sensitive discipline module and those that didn't (Juffer et al., 2018) strengthens our confidence in the key role played by the parental sensitivity training.

Attachment and Biobehavioral Catch-Up

Attachment and Biobehavioral Catch-Up (ABC; Dozier & Bernard, 2019; Dozier et al., 2005, 2014) is a home-visit program implemented with parents of children ages 6 to 28 months. It includes a standardized protocol of 10 weekly, 1-hour sessions with one of the parents and his or her child, targeting core components of Ainsworth's construct of parental sensitivity: mutual delight, responsiveness, and nonintrusiveness. The ABC program has three main goals: (1) to encourage parents to follow the child's lead with delight; (2) to heighten parents' provision of comfort and support when a child is distressed; and (3) to reduce parents' intrusive and frightening behaviors while interacting with the child. Unlike the VIPP-SD, the ABC program includes one module dealing with parents' own attachment insecurities, which can interfere with the provision of sensitive and responsive care to the child ("voices from the past").

The most important technique used in the ABC program is what Dozier et al. (2014) call "in-the-moment" comments, in which the intervener (or "parent coach," as this person is called in the program) observes ongoing parent–child interactions and makes spontaneous comments about the parent's behavior. The comments may contain a description of either a parental behavior (e.g., "He cried and you picked him right up"), an intervention target (e.g., "That's such a good example of following the child's lead"), or a behavior's outcome for the child (e.g., "That will let him know he can be confident you will be there for him when he's upset"). According to Dozier et al., these comments increase parents' awareness of their own sensitive behaviors and encourage them to reflect on these responses and their effects on the child. As in VIPP-SD, the comments are positive and constructive, celebrate parents' sensitivity, build on their strengths, and thereby enhance parental self-efficacy and openness to the intervener's feedback in moments of insensitive behavior. Caron et al. (2018) found that both the frequency and quality of in-the-moment comments made by ABC interveners were associated with greater improvement in postintervention parental sensitivity, highlighting their important role in effecting change.

The ABC program also includes a psychoeducation component dealing with basic attachment principles, guided practice of the three targeted behaviors, and provision of video feedback concerning these behaviors. As in VVIP-SD, parent–child interactions are video-recorded, allowing the intervener to show parents brief clips from a previous session, clips in which they provided comfort and support to the child, followed the child's lead with delight, or avoided intrusive or frightening behaviors.

The intervention is manualized, and the manual specifies the content of each of the 10 sessions. Sessions 1 and 2 focus on provision of affection, comfort, and support to a distressed child. Across these sessions, the intervener's comments are constructed to communicate three messages: (1) All children want to be cared for, even if they don't explicitly ask for support; (2) parents need to respond appropriately to children's feelings and needs; and (3) parents need to be aware of their children's distress and respond with care and affection, even if a child turns away or continues to cry. The intervener also shows video clips of children in the laboratory Strange Situation procedure and talks with parents about children's feelings and needs, as well as parents' sensitive responses to anxious and avoidant children.

Sessions 3 and 4 focus on following the child's lead with delight. The intervener talks with parents about the importance of this behavior, shows them videos of a parent following a child's lead and a parent not following a child's lead, asks them to interact with their child while trying to follow the child's lead, and coaches them through the interactions with empowering in-the-moment comments.

Sessions 5 and 6 focus on avoidance of intrusive and frightening behaviors, which research has connected with a child's disorganized attachment pattern (e.g., Lyons-Ruth et al., 1999). The intervener talks with parents about behaviors that can be scary to children and shows them videos of parents and children interacting with puppets (in some of which the parent behaves in an intrusive or frightening manner toward the puppet). Then, the intervener provides parents with puppets and coaches the parents to follow the child's lead and to refrain from engaging in intrusive or frightening behaviors. The intervener also asks parents to reflect on their feelings when they are frightened and discuss the negative effects of frightening behaviors on their child's experience.

Sessions 7 and 8 focus on the ways in which parents' negative experiences with their own parents, and their attachment insecurities, influence their responses to their child. The intervener uses video feedback to contrast times when parents' attachment insecurities intrude into interactions with their child and times when they are able to override these insecurities and behave in a more sensitive manner. Interveners' comments are aimed at helping parents recognize and override voices from the past during parent–child interactions. Sessions 9 and 10 are devoted to reviewing and consolidating the gains and discussing remaining challenges. In the final session, the intervener presents a montage video of the parent nurturing and following his or her child with delight.

The effectiveness of ABC has been examined in eight published RCTs (see Table 4.2 for a summary of these studies' methods). Samples included infants and toddlers in foster care, infants living with neglectful parents or a mother with substance-abuse problems, infants adopted internationally, infants from low-income families, and infants living in intact, normative families (see Table 4.2). In all of these cases, the biological, foster, or adoptive mother received the intervention together with her child. As can be seen in Table 4.2, in most of these studies, the ABC program was compared to a well-matched control intervention that was also guided by a manual, involved 10 one-hour sessions, and was implemented in parents' homes. (The control intervention was the Developmental Education for Families Intervention, which was designed to enhance children's cognitive development.)

The contribution of the ABC program to parental sensitivity has been examined in the eight RCTs (see Table 4.2). In all of them, mothers in the ABC program, compared with mothers in the control condition, exhibited higher levels of postintervention sensitive responsiveness, positive affect, and nonintrusiveness during interactions with their children. These positive effects have been found both immediately after the intervention and at follow-ups varying from 3 months to 6–8 years. In addition, Bernard, Simons, et al. (2015) found that, as compared to maltreating mothers in a control condition, maltreating mothers who underwent the ABC program showed a larger postintervention enhancement of evoked-potential neural responses for pictures of crying or laughing children (relative to neutral children's faces)—a neural sign of improved sensitive responsiveness. Moreover, these mothers (vs. control mothers) were found to hold more secure representations (richer secure-base script knowledge) 6–8 years after the intervention (Raby et al., 2021).

TABLE 4.2. Summary of RCTs on Effectiveness of the ABC Intervention

			Pre- and postintervention assessments	
Authors	Sample	Conditions	Parent	Child
Dozier et al. (2006, 2008); Bick & Dozier (2013) Follow-ups: Bernard et al. (2017); Labella et al. (2020); Lewis-Morrarty et al. (2012) (2–3 years later)	60–96 foster mothers with their 4- to 24-month-old infants	10-session ABC vs. a 10-session educational program (DEFI)	• Behavioral observations of parental sensitivity	• Diurnal cortisol regulation • Stress-related cortisol regulation and recovery during the Strange Situation • Caregiver's reports of child's problem behaviors • Vocabulary development, cognitive flexibility, and theory-of-mind skills (2–3 years later) • Anger regulation during frustrating task (2–3 years later)
Bernard et al. (2012); Bernard, Dozier, et al. (2015); Bernard, Simons, et al. (2015); Lind et al. (2014) Follow-ups: Bernard, Hostinar, et al. (2015); Bernard et al. (2018); Labella et al. (2020), Lind et al. (2020) (2–3 years later); Bick et al. (2019); Garnett et al. (2020); Korom et al. (2021); Raby et al. (2021); Tabachnick et al. (2019); Valadez et al. (2020); Zajac et al. (2020) (6–8 years later)	113 maltreating mothers and their 2- to 21-month-old infants	10-session ABC vs. a 10-session educational program (DEFI)	• Evoked potentials to emotional children's faces • Behavioral observations of parental sensitivity to the 4- to 5-year-old children's distress • Behavioral observations of parental sensitivity with their 7- to 8-year-old children • Secure-base script knowledge (6–8 years later)	• Attachment security • Positive affect during challenging task • Diurnal cortisol regulation • Cortisol regulation (2–3 years later and 6–8 years later) • Anger regulation, compliance with parents (2–3 years later) • Felt security, inhibitory control, resting brain activity, neural responses to maternal cues, and autonomic regulation (6–8 years later)
Berlin et al. (2014)	16 mothers with substance abuse disorder and their 1- to 20-month-old children	10-session ABC vs. 10 sessions of "Book-of-the-Week" program	• Behavioral observations of parental sensitivity	—

Yarger et al. (2016)	24 highly deprived, high-risk mothers and their 8- to 18-month-old children	10-session ABC vs. a 10-session educational program (DEFI)	• Behavioral observations of parental sensitivity	—
Lind et al. (2017) Follow-up: Raby et al. (2019) (1 and 2 years later)	121 foster mothers with their 2- to 3-year-old children	10-session ABC vs. a 10-session educational program (DEFI)	• Behavioral observations of parental sensitivity	• Attention regulation problems • Cognitive flexibility • At follow-up: vocabulary development
Berlin et al. (2018, 2019); Hepworth et al. (2020, 2021); Harden et al. (2021)	202 low-income mothers and their 6- to 18-month-old children	10-session ABC vs. 10 sessions of "Book-of-the-Week" program	• Behavioral observations of parental sensitivity and dyadic mutuality during parent-child interactions • Behavioral observations of parental responsiveness to children's distress	• Stress-related cortisol release and recovery • Reliance on mother for soothing distress (proximity seeking) • Externalizing behavioral problems
Yarger et al. (2020); Lind et al. (2021)	114 adoptive mothers and their 6- to 48-month-old adopted children	10-session ABC vs. a 10-session educational program (DEFI)	• Behavioral observations of parental sensitivity (immediately after intervention and 2 years later)	• Parents' reports and behavioral observations of socioemotional competence (immediately after intervention and 1 and 2 years later)
Perrone et al. (2021)	158 mothers and their 5- to 21-month-old children	10-session ABC vs. a waiting-list control group	• Behavioral observations of parental sensitivity • Depression	—

Note. DEFI, Developmental Education for Families Intervention.

The impact of the ABC program on children's attachment security, however, has been tested in only one RCT. Bernard et al. (2012) found that, as compared to controls, children in the ABC program showed higher rates of attachment security in the Strange Situation 1 month after the intervention. Zajac et al. (2020) found that heightened attachment security (assessed with the Security Scale) was still evident when these children reached 9 years of age. Lamentably, no data were collected on the extent to which children's increased security was predicted by postintervention increases in mothers' sensitivity.

More evidence has been collected with regard to the effects of the ABC program on other child outcomes (see Table 4.2). As compared to control conditions, ABC results in lower levels of externalizing behavioral problems, better regulation of cortisol production, more expression of positive affect during challenging tasks, and better anger regulation during frustrating tasks (e.g., Bernard, Dozier, et al., 2015; Dozier et al., 2006; Labella et al., 2020; Lind et al., 2014). These improvements in socioemotional development have been observed at both preschool age and middle childhood. For example, 3- and 5-year-old children who were assigned to the ABC program in infancy exhibited greater socioemotional competence and more compliance with parents' requests than controls (Lind et al., 2020, 2021). Moreover, 8- to 9-year-old children who were assigned to the ABC program during early childhood showed stronger parasympathetic (calming) responses during a stressful episode than controls (Tabachnick et al., 2019), and their electrophysiological profile was more indicative of cortical maturity (Bick et al., 2019).

There is also evidence that ABC contributes to linguistic development (Bernard et al., 2017; Raby et al., 2019) and has positive effects on children's cognitive flexibility and theory-of-mind skills (Lewis-Morrarty et al., 2012; Lind et al., 2017). These cognitive benefits of the ABC program have been found to persist 2–3 years after the intervention. Raby et al. (2019) also found that the positive effect of ABC on linguistic development was mediated by increases in postintervention parental sensitivity.

Pre- and postassessment studies (without a control group) have also yielded encouraging findings regarding the effectiveness of implementations of ABC in community practice. For example, Caron et al. (2016) found significant pre- to postintervention increases in parental "following the lead with delight" and decreases in parental intrusiveness among Hawaiian mothers who completed the ABC in diverse community settings. Roben et al. (2017) also found significant pre- to postintervention increases in the parental sensitivity of 108 mothers who completed the ABC with 37 different interveners in five community sites. Importantly, the strength of the postintervention changes in maternal behavior in these community settings was comparable to effect sizes observed in RCTs conducted in well-controlled settings.

Overall, there is good evidence that ABC is an effective intervention for increasing parental sensitivity, but only one RCT has tested the intervention's effect on children's attachment security. In addition, there is encouraging evidence concerning the therapeutic impact of in-the-moment comments (Caron et al., 2018). However, more systematic research is needed on the specific intervention elements that contribute to ABC's effectiveness in increasing parental sensitivity and children's attachment security.

The Circle of Security Intervention

The Circle of Security intervention (COS; Hoffman et al., 2006; Powell et al., 2014; Woodhouse et al., 2018), a widely used, manualized intervention for parents of children ages 0–5 years, does not include the child in the therapeutic sessions (except for being included in videotaped interactions with a parent, which are examined in intervention sessions with the parent). It integrates psychoeducation regarding attachment theory and psychotherapeutic techniques aimed at addressing a parent's insecurities. It is an effort to enhance parental sensitivity by targeting parents' actual behavior and mentalization during parent–child interactions. At the behavioral level, parents learn more effective ways of serving as a safe haven and secure base for their child and how to repair inevitable empathic failures in meeting the child's needs. With respect to mentalization, parents are assisted in (1) developing a better understanding of their child's feelings and needs, (2) recognizing how their own working models affect their responses to the child's needs, and (3) reflecting on how these responses affect the child and how the parents can regulate their emotions for the benefit of the child. In Woodhouse et al.'s (2018) words, COS offers "a relational environment within which the parent feels safe enough to engage in a reflective dialogue that ultimately leads to better parental regulation and parental provision of a secure base/safe haven" (p. 53).

COS begins with a preintervention assessment of the parent–child relationship, which helps the intervener create an individualized treatment plan for each parent. In this way, the intervention is tailored to the specific parent's attachment-related representations, fears, and difficulties, as well as the specific relationship he or she has with the child in question. In this assessment, parents are interviewed about their working models (COS-Interview; Powell et al., 2014) and are observed during actual interactions with their child (e.g., reading a book, directing the child to return toys to a box). For children ages 12 months or older, parent–child dyads are also observed during the Strange Situation procedure. All of these interactions are video-recorded and used during the intervention to allow parents to review and reflect on what Powell et al. (2014) call each parent's *linchpin struggle*—the central interaction pattern that most interferes with secure-base provision. The term *linchpin* was chosen because it refers to a parent's central relational problem that defines and shapes the larger pattern of his or her interactions with the child.

During the intervention, parents learn to use the COS vocabulary and graphics (see Figure 4.1), in which the parents' actions are represented by the *hands on the circle*—the secure base from which the child explores the world and the safe haven to which the child returns when distressed. The top half of the circle represents children's exploration activities and their need for a secure base; the bottom half represents children's proximity-seeking bids and their need for a safe haven (see Figure 4.1). Using COS graphics, parents learn about a child's needs, how to use "hands" in an effective manner, and specific difficulties the parents might experience in meeting their child's needs. They are also encouraged to reflect on their own attachment history and working models in an effort to see how these can instigate linchpin struggles in each half of the circle. On this basis, parents can reflect on what Powell et al. (2014) call *limited hands and limited circles*—the ways in which parents' own fears, attitudes, and behavior can move children toward insecurity and increase children's difficulties in comfortably and independently exploring the world and/or relying on parents for protection and comfort.

The most important COS technique involves parents' viewing and reviewing video-recorded interactions between themselves and their children. In these reviews, the intervener encourages parents to provide behavioral descriptions of the interactions and to create hypotheses about the child's needs, the parents' own emotions and struggles, and how their working models influence their responses (what Powell et al. [2014] call *seeing and guessing*). There are three phases of tape review.

Phase 1 tape review focuses on helping parents track, moment by moment, their children's signals and needs, and reflect, with the help of the COS graphics and vocabulary, on their own struggles in meeting these needs. Phase 2 tape review occurs after the intervener introduces the metaphor of *shark music*—the idea, influenced by ominous background music

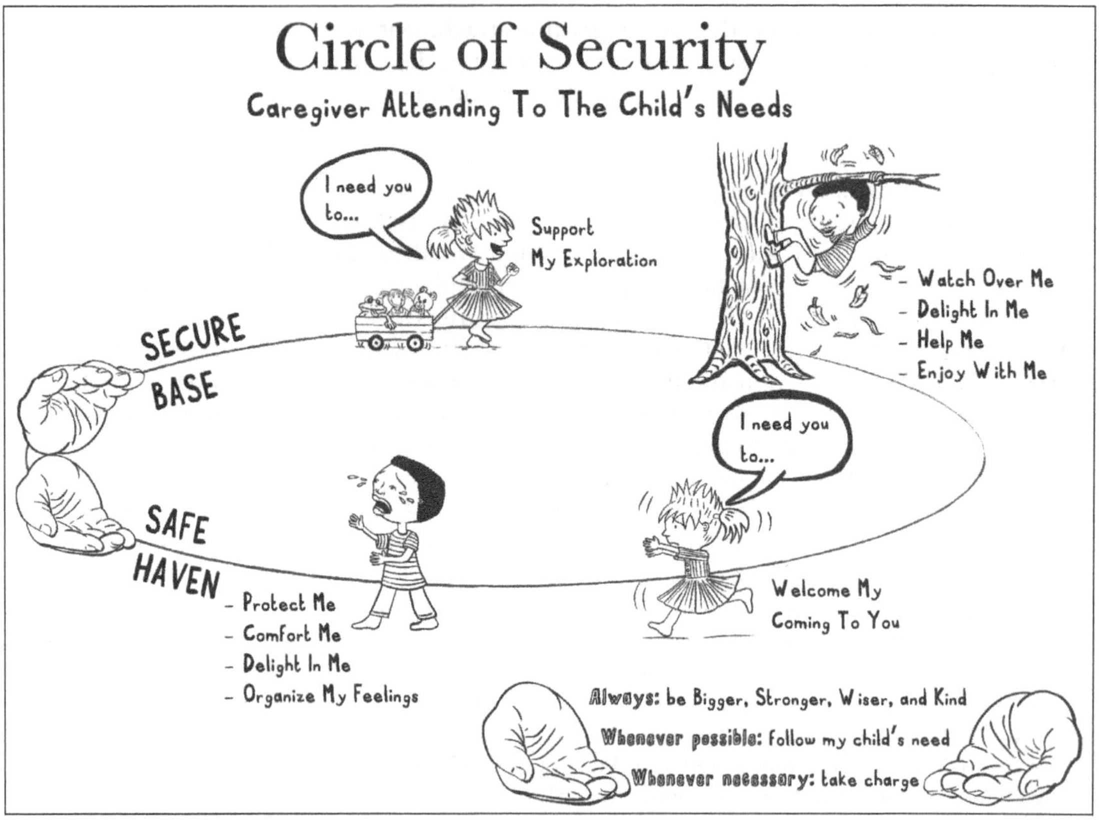

FIGURE 4.1. Circle of Security graphics. Copyright © 2018 Glen Cooper, Kent Hoffman, and Bert Powell; Circle of Security International. Reprinted by permission.

in the movie *Jaws,* that painful past experiences with attachment figures can loom in memory and lead a parent to feel threatened or frightened during certain interactions with his or her child. The Phase 2 tape review focuses on helping parents reflect on and talk about their own shark music and realize how it can lead to linchpin struggles and limited or disrupted circles of security. After the Phase 2 review, parents and children are again video-recorded, so that any new parenting capacity can be observed. The subsequent Phase 3 tape review focuses on celebrating positive changes in the parent–child relationship and reflecting on newly acquired behaviors for effectively meeting children's needs.

The COS protocol (Hoffman et al., 2006; Powell et al., 2014) includes a preintervention assessment and a 20-week period in which groups of approximately six parents (without their children) meet on a weekly basis for 75 minutes. Weeks 1 and 2 are devoted to creating a trusting relationship between intervener and group members, and introducing the COS graphics and vocabulary with videos depicting successful moments of group members meeting their children's needs. Weeks 3–8 are devoted to Phase 1 tape review. Each week, one parent (the focal parent) engages in "seeing and guessing" with reference to video clips from his or her preintervention assessment, and the other group members are encouraged to support the parent and learn from his or her observations and insights.

In Week 9, the shark music metaphor is introduced, and the group discussion focuses on how parents' attachment history and working models can create linchpin struggles and insufficient circles of security. Weeks 10–15 are devoted to Phase 2 tape review. Each week, one parent watches video clips from his or her preintervention assessment, and the intervener helps the parent identify and soften his or her shark music and mitigate linchpin struggles. Then, parent–child interactions are video-recorded again, and clips are edited for Phase 3 reviews (Weeks 16–19). During these sessions, each parent is given an opportunity to review the new clips and reflect on newly acquired strengths and current struggles. Week 20 is reserved for a graduation celebration.

Since its creation, other versions of the COS protocol have been implemented, but all involve the same goals, graphics, vocabulary, techniques, and phases as the original version. For example, the COS Perinatal Protocol (COS-PP; Cooper et al., 2003) transformed the COS protocol into a 15-month jail-diversion intervention for pregnant, nonviolent offender women, starting during the third trimester of pregnancy and ending when the infants were 12 months old. The COS–Home Visiting–4 intervention (COS-HV4; Cooper et al., 2000) incorporated the core COS elements into a protocol that can be delivered in a brief, four-session, home-visiting program with parents of infants ages 0–1 years.

To facilitate implementation and dissemination of the COS approach in the community, Cooper et al. (2009) developed the COS–Parenting protocol (COS-P). This protocol is similar to the original, with one critical difference: Instead of watching and reviewing video clips from their preintervention assessment, parents work on video clips that were previously created by the developers (currently provided in DVD format) in which other parents, children, and sometimes actors interact. In addition, parents are invited at each session to present descriptions of particular interactions with their own child as a means of personalizing the impersonal video material. The stories are framed as *Circle Stories* and the intervener encourages parents to link what they watch in the video clip with their own personal experiences. The COS-P protocol is delivered in eight 90-minute, weekly sessions and it targets the same parental capacities as the original COS protocol.

The effectiveness of the COS intervention has been examined in five published RCTs (see Table 4.3 for a summary of these studies' methods). One was conducted with mothers diagnosed with postpartum depression and randomly assigned to the original COS protocol or treatment as usual (Ramsauer et al., 2020). A second study was conducted with low-SES mothers of irritable infants randomly assigned to the COS-HV4 protocol or three home visits focused on child development (Cassidy et al., 2011). Three studies examined the effectiveness of the COS-P protocol as compared to treatment as usual or a waiting-list control condition. The samples included low-SES American mothers of preschool children (Cassidy et al., 2017) and Swedish and Australian mothers at risk for parenting problems (Risholm Mothander et al., 2018; Zimmer-Gembeck et al., 2022).

With regard to mothers, those who received the COS-P protocol reported more positive self-representations as a mother, less parenting stress, and less attachment anxiety (in the ECR) after the intervention than did mothers in control conditions (Risholm Mothander et al., 2018; Zimmer-Gembeck et al., 2022). Cassidy et al. (2017) also found that the COS-P intervention reduced mothers' unsupportive responses to child distress but failed to alter mother's supportive responses. However, Ramsauer et al. (2020) found no significant effect of the original 20-session COS protocol on mothers' sensitivity during mother–child interactions (although some improvement was found among mothers with unresolved states of mind on the AAI, an important predictor of a child's disorganized attachment).

Findings were less consistent with regard to children's outcomes. The three RCTs that assessed children's attachment (Cassidy et al., 2011, 2017; Ramsauer et al., 2020) failed to find higher rates of security following the COS intervention than following the control conditions. However, such an effect was found among infants or children who were most at risk

TABLE 4.3. Summary of RCTs on Effectiveness of the COS Intervention

			Pre- and postintervention assessments	
Authors	Sample	Conditions	Parent	Child
Cassidy et al. (2011)	220 low-income mothers and their highly irritable 6- to 9-month-old infants	Three-session COS-HV4 vs. three home visits focused on child development	—	• Attachment security (3 months after intervention)
Cassidy et al. (2017)	141 low-income mothers and their 3- to 5-year-old children	10-session COS-P vs. waiting-list control	• Self-reported coping responses to children's distress and anger	• Attachment security • Behavioral observations of children's self-regulation and cognitive flexibility • Internalizing and externalizing behavioral problems
Risholm Mothander et al. (2018)	52 at-risk mothers for parenting-related problems and their 1- to 48-month-old children	Eight-session COS-P vs. treatment as usual	• Behavioral observations of parental sensitivity • Interview about mental representations of the child and relationship with him or her (WMCI)	• Behavioral observations of involvement and positive affect during mother–child interactions
Ramsauer et al. (2020)	72 depressed mothers and their 4- to 9-month-old infants	20-session COS vs. treatment as usual	• Behavioral observations of parental sensitivity	• Attachment security
Zimmer-Gembeck et al. (2022)	85 at-risk mothers for parenting-related problems and their 1–7-year-old children	10-session COS-P vs. waiting-list control	• Reported parenting stress and parenting practices • Attachment orientations • Depressive symptoms	—

Note. WMCI, Working Model of the Child Interview.

for developing insecure attachment, such as highly irritable infants (Cassidy et al., 2011) or children whose mothers were avoidant with respect to attachment and therefore less willing and able to provide love and care (Cassidy et al., 2017). Cassidy et al. also found that, as compared to the control condition, COS-P improved children's self-regulation (inhibitory control) skills. However, this improvement was not significantly associated with changes in child's felt security or maternal responses to children's distress.

Beyond these RCTs, studies using a pre- and postintervention design without a control condition have found significant reductions in parenting stress and psychological symptoms among biological and foster mothers who participated in the COS or COS-P interventions (Cassidy, Ziv, et al., 2010; Huber et al., 2016; Kitagawa et al., 2022; Krishnamoorthy et al., 2020; Maxwell et al., 2021). Moreover, as compared to a preintervention assessment, mothers showed improvements in emotion regulation, mentalization, and the positivity of representations of the child following the intervention (Horton & Murray, 2015; Huber et al., 2015a; Krishnamoorthy et al., 2020; Maxwell et al., 2021). Interestingly, these benefits were most notable among mothers who showed relatively high levels of distress prior to the intervention.

With regard to child outcomes, findings indicate that children whose parents were in the COS or COS-P intervention condition showed significant pre- to postassessment increases in attachment security and decreases in attachment disorganization and emotional and behavioral problems (Hoffman et al., 2006; Huber et al., 2015a, 2015b; Kitagawa et al., 2022). In addition, Cassidy, Ziv, et al. (2010) found that infants of 20 incarcerated mothers who completed the COS-PP intervention displayed rates of attachment security comparable to those of low-risk, middle-class samples and better than typical high-risk samples. However, the lack of a control group and small sample sizes raise doubts about the validity of these findings.

Overall, research attests to the promise of the COS intervention, but more research is needed before we can have confidence in its effectiveness for increasing children's attachment security. Moreover, no data have been collected on two parental variables that are directly targeted by the COS protocol: parents' mentalization capacities and internal working models.

Future RCTs might take advantage of the COS Interview, which was designed to assess parents' preintervention working models, mentalization, and attachment insecurities but could also be administered again immediately after the intervention and at different follow-ups in order to examine changes in these important parental variables. Future studies might also build on the COS vocabulary and create reliable and valid assessment tools to measure common parenting difficulties (e.g., linchpin struggles, shark music, limited circles, limited hands). In this way, researchers could examine the effectiveness of the COS protocol in altering each of these difficulties during parent–child interactions and the extent to which each of these improvements is associated with beneficial COS intervention influences on children's attachment security.

Minding the Baby

Minding the Baby (MTB; Sadler et al., 2006; Slade et al., 2018) is a 27-month home-visiting program aimed at enhancing parental mentalization and improving the quality of parent–child relationships in first-time vulnerable mothers (mothers who are at moderate-to-high risk for developing mental health problems). MTB has two main goals: (1) to provide mothers with a safe haven and secure base (a trusting relationship with a responsive intervener) that can help them in mitigating parenting-related distress and regulating themselves during interactions with their baby; and (2) to enhance parental mentalization so that mothers can direct attention to their own and their child's mental states and sensitively respond to the child's needs.

The program is built on the strengths of two prominent home-visiting models: the Nurse–Family Partnership Program (Olds, 2002) and child–parent psychotherapy (see next section). Nurse–Family Partnership, the most widely implemented and tested home-visiting intervention in the United States, is delivered by public health nurses who address health care needs of vulnerable families. However, nurses are not prepared to address parents' mental health difficulties and the negative repercussions of these problems on parent–child relationships. Child–parent psychotherapy was designed specifically to address these difficulties and to improve parental sensitivity and children's felt security. However, clinicians cannot effectively deal with a family's health care needs and replace nurses. Therefore, in addressing these limitations, MTB creates interdisciplinary teams of nurses and clinicians working together, engaging mothers as part of a team, and meeting the multiple needs of a family in a collaborative way.

The program begins during the third trimester of pregnancy and continues until the child is 24 months old. It includes regular home visits with mother, and most of the visits following the birth of the child are conducted with mother and infant together. Families are visited weekly for 1 hour until the child's first birthday, then every other week until the child is 2 years old. Visits are carried out on an alternating basis by a team that comprises an advanced practice nurse and a licensed clinical social worker who has passed a 3-day MTB training course (the nurse sees a family one week, the social worker the next). Although the MTB approach has been manualized based on a well-developed set of principles, protocols, and guidelines (Slade, Sadler, & Mayes, 2005), it is highly individualized according to the needs and circumstances of a particular family.

The roles of the nurses and clinicians are both distinct and overlapping. The nurses' roles include reinforcing prenatal care and health education (e.g., informing mothers about nutrition and fetal brain development, developing a labor plan) and supporting the child's health and development (e.g., assessing a child's development, diagnosing and treating illness, attending to the mother's health). The social workers' roles include ongoing assessment of both mother and child, diagnosing the mother's psychological distress and mental health problems, providing a range of potential treatments when needed, and helping mothers negotiate legal and court-related issues. Both nurses and social workers make efforts to enhance a mother's mind-mindedness, fostering parental sensitivity, and improving the quality of mother–infant interactions.

The first stage of MTB involves building a trusting relationship with mothers so they can gradually regard the nurse and social worker as effective safe havens when distressed and as secure bases when challenged by parenting and other duties. The goal is to help the mothers feel protected, calm, and secure in the interveners' presence. This stage includes sensitive provision of support and praise for the mother's strengths and competencies, which by itself can move mothers toward a more open and curious attitude toward their inner experiences and facilitate mentalization. According to Sadler et al. (2006), "Mentalization arises out of the relationship. . . . The mothers experience themselves as *meaningful* in the eyes of the home visitors; the experience of being held in mind as a coherent, intentional person who is trying to do her best allows mothers to start experiencing themselves and the baby in the same way" (p. 278).

After the nurses and social workers become a secure base for mothers, their reflective stance during home visits can improve a mother's mentalization. This involves being curious about the mother's and child's thoughts and feelings, and using "wondering" statements and questions (e.g., "I wonder what it feels like to you when your child cries and you don't know why he is crying?"; "What do you imagine your child feels when he is in pain and you are out of sight?"). In this way, mothers are encouraged to talk about their own feelings and explore the child's feelings and needs. Other techniques involve (1) the intervener's description or interpretation of mother's or child's behaviors in terms of beliefs, feelings, and intentions; and (2) the intervener's disclosure of his or her own feelings and thoughts during their interactions with mothers and infants. Interveners can also video-record mother–infant interactions and watch the video clips with mothers while encouraging them to explore their own and their child's inner experience during the recorded episode. In addition, they can offer mothers activities such as journaling and scrapbooking, which provide opportunities for mothers to explore and verbalize their feelings and thoughts, and develop curiosity concerning their babies' mental states.

To date, the effectiveness of the MTB intervention has been examined in two published RCTs (Sadler et al., 2013; Slade et al., 2020). In both studies, the MTB program was compared with a well-matched control group of mothers who received routine prenatal and postnatal health-focused home visits. With regard to mothers' outcomes, the findings are not very consistent across the two studies. Whereas Slade et al. found that, as compared to their control group, mothers in the MTB group had higher levels of parental mentalization at the end of the intervention (as assessed by the PDI), Sadler et al. (2013) failed to find a significant group difference on this measure. Moreover, Sadler et al. found that mothers in the MTB group displayed higher-quality mother–child interactions when their infants were 4 months old than did controls (lower rates of disrupted, atypical interactions), but Slade et al. (2020) failed to replicate this finding. Follow-up assessments of mothers in these RCTs 2–8 years after the intervention revealed that, as compared to controls, mothers in the MTB group exhibited higher levels of mentalizing and lower levels of hostile and coercive parenting (Londono Tobon et al., 2022; Ordway et al., 2014).

With regard to children's outcomes, the findings are more consistent. In both studies, children in the MTB group had significantly higher rates of secure attachment and lower rates of disorganized attachment (assessed in the Strange Situation) after the intervention than did control children. Follow-ups of the RCTs when the children were 4 to 5 years old revealed that, as compared to controls, children in the MTB group had fewer emotional and behavioral problems (Londono Tobon et al., 2022; Ordway et al., 2014) and lower rates of obesity (Ordway et al., 2018). These findings strengthen our confidence in MTB's effectiveness, but we need more RCTs to further examine the effects of the intervention with different kinds of parent–child dyads to understand the observed inconsistencies in mothers' postintervention parenting skills, and to replicate the observed effects on children's attachment security.

Child–Parent Psychotherapy

Child-parent psychotherapy (CPP; Lieberman & Van Horn, 2005, 2008) is a manualized intervention designed to improve parental caregiving by working through parents' painful childhood experiences and attachment insecurities. CPP has four main goals (Toth et al., 2018). First, it attempts to foster parents' sensitivity to children's signals and needs. Second, it aims to promote parents' ability to provide a safe haven and secure base while balancing their own and their children's needs (creating what Bowlby [1969/1982] called a *goal-corrected partnership*). Third, CPP is designed to cultivate parents' feelings of safety and security by helping them cope with stress and regulate distress during parent–child interactions. Fourth, the intervention attempts to modify parents' maladaptive perceptions of, and inappropriate reactions to, their child stemming from their own attachment history and insecure working models. In summing up these goals, Lieberman and Van Horn (2008) concluded that CPP might effectively help parents to recognize and control the intrusion of attachment-related negative thoughts and feelings into the relationship with their child, and to foster more reality-attuned, sensitive parental responses.

CPP is implemented on a dyadic basis with children ages 0–5 years and one of their caregivers (usually the mother) in weekly, hour-long sessions conducted over a period of approximately 10–12 months (for a total of 40–50 sessions). Therapists are licensed psychologists, clinical social workers, or psychiatrists who take university-level courses and training in the use of the CPP manual (Lieberman et al., 2015). CPP may be conducted in home or clinic settings given that there are toys for the child to play with and enough space to allow for parent–child interactions. Parents freely interact with their child during the therapeutic session, and the therapist reflects on what he or she observes during the interactions.

Due to this approach's psychoanalytic origins (Fraiberg, 1980), most of the therapist's reflections focus on exploring and addressing parents' painful childhood experiences and insecure working models, and on how these affect their feelings and responses to their child (Lieberman & Van Horn, 2008). However, Toth et al. (2018) noted that therapists can also "flexibly adapt behavioral interventions contributed by cognitive-behavioral therapy and other approaches in order to guide parental and child behavior toward more adaptive manifestations, never losing sight of the emotional meanings of the behaviors targeted for change" (p. 299).

Establishing a trusting, supportive, and secure relationship between the therapist and the parent is a crucial stage in CPP (Toth et al., 2018). The therapist strives to provide parents a safe haven that comforts, calms, and reassures them when they feel threatened or are distressed, as well as a secure base for exploring and reflecting on their painful memories and maladaptive patterns of relating—both in general and with regard to their child in particular. In this way, parents gradually form something like a secure attachment to the therapist, which allows the parents to explore their memories, feelings, thoughts, and relational behaviors with confidence that the therapist will be available and responsive when needed. In addition, the therapist aims to create an emotionally corrective experience for parents by acknowledging their attachment-related wishes and fears, and supporting and encouraging them to be emotionally available and engaged during parent–child interactions. The therapist also (1) verbalizes the child's feelings and needs as a means of increasing the parent's awareness and sensitivity to the child's inner life (mentalization, again), and (2) provides gentle modeling of appropriate behavior when interacting with the child so that the parent can learn more effective patterns of relating.

CPP begins with a thorough assessment of the child, the parent, and their relationship. This initial phase provides an opportunity to begin building a trusting relationship with the parent and gain knowledge about the family's concrete circumstances, the parent's attachment history and working models, and the ways in which he or she understands the child's problems. It culminates in a feedback session in which the clinician and parent discuss what they learned during the process and co-create a treatment plan for working through parent's working models and difficulties, improving the quality of parent–child interactions, then supporting their child's healthy development.

The effectiveness of CPP has been examined in five RCTs, with children who are at risk for developing insecure attachment (see Table 4.4 for a summary of these studies' methods). These RCTs were conducted with attachment-anxious infants and their mothers; infants and preschoolers from maltreating families and their mothers; clinically referred preschoolers and their mothers; and toddlers and their depressed mothers (see Table 4.4). In these

TABLE 4.4. Summary of RCTs on CPP

			Pre- and postintervention assessments	
Authors	Sample	Conditions	Parent	Child
Lieberman et al. (1991)	59 low-income mothers and their 1-year-old attachment-anxious children	1 year of weekly CPP sessions vs. no treatment	• Behavioral observations of parental sensitivity • Reports of maternal childrearing attitudes	• Attachment security • Behavioral observations of affect expression, angry behavior, and avoidance
Toth et al. (2002)	87 maltreating mothers and their 4-year-old children	1 year of weekly CPP sessions vs. educational home visits or community standard intervention	—	• Narrative-coded scores of representations of the self and mother
Lieberman et al. (2005); Ghosh Ippen et al. (2011); Bernstein et al., 2019 Follow-up: Lieberman et al. (2006) (6 months later)	75 clinically referred mothers with their 3- to 5-year-old children	1 year of weekly CPP sessions vs. case management plus individual treatment	• Posttraumatic stress disorder symptomatology • Biases toward anger and fear in interpreting children's facial expression • At follow-up: psychiatric symptomatology	• Mother's report of traumatic stress disorder • Mother's report of internalizing and externalizing problems • At follow-up: internalizing and externalizing problems
Cicchetti et al. (2006); Cicchetti, Rogosch, Toth, & Sturge-Apple (2011) Follow-ups: Cicchetti, Rogosch, & Toth (2011); ; Stronach et al. (2013) (1 year later)	137 maltreating mothers and their 1-year-old infants	1 year of weekly CPP sessions vs. educational home visits or community standard intervention		• Attachment security • Diurnal cortisol
Cicchetti et al. (2000); Toth et al. (2006) Follow-ups: Peltz et al. (2015) (1 and 2 years later); Guild et al. (2017, 2021) (6 years later)	97–130 depressed mothers and their 18- to 24-month-old children	1 year of weekly CPP sessions vs. no treatment	• Depression severity • Marital satisfaction • Behavioral observations of responses to the child during a mother–child conflict conversation (6 years later)	• Attachment security • Behavioral observations of responses to mother during a mother–child conflict conversation; teacher's report of peer relationships (6 years later)

Note. WPPSI, Wechsler Preschool and Primary Scale of Intelligence.

studies, CPP was compared to a no-intervention condition, a psychoeducational parenting intervention, a community standard treatment, or individual psychotherapy (see Table 4.4). Whereas children's outcomes were assessed in all five of the RCTs, mothers' outcomes were assessed in only three studies (see Table 4.4).

With regard to mothers' outcomes following the intervention, those in the CPP group, compared with controls, showed higher levels of sensitive responsiveness during mother–child interactions, reported more positive attitudes toward childrearing and lower levels of trauma-related distress and psychiatric symptomatology, and were less likely to misinterpret ambiguous infant expressions as communicating fear (Bernstein et al., 2019; Lieberman et al., 1991, 2005). Lieberman et al. (2006) reported that the positive effects of CPP on mothers' postintervention distress were sustained 6 months later. In their sample of depressed mothers, Toth et al. (2006) reported that CPP failed to reduce mothers' depression, but follow-ups revealed that mothers in the CPP group reported higher marital satisfaction immediately after the intervention and 1 and 2 years later (Peltz et al., 2015). Moreover, Guild et al. (2021) reported that CPP, as compared to a control condition, resulted in more maternal warmth during a mother–child conflict conversation 6 years after the intervention.

Unfortunately, these studies failed to assess whether CPP actually produced the expected positive changes in mothers' mentalization skills and working models. Thus, the researchers could not examine whether these changes were responsible for the observed CPP effects on mothers' attitudes and behaviors toward their child. In addition, the RCTs do not provide support for the hypothesis that postintervention increases in maternal sensitivity contribute to the enhancement of children's attachment security.

With regard to the children's outcomes, the findings are strong, indicating that, as compared to control conditions, CPP increased children's attachment security immediately after the intervention and 1 year later (Cicchetti et al., 2006; Lieberman et al., 1991; Stronach et al., 2013; Toth et al., 2006). In addition, children in the CPP group showed more positive representations of self and mother, improved cortisol regulation, and lower levels of emotional and behavioral problems after the intervention than control children (Cicchetti et al., 2000, 2011; Lieberman et al., 2005; Toth et al., 2002). Lieberman et al. (2006) reported that the positive effects of CPP on children's mental health were sustained 6 months later.

Importantly, Ghosh Ippen et al. (2011) found that the strongest beneficial mental health effects of CPP were found in high-risk children (children who had frequently experienced traumatic life events). CPP has also been found to have long-term benefits years after the intervention, such as better peer relationships and lower levels of anger during a mother–child conflict discussion at age 9, which were statistically dependent on the child's increased attachment security following the intervention (Guild et al., 2017, 2021).

Findings from studies that have relied on a pre- and postassessment design without a control condition also provide evidence of CPP's effectiveness. For example, Hagan et al. (2017) found that mothers' posttraumatic stress symptomatology (PTSS) decreased after CPP. Importantly, this positive change explained reductions in children's postintervention PTSS. In addition, Lavi et al. (2015) found decreases in mothers' depression, as well as increases in positive attitudes toward their children after CPP (relative to a preintervention assessment).

Studies that have examined the implementation of CPP in community settings have also provided evidence for the effectiveness of the intervention (Toth & Gravener, 2012). For example, Lowell et al. (2011) conducted an RCT comparing Child FIRST (Child and Family Interagency, Resource, Support, and Training), a community intervention that combines CPP with the provision of welfare services, with a usual care condition. Results indicated that children assigned to the Child FIRST intervention showed significant improvements immediately after the intervention compared with children in the usual care group in linguistic development and mental health. Moreover, mothers in the Child FIRST group experienced less parenting stress and lower levels of psychopathology than controls. Of course, we cannot discern whether CPP, the welfare services provided by Child FIRST, or both working together are responsible for the positive outcomes. However, this is encouraging evidence regarding the positive implications of using CPP in community services.

Comparison of the Interventions and Future Considerations

The five reviewed attachment-based interventions are well grounded in attachment theory and research, involve carefully developed and standardized protocols and techniques for facilitating the formation of a secure parent–child relationship, and have been shown by rigorous RCTs to be successful in moving a child toward heightened security and healthy development. Most of these interventions are conducted with parents and children together, allowing parents to observe their own reactions to their children's behaviors (*in vivo* or via video clips), receive feedback on their parenting behavior, and practice more appropriate patterns of relating. An early meta-analysis (Bakermans-Kranenburg et al., 2003) revealed that parenting interventions after the birth of children were more effective than those conducted prenatally. Probably, interventions that rely exclusively on a psychoeducational, didactic approach (e.g., preparing pregnant women for future parenting tasks) are less effective in changing children's felt security than those that also provide parents with an opportunity to review and practice sensitive parental behaviors with their own child.

In an integrative analysis of attachment-based interventions, Pitillas (2020) concluded that they share four common therapeutic elements. First, all of the interventions emphasize the importance of enhancing parents' feelings of safety and security. This emphasis is evident in interveners' efforts to create a trusting and solid working alliance with parents, being a reliable source of a safe haven and secure base for parents, and encouraging parents' positive transference to the intervener (admiring and identifying with the intervener). The accepting, reassuring, and empowering in-session climate that characterizes attachment-based interventions probably act as a corrective emotional experience for attachment-insecure parents and arouse in them a strengthened sense of attachment security. This corrective experience can calm parents' attachment-related worries and fears, thereby increasing their sensitivity and responsiveness to their children's needs. In Pitillas's view, an intervener's provision of security to parents creates a "chain of security" in which the final link is a more secure child. This rationale is supported by findings we reviewed earlier in this chapter that parents who feel safer and more secure are more sensitive and responsive to their children's needs. (As will be seen in subsequent chapters, this "chain of security" is important for many kinds of nonparental attachment figures as well.)

Second, all of the attachment-based interventions encourage parents to explore and reflect on the mental states that underlie children's behavior as well as their own reactions during parent–child interactions. Although some of the interventions are designed primarily to strengthen parents' mentalization skills (MTB, CPP) while others are more behaviorally oriented (VVIP-SD, ABC), interveners' comments and feedback in all of the interventions direct parents' attention not only to the observed behavior but also to the needs and feelings it reveals and expresses. In this way, all of the attachment-based interventions are attempts to increase parents' awareness of and sensitivity to their children's feelings and needs.

Third, all of the attachment-based interventions involve promoting parenting skills (sensitivity, mentalization, secure-base provision) through observation and understanding of what happens during interactions with the child. In all of these interventions, interveners encourage what Cohen et al. (1999) called cycles of watching, waiting, and "wondering about" during parent–child interactions (e.g., ABC's in-the-moment comments, VIPP-SD's speaking for the child, COS's seeing and guessing). According to Woodhead et al. (2006), these cycles provide parents an opportunity to keep their child in mind and understand what the child sees and experiences when interacting with them, and then improve their sensitivity and secure-base provision.

Fourth, all of the attachment-based interventions involve attempting to enhance parents' positive representations of themselves as caregivers. Through the intervener's accepting and empowering comments and feedback, parents gradually create a new, more positive image of themselves as reflected in the eyes of the intervener. This positive representation can challenge previous negative representations of parents as caregivers (models of others) and allow them to appreciate their strengths and the positive influence they can exert on their child's development (models of self). According to Pitillas (2020), "The way the therapist looks at the parent–child dyad constitutes a fundamental instrument of change. The parent needs to *be seen* in new ways to be able to change his or her self-image" (p. 33, emphasis in original).

Unfortunately, to date, no study has assessed these theoretically derived therapeutic elements in attachment-based interventions and the extent to which each of them does or does not enhance children's attachment security. Specifically, we don't yet have evidence regarding the formation of a trusting and secure intervener–parent relationship during an intervention; parents' appraisal and use of the intervener as a security-enhancing attachment figure; interveners' use of watching, waiting, and wondering cycles; parents' increasing understanding of parent–child interactions; and parents' beliefs about how the intervener sees them as a caregiver. Such assessments might allow researchers to empirically compare different attachment-based interventions with respect to these therapeutic elements and determine which are the most important mechanisms of change in each of the interventions.

Another commonality among attachment-based interventions is their focus on the dyadic relationship between the child and one of his or her parents. There is little or no attention paid to the quality of the parents' couple relationship as a potential intervention target (with the exception of referrals of severely disturbed couples to couple counseling). However, there is accumulating evidence for a family-systems perspective on the development of children's attachment orientations (Cowan & Cowan, 2002; Cummings & Davies, 2002). Indeed, findings indicate that problems in the couple relationship seem to interfere with parental sensitivity to the child (e.g., Cross et al., 2021).

Therefore, attachment-based interveners might devote more energy to evaluating the quality of the parents' couple relationship as part of preintervention assessments, and to addressing couple conflicts and the ways in which they affect parenting. When a couple's conflict focuses on parenting, interveners can adopt a triadic, coparenting approach and work with both parents while they interact with the child. This kind of intervention might neutralize the spillover of couple conflicts into the parenting domain, increasing the chances of moving the child toward greater attachment security.

Despite these commonalities, attachment-based interventions differ in several important ways. First, they differ in length. Whereas some are short-term interventions, ranging from 2 to 5 months (VIPP-SD, COS, COS-P, ABC), the MTB and CPP are longer interventions that range from 1 to 2 years. In addition, they differ in focus. Whereas the VIPP-SD and ABC interventions explicitly focus on changing parenting behaviors, the other interventions also target parents' mentalization skills or their internal working models of self and others. The interventions also differ in their use of *in vivo* or video-recorded parent–child interactions, the inclusion of modules that are not derived from attachment theory (e.g., sensitive discipline in VIPP-SD, health care needs in MTB), and the presence of the child during the intervention sessions (the child is not present, except in video recordings, in COS sessions, but is included in sessions of the other interventions).

In the meta-analysis that Bakermans-Kranenburg et al. conducted in 2003, the findings surprisingly indicated that attachment-based interventions with shorter durations (less than 16 sessions) were actually more effective than longer interventions in enhancing children's attachment security. Additional meta-analytic findings indicated that attachment-based interventions that focused specifically on changing parents' behaviors were more effective than interventions that focused on changing parents' mental representations (Bakermans-Kranenburg et al., 2003). However, these meta-analyses reflected the state of the art 18 years ago, before most of the RCTs reviewed in this chapter were conducted. Today, dozens of RCTs and pre- and postassessment studies have been conducted on the various attachment-based interventions. Therefore, it would be worthwhile to conduct new meta-analyses and examine differences in the effectiveness of the interventions as a function of their length, intervention focus, specific techniques (e.g., reliance on *in vivo* or video-recorded parent–child interactions), targeted population of parent–child dyads, age of the child at the time of the intervention, and other characteristics of the sample.

With regard to the evidence base concerning the effectiveness of the reviewed interventions, we agree with Berlin et al.'s (2016) conclusion that "attachment-based interventions can indeed support the development of attachment security and can reduce the risk of developing or maintaining attachment insecurity" (p. 747). Specifically, the effectiveness of VIPP-SD is supported by a robust body of evidence (including meta-analyses of 27 RCTs) in a wide variety of parent–child dyads. Moreover, the California Evidence-Based Clearing House for Child Welfare (2014, 2019) concluded that ABC and CPP are well supported by research evidence, and that the COS program has garnered promising research evidence.

There are, however, some important limitations to this evidence base. First, the vast majority of the RCTs have been conducted with mothers or child-center caregivers, not with fathers. Second, beyond a single study conducted by Caron et al. (2018) on the therapeutic impact of ABC interveners' in-the-moment comments, we do not have much insight into the specific therapeutic elements that contribute to the success of attachment-based interventions. Third, no RCT has been conducted comparing the effectiveness of different attachment-based interventions (beyond comparing each of them to a control condition), so we do not know what works better overall or with a particular type of parent–child dyad.

We have preliminary findings on the question of what works for whom, showing that attachment-based interventions are most effective with children who are at risk of developing attachment insecurities, such as children who have experienced frequent and intense stressful events, highly irritable children, and genetically vulnerable children with the dopamine receptor D4 (*DRD4*) 7-repeat allele (e.g., Bakermans-Kranenburg, van IJzendoorn, et al., 2008; Cassidy et al., 2011; Ghosh Ippen et al., 2011). However, more research is needed comparing the effectiveness of the various attachment-based interventions when applied to different kinds of mothers and children. At present we do not know what is the most effective intervention for a particular parent–child dyad.

With increasing implementation of attachment-based interventions in large community settings, we need more research examining the effectiveness of these initiatives. As reviewed earlier, some studies have examined the effectiveness of community implementations of the ABC, COS, and CPP protocols (e.g., Berlin et al., 2018; Cassidy, Ziv, et al., 2010; Lowell et al., 2011), but they do not cover the full spectrum of the eventual integration of attachment-based intervention protocols into comprehensive community services. For example, the VIPP-SD is being offered to all adoptive parents in Holland and to all foster parents in Flemish Belgium, but the effectiveness of these services has not yet been examined. In addition, these community implementations raise issues of interveners' fidelity and quality of control of the intervention protocol. Although both CPP and ABC have been implemented in community settings through the learning collaborative model developed by the National Center of Child Traumatic Stress for promoting fidelity and sustainable practice, research should be conducted on fidelity-related issues in order to facilitate the scaling up of attachment-based interventions to large community settings (for encouraging findings, see Caron & Dozier, 2019; Costello et al., 2019).

Concluding Remarks

Given the origins of attachment theory in the context of psychoanalysis, which was long criticized for being impervious to empirical testing, it is amazing how thoroughly many aspects of attachment theory and attachment-related clinical interventions have been examined empirically. As seen in this chapter, the resulting research has led to ambitious, societally significant interventions designed to improve parenting and increase the frequency of secure child-parent attachments. Although we have listed some of the remaining gaps in the research base, we are extremely impressed by the research efforts undertaken to date. In general, the measures have been carefully designed and validated, and the intervention procedures have been carefully conveyed to the various interveners. These studies are expensive, time-consuming, and difficult to manage, especially when they are carried out over periods of years. But the results make a huge contribution to refining theory, empirically shaping optimal interventions, and contributing to human welfare. Psychodynamic theory, at least Bowlby and Ainsworth's version of it, has proven to be empirically testable and systematically applicable—a great achievement!

CHAPTER 5

Enhancing Attachment Security in Relationships between Parents and Adolescents

During the past 20 years, attachment-based interventions have been developed to increase adolescents' secure attachment to parents and support their healthy development during what is often a very challenging life transition (Kobak & Kerig, 2015; Steele & Steele, 2018). Some of the interventions have been tested in RCTs, and research has provided encouraging evidence regarding their effectiveness in promoting more secure parent–adolescent relationships and enhancing adolescents' mental health. The interventions parallel the two main therapeutic tasks of attachment-based interventions in early childhood (see Chapter 4). First, they are designed to enhance parents' sensitive responsiveness to their offspring's needs and feelings, and improve their provision of a safe haven and secure base. Second, they are an attempt to cultivate parents' exploration and reflection (mentalization) on the ways their own attachment insecurities and negative attachment experiences may be impairing the quality of interactions with their adolescent offspring, putting him or her at risk for emotional or behavioral problems.

But attachment-based interventions during adolescence include additional components that reflect the unique characteristics of the parent–adolescent relationship. Unlike young children, adolescents are strongly motivated to expand their own competences and autonomy, and to explore and discover their unique subjectivity and identity even at the expense of temporary conflicts with, or detachment from, parents (Allen & Tan, 2016). In addition, adolescents gradually become active, autonomous, and relatively equal partners in shaping the quality of parent–adolescent interactions (Ainsworth, 1989; Kobak et al., 2017).

Hence, attachment-based interventions are designed to improve parents' ability to maintain a warm, close relationship with their offspring and provide comfort and relief in times of need (safe-haven support) while at the same time accepting, supporting, and encouraging the adolescent's needs for privacy, autonomy, and uniqueness (secure-base support). The interventions also cultivate parents' ability to maintain cooperative and mutually satisfying conversations with their adolescent offspring in a respectful and fairly equalitarian manner. In addition, some of the interventions include individual therapy sessions with the adolescent, designed to work through, if warranted, his or her painful attachment experiences and insecure working models while encouraging more positive attitudes toward parents and more constructive patterns of communication and conflict resolution.

In this chapter, we first review research showing that parents often can still serve as safe havens and secure bases for their offspring during adolescence. We also consider evidence concerning (1) the particular parental attitudes and behavior that sustain adolescents' broaden-and-build cycle of attachment security, and (2) the ways in which these security-enhancing attitudes and behaviors can be disrupted by the attachment insecurities of both parents and offspring. We then show how this growing body of evidence is being applied in two attachment-based interventions, the Connect Parenting Program (Moretti & Obsuth, 2009; Moretti et al., 2018) and attachment-based family therapy (ABFT; G. S. Diamond et al., 2014, 2021), and we evaluate each of them with respect to their efficacy in promoting adolescents' felt security and mental health.

Security Enhancement Processes in the Parent–Adolescent Relationship

In their comprehensive review of attachment in adolescence, Allen and Tan (2016) discussed normative changes in the ways in which adolescents relate to parents and peers (friends, romantic partners) that raise serious questions about the extent to which they still regard and rely on parents as safe havens and secure bases in times of need. From a clinical perspective, this issue is critical, because most attachment-based interventions during adolescence explicitly assume that improving parents' sensitive provision of a safe haven and secure base is crucial for maintaining and enhancing adolescents' felt security and healthy development. However, if adolescents no longer turn to parents for comfort, support, and encouragement when facing threats and challenges, improving parents' willingness and ability to provide these attachment-related resources might have no positive effects on adolescents' felt security or mental health. Unlike young children, who need parents' availability, responsiveness, and supportiveness to feel safe and secure (Ainsworth, 1991), adolescents may attempt to manage distressing experiences and cope with novel, uncertain, and challenging circumstances without relying on parents' protection and support. Their evolving self-soothing skills and mental representations of themselves as strong and competent might make parental protection and support less necessary, and even embarrassing or intrusive. According to Allen and Tan (2016),

> During adolescence, rapidly developing competencies decrease the need for dependence on parental attachment figures, and the strong need to explore and master new environments promotes healthy growth in the exploratory system. These changes necessitate a new balance between attachment behaviors and exploratory needs, with exploration taking an increasingly central role. (p. 400)

In other words, adolescents might prefer to cope with threats and challenges on their own rather that asking parents to meet their needs for safety and security.

This emphasis on self-reliance is particularly evident in the ways adolescents mentally represent their parents in the AAI. In a review of the first 10,000 AAIs, Bakermans-Kranenburg and van IJzendoorn (2009) found that adolescents were more likely than adults to be classified as having a dismissing (avoidant) state of mind with respect to parents. Longitudinal data indicate that derogating attitudes toward parents and negative perceptions of parents in the AAI gradually increase from ages 10 to 14 (Ammaniti et al., 2000). And adolescents classified as secure in the AAI tend to show restricted expressions of affection and warmth toward parents even when talking coherently about their relationship with them (Scharf et al., 2004). (This coherence is one of the major characteristics that get them classified as secure [Hesse, 2016].) But these findings do not necessarily imply that adolescents tend to become insecure with respect to parents. Rather, they indicate that even attachment-secure adolescents tend to direct attention away from childhood memories of dependency on parents, which is part of a healthy and adaptive means for sustaining their emerging sense of autonomy.

The AAI findings also do not necessarily mean that adolescents completely give up parental support or that parental sensitivity is no longer relevant for sustaining their felt security. In fact, there is evidence that parental sensitivity remains central for predicting when adolescents feel loved (Coffey et al., 2022; McNeely & Barber, 2010) and that the quality of the parent–child relationship is still important for understanding individual differences in adolescents' well-being, mental health, and functioning in interpersonal, social, and academic domains (Steinberg, 2019).

What the research findings seem to imply is that parents' attachment-related roles may become redefined or reorganized during their children's adolescence. Many adolescents may not explicitly ask parents to hold, comfort, and soothe them when distressed (although many do). But they may still ask parents to support and not interfere with their emerging autonomy, to accept their desire to cope with threats and challenges on their own, and to understand that they want to maintain optimal closeness and distance as they explore new opportunities and construct their own unique identity (Allen & Tan, 2016). According to Allen (2021, p. 165), "If the infant's working model of self-in-relationship asks, 'Can I get help from my caregiver when I'm threatened or distressed?', the adolescent's model likely adds an element: 'Can I get help when I need it in a way that doesn't threaten my growing need for autonomy?' "

Hence, parents may still serve as attachment figures for their adolescent children. However, their main task is to provide secure-base forms of support as their adolescent moves confidently outside his or her comfort zone (the immediate vicinity of parents) to deal autonomously with new experiences and challenges in a well-regulated manner. During this developmental period, parents' sensitivity is defined not just by their capacity to accept and validate their teen's proximity-seeking bids and to provide comfort and relief when needed (safe-haven support). It is defined primarily by their capacity to react in an accepting, loving, and supportive manner in response to their teen's requests for distance, privacy, and autonomy. Both of them—safe-haven support and secure-base support—are probably crucial for sustaining offspring's felt security during adolescence (see next section for a review).

Just as adolescents attempt to refrain from frequently turning to parents for protection and support, they seem to choose close friends and romantic partners as alternative sources of a safe haven and secure base, and to seek proximity to these people in times of need (Rosenthal & Kobak, 2010). According to Allen and Tan (2016), a good friend might play a much larger role than parents in helping to regulate distress in threatening and fear-inducing situations during adolescence. Adolescents may also feel confident to explore the world, in particular romantic and sexual relationships, in the company of a good friend. As a friend is also building and broadening his or her own evolving competencies and identity, the friend is likely to be appraised as a good partner with whom to explore new situations, ideas, and activities.

In addition, being involved in an attachment relationship with a good friend allows adolescents to learn and practice interpersonal skills necessary for forming and maintaining reciprocal, equalitarian relationships, in which each partner may at different times be a care seeker or a care provider, which is characteristic of adult–adult pair bonds (Zeifman & Hazan, 2016). These interpersonal skills are less likely to be learned within the parent–child relationship, in which parents typically occupy the caregiver role most of the time.

In a pioneering study, Hazan and Zeifman (1994) provided evidence concerning the developmental trajectory according to which friends and romantic partners gradually replace parents as principal attachment figures during the period from middle-childhood to young adulthood. In this study, participants were explicitly asked to nominate people to whom they turned for closeness, protection, and security (proximity, safe haven, and secure base, in attachment theory's terms).

Specifically, participants completed the WHOTO scale, which identifies a person's primary attachment figures by asking for the names of people who are preferred as providers of proximity, a safe haven, and a secure base (see Chapter 3). Hazan and Zeifman (1994) found that participants ages 6–17 preferred to spend time with (maintain proximity to) peers rather than parents, regardless of age. In other words, proximity seeking was already targeted at peers during elementary school. However, the targeting of peers as principal providers of a safe haven and secure base typically occurred later, during adolescence and young adulthood. Specifically, peers replaced parents as a safe haven between the ages of 8 and 14, and replaced them as a secure base only late in adolescence. These developmental transitions were also found in other studies that employed the WHOTO measure (e.g., Fraley & Davis, 1997) or other self-report scales (e.g., Rosenthal & Kobak, 2010).

Again, these findings do not necessarily imply that parents no longer accomplish any attachment functions during adolescence. Although close friends are often nominated as a safe haven, adolescents still seek parents' protection and support following painful separations and losses (Rosenthal & Kobak, 2010). Reliance on parents' support also seems to increase during demanding periods (e.g., the birth of a first child) even during young adulthood (Feeney et al., 2001). These findings fit with Weiss's (1993) idea that parents serve as "attachment figures in reserve" and are called into active service whenever their adolescent or young adult offspring passes a developmental milestone or encounters serious difficulties. There is also evidence that if adolescents and young adults are not involved in a long-term romantic relationship or marriage, they still prefer parents rather than friends or siblings as a secure base for dealing with threats and challenges (Hazan & Zeifman, 1994).

Overall, the answer to the question "Do parents still function as attachment figures during adolescence?" seems to be yes. However, the answer is qualified by developmental transformations in parents' attachment-related roles and the adolescent's network of attachment figures. First, although parents may still function as attachment figures during adolescence, their main role is to manage in a sensitive, comforting, and empowering manner their offspring's needs for distance, autonomy, privacy, and uniqueness. Second, parents should understand and accept that their adolescent's network of attachment figures now includes friends and romantic partners who can accomplish attachment functions and gradually replace parents as principal attachment figures. With these two qualifications in mind, we can review studies examining the extent to which (1) parental sensitive responsiveness to an adolescent offspring's needs and feelings contributes to his or her felt security and mental health, and (2) parents' and adolescents' attachment insecurities interfere with the formation of a secure parent–adolescent relationship.

The Contribution of Parental Attitudes and Behavior to Adolescents' Attachment Security

In Chapter 4, we reviewed evidence that parental sensitivity during infancy contributes to children's security with respect to parents and sustains their felt security during childhood, adolescence, and even young adulthood. These findings provided the empirical basis and impetus for the design of attachment-based interventions with parents of young children (see Chapter 4). However, this body of research is less relevant for informing attachment-based interventions during adolescence. For this kind of intervention, we need evidence showing that parents' sensitivity to their adolescent offspring's current needs and feelings can sustain or even increase felt security over time.

Fortunately, parental sensitivity has been assessed within parent–adolescent interactions, with results consistently showing that adolescents whose parents exhibit greater sensitive responsiveness are more likely to possess a strong sense of attachment security (e.g., Allen et al., 2003; Brenning et al., 2012a, 2012b; Waslin et al., 2022). In these studies, parental sensitivity was measured with self-report scales and with behavioral observations of parental warmth, acceptance, positive engagement, responsiveness to the adolescent offspring's needs, and support provision. Offspring's felt security was assessed with the Security Scale (Kerns et al., 2001), which measures the perceived quality of attachment to parents, self-report scales measuring attachment anxiety and avoidance in close relationships, or interviews (AAI, Child Attachment Interview, Friends and Family Interview) tapping states of mind regarding attachment to parents. Koehn and Kerns (2018) meta-analyzed 24 of these studies ($N = 17{,}315$) and found a significant moderate association linking parental sensitivity during middle childhood and adolescence with offspring's attachment security.

Prospective longitudinal studies that map the trajectory of felt security during adolescence and young adulthood also provide important evidence concerning the security-enhancing effects of parental sensitivity. For example, parents' approval and support during early adolescence (as reported by parents and their offspring) predicted increases in offspring's self-reports of attachment security over a 4-year study period (Ruhl et al., 2015). And behavioral observations of parental responsiveness at child age 15 were associated with lower scores on attachment anxiety and avoidance scales (indicating greater security) at age 25 (Dinero et al., 2008). In another rigorously conducted prospective study, mothers' provision of safe-haven and secure-base forms of support (as rated by trained coders) when their offspring were 13 and 16 years old predicted increases in attachment security (measured with the AAI) from ages 14 to 24 (Allen et al., 2018).

From a clinical perspective, these research findings need to be complemented by studies examining whether spontaneous or therapeutically induced increases in parental sensitivity during adolescence can transform insecure children into secure ones. Fortunately, longitudinal findings provide an affirmative answer to this crucial question. In a longitudinal study of early adopted children, for example, Beijersbergen et al. (2012) found that increases in mothers' sensitive provision of support during the study period (less support in early childhood but more support in adolescence) predicted children's change from insecurity at 12 months (in the Strange Situation) to security at 14 years (according to the AAI). Similarly, Booth-LaForce et al. (2014) found that children shifted from insecurity in early childhood to security in adolescence as a function of increases in mothers' sensitivity during early adolescence (relative to their sensitivity in early childhood). Similar positive changes in attachment security have been noted among adolescents with a history of maltreatment who were placed in foster care at age 7: The greater the foster mother's sensitivity, the greater the likelihood of insecure children becoming secure adolescents (Joseph et al., 2014). These findings indicate that positive changes in the quality of parenting during adolescence can enhance felt security even among children exposed to early adversity and trauma.

As discussed in the previous section, parental sensitivity during adolescence also involves sensitively providing a secure base that is helpful but does not threaten or interfere with a teen's emerging autonomy. Several cross-sectional and prospective longitudinal studies that have focused on this core aspect of parental sensitivity show that adolescents feel more secure with respect to a parent when he or she is more likely to accept, respect, support, encourage, and genuinely celebrate their autonomy and individuality (e.g., Allen et al., 2003, 2004; Brenning et al., 2012a, 2012b).

Conversely, adolescents tend to be more distressed, angry, and helpless, and to feel less secure with regard to a parent when he or she disrespects their choices and decisions, restricts or punishes autonomy, or provides support that is not needed or not wanted in intrusive, overcontrolling, or emotionally overinvolved ways (e.g., Allen & Hauser, 1996; Doyle & Markiewicz, 2005; Van der Vorst et al., 2006). We also know that adolescents' perceptions of parental disapproval, criticism, and verbal, physical, or psychological pressure are related to less felt security with respect to the parent (e.g., Gallarin & Alonso-Arbiol, 2012; Scott et al., 2011). In a meta-analysis of 10 relevant studies ($N = 3{,}185$), Koehn and Kerns (2018) found a significant small-to-medium association between parental autonomy (secure-base) support during adolescence and offspring's felt security.

Parental sensitivity during adolescence also contributes to the broaden-and-build cycle of healthy development. As expected, self-reports and behavioral observations of parents' warmth, acceptance, and provision of safe-haven and secure-base forms of support during middle childhood and adolescence have been implicated in a broad range of positive adolescent outcomes, such as greater well-being and improved self-control and adaptive emotion regulation (for meta-analyses, see Goagoses et al., 2022; Li et al., 2019; Vasquez et al., 2016).

In addition, lack of parental sensitivity in the form of negligent, overcontrolling, or harsh/punitive parental behaviors (as assessed in parents' own reports or adolescents' perceptions) is associated with adolescents' emotional and behavioral problems (e.g., anxiety, depression, antisocial behavior) and academic difficulties. And it predicts increases in these problems over time (see Pinquart, 2016, 2017a, 2017b, for reviews and meta-analyses). Overcontrolling maternal behavior during early adolescence also predicts problems in adolescents' capacity for autonomy in interpersonal relationships 3 years later (Hare et al., 2015) as well as lower likelihood of being in a romantic relationship and lower academic achievement by age 32 (Loeb et al., 2021).

Kobak et al. (2017) described three categories of parenting practices that can increase the beneficial impact of parental sensitivity on adolescents' felt security. The first category involves creating parent–adolescent interactions marked by affection, respect, and positive feelings (*parental positive engagement*). While interacting with positively engaged parents, adolescents learn that emotional closeness to parents can be an enjoyable experience, and that they don't need to be afraid of parents' advice and guidance. This positive relational climate can soften adolescents' defensive distancing from parents and allow them to benefit from parental sensitivity. Indeed, research indicates that parental positive engagement is associated with positive adolescent outcomes, including increased self-worth and adaptive emotion regulation and reduced risk for substance abuse and unprotected sex (see Kobak et al., 2017, for a review).

The second category of security-enhancing parenting practices includes sensitive monitoring and supervision of a teen's behavior without intruding on his or her privacy or controlling his or her behavior. This kind of monitoring and the improved knowledge about one's offspring's behavior might allow parents to "make well-attuned decisions about how to balance supervision and guidance with support for autonomous decision-making" (Kobak et al., 2017, p. 139). When this is done well, adolescents feel that parents "see," understand, and care for them, and that parents' guidance does not entail a threat to their sense of autonomy.

The third category of security-enhancing parenting practices involves collaborative communication and cooperative negotiation around autonomy-related conflicts. In this collaborative position, parents attend to and mentalize offspring's needs, maintain a mindful stance during the conflictual interaction, rely on pro-relational strategies of conflict resolution (e.g., compromising and integrating one's own and the offspring's needs), and refrain from escalating anger, hostility, and distress. These parental practices contribute to a teen's felt security, because he or she feels loved, valued, and respected by parents even during conflictual interactions. In support of this view, Kobak et al. (2017) reviewed studies showing that both parental sensitive monitoring and cooperative negotiation have positive effects on adolescents' healthy development.

The Interfering Effects of Parents' and Adolescents' Attachment Insecurities

In Chapter 4, we reviewed research showing that parents' own attachment insecurities interfere with parental sensitivity to their young child's needs and feelings, which in turn can prevent the development of attachment security in the child. Similar kinds of interference have been observed in studies assessing attachment-related differences in parental sensitive, responsive, and supportive responses during parent–adolescent interactions (see Jones et al., 2015a, 2015b, for reviews). For example, in a study of maternal responses during video-recorded mother–adolescent conversations about the adolescent's leaving home for college, attachment-anxious mothers had greater difficulty providing a secure base for their offspring's exploration. And they were more intrusive (as rated by observers) than secure mothers (Kobak et al., 1994). In addition, mothers who scored higher on an avoidant attachment scale were rated by observers as less supportive and more hostile during a conflict management discussion with their adolescent offspring (Jones & Cassidy, 2014).

Studies assessing parents' reports of their own parental behavior, attitudes, and emotions have also revealed attachment-related difficulties. More attachment-insecure parents (those with higher scores on attachment anxiety or avoidance scales) report more destructive responses during parent–adolescent conflicts, such as greater anger, more yelling, and fewer attempts to compromise and integrate their own and their teen's needs (e.g., Feeney, 2006; García-Ruiz et al., 2013; La Valley & Guerrero, 2012). Attachment-insecure parents also tend to report less supportive and more disapproving, overcontrolling, and punitive responses to their teen's expressions of vulnerability and distress (Jones et al., 2014). Parental attachment insecurities are also associated with less autonomy-granting attitudes toward their adolescent child (Kilmann et al., 2009), less knowledge about the teen's whereabouts and activities (Jones et al., 2015c), and greater endorsement of harsh disciplinary measures, including physical punishment (Goldberg & Scharf, 2020). In addition, more attachment-insecure parents tend to report higher levels of stress and distress during interactions with their adolescent child and to hold more negative views of their offspring and their own functioning as a parent (Caldwell et al., 2011; Cohen et al., 2011; Kor et al., 2012).

The ability of parents to effectively provide a safe haven and secure base can also be disrupted by the teen's attachment insecurities. Notably absent from studies of parental sensitivity during early childhood are assessments of the interfering effects of the child's insecure working models. At this early age, children's beliefs about the self and others are in a formative stage, and they are being gradually shaped by their parents' attachment working models and caregiving patterns. In other words, during early childhood, children's attachment patterns are viewed as an outcome of parental sensitivity (see Chapter 4) and not as a separate factor that can shape the quality of the early parent–child relationship.

The situation is completely different during middle childhood and adolescence, because insecure children have already developed fairly stable negative working models of the self and others (during interactions with inadequately responsive parents and other relationship partners) that can negatively bias their relational feelings, cognitions, and behavior with regard to a parent. As a result, their pessimistic beliefs about parental attitudes and behavior can lead them to reject parental support or adopt a combative, destructive stance during conflictual interactions. Even if a parent can sometimes try to be sensitive and responsive, the adolescent's negative feelings may cancel the benefits that could be derived from positive interactions with a responsive and supportive parent.

Adolescents' attachment insecurities can inhibit proximity- and support-seeking from parents in times of need and work against reliance on parents as safe havens and secure bases. For attachment-insecure adolescents, painful interactions with cold and rejecting or unreliably supportive parents during early childhood may have formed associative links in memory between proximity-seeking impulses and worries about being rejected and abandoned. As a result, both attachment-anxious and avoidant adolescents might be wary and tense when entertaining the possibility of seeking proximity to and support from parents. However, anxious and avoidant adolescents may differ in how they cope with these attachment-related worries.

Adolescents high on attachment-related avoidance, who typically deactivate attachment needs and behaviors, may inhibit proximity seeking and maintain distance from parents even when distressed and in need of support. Adolescents high in attachment anxiety, who typically tend to hyperactivate attachment worries, may engage in intrusive, ambivalent, tense, angry, and ineffective forms of relating to parents, which can exacerbate tensions and conflicts.

In support of these theoretical expectations, Dujardin et al. (2016) presented 8- to 12-year-old children with a stressful task and found that more anxiously or avoidantly attached children waited longer before calling for their mother's help. In a recent study, Borelli, Gaskin, et al. (2021) asked 8- to 12-year-old children to read and reflect on vignettes that described a hypothetical child experiencing physical vulnerability (e.g., being hurt, being ill), with some of the vignettes describing only the vulnerability and others also describing the child seeking parents' support. Autonomic nervous system reactivity (measured as galvanic skin response [GSR], an index of physiological arousal; and respiratory sinus arrhythmia [RSA], an index of distress regulation) was assessed at baseline and during each of the vignettes. Attachment-insecure children reacted to the support-seeking vignettes (but not to other vignettes) with higher levels of autonomic arousal and lower indications of distress regulation (relative to baseline measures). These findings imply that support seeking among attachment-insecure children is associated with physiological indicators of distress.

Their negative working models of others might cause attachment-insecure adolescents to have difficulty perceiving a parent as responsive and supportive, or trusting his or her good intentions and kindness (Allen et al., 2003). This distrust might in turn contribute to the formation of more defensive, and even aggressive, attitudes and responses when interacting with parents, mainly when these interactions include conflicts related to closeness–distance or dependence–autonomy.

Indeed, attachment-insecure adolescents (assessed with the AAI) do exhibit less open and constructive patterns of communication with parents than do secure adolescents and display fewer positive behaviors (e.g., mutual validation, empathy, engagement) and more negative behaviors (e.g., anger, avoidance) in observed parent–adolescent interactions (see Allen & Tan, 2016, for a review). For example, during conversations with their mothers about topics they disagree on, attachment-insecure adolescents (assessed with the AAI) exhibit more dysfunctional anger and fewer attempts to deal constructively with the disagreement (as rated by trained observers) than do secure adolescents (Kobak et al., 1993).

They are also rated by observers as exhibiting less agreeable autonomy (attempts to assert autonomy without creating distance or escalating conflict with the mother) and more hostile autonomy (e.g., dismissing the mother's question, arguing against it) during conflictual interactions with the mother (Zimmermann et al., 2009).

With regard to the differential interfering effects of specific types of attachment insecurities (anxiety, avoidance), avoidant adolescents are detached from parents and experience serious problems in talking with them about their needs and feelings (Becker-Stoll et al., 2008). In contrast, attachment-anxious adolescents tend to overengage in repetitive and futile, sometimes angry and bitter, arguments with parents around conflictual issues that undermine relationship quality and their own autonomy (Allen & Hauser, 1996). Interestingly, during late adolescence, this unproductive pattern of parent–adolescent interactions contributes to attachment-anxious adolescents' difficulties in leaving home for college and effectively adjusting to the college transition (Bernier et al., 2005).

Overall, the research we have reviewed implies that security enhancement in relationships between parents and adolescents can be disrupted by attachment insecurities that both parents and adolescents bring to the relationship. These insecurities can interfere with parental sensitivity, militate against collaborative and constructive relational behaviors of both parents and adolescents, and either damage the secure attachment that some adolescents have formed with parents during childhood or prevent security enhancement from occurring among more insecurely attached adolescents. Hopefully, a skillful attachment-oriented intervener can help by sensitively managing both parents' and adolescents' insecurities, soften their destructive patterns of relating, assist insecure parents in cultivating sensitive and responsive parenting practices, coach insecure adolescents to accept and enjoy their parents' love and care, and then help move all parties toward greater security and healthy autonomy. These challenging therapeutic steps are the main focus of the remainder of this chapter.

Attachment-Based Interventions Focused on Parent–Adolescent Relationships

The data showing that felt security remains malleable during adolescence and has long-term benefits for mental health, interpersonal functioning, and relationship quality (see Chapter 2) helps to explain the proliferation of attachment-based interventions aimed at enhancing adolescents' felt security and its broaden-and-build effects. Some of these interventions are attempts to enhance adolescents' felt security within individual psychotherapy, such as interpersonal therapy or mentalization-based treatment for adolescents (Klerman et al., 1984; Rossouw, 2018). Other interventions work on enhancing teens' felt security in group relationships with peers, such as the Connection Program (Allen et al., 2021). Still others focus on the quality of parent–adolescent relationships with the aim of improving parents' provision of a safe haven and secure base and enhancing teens' felt security toward parents, such as the Connect Parenting Program and ABFT (G. S. Diamond et al., 2014; Moretti et al., 2018).

In this section, we focus on the Connect Parenting Program and ABFT. These interventions devote most of their therapeutic efforts to improving parents' sensitive responsiveness to their adolescent's needs and feelings as a means of enhancing the adolescent's felt security and improving his or her mental health. We consider individual (rather than dyadic) interventions with adolescents in the chapter devoted to attachment-informed individual psychotherapies (Chapter 7). We deal with the Connection Program in our review of attachment-based interventions aimed at enhancing felt security within relationships with groups (Chapter 9).

The Connect Parenting Program

Connect is a 10-week manualized program for parents or alternative caregivers of preadolescents and adolescents with emotional or behavioral problems. It does not include the adolescent in the therapeutic sessions (Moretti & Obsuth, 2009; Moretti et al., 2018). The main goal of the program is to enhance parental attitudes and behaviors that ensure adolescents' felt security and broaden-and-build processes. For this purpose, the program targets four parenting skills associated with attachment security during adolescence (see previous section). First, interveners assist parents' in attending to, understanding, validating, and caring for their offspring's needs (*caregiver sensitive responsiveness*). Second, the intervention cultivates parents' ability to take their teen's perspective and hold in mind his or her needs and feelings, while simultaneously reflecting on their own parental feelings and thoughts (*reflective function*, another name for *mentalization*). Third, therapeutic efforts are invested in strengthening parents' ability to constructively regulate the emotional tone of interactions with their teen, while assisting the teen in down-regulating distress during these interactions (*dyadic affect regulation*). Fourth, parents are encouraged to respect their offspring's emerging autonomy and to adopt mutually satisfying modes of communication and cooperative negotiation around autonomy-related goals (*shared partnership and mutuality*).

During the program, interveners support and encourage parents to step back from coercive, intrusive, or overcontrolling parenting strategies, down-regulate strong negative emotional reactions to their teen's behavior (e.g., anger, contempt), and reflect on how these reactions fuel distress, hostility, and detachment. In addition, interveners provide parents with alternative, more constructive parental attitudes and behaviors, such as empathizing with their teen's needs and feelings, reflecting on the attachment needs underlying the teen's behavior, and sensitively responding to challenging behavior while maintaining clear expectations and limits (i.e., not accepting every instance of destructive or aggressive behavior). According to Moretti et al. (2018),

> Connect promotes parental autonomy in understanding and responding to parent-teen problems by adopting a collaborative stance in which parents are supported as they develop skills to effectively identify and respond to problems that arise with their teen. This decreases parental sense of blame and increases their engagement in, and their sense of efficacy and ownership of, new learning. (p. 380)

The Connect program includes a preintervention assessment and a 10-week period in which groups of approximately eight to 14 parents meet on a weekly basis for 90 minutes with two certified, trained interveners. The preintervention assessment is designed to identify parental strengths and difficulties, increase parents' commitment to the program, and transmit a message of hope regarding their relationship with their teen. Each of the 10 sessions begins with a brief presentation of a key attachment theory principle related to parenting and the parent–adolescent relationship. This presentation is followed by a variety of experiential activities, including role plays and reflection exercises aimed at building the four targeted parenting skills.

Role plays of typical parent–adolescent conflictual interactions allow parents to be emotionally engaged with the depicted conflict. At the same time, they can remain calm and well regulated, because the role play is similar but not identical to what they are experiencing at home. This engaged but mindful state allows parents to calmly recognize and reflect on their own feelings and behavior, and to mentalize their teen's needs. Subsequent reflection exercises related to what happened in the role play assist parents in considering more constructive options for responding sensitively to their teen's needs and increasing the teen's safety and personal growth. These exercises follow a three-step process. First, interveners encourage parents to reflect on the feelings and behavior of the teen in the role play, and on the attachment needs that he or she is communicating during the conflict. Second, interveners ask parents to reflect on the feelings and thoughts of the parent in the role play, whether he or she was aware of the teen's attachment needs, and how the parent's behavior affected the course and outcome of the conversation. Third, parents are invited to consider alternative options for responding more constructively to the teen's behavior in the role play. Following these three steps, the group engages in a "reconstructed" version of the role play, which integrates parents' reflections, insights, and suggestions.

During the first three sessions, the parent–adolescent conflictual interaction is role-played by the two interveners, and the parents are invited to watch and reflect on the thoughts, feelings, and behavior of the two actors. From the fourth session forward, parents are invited to take the role of the adolescent in the "reconstructed" role play, which integrates parents' suggestions about more sensitive and constructive parental responses. "By stepping into the role of the teen, parents experience firsthand the powerful impact of parental sensitivity and support. Many parents are surprised by the experience, commenting, 'The way you responded changed how I felt' or 'I didn't understand how my teen might feel until now' " (Moretti et al., 2018, p. 382).

The Connect protocol includes three phases. The first phase (Sessions 1–3) is intended to build trust in the group and the interveners, help parents down-regulate their distress, and engage parents in structured reflection exercises. Session 1 deals with the principle that *all behavior has meaning* and parents learn through role plays and reflection exercises that adolescents' challenging behavior is an expression of their feelings (e.g., frustration, sadness) and core needs for safe-haven and secure-base forms of support. In Session 2, parents learn about how attachment needs are expressed differently during infancy, childhood, and adolescence (*attachment is for life*) and are encouraged to reflect on their own attachment needs, how they expressed these needs to their parents during adolescence, and how they were affected by their parents' responses. Session 3 focuses on the principle that *conflict is part of attachment* and parents are encouraged to reappraise conflicts as an opportunity for dealing with unresolved relational issues and strengthening relational closeness and satisfaction. Interveners also invite parents to reflect on how maintaining emotional composure during conflicts, respecting and empathizing with their teen's needs and feelings, and engaging in cooperative negotiation can transform a potentially harmful conflict into an empowering relational experience.

The second phase of the program (Sessions 4–6) is aimed at building the four targeted parenting skills. Session 4 is guided by the principle that *autonomy includes connection.* Interveners support and encourage parents to reflect on the importance of autonomy during adolescence, to recognize that their teen still needs them as a secure base for developing autonomy and personal identity, and to learn sensitive ways of providing support while respecting and not interfering with autonomy strivings. Session 5 is guided by the principle that *empathy is the heartbeat of attachment.* Parents reflect on and practice how to attend to and care for their teen's needs in an accepting, compassionate, and nonjudgmental manner. Session 6 deals with the principle of *balancing our needs with the needs of others,* and parents are encouraged to develop empathy and feel compassion for themselves. Interveners also help parents reflect on their own needs for a safe haven and secure base, and on the best ways to balance these needs with those of their teen.

The third and final phase of the program (Sessions 7–10) is aimed at consolidating the skills parents have already acquired and improving their ability to identify, understand, and sensitively respond to challenges posed by their teen's behavior. The key principle of Session 7 is that *growth and change are part of relationships.* Interveners encourage parents to understand that changes are inevitable in a parent–adolescent relationship and to reflect on how to flexibly adjust to these changes and sensitively respond to their growing teen's fluctuating needs.

Session 8 deals with the principle that *in celebrating attachment, attachment brings joy and pain.* Parents are encouraged to reflect on positive interactions with their teen and how these interactions promote mutual affection, joy, and relational satisfaction. Session 9 is organized by the principle *two steps forward, one step back* and focuses on relapse prevention. Interveners "weave all the principles together, integrating comments made by parents over the course of the therapy group and discussing the principles as a toolkit for weathering the inevitable storms that will occur as they move forward" (Moretti et al., 2018, p. 385). The last session (Session 10) is a feedback and integration session in which parents are encouraged to reflect on their experiences during the program and to share their feelings and thoughts with the group.

The effectiveness of the Connect program has been examined in six RCTs with parents of preadolescents and adolescents (see Table 5.1 for a summary of these studies' methods). These RCTs were conducted in Italy, Sweden (with Swedish and Somali-born parents), and Australia (with kinship caregivers of children who were in out-of-home care due to maltreatment). In these studies, the Connect program was compared to a no-intervention condition (waiting list) or a treatment-as-usual group (see Table 5.1). In only one study (Stattin et al., 2015) was Connect also compared to other psychoeducational parenting interventions (Comet; Community Parent Education Program [COPE]) that provide parents with specific practices aimed at reinforcing a teen's compliance with parental norms and expectations and managing the teen's misbehavior.

Five of the six RCTs assessed parents' self-reports of parental attitudes and behavior before and after the intervention, and the results were, unfortunately, weak and inconsistent. Four studies assessed parents' appraisals of their competence as parents (see Table 5.1), but only two of them found that Connect led to more positive changes in these appraisals than a waiting-list condition (Osman, Flacking, et al., 2017; Stattin et al., 2015). Three studies assessed parents' reports of negative reactions to their child's misbehavior (coldness/rejection, angry responding, aggression). One study found no significant effect of Connect on any of these reactions (Stattin et al., 2015); another study found that Connect (vs. waiting list) led to a greater reduction in parents' coldness/rejection (Giannotta et al., 2013); and the remaining study found a significant effect of Connect on decreased parental aggression after the intervention (Pasalich et al., 2021).

Of the two studies that assessed parents' positive reactions to their child's misbehavior, only one found that Connect was more effective than a waiting-list condition in increasing sensitive parenting (Stattin et al., 2015). However, this study also found that Connect was not more effective than other psychoeducational parenting interventions (Comet, COPE) in increasing parental sensitivity. More consistent findings were obtained in the four studies that assessed parents' reports of stress, depression, and mental health. In three of them, Connect led to more positive postintervention changes than waiting-list or treatment-as-usual conditions (Osman, Flacking, et al., 2017; Pasalich et al., 2021; Stattin et al., 2015).

TABLE 5.1. Summary of RCTs on the Connect Program

			Pre- and postintervention assessments	
Authors	Sample	Conditions	Parent	Adolescent
Giannotta et al. (2013)	147 Italian mothers of 11- to 14-year-old adolescents	Connect (10 weeks) vs. a waiting-list group	• Parental competence • Negative and positive reactions to children's misbehavior • Parental monitoring	• Parents' reports of behavioral problems • Self-reports of smoking and alcohol consumption
Stattin et al. (2015); Högström et al. (2017) (1- and 2-year follow-ups)	661 Swedish parents of 9- to 12-year-old adolescents	Connect (10 weeks) vs. Comet, COPE, and a waiting-list group	• Parental competence • Negative and positive reactions to children's misbehavior • Depression and stress	• Parents' reports of behavioral problems and symptoms of attention-deficit/hyperactivity disorder
Osman, Flacking, et al. (2017); Osman, Salari, et al. (2017)	120 Somali-born parents of 11- to 16-year-old adolescents	Connect (12 weeks) vs. a waiting-list group	• Parental competence • Mental health	• Parents' reports of behavioral problems
Ozturk et al. (2019)	44 Italian parents of 13- to 16-year-old adolescents	Connect (10 weeks) vs. a waiting-list group	• Parenting stress	• Parents' reports of emotional and behavioral problems
Barone, Carone, Costantino, et al. (2021)	100 Italian mothers of 12- to 18-year-old adolescents	Connect (10 weeks) vs. a waiting-list group	—	• Mothers' reports of reports of emotional and behavioral problems and anxious and avoidant attachment after the intervention and 4 months later
Pasalich et al. (2021)	26 Australian kinship caregivers of 8- to 12-year-old abused children	Connect (10 weeks) vs. a care-as-usual group	• Caregiver competence, strain, and aggression after the intervention and 6 months later	• Caregivers' reports of affect regulation, emotional and behavioral problems, and anxious and avoidant attachment after the intervention and 6 months later

With regard to adolescents' outcomes, two of the six RCTs collected data on teens' felt security before and after the intervention (see Table 5.1). However, the studies relied exclusively on parents' reports of their teen's attachment anxiety and avoidance rather than conducting attachment interviews with adolescents or asking them to complete self-report attachment scales. Moreover, the findings were weak and inconsistent. On the one hand, Barone, Carone, Constantino, et al. (2021) found that Connect (vs. a wait-list control) produced a greater reduction in mothers' reports of teens' attachment anxiety and avoidance, and it was maintained 4 months after the end of the intervention. On the other hand, Pasalich et al. (2021) found no significant difference between Connect and a treatment-as-usual condition in bringing about positive changes in teens' felt security immediately after the intervention or 6 months later. However, it's important to recall that adolescents in Pasalich et al.'s study were taken away from home due to maltreatment and cared for by a kinship caregiver, so their attachment injuries may well have been more severe than those of the low-risk teens sampled by Barone, Carone, Constantino, et al. (2021).

With regard to other adolescent outcomes, four of the six RCTs that assessed parents' reports of teens' behavioral problems found that Connect led to greater reductions in behavioral problems than a waiting-list condition (Barone, Carone, Constantino, et al., 2021; Osman, Salari, et al., 2017; Ozturk et al., 2019; Stattin et al., 2015). Importantly, Connect was also more effective than other psychoeducational parenting interventions (Comet, COPE) in reducing parents' reports of teens' behavioral problems one and two years after the intervention (Högström et al., 2017). Moreover, Connect (vs. waiting-list or treatment-as-usual conditions) led to greater reductions in teens' self-reported consumption of wine and beer (Giannotta et al., 2013) and yielded greater improvement in teens' affect regulation, at least as reported by parents (Pasalich et al., 2021). However, only one of the three RCTs that assessed parents' reports of teens' emotional problems found that Connect (vs. waiting list) was more effective in reducing mothers' reports of teens' emotional problems (Barone, Carone, Constantino, et al., 2021). Overall, the findings indicate that Connect is more effective in reducing teens' behavioral than emotional problems. However, we need more RCTs assessing adolescents' own reports and clinicians' ratings of these problems.

Findings from six studies that relied on a pre- and postassessment design, without a control condition, provided stronger and more consistent evidence concerning the effectiveness of the program (Moretti et al., 2004, 2012, 2015; Moretti & Obsuth, 2009; Obsuth et al., 2006; Osman et al., 2021). All six studies found that parents' reports of their teens' behavioral problems decreased after the Connect program, and five of them found a similar significant decrease in parents' reports of teens' emotional problems. Importantly, these positive changes were observed even 1 and 3 years after the intervention (Moretti & Obsuth, 2009; Osman et al., 2021). And Obsuth et al. (2006) found that teens themselves reported fewer emotional and behavioral problems after the program (relative to a preintervention assessment).

Two studies assessed parents' reports of teens' attachment insecurities, and both found a significant pre- to postintervention decrease in insecurities (Moretti et al., 2015; Obsuth et al., 2006). In addition, two studies that assessed parental attitudes and behaviors found significant pre- to postintervention effects on reports of parental competence and parental sensitivity (Moretti et al., 2012; Obsuth et al., 2006). Overall, then, participation in the Connect program does seem to be associated with positive changes in parenting and in teens' felt security and mental health. However, because none of the studies with a pre- to postassessment design included control groups, we can't be certain that the changes attributed to the intervention were not due to something other than the Connect program itself.

Interestingly, the studies with a pre- and postassessment design provide stronger support for Connect program's effectiveness than the six RCTs described in Table 5.1. However, whereas five of the six studies with a pre- and postassessment design were conducted with high-risk adolescents referred by authorities for severe behavioral problems, the sample of five of the six RCTs included only low-risk, normative adolescents. Therefore, we might speculate that Connect is a more effective intervention for parents of high-risk than low-risk adolescents. This possibility is consistent with research findings that prevention programs in general and the Connect program in particular are typically most effective for high-risk adolescents who show severe behavior problems before the intervention (Conduct Problems Prevention Research Group, 2011; Pasalich et al., 2022). This may be the case because they have a greater magnitude of problems on which to improve. However, we should regard this possibility with caution until more RCTs are conducted with samples of high-risk teens.

The hypothesized mechanisms of change underlying the effects of the Connect program on adolescents' mental health (increased parental sensitivity and teens' felt security) have been examined in two studies. In one study, Moretti et al. (2012) found that positive shifts in parental competence and sensitivity after Connect were associated with pre- to postintervention reductions in adolescents' emotional and behavioral problems. In a later study, Moretti et al. (2015) linked this improvement in adolescents' mental health to the enhancement of their sense of attachment security (at least as reported by parents) after Connect. Specifically, pre- to postintervention reductions in attachment-related avoidance were associated with decreases in behavioral problems, whereas reductions in attachment anxiety were associated with decreases in emotional problems. Overall, these studies are encouraging initial steps in supporting a model of change by which Connect might reduce adolescents' emotional and behavioral problems by improving parental sensitive responsiveness to teens' needs, which is key for enhancing their felt security.

Taken as a whole, the reviewed RCTs fail to provide strong and consistent evidence supporting the hypothesized effects of the Connect program on parents' sensitive responsiveness and adolescents' felt security and mental health. However, we should remember that these RCTs were conducted mostly with low-risk adolescents. And all of them relied on parents' reports of their beliefs and attitudes rather than on observations of parents' sensitive responsiveness during actual interactions with their teen, or on interview-based measures of parents' reflective functioning (mentalization). In addition, researchers have assessed parents' reports of teens' felt security and mental health rather than assessing adolescents' own reports of felt security and mental health, or clinicians' ratings of teens' emotional and behavioral problems.

Future RCTs should test the effectiveness of this promising attachment-based program by sampling high-risk adolescents, assessing specific changes in the four targeted parenting skills (with behavioral observations and interview measures), and relying on teens' own reports (or clinical interviews) of their felt security and mental health. These RCTs should also examine the short- and long-term effectiveness of Connect relative to other, alternative parenting programs while studying which practices (e.g., role plays, reflection exercises) and attachment principles (guiding each of the sessions) contribute most to therapeutic outcomes. In particular, it would be worthwhile to compare the effectiveness of the Connect program with other attachment-based interventions that work with both parents and adolescents (e.g., ABFT; see next section). In fact, there is evidence that interventions designed to improve relational feelings and behaviors of both parents and children tend to be more effective than those that work with parents alone (Cook et al., 2007).

Attachment-Based Family Therapy

ABFT (G. S. Diamond et al., 2003, 2014, 2021) is a manualized family therapy for at-risk adolescents and their parents. It includes individual sessions with adolescents, individual sessions with parents, and joint sessions with both parents and adolescents. ABFT is designed to enhance adolescents' felt security with respect to parents by facilitating comforting and empowering parent–adolescent interactions.

For this purpose, the therapist first helps both adolescents and parents to reframe the adolescents' problems (e.g., suicidal ideation) as relational rather than solely personal issues (*relational reframe*) and to constructively process painful emotions typically experienced during interactions (*emotional processing*). The therapist then supports and coaches (1) adolescents to openly share their feelings with parents and (2) parents to attend to and empathize with their teen's feelings in a calm, nondefensive, and reassuring fashion. The therapist also encourages family members to engage in cooperative negotiation around autonomy-related issues while trying to understand each other's needs and integrate them in a mutually satisfactory solution. In this way, ABFT is an attempt to provide *corrective attachment experiences,* which might increase a teen's reliance on parents as safe havens and secure bases, and move the teen toward greater felt security and healthier development.

ABFT is implemented in weekly hour-long sessions conducted over a period of approximately 12–16 weeks (but G. M. Diamond et al., 2022, extended ABFT to 6 months). It includes five distinct therapeutic tasks: (1) relational frame, (2) adolescent alliance, (3) parent alliance, (4) repairing attachment, and (5) promoting autonomy. Whereas the first task typically involves only one session, each of the other tasks require between two and eight sessions. Each task includes a distinct set of procedures, processes, and goals, but all of them involve conversations about the parent–adolescent relationship and the typical wishes, thoughts, feelings, and behaviors that conflictual interactions arouse in each family member.

The first, fourth, and fifth tasks are carried out in joint sessions with adolescents and their parents. The second task (individual sessions with adolescents) and third task (individual sessions with parents) are necessary preparatory stages for encouraging comfortable and empowering parent–adolescent interactions during the fourth and fifth tasks. Therefore, the therapist does not move to the fourth task until he or she is confident that both parents and teens are well prepared to engage in mutually satisfying conversations. The five tasks serve as a road map guiding therapists' efforts to strengthen parental sensitivity, provide corrective attachment experiences, and increase teens' confidence that parents' support will be available when needed.

In the first task (*relational reframe*), the therapist attempts to create a strong therapeutic alliance with both adolescents and parents around the goal of improving the quality of their relationship. Parents may come to therapy with the belief that their offspring's problem is an individual issue (e.g., "Can you help him with his depression?"). During the first session, the therapist works to reframe the problem as relational: He or she elicits information from the adolescent and the parent or parents about how conflictual interactions between them might have contributed to the current impasse or crisis, while showing them how mutually comfortable interactions can help to resolve the crisis.

According to G. S. Diamond et al. (2021), "The therapist focuses on resuscitating the adolescent's desire for protection and support and the caregivers' longing to provide love and protection to their child. The therapist promotes the caregivers as the medicine (not the problem) to help adolescents cope with and recover from depression and suicide risk"

(p. 288). This reframing of the therapy's goals in relational terms is a necessary precondition for guaranteeing family members' compliance and engagement with the next four therapeutic tasks.

In the second task (*adolescent alliance*), the therapist works individually with adolescents with the aim of increasing their mentalization and mindful processing of painful attachment injuries (e.g., experiences of parental rejection, neglect, abuse, criticism, or overcontrol). The therapist supports and encourages adolescents to access painful memories of frustrating and painful interactions with parents and to connect to, calmly reflect on, and regulate vulnerability-related emotions (e.g., despair, sadness, fear) aroused by these interactions. The therapist also helps adolescents to mentalize (reflect on and articulate) their own needs for comfort and support and to think about parents' intentions and difficulties during these interactions. The therapist also prepares adolescents to discuss these hurtful attachment injuries with parents (in the fourth task) and to share their feelings and reflections in a well-regulated and constructive manner.

During the second task, adolescents learn to identify, articulate, and regulate painful feelings without being overwhelmed by them or engaging in interaction patterns that prevent parents from responding in a sensitive and constructive manner. Specifically, the therapist encourages adolescents to deal with their own concerns and distress without necessarily accusing parents and demanding reparation in a hostile and dysregulated manner (in the case of attachment-anxious adolescents) or emotionally and behaviorally withdrawing from parents (in the case of attachment-avoidant adolescents). Instead, the therapist coaches adolescents to share their painful feelings with parents in a way that allows parents to be engaged and responsive rather than defensive and hostile. According to G. S. Diamond et al. (2021), "These feelings may or may not fuel the depression, but, certainly, expressing them and feeling heard and supported can alleviate the depression and make adolescents feel less alone in their pain" (p. 288).

In the third task (*parent alliance*), the therapist works individually with parents to cultivate curiosity and engagement with their child's experiences, the adoption of a more understanding and validating (less defensive and critical) parental stance, and respect and support of their teen's autonomy strivings. Parents are encouraged to think about (mentalize) and reach a more accurate understanding of the ways in which their own attachment injuries may have eroded the affection and love they once felt for their child and how these injuries may fuel relationship distress and conflictual interactions. Parents are encouraged to develop greater empathy and compassion for themselves and their teen, and to reappraise their teen in a kinder, more favorable way rather than blaming him or her for the current crisis, perceiving him or her as difficult or burdensome, or defensively detaching from the teen. Ideally, they become more motivated to repair past parenting failures and to try new approaches for interacting with their child in a more responsive and constructive manner. These transformations provide the basis for moving to the fourth task: asking parents to implement their new sensitive responsiveness during actual conversations with their child.

In the fourth task (*attachment repair*), the therapist attempts to shape and facilitate *corrective attachment experiences* during in-session parent–adolescent conversations about attachment injuries that have damaged the quality of their relationship. The therapist helps and coaches adolescents to talk openly and calmly about attachment injuries, to express their needs for comfort and support, and to feel safe enough to ask parents to try to meet these needs. At the same time, parents are encouraged to attend and listen to their teen's disclosure in a calm, accepting, responsive, and supportive manner, even if they find inaccuracies in the discourse. In this way, adolescents realize that they can openly express their needs and feelings, and that they are understood, validated, and cared for by parents. They may then reduce their defensiveness and hostility, and recognize their own contribution to possible collaborative, comforting, and empowering conversations with parents. Through repeated conversations like this during the fourth-task sessions, adolescents come to feel more secure with respect to parents, and parents to feel closer to their child and more capable of accomplishing the role of security provider.

G. S. Diamond et al. (2021, p. 288) eloquently described the crucial role that these corrective attachment experiences play in reviving and revitalizing a mutually satisfying parent–adolescent relationship and renewing adolescents' felt security toward parents:

> Engineering these attachment-promoting conversations experientially (e.g., exposure) challenges the views and expectations of self and others ("Oh, maybe my parents can listen to me"). When adolescents are more direct, honest, and regulated, it revises caregivers' view of them as autonomous people needing respect, love, and support. . . . Learning to express these more vulnerable feelings directly frees adolescents from the constrained and guarded insecure attachment strategies they have developed to protect themselves. When adolescents express vulnerability in family sessions, it activates caregiving instincts. As parents connect to their worry or fear, as opposed to their frustration and anger, they respond in a softer, more caring, and attuned manner. The therapist might say to an angry father, "Dad, I know you are angry for all the trouble Johnny is causing, but I imagine that you must have been scared when you took him to the hospital. Did you worry he was going to die?" Accessing these primary, vulnerable, adaptive emotions provides adolescents and parents with better information about their needs and activates healthier, more effective, interpersonal exchanges: the father stops shaming the son for his depression and begins to provide more support.

After restoring adolescents' confidence in parents' responsiveness, therapists move to the fifth and final ABFT task (*promoting autonomy*), which involves in-session parent–adolescent conversations about other areas of life (e.g., school, friendships, dating). During these conversations, the therapist encourages adolescents to use parents as a secure base for dealing with practical issues and making autonomous decisions. Parents are encouraged to attend, empathize, and respect their offspring's strivings, and to be responsive and supportive without threatening or interfering with his or her emerging autonomy. Over time and through repeated conversations, adolescents become more confident in using their parents as effective secure bases and learn to consider their guidance and advice when making decisions about school, social life, or identity-related issues. At the same time, parents practice and improve their sensitive attunement to their teen's feelings and needs, and learn how to offer a secure base for his or her healthy development.

The effectiveness of ABFT has been examined in seven published RCTs (see Table 5.2 for a summary of these studies' methods). Samples included adolescents with symptoms of depression or anxiety, suicidal ideation, or unresolved anger toward parents (see Table 5.2). In all of these studies, biological parents underwent the intervention together with their offspring. The effectiveness of ABFT was compared to waiting-list or treatment-as-usual conditions, or well-known therapies for treating depression (cognitive-behavioral therapy, family-enhanced nondirective supportive therapy) or dysregulated emotions (individual emotion-focused therapy).

Unfortunately, none of the seven published RCTs examined the contribution of ABFT to parents' sensitive responsiveness or their provision of safe-haven or secure-base forms of support (see Table 5.2). In three RCTs, data were collected on adolescents' reports of family conflict and functioning (see Table 5.2): Adolescents who underwent ABFT reported lower levels of family conflict and better family functioning after treatment than those who were

TABLE 5.2. Summary of RCTs on ABFT

			Pre- and postintervention assessments	
Authors	Sample	Conditions	Parent	Adolescent
G. S. Diamond et al. (2002)	32 depressed adolescents	ABFT (12 weeks) vs. a 6-week waiting-list group	—	• Self-reports and clinician ratings of depression • Self-reports of family conflict and cohesion, emotional closeness to parents, and hopelessness
Siqueland et al. (2005)	11 anxious adolescents	ABFT (16 weeks) vs. cognitive-behavioral therapy (16 weeks)	—	• Self-reports and clinician ratings of anxiety and depression • Self-reports of family functioning
G. S. Diamond et al. (2010, 2012)	66 depressed adolescents with suicidal ideation	ABFT (M = 10 sessions) vs. enhanced usual care (M = 3 sessions)	—	• Self-reports and clinician ratings of suicidal ideation • Self-reports of depression
Israel & Diamond (2013)	20 depressed adolescents	ABFT (12 weeks) vs. a treatment-as-usual during 12 weeks	—	• Self-reports and clinical ratings of depression
G. M. Diamond et al. (2016)	32 adolescents with unresolved anger	ABFT (10 weeks) vs. individual emotion-focused therapy (10 weeks)	—	• Self-reports of anger, attachment anxiety and avoidance, and psychological symptoms
G. S. Diamond et al. (2019); Zisk et al. (2019)	129 depressed adolescents with suicidal ideation	ABFT (16 weeks) vs. family-enhanced nondirective supportive therapy (16 weeks)	—	• Self-reports of depression and suicidal ideation • Self-reports of family conflict and cohesion
Rognli et al. (2020); Waraan et al. (2021)	60 depressed adolescents	ABFT (16 weeks) vs. treatment as usual (16 weeks)	—	• Self-reports and clinician ratings of depression

in a waiting-list condition or underwent other kinds of therapy. However, these findings are far from strongly supporting the effectiveness of ABFT in bringing about positive changes in parental sensitivity.

As can be seen in Table 5.2, pre- and postintervention assessments have focused mainly on adolescent's mental health, which is obviously an important outcome variable. In the seven RCTs, adolescents who underwent ABFT reported a significant pre- to posttherapy improvement in mental health (e.g., less intense symptoms of anxiety or depression; less frequent suicidal thoughts; better regulation of anger toward parents). These positive changes in mental health were stronger than those observed in waiting-list or treatment-as-usual conditions (but see Waraan et al., 2021, for an exception), and they were most notable among adolescents who engaged in less cooperative communication and more conflicts with parents at the beginning of therapy (Rognli et al., 2020; Zisk et al., 2019). No difference was observed, however, between ABFT and other kinds of therapy (cognitive-behavioral therapy, family-enhanced nondirective supportive therapy, individual emotion-focused therapy). Overall, ABFT seems to be an effective treatment for improving mental health among at-risk adolescents involved in destructive relational patterns with parents, although it seems not to be more effective than other kinds of individual and family therapy.

The impact of ABFT on adolescents' felt security with respect to parents has been tested in only one RCT. G. M. Diamond et al (2016) found that adolescents with unresolved anger toward parents showed a significant decrease in self-reports of attachment anxiety and avoidance after ABFT (as compared to a preintervention assessment). Importantly, control adolescents who underwent individual emotion-focused therapy also showed a significant pre- to postintervention decrease in self-reports of attachment anxiety but failed to show any change in avoidant attachment. In other words, whereas the two kinds of therapy reduced adolescents' anxious attachment, only ABFT was effective in reducing attachment-related avoidance. It is important to note, however, that G. M. Diamond et al. implemented ABFT only among 16 adolescents who suffered from unresolved anger toward parents. So their finding can't be taken as strong support for the effects of ABFT on security enhancement. We need more RCTs with larger and more representative samples of at-risk adolescents.

Beyond these RCTs, four studies used a pre- and postintervention design without a control condition in samples of suicidal lesbian, gay, and bisexual adolescents, as well as sexual/gender minority adolescents (G. M. Diamond et al., 2012, 2019, 2022; Russon et al., 2022). As compared to a preintervention assessment, adolescents who underwent ABFT reported improved mental health (lower levels of depression and suicidal ideation) immediately at the end of therapy and 2 months later. Moreover, adolescents who underwent ABFT reported significant increases in feelings of parental acceptance after therapy, and their parents also showed a parallel increase in the extent to which they accepted their offspring's sexual identity. This finding is the single, direct indication that ABFT is associated with increased parental acceptance. Hence, more research is needed to substantiate the claim that ABFT makes parents more sensitive and responsive to their adolescents' needs and feelings.

Two of these studies (G. M. Diamond et al., 2012, 2022) included pre- and postintervention assessments of adolescents' self-reports of attachment anxiety and avoidance with respect to parents. These studies documented significant decreases in adolescents' attachment-related avoidance immediately at the end of therapy and 2–3 months later. However, whereas G. M. Diamond et al. (2012) found a similar decrease in reports of attachment anxiety, G. M. Diamond et al. (2022) did not find a significant change. Together, these studies suggest that ABFT is associated with increased felt security on the part of lesbian, gay, bisexual, transgender, queer, or sometimes questioning), and others (LGBTQ+) adolescents with respect to their parents.

Although the reviewed RCTs and pre- and postintervention studies haven't directly tested the effects of ABFT on parental behavior, process-oriented studies examining the mechanisms through which ABFT works provide initial evidence regarding the changes that parents experience over the course of therapy. For example, G. S. Diamond et al. (2003) interviewed parents who underwent ABFT. Their qualitative analyses of parents' retrospective accounts revealed that their adolescents' in-session expressions of vulnerability and pain, as expected, softened parents' defensive and hostile attitudes and motivated them to commit to relationship repair. This positive parental change was also found in a study of ABFT therapists' relational reframe interventions (Moran et al., 2005). Microanalyses of five early therapy sessions with parents of depressed adolescents revealed that after therapists addressed the depression in terms of disruptions in the parent–adolescent relationship (*relational reframe*), parents were more likely to talk openly and constructively about relational problems in at least two of their six immediately subsequent speech turns.

Subsequent studies have provided additional evidence concerning parents' in-session changes in sensitive responsiveness over the course of ABFT. For example, an analysis of 13 sessions with parents revealed that after a therapist's expression of positive regard or an attachment-oriented intervention (e.g., addressing parents' insecurities), parents were less likely to express negative attitudes about their child (Moran & Diamond, 2008). Also, parents who formed a stronger alliance with a therapist during individual sessions (the third task) were more empathic and less defensive during joint attachment-repair sessions with their child (the fourth task) and were more likely to encourage the adolescent to share painful feelings (Feder & Diamond, 2016).

In another study of 18 suicidal adolescents, Shpigel et al. (2012) found that mothers' in-session autonomy (secure-base) support (as rated by observers) increased across the first four ABFT sessions. Moreover, increases in mothers' provision of autonomy support over the ABFT sessions was associated with decreases in adolescents' self-reports of attachment anxiety and avoidance over the course of therapy, which in turn contributed to reduced depression at discharge. As a whole, these findings are in line with the core premise of attachment-based interventions: ABFT can bring about positive changes in parental sensitivity, which in turn contributes to adolescents' felt security and mental health.

Process-oriented studies have examined the role that emotional processing plays in ABFT. Two studies have found that therapists' relational reframes and focus on vulnerability-related emotions (e.g., sadness, helplessness) in a given session are associated with adolescents' engagement in productive processing of these emotions in subsequent portions of the session (Tsvieli & Diamond, 2018; Tsvieli et al., 2020). There is also evidence that adolescents' engagement in this kind of emotional processing is associated with better psychological outcomes at the end of therapy (G. M. Diamond et al., 2016; Lifshitz et al., 2021).

There is also evidence that the occurrence of corrective attachment experiences during joint parent–adolescent sessions contributes to ABFT effectiveness (Tsvieli et al., 2022). Specifically, as compared to cases with poor outcomes, adolescents who showed posttherapy mental health improvement were more likely to experience corrective attachment experiences during the fourth task (attachment repair). These experiences are initiated by the therapist's focus on the adolescent's unmet attachment needs, followed by the adolescent's constructive sharing of his or her painful feelings, and followed by parents' expression of warmth and willingness to meet their offspring's attachment needs. This sequence of adolescents' proximity seeking and parents' responsiveness might lead adolescents to feel more secure, with resulting mental health benefits.

Overall, an impressive body of research attests to the promise of ABFT, but as research evaluators, we still cannot draw firm conclusions about its effectiveness in bringing about the desired changes in both parents and teens. First, although process-oriented studies have shown that parents' attitudes and responses change within ABFT sessions, we need further RCTs examining the effects of ABFT on parents' sensitive responsiveness after therapy. Second, the reviewed RCTs and pre- and postintervention studies provide compelling evidence regarding the positive effects of ABFT on adolescents' mental health, but evidence on pre- to postintervention enhancement of adolescents' felt security is scarce. Future RCTs should focus on adolescents' felt security and provide evidence concerning the expected posttherapy increases in adolescents' reliance on parents as safe havens and secure bases. We also need more data on the extent to which ABFT strengthens adolescents' positive feelings toward parents and fosters the adoption of a collaborative stance and pro-relational strategies of conflict resolution. Of course, these are high standards—easy for basic researchers like us to recommend—for what is clearly already an ambitious research and intervention program.

Concluding Remarks

In this chapter, we have focused on interventions based on attachment theory that have been developed to increase teens' secure attachment to parents and support teens' healthy development. The two interventions we reviewed (Connect and ABFT) are well grounded in attachment theory and research, and involve carefully developed and standardized protocols and techniques for strengthening parents' sensitive responsiveness and facilitating the formation of a secure parent–teen relationship. Research findings concerning the effectiveness of these interventions are promising, but we still lack systematic information on the extent to which the interventions positively affect the entire cycle of security enhancement in the relationship between parents and teen.

In addition, we think that attachment-informed clinicians and practitioners working with adolescents and their parents should devote more attention to two important issues that both the Connect program and ABFT seem to slight. First, as explained in the first section of this chapter, adolescents gradually transfer their search for a safe haven and a secure base to close friends and romantic partners. Moreover, the quality of their friendships and romantic relationships tend to have stronger long-term psychological effects than the quality of their relationship with parents (Allen et al., 2022). Therefore, every intervention aimed at increasing adolescents' sense of attachment security and facilitating healthy development should target not only their relationships with parents but also their needs, feelings, thoughts, and behavior in interactions and relationships with friends and romantic partners. As we show in Chapter 9, the Connection program (Allen et al., 2021) deals to some extent with this limitation by focusing on adolescents' peer relationships, but without addressing attachment injuries and insecurities experienced in conflictual parent–teen relationships.

Second, neither the Connect program nor ABFT take into consideration that adolescents, unlike young children, have developed substantial working models of self and others and have a dominant attachment orientation that may bias their reactions to a therapist's or intervener's comments and interventions (Zilberstein, 2014). The interventions so far do not customize therapeutic tasks and techniques according to the relative dominance of teens' anxious or avoidant patterns of relating. We suspect that this kind of customization is important for anticipating treatment obstacles, identifying useful targets for therapeutic change, and providing the most effective intervention for handling teens' relational worries and defenses and softening their destructive consequences (McBride et al., 2006). This is a demanding but promising challenge for improving the effectiveness of both the Connect program and ABFT.

Despite these limitations and challenges, we remain hopeful and confident that applications of attachment theory and research can contribute immensely to improving teens' relationships with parents and peers, treating their behavioral and emotional problems, and sustaining their healthy development. In fact, both the Connect program and ABFT have successfully implemented the defining principle of attachment-based interventions (enhancement of an attachment figure's provision of a safe haven and secure base as a means of increasing a person's felt security and promoting broaden-and-build processes). And although empirical questions remain with respect to their effectiveness, the two reviewed interventions are promising methods of enhancing adolescents' mental health and interpersonal functioning. They reflect an incredible amount of difficult and illuminating clinical research.

CHAPTER 6

Enhancing Attachment Security within Couple Relationships

In his 1979 volume, *The Making and Breaking of Affectional Bonds*, Bowlby wrote that romantic relationships and marriages are among an adult's most important attachment relationships and that a romantic or marital partner is often an adult's primary attachment figure. Following Bowlby's lead, Shaver et al. (1988) proposed that sustained romantic love in adulthood involves an emotional attachment that is conceptually similar to an infant's emotional bond with a primary caregiver, often a parent.

For example, love in both infancy and adulthood includes a desire to be comforted by one's relationship partner when distressed; the experience of anger, anxiety, and sorrow following separation or loss; and the experience of happiness and joy upon reunion. Moreover, formation of a secure relationship with either a primary caregiver during childhood or a mate during adulthood depends on the caregiver/mates' responsiveness to one's bids for proximity, and this responsiveness causes the attached person to feel safer, more confident, happier, more outgoing, and kinder to others. Furthermore, in both kinds of relationships, when the partner is not responsive to one's bids for proximity and care, one can become anxious and hypersensitive to signs of (or the absence of) love, approval, or rejection, or can defensively distance from the partner to avoid the pain of repeated frustration. These kinds of parallels led Shaver et al. (1988) to conclude that infants' bonds with parents and romantic partners' bonds with partners in adulthood are variants of a single underlying process.

Today, more than 30 years after Shaver et al.'s extension of Bowlby's theory, there is ample evidence that couple relationships can be fruitfully viewed as attachments, that mates often function as a safe haven and secure base for one another, and that a person's sense of attachment security can be enhanced within the context of a pair-bond relationship (*pair bonding* being the biological term for stable mating).

This growing body of evidence for adult attachment to a mate led Susan Johnson (2004, 2008) to apply attachment theory in the domains of couple therapy and couple relationship education. She and her colleagues have developed attachment-based interventions designed to enhance partners' attachment security (hence fostering couple stability and satisfaction). In this chapter, we consider such attachment-based interventions, explain their basis in research, describe their key features, and review evidence regarding their effectiveness. We also offer suggestions for strengthening the application of attachment theory to repairing and strengthening couple relationships.

Security-Enhancement Processes in Couple Relationships

In this section, we present the empirical basis for applying attachment theory to couple relationships. We first review evidence that romantic partners or spouses can provide a safe haven and secure base for each another, thereby facilitating the construction and maintenance of a secure emotional bond. We also review evidence that partners' attachment insecurities can interfere with the formation of a secure emotional bond within a couple. We then summarize theoretical ideas and empirical data concerning the attitudes and behaviors of one romantic partner that enhance the other partner's felt security and can move even attachment-insecure partners toward greater security. For couple counselors and educators, these research findings provide a road map for attachment-based interventions.

To wit, if one wishes to enhance a person's felt security and foster the associated broaden-and-build cycle of attachment security within a couple, one should (1) increase the exchange and flow of safe-haven and secure-base provisions during couple interactions; (2) address partners' attachment insecurities, which can interfere with security enhancement and reduce the effectiveness of attachment-based interventions; and (3) cultivate couple members' security-enhancing attitudes and behaviors.

Romantic Partners and Spouses as Sources of Security

In considering whether couple relationships can be sensibly viewed as attachments, adult attachment researchers have dealt with two main questions. First, are romantic partners or spouses nominated, when asked, as principal sources of security in adulthood? Second, are they capable of alleviating each other's distress (safe-haven support) and empowering each other's exploration and autonomous pursuit of personal goals (secure-base support)? With regard to the first question, we have already shown in Chapter 5 that adolescents and young adults typically choose romantic partners as their principal security providers (Hazan & Zeifman, 1994). This finding has been replicated in a sample of married midlife adults and a broad sample of 812 adults ranging in age from 16 to 90 (Doherty & Feeney, 2004; Schachner et al., 2008). Therefore, we focus here on the second question and consider studies dealing with the safe-haven and secure-base functions of romantic partners and spouses.

The Safe-Haven Function of Romantic Partners and Spouses

Because adults regard their romantic partner/spouse as a principal source of security, they typically seek proximity to this person in times of need and rely on his or her responsiveness and support for alleviating distress. In a naturalistic study conducted in the departure lounges of a large airport, Fraley and Shaver (1998) found that couples who were about to separate from each other (because one partner was flying to another city) were more likely to seek and maintain physical contact (e.g., by mutually gazing at each other's faces, holding hands) than did couples who were about to fly somewhere together. Conceptually similar findings were reported by Collins and Feeney (2000) based on a laboratory observational study of support-seeking behaviors during a couple interaction in which one partner disclosed a personal concern to the other. Participants who evaluated the problem as more serious and distressing were more likely to seek emotional support from their partner during the conversation (as rated by trained coders). Seeking proximity to a romantic partner in times of need was also documented in Campa et al.'s (2009) 28-day diary study of dating couples: During days on which participants reported more stressful events, they also reported seeking more instrumental and emotional support from their partners.

More important, when these desires and expectations for attention and care in times of need are effectively met by responsive and supportive gestures and responses of a romantic partner or spouse, a person's distress is likely to be alleviated, and he or she feels safer and more relaxed. In two observational studies of dating couples who were video-recorded while one partner shared a personal problem with the other, study participants whose romantic partner provided more responsive support or more affectionate touch during the interaction (as judged by independent coders) felt calmer and more competent after sharing their personal concern (Collins & Feeney, 2000; Jakubiak & Feeney, 2019). Similarly, women who were waiting to take a challenging math test were more calmed and relaxed when their romantic partner made more supportive remarks (Simpson et al., 1992). In another observational study of dating couples who were video-recorded while trying to resolve a relationship problem, participants were rated by external observers as calmer during peak distress points in the discussion if their partner was coded as more supportive (Simpson, Winterheld, et al., 2007).

Beyond these correlational studies, experimental manipulations of a romantic partner's responsiveness and support have been found to calm study participants who were facing a stressful experience (see Mikulincer & Shaver, 2023, for a review). For example, Coan et al. (2006) examined brain responses (using fMRI) of married women who received a threat of electric shock while they were holding their husband's hand, holding the hand of an otherwise unfamiliar male experimenter, or holding no hand at all. Spousal hand-holding, as compared to the other conditions, reduced activation in brain regions associated with stress and distress (right anterior insula, superior frontal gyrus, and hypothalamus). Coan et al. (2013) reanalyzed the original Coan et al. (2006) data set and found that the soothing effects of spousal hand-holding were particularly strong when each spouse showed interest in the feelings, thoughts, and aspirations of the other. This finding implies that a partner's responsiveness is a key ingredient of the safe-haven effect created by spousal hand-holding.

The Secure-Base Function of Romantic Partners and Spouses

Are romantic partners and spouses capable of providing each other with a secure base for exploration and thriving (maintaining a broaden-and-build cycle)? Findings from several studies provide an affirmative answer to this question. For example, B. Feeney (2004) video-recorded dating couples during discussions of each partner's personal goals and found that participants were more likely to discuss personal goals openly and explore alternative ways to achieve these goals when their partner was coded by independent observers as more supportive. Similarly, B. Feeney et al. (2017) videotaped married couples while each spouse was presented with a challenging opportunity and found that decision makers were more likely to embrace the opportunity when their spouse accepted and validated their goal strivings (as coded by independent judges). In diary studies, spousal acceptance and validation of participants' goal strivings on a given day fostered same-day and next-day progress in goal pursuit (Jakubiak & Feeney, 2016). Longitudinal studies also indicate that individuals whose romantic partner is more responsive and supportive (as reported by the partners or coded by external judges) report increased autonomous exploration and feelings of mastery and accomplishment over time (e.g., B. Feeney, 2007; Tomlinson et al., 2016, 2020).

Overall, these and similar findings indicate that romantic partners and spouses can serve as not only a safe haven but also a secure base for each other. The research also indicates that a partner's mere presence is not sufficient to optimally reduce distress or promote exploration and goal pursuit. Rather, partners' *responsiveness* seems to be the key ingredient underlying the experience of a couple relationship as a safe haven and secure base. This finding parallels what is known about the key ingredient in parental provision of a safe haven and secure base for infants and children (see Chapter 4).

The Interfering Effects of Attachment Insecurities

Although the research we've just reviewed highlights the potential for responsive and caring romantic partners/spouses to serve as a safe haven and secure base for each other, we should bear in mind that the accomplishment of these attachment functions can be disrupted by the attachment insecurities that some partners bring into their relationships. These insecurities can discourage engagement in couple interactions that involve support seeking or support provision, or can distort the perception of a partner's responsiveness and supportiveness.

Difficulties with Proximity Seeking and Intimacy

People suffering from attachment insecurities of either the anxious or the avoidant variety often have difficulty relying on a romantic partner or spouse in times of need or being open to engaging in intimacy-promoting activities. Throughout their history of frustrating, disappointing, or painful interactions with cold and rejecting or unreliably supportive attachment figures, insecure adults may have long ago learned that proximity seeking and reliance on others can be dangerous and painful. As a result, they are worried and apprehensive when considering the possibility of seeking proximity to a romantic partner. However, people with different attachment histories, and resulting attachment orientations, differ in how they cope with these concerns. Those who score high on attachment-related avoidance, who typically try to deactivate attachment needs and behaviors, tend to maintain distance from a partner even when distressed. In contrast, attachment-anxious people, who typically tend to hyperactivate attachment needs and worries, may engage in intrusive, ambivalent, tense, or other ineffective forms of proximity seeking that often irritate, overwhelm, or alienate their partner. Both kinds of responses can lead insecure people to miss opportunities to learn about their partner's responsiveness and to savor the joy of being loved and supported, thus decreasing the possibility of security enhancement within a couple relationship.

Observational studies of seeking support from romantic partners reveal the interfering effect of attachment-related avoidance. For example, Simpson et al. (1992) told female members of heterosexual dating couples that they were about to endure a stressful task after waiting with their partner for 5 minutes. During this period, the couple's behavior was unobtrusively video-recorded and later coded regarding the extent to which each participant sought the other's support. Women who scored relatively high on attachment-related avoidance were rated as seeking less support from their partner mainly when their level of distress was high. In such cases, avoidant women often attempted to distract themselves by reading magazines (provided in the waiting area) instead of asking for support.

Further evidence for avoidance-related inhibition of proximity seeking can be found in Fraley and Shaver's (1998) unobtrusive assessment of proximity-seeking behaviors when romantic or marital partners were about to separate from each other at a large airport, and in Collins and Feeney's (2000) coding of support-seeking behavior while members of dating couples talked about a personal problem in the laboratory. In both studies, attachment-related avoidance was associated with less frequent seeking of proximity or support. In addition, although attachment anxiety did not affect direct requests for partner support, Collins and Feeney found that more attachment-anxious people were more likely to ask for help through nonverbal distress signals (crying, pouting, or sulking).

Additional evidence can be found in studies assessing self-reports of couple intimacy (see Table 10.2 in Mikulincer & Shaver, 2016, for a summary of these studies). Across numerous cross-sectional and prospective longitudinal studies, both attachment anxiety and avoidance are associated with lower levels of intimacy in couple relationships. Attachment insecurities have also been found to be related to less desire for affectionate touch (e.g., Jakubiak et al., 2021) and lower levels of synchrony in emotional experiences between romantic partners (e.g., Randall & Butler, 2013). It seems that attachment insecurities interfere with emotional closeness within couples and prevent partners from comfortably expressing and sharing emotions.

There is also evidence concerning attachment-anxious individuals' tendency to engage in intrusive behaviors during couple interactions. In a 14-day diary study, Lavy et al. (2013) found that more attachment-anxious people were more likely to engage in daily intrusive behaviors. Moreover, attachment-anxious people reported more intrusive behavior mainly when they had been dissatisfied with their relationship the previous day, implying that intrusiveness may be part of their effort to restore closeness. Like other anxious behaviors, however, these efforts to restore closeness can backfire if they cause a partner to feel imposed or intruded upon.

Difficulties in Perceiving a Partner's Responsiveness

Insecure attachment working models, like other kinds of cognitive–affective mental schemas, can distort appraisals of a partner's responsiveness, leading attachment-insecure people to ignore, dismiss, or forget positive instances of partner responsiveness (Mikulincer & Shaver, 2023). As a result, insecure individuals can be less likely to benefit from positive partner attitudes and behaviors that could potentially calm them and provide a secure base for exploration and thriving. Indeed, dozens of cross-sectional and prospective longitudinal studies confirm that insecure couple members report receiving less support from their partners and feeling less satisfied with the support they receive (see Mikulincer & Shaver, 2016, Table 6.4, for a summary of these studies).

In an effort to assess the cognitive biases associated with attachment insecurities, Collins and Feeney (2004, Study 1) informed one member of each of a group of dating couples that he or she would perform a stressful task (give a video-recorded speech), manipulated his or her partner's supportiveness, and assessed perceptions of the partner's support. Support was manipulated by having the non-speech-making partner copy either two clearly supportive notes (e.g., "Don't worry–just say how you feel and what you think and you'll do great") or two ambiguously supportive notes (e.g., "Try not to say anything too embarrassing–especially since so many people will be watching your tape") to send to the partner who had to give a speech. The speech-giver then read the notes and rated their supportiveness. No significant attachment-style differences were found in appraisals of clearly supportive notes, but less secure individuals rated the ambiguous notes as less supportive and more upsetting, and they inferred more negative intent on the part of their partner. These findings were replicated in a second study (Collins & Feeney, 2004, Study 2) in which partners were allowed to write authentic notes: More attachment-insecure people rated the notes as less supportive mainly when the notes were more ambiguous (as rated by independent judges).

Taken together, the findings indicate that insecurely attached people are predisposed to perceive a partner's supportive behavior as less responsive and helpful. However, it's important to note that clear-cut signs of a partner's responsiveness (e.g., a clearly supportive note) can be appraised as supportive even by attachment-insecure people, which might be a first small step in disconfirming their negative working models. This is an initial indication that the quality of a partner's sensitivity and responsiveness matters (see the next section for more indications).

Although attachment-insecure people tend to experience biased perceptions of their partner's behavior, there are also times, of course, when the partner of an insecure individual actually fails to be supportive. Moreover, partners of insecure individuals may in fact be less supportive than partners of secure people. Rholes et al. (2001) proposed that, beyond choosing less supportive partners, insecure people may actively interfere with their partner's supportive behavior, thus confirming and strengthening their negative working models. In particular, insecure people's disbelief in others' supportiveness may cause them to be suspicious concerning a romantic partner's helpful actions, which in turn may induce the partner to withdraw support over time. Or insecure people may repeatedly claim that a partner is unsupportive, until the partner accepts this view and begins to behave nonsupportively. However, if a romantic partner is secure and resilient enough to resist an insecure partner's doubts and complaints, he or she may still be able to provide clear-cut signs of love and care that foster felt security.

Difficulties in Support Provision

Attachment-insecure people often have difficulty being responsive to their romantic partner's needs and providing effective support when called upon to do so (Shaver et al., 2016). These difficulties are especially notable in the case of avoidant individuals, who hold negative views of others and feel uncomfortable expressing needs or being dependent. However, attachment-anxious people also tend to experience problems in providing effective support. Their tendency to become distressed in a self-focused, ruminative way can cause them to react to a romantic partner's needs or suffering with their own personal distress rather than effective helping. Moreover, they sometimes use support provision as a means of satisfying their own unmet needs for approval and reassurance (Feeney & Collins, 2003; Feeney et al., 2013). This self-centered motivation can yield insensitive and intrusive caregiving efforts. Such difficulties can prevent attachment-insecure people and their partners (as support recipients) from enjoying comforting and empowering interactions.

Several cross-sectional and prospective longitudinal studies have involved collecting self-reports of support provision in couples and found that attachment-insecure people are less likely to provide support to a needy partner and less likely to be sensitive to the partner's needs (e.g., Davila & Kashy, 2009; Kunce & Shaver, 1994; Millings et al., 2013). Similar results have been obtained in observational studies of support provision in the laboratory. Using a laboratory paradigm described earlier, Simpson et al. (1992) video-recorded dating couples while the female partner waited to endure a stressful task, and judges then rated the male partner's supportive behavior. Whereas secure men recognized their partner's worries and provided greater support if their partner showed higher levels of distress, men who scored high on avoidance provided less support, especially as their partner's distress increased. Collins and Feeney (2000) video-recorded dating couples while one partner disclosed a personal problem to the other and found that more attachment-anxious participants were rated by judges as less supportive, less responsive, and more negative toward the distressed partner.

In another laboratory experiment, Feeney and Collins (2001) brought dating couples to the laboratory and informed one member of the couple that he or she would perform a stressful task—preparing and delivering a speech that would be video-recorded. The other member of the couple was led to believe that his or her partner was either extremely nervous (the high-need condition) or not at all nervous (the low-need condition) about the speech task, and was given the opportunity to write a private note to the partner. More attachment-insecure participants wrote less emotionally supportive notes (as rated by judges) in both the high- and low-need conditions, and they provided less instrumental support in the high- than in the low-need condition, precisely when the partner most needed support. Moreover, they reported having less empathic feelings for their partner and were less willing to altruistically switch tasks with the partner.

The negative effects of attachment insecurities on support provision have also been observed when a romantic partner is exploring new career opportunities or personal plans. This is important with respect to the notion of secure-base provision and support for a broaden-and-build cycle. In an observational study of married couples discussing each partner's personal goals, Feeney and Thrush (2010) found that attachment-insecure participants were less likely to provide effective support for a partner's exploration (as judged by observers). Specifically, spouses' avoidant attachment was predictive of being less available to their partner, and spouses' attachment anxiety was predictive of greater interference in their partner's exploration.

Relational Attitudes and Behaviors That Move Insecure Partners' to Heightened Security

In the two previous sections, we reviewed evidence that romantic partners and spouses are a potential source of a safe haven and a secure base for one another, but that their attachment insecurities can interfere with the creation of a secure and efficacious bond between them. In this section, we consider evidence that, despite the projection of previously established insecure working models onto a current partner, sensitive and responsive behavior by the partner can gradually reduce the interfering effects of attachment insecurity.

Based on the kinds of research we have reviewed briefly here, Arriaga et al. (2018) created the attachment security enhancement model (ASEM), a dual-process model focused on the ability of romantic partners and spouses to produce positive attachment-related change within their relationship. Regarding the first process, partners' responsive behaviors can weaken the destructive relational tendencies aroused by attachment insecurities during couple interactions (see previous section). These behaviors (*safe/softening strategies*) can reduce distress and promote a calm relational climate in which each partner can benefit from the other's responsiveness. Regarding the second process, partners' ongoing provision of a safe haven and a secure base can foster the revision of deeply rooted insecure working models, which increases the possibility of sustained felt security in the long run.

Managing Attachment Insecurities during Couple Interactions

According to Arriaga et al. (2018), partners who are sensitive and responsive to each other's needs, fears, and defenses can effectively manage the dysfunctional manifestations of attachment insecurities during couple interactions. In the case of attachment-anxious people, who tend to doubt their value and lovability, and experience intense fears of rejection and abandonment, a sensitive and responsive partner/spouse can allay these concerns by providing unwavering reassurance, love, and commitment. This kind of behavior signals safety in the relationship (*safe strategies*), which can reduce attachment-anxious individuals' worries and counter their need to cling, monitor, intrude, and demand care. In the case of people who score high on attachment-related avoidance, who distrust a partner's intentions and feel uncomfortable with intimacy and interdependence, a responsive partner/spouse can soften these concerns by understanding and validating the person's need for self-reliance and conveying a sense that it is possible to feel unconstrained and autonomous even during intimate interactions (*softening strategies*). By being empathic with, and respectful of, an avoidant partner's need to feel self-reliant, the other partner can make it feel less dangerous to engage in intimate, emotion-laden interactions.

Research has shown that a partner's display of affection, commitment, and love can reduce attachment-anxious people's self-focused worries and destructive relational tendencies during couple interactions. For example, in a study of married couples asked to discuss a major conflict, the well-known tendency of attachment-anxious people to display intense relational distress and their reluctance to rely on effective conflict management strategies (e.g., compromising and integrating their own and their spouse's positions) were softened when their spouse expressed stronger commitment to the relationship (Tran & Simpson, 2009). Attachment-anxious people are also less likely to express intense romantic jealousy after an experimental manipulation of affectionate touch in the laboratory (a romantic partner was instructed to place his or her arm around the focal participant's shoulder) than after a no-touch condition (Kim et al., 2018). Similarly, in a 10-day diary study of dating couples, the link between attachment anxiety and relational distress on a given day was weaker in couples who reported more physical touch during that day (Carmichael et al., 2021).

Additional findings from diary studies of dating couples indicate that affectionate sexual experiences on a given day reduce attachment-anxious people's following-day relational distress and doubts about their partner's love (Birnbaum et al., 2006; Little et al., 2010, Raposo & Muise, 2021). For example, Raposo and Muise conducted a 21-day diary study of romantic couples and found that on days when a partner was perceived as responsive to their sexual needs, people scoring high on attachment anxiety reported similar levels of relationship satisfaction, trust, and commitment as people who scored relatively low on anxiety. Only on days when a partner was perceived as unresponsive to their sexual needs did attachment-anxious people show the typical pattern of relationship dissatisfaction and lack of trust and commitment. In addition, the study indicated that perceived partner sexual responsiveness increased attachment-anxious people's commitment to their relationship over time.

There is also evidence that a partner's softening strategies can weaken avoidant defenses during couple interactions. For example, avoidant people's tendency to respond with anger and emotional distancing after being asked by a romantic partner to make a change in their attitude or behavior was dramatically reduced when their partner showed respect for their need for self-reliance (Overall et al., 2013). And Farrell et al. (2016) found that more avoidant individuals were more likely than less avoidant ones to reject their romantic partner's request to make a sacrifice to support his or her plans and to experience lower trust and commitment following the request. However, these negative reactions did not occur if the requesting partner presented the request as reasonable, respected the partner's autonomy, and appreciated the partner's efforts in making a personal sacrifice. Recently, findings from two daily experience studies revealed that attachment-avoidant people's reluctance to make personal sacrifices in order to benefit their partner was softened on days when they felt highly appreciated by their partner (Schrage et al., 2022).

In observational studies of married couples asked to discuss relationship problems, more avoidant individuals responded with greater hostility and relational disengagement except in couples in which their spouse respected their discomfort with emotion-laden interactions and provided practical advice and suggestions without demanding emotional sharing or self-disclosure (Girme et al., 2015; Simpson et al., 2007). In a recent study, Schrage et al. (2020) found that avoidant people's tendency to respond with negative affect and disengagement to their dating partner's disclosure of a time he or she felt strong love for them was dramatically reduced when this disclosure included more nonverbal expressions of affection (e.g., smiling, leaning, gazing) rather than emotion-laded words or phrases (e.g., "I love you"). It seems that avoidant people feel comfortable when their romantic partner's disclosure is tailored to their unique needs and inclinations (e.g., avoidance of direct verbal expressions of love and affection) and does not imply a burdensome request to reciprocate intimacy.

Research also confirms that romantic partners or spouses who maintain positive and lighthearted exchanges that "ease the burden" of relationship stresses can reduce avoidant defenses. For example, avoidant people's distress and emotional distancing during and after a discussion about a relationship problem were dramatically reduced if their romantic partner was rated (by external raters) as overtly calm and accepting rather than angry and demanding (Barry & Lawrence, 2013; Salvatore et al., 2011). Moreover, playful, carefree couple interactions and perceived expressions of gratitude and appreciation from a romantic partner can weaken the typical association between attachment-related avoidance and reduced levels of self-disclosure and relational commitment (Park, Impett, et al., 2019; Stanton et al., 2017).

Fostering Felt Security within a Couple

The studies we've reviewed thus far deal mostly with short-term interactions and interventions. What about longer-term change in couple functioning? In an 8-month study of newly committed couples, Lavi (2007) obtained preliminary evidence for the long-term effects of a partner's sensitive responsiveness on security enhancement. Specifically, participants' self-reports of attachment anxiety and avoidance within a new relationship were more likely to decrease during the 8-month study if a partner was more sensitive (more accurate in decoding emotions displayed by participants during a nonverbal communication task) and more responsive (more supportive, as coded by independent judges, to participants' disclosure of a personal problem) at the beginning of the study. Of clinical importance, these positive changes in within-relationship attachment orientations were found even among people who reported relatively high levels of attachment anxiety or avoidance in close relationships (i.e., who were dispositionally insecure) at the beginning of the study.

Although a partner's responsiveness might lead to positive changes in the other partner's felt security, the mechanism of change seems to be somewhat different for attachment-anxious and attachment-avoidant partners. According to Arriaga et al. (2018), moving an attachment-anxious person toward longer-term security within a couple requires not only the partner's expression of love and affection but also the provision of opportunities to disconfirm the anxious person's negative models of self and replace them with a sense of competence and self-worth. Attachment anxiety, bound up with negative self-views, is likely to decline as anxious people experience their partner's encouragement, support, and confidence in their strength and competence (secure-base support). Arriaga et al. suggested that "partners can facilitate this process by creating or amplifying moments that (1) affirm an anxious person's strengths, goals, interests, and positive qualities; or (2) result in an anxious person gaining confidence, self-efficacy, or autonomy in contexts outside of the relationship. Anxious individuals may benefit the most when (3) partners help them infer broader meaning into these situations that bolster their self-models" (p. 85).

Recent studies confirm that relational experiences that bolster the sense of personal value and competence are critical for reducing attachment anxiety within a couple relationship. In a study of a newlywed couples, participants who were more likely to perceive their partner as accepting and valuing of their personal goals reported less attachment anxiety 12 months later (Arriaga et al., 2014). Also, data from a 7-year longitudinal study revealed that participants' attachment anxiety in a given year declined when they perceived a romantic partner as bolstering their sense of personal value during the previous year by appreciating their qualities or expressing gratitude to them (Park, Johnson, et al., 2019). In a recent 2-year longitudinal study, Arriaga et al. (2020) found that attachment anxiety decreased during the transition to parenthood as spouses perceived themselves as more competent in their parenting role.

In the case of people who score high on attachment-related avoidance, moving them toward greater security in the context of a couple relationship requires not only respecting their need for self-reliance but also creating positive relational experiences involving heightened intimacy and interdependence, which can disconfirm their negative working models of others and of close relationships (Arriaga et al., 2018). During such positive experiences, avoidant individuals gradually learn that interdependence is not as frightening as they feared (based on earlier relationships) and that they can trust their loving partner. According to Arriaga et al. (2018), "avoidant individuals are likely to benefit the most when they . . . reflect on the positive aspects of these situations (e.g., enjoyment, fulfillment, an authentic and comfortable feeling of belonging), which is more likely to occur when partners directly or indirectly guide such perceptions" (p. 87).

Research also provides preliminary support for the possibility that a person's attachment-related avoidance can decrease as a result of positive relational experiences. In longitudinal studies of couples transitioning to parenthood, for example, participants who reported being engaged in more comfortable support-seeking or support-providing interactions with their partner during the study period exhibited a steeper decline in self-reported avoidant attachment over time (Rholes et al., 2021; Simpson et al., 2003). In an experimental study, Stanton et al. (2017) found that participants who were randomly assigned to engage in a nonthreatening intimate interaction (a mixture of disclosure of personal information and engagement in a relaxing dyadic activity) reported lower attachment-related avoidance after the interaction and 1 month later than participants who engaged in a neutral couple interaction (e.g., reading excerpts from texts).

Research Summary

Research on attachment-related processes within couple relationships consistently shows that partners' responsiveness to each other's needs and the sharing of comforting intimate experiences can bring about a revision of insecure working models and enhance felt security. However, the studies we've just reviewed also indicate that attachment insecurities brought by partners into their relationship can interfere with security-enhancement processes, often leading to relational instability and dissatisfaction, and impairing the effectiveness of couple therapy. Indeed, Callaci et al. (2021) found that although 15 sessions of couple therapy led to a decrease in partners' relational disengagement, their attachment insecurities (as assessed prior to therapy) were found to weaken this pro-relational change over the course of therapy.

Influenced by this large body of theory and research, Johnson (2004, 2008) developed and evaluated two important attachment-focused interventions for couples: emotionally focused therapy (EFT) for distressed couples and the Hold Me Tight (HmT) couple relationship education program. These interventions provide practitioners with a clear map concerning the steps they need to take to enhance felt security within a couple context. These steps correspond closely to the ASEM processes we have discussed: Increase partners' ability to soften the destructive consequences of attachment insecurities; promote partners' sensitive responsiveness to each other's needs and feelings; and encourage comforting relational experiences.

Emotionally Focused Therapy for Couples

EFT for couples was originally developed by Greenberg and Johnson (1988), but its articulation as an attachment-focused intervention was made by Johnson in the second edition of her book *The Practice of Emotionally Focused Marital Therapy* (2004). EFT is an evidence-based, short-term therapy for distressed couples that involves eight to 20 sessions (Johnson, 2019a). It is applied mainly to couples who seek therapy because of relational conflicts and distress, but it has also been applied to distressed couples in which one partner is suffering from a major psychological or physical problem, such as depression (e.g., Denton et al., 2012), posttraumatic stress disorder (PTSD; e.g., Dalton et al., 2013), or cancer (e.g., McLean et al., 2013).

The goal of EFT is to enhance partners' attachment security and sustain their broaden-and-build cycles of security, thereby enhancing the well-being of the individual partners and the success of their long-term relationship. Like Arriaga et al. (2018), Johnson (2004) views security enhancement as involving two main processes: (1) addressing partners' attachment insecurities and associated disturbing emotions, and softening the destructive patterns of couple interaction fueled by these insecurities, and (2) cultivating partners' sensitivity and responsiveness to each other. In Johnson's view, these two processes can shape more positive interaction patterns and increase feelings of being loved, accepted, understood, and validated, which in turn can disconfirm negative working models and promote felt security.

Following attachment theory and research, Johnson (2004) emphasizes that attachment insecurities and secondary attachment strategies (hyperactivation or deactivation of the attachment system) are key contributors to relationship distress and lack of sensitive responsiveness to one's partner. During couple interactions, attachment-insecure partners attempt to deal with their own concerns and distress by either hyperactivating proximity seeking and engaging in needy, intrusive, critical demands for attention and love (in the case of attachment-anxious people) or deactivating attachment needs and maintaining distance from intimate, interdependent interactions (in the case of people who score high on attachment-related avoidance).

In both cases, these secondary attachment strategies exacerbate rather than reduce relationship distress and prevent partners from responding constructively to each other. It's obviously difficult to respond constructively to an attachment-anxious partner's criticism and blame-casting or to an avoidant partner's distancing and stonewalling. Therefore, Johnson (2004) believes that the first step in healing distressed couples is to encourage partners to express their demoralization, needs, and vulnerability in a constructive manner instead of angrily criticizing or withdrawing, and to soften their potentially destructive tendencies. Only then can partners feel less attacked or rejected, giving the therapist an opportunity to explain and encourage the adoption of more empathic and responsive stances that promote increases in felt security.

In EFT training, therapists are instructed to focus on attachment concerns and emotions that underlie frustrating and discouraging couple interactions and that interfere with, or preclude, sensitive responsiveness (Johnson, 2004). The EFT therapist helps partners to identify, explore, and accept the sadness, fear, and shame (which Johnson calls *primary emotions*) aroused by the frustration of attachment needs. Moreover, the therapist encourages partners to explore how these primary painful emotions (associated with vulnerabilities) can be masked by feelings of anger, frustration, and contempt (*secondary emotions*) and how they shape angry, critical, demanding responses (*pursuer/blaming position*) or emotional distancing and stonewalling (*withdrawal position*). An EFT therapist also helps partners understand how their pursuer/blaming or withdrawing responses push them away each from the other and exacerbate their primary vulnerability-related emotions and relationship distress.

With partners' increasing awareness of the ways in which unmet attachment needs and primary emotions underlie their distressed relationship, the therapist can help them experiment and use more constructive ways of communicating their needs and emotions. For example, "a person with a tendency to make accusations and to criticize his or her partner learns to identify the needs and fears beneath the criticism. Instead of expressing secondary anger, the person develops an ability to speak of his or her loneliness and desire for emotional connection" (Greenman et al., 2019, p. 294). This makes it easier for the therapist to help both partners understand and empathize with each other's pain, opening the door to more supportive responses and constructive dialogue. Repeatedly, the therapist encourages one partner to disclose his or her primary emotions and needs (which often have to do with what Johnson [2004] calls *attachment injuries*) while guiding the other partner to respond in a sensitive and comforting manner. These episodes, which Johnson calls *in-session enactments*, are essential for each partner to experience the other as a safe haven and secure base.

EFT therapists are also trained to be emotionally present, accepting, and responsive to both partners' current relational wishes and fears, and to provide a secure base for exploring and reprocessing their primary and secondary emotions and destructive patterns of relational responses. (In this sense, the therapist acts, for the couple members, as a safe haven and secure base for exploration.) In addition, the therapists plan couple-specific interactions to provide the partners opportunities to cultivate sensitive responsiveness and to feel loved, accepted, and cared for (Greenman et al., 2019). This involves the use of a wide variety of techniques, such as empathic reflections of partners' emotions, evocative questions (e.g., "What happens to you when your partner is angry and complains about your faults?"), empathic conjectures (e.g., "That sounds like you are afraid"), reframes (e.g., "The problem is that both of you feel alone, not that you are bad persons"), and emotional coaching during in-session enactments (Johnson, 2004).

Johnson (2019b), an enthusiastic dance student, views the therapist as a choreographer of an *EFT Tango;* making the following steps continuously throughout therapy, he or she

> reflects patterns of emotional processing and interpersonal responses ("You sound angry but then lapse into 'lonely' tears, but he only hears the anger and then he withdraws, priming your sense of loss and anger"); deepens emotion with clients ("Underneath the anger there is this 'desperation' and sense of not mattering"); sets up new interactions using the deepened emotional cues ("Can you tell him, 'I get so scared that I don't matter to you—you can just shut me out—that I yell to try to reach you'?"); processes these new interactions and fosters empathic connection ("How does it feel to say this?" "How does it feel to hear this"—"Can you let that in—help her with this feeling?"); and validates and integrates this new experience ("Look how well you did. You risked and reached, put your emotions together in a new way, responded to each other. You can do this. You can make sense of your relationship and find a way home.") (p. 103)

EFT involves three stages that resemble the two processes proposed by Arriaga et al. (2018)—management of attachment insecurities and promotion of felt security. The first stage, *assessment and deescalation*, includes four steps: (1) building a solid working alliance between the therapist and the couple; (2) making partners aware of the problematic pattern of interaction that underlies their relationship distress; (3) identifying and accessing partners' primary emotions and unmet attachment needs; and (4) helping the couple reframe their distress as the result of their unmet attachment needs, primary and secondary emotions, and behavioral tendencies. In this way, attachment-anxious partners learn to recognize and deescalate their pursuer/blaming position, and attachment-avoidant partners to soften their tendency to withdraw and stonewall. According to Greenman et al. (2019), "At the end of Stage I, couples reach de-escalation, which means that . . . they understand that each person's position in the cycle stems from a desire to feel emotionally connected to the other and the strong feelings that are triggered when this connection is under siege" (p. 295).

The second stage, *restructuring attachment interactions*, includes three steps: (1) helping partners openly express their attachment wishes and feel safe enough to ask each other to meet them; (2) fostering partners' sensitive responsiveness to each other's needs and bids for proximity; and (3) shaping interactions of responsiveness and emotional engagement during in-session enactments. Through these steps, partners learn to replace their conflictual interactions with more mutually empathic, responsive interactions, in which each partner feels that his or her attachment needs are accepted, understood, and validated by the other. The EFT therapist facilitates this restructuring process by validating and amplifying partners' primary emotions (often, hurt feelings) and helping them to practice safe self-disclosure and responsiveness. In Greenman et al.'s (2019) words, "The key is not to simply discuss feelings and needs on a cognitive level, but to provoke vulnerable emotional responses in session. The rationale behind this type of intervention is the notion that comforting responses to clear expressions of vulnerability strengthen emotional connections between relationship partners" (p. 296).

During this stage, the therapist's interventions facilitate what Johnson (2004) calls *softenings*. An attachment-avoidant person might be helped to feel understood by his or her partner, calm his or her relational fears, and then be able to remain emotionally engaged during couple interactions (*withdrawer reengagement*). And an attachment-anxious partner might soften his or her anger and demands and express neediness and vulnerability in a more constructive manner (*pursuer/blamer softening*). According to Johnson and Greenman (2006), these softenings are key for enhancing partners' responsiveness and sense of connection.

In the third stage, *consolidation and integration*, partners learn to apply security-enhancing patterns of interaction in everyday life and to consolidate a secure emotional bond. This stage includes two steps: (1) fostering patterns of positive interaction based on emotional engagement and responsiveness, and (2) helping partners deal with practical issues (e.g., financial decisions) through these positive interactional patterns. In addition, "therapists discuss future challenges the couple might face, assist them in making time for 'attachment rituals' (i.e., activities and behaviors that help partners feel close and connected to each other), and address the importance of recognizing when they might have fallen back into their negative cycle as the first, most powerful tool for stepping out of it" (Greenman et al., 2019, p. 296).

EFT is now taught in over 65 training centers around the world, which provide systematic training that leads to certification as an EFT therapist. EFT certification is open to licensed psychotherapists with expertise in couple therapy and includes 48 hours of core skills training, 8 hours of individual supervision led by an EFT supervisor, and submission of two therapy excerpts. More information and numerous demonstrations are available at *www.iceeft.com.*

Research Evidence on EFT Effectiveness

The effectiveness of EFT has been examined in 13 published RCTs, with samples ranging from 12 to 80 couples (see Table 6.1 for a summary of these studies' methods). Most of the studied couples came to therapy because of relationship distress. But samples have also included parents of children with a chronic disease, couples with one partner diagnosed with major depression, couples with the female partner having experienced childhood abuse or suffering from inhibited sexual desire, and couples with one partner in the end stage of metastatic cancer. In all 13 RCTs, couples who received EFT have been compared either to couples in a waiting-list control group or to couples who received treatment as usual (not EFT). A few studies have examined whether EFT is more effective than other specific couple therapies, such as behavioral problem-solving therapy, cognitive marital therapy, and a combination of acceptance and commitment therapy and mindfulness-based therapy for couples. Most of the RCTs have tested the effectiveness of eight EFT sessions. However, couples in six RCTs received between 10 and 24 sessions.

As can be seen in Table 6.1, 11 of the 13 RCTs examined EFT effectiveness in improving pretreatment levels of relationship quality (intimacy, commitment, patterns of communication, relationship satisfaction). Data have also been collected on EFT effectiveness in improving depression, trauma-related symptoms, and sexual satisfaction. In seven RCTs, these outcome assessments have been conducted only immediately after the end of therapy. But six studies followed up couples for periods of 2 to 6 months after therapy.

In all 11 RCTs that included measures of relationship quality, the findings indicate that EFT produced a higher posttherapy level of these quality measures than a control condition. In addition, EFT led to better relational outcomes than behavioral problem-solving therapy (Johnson & Greenberg, 1985a) and cognitive marital therapy (Dandeneu & Johnson, 1994), but it failed to outperform a combination of acceptance and commitment therapy and mindfulness-based therapy for couples (Ghochani et al., 2020). In addition, as compared to a control condition, EFT was more effective in reducing depression and PTSD, and increasing sexual desire. These positive effects have been found both immediately after therapy and at follow-ups varying from 2 to 6 months. However, James (1991) found that the effects of EFT on relationship satisfaction had disappeared 4 months after ending therapy.

A meta-analysis conducted by Johnson et al. (1999) of four of these studies (N = 120 couples) revealed a robust effect of EFT in improving relationship quality (relative to control conditions). This large-size effect of EFT on postintervention measures of relationship quality was fully replicated in a recent meta-analysis of the nine RCTs conducted since the publication of the initial meta-analysis (Beasley & Ager, 2019). It's worth noting, however, that many of the reviewed RCTs were underpowered (having small sample sizes), and most did not compare EFT with other non-attachment-based couple therapies. In addition, lamentably, none of the 13 RCTs examined the hypothesized effects of EFT on attachment-related constructs, such as felt security, attachment orientations (anxiety and avoidance), working models, or construal of a relationship as a safe haven and secure base. Therefore, we do not have rigorous RCTs confirming that partners' sense of attachment security is enhanced by EFT.

Studies that rely on a pre- and posttherapy assessment without a control group have also provided evidence for the effectiveness of EFT in improving relationship quality (see

TABLE 6.1. Summary of RCTs on Effectiveness of EFT for Couples

Authors	Sample	Control conditions	Number of sessions	Timing of assessment	Assessed variables
Johnson & Greenberg (1985a)	45 distressed couples	Waiting list, BPST	8	Before therapy After therapy 2-month follow-up	Relationship quality, relational intimacy
James (1991)	42 distressed couples (14 per condition)	Waiting list, EFT + 4 CT sessions	8	Before therapy After therapy 4-month follow-up	Relationship quality, relational intimacy, romantic love
Dandeneau & Johnson (1994)	36 couples from general population	Waiting list, CMT	6	Before therapy After therapy	Relationship quality, relational intimacy, relational trust, self-disclosure
MacPhee et al. (1995)	49 couples in which woman reported sexual problems	Waiting list	12	Before therapy After therapy	Sexual desire, sexual satisfaction, depression
Walker et al. (1996)	32 parents of children with chronic illnesses	Waiting list	10	Before therapy After therapy 5-month follow-up	Relationship quality, relational intimacy, Communication skills
Denton et al. (2000)	36 distressed couples	Waiting list	8	Before therapy After therapy	Relationship quality, relational intimacy, positive feelings toward spouse
Dessaulles et al. (2003)	12 couples with woman diagnosed with depression	Medication treatment as usual	16	Before therapy After therapy	Relationship quality, depression

				3-month follow-up 6-month follow-up	
Denton et al. (2012)	24 couples with woman diagnosed with depression	Medication treatment as usual	15	Before therapy After therapy 3-month follow up 6-month follow up	Relationship quality, clinician-rated depression, communication skills
Dalton et al. (2013)	22 couples in which woman experienced childhood abuse	Waiting list	24	Before therapy After therapy	Relationship quality, trauma-related symptoms
McLean et al. (2013)	42 couples with one partner diagnosed with cancer	Treatment as usual	8	Before therapy After therapy 3-month follow-up	Relationship quality, depression, caregiver burden
Alder et al. (2018)	80 couples with one partner diagnosed with depression	Treatment as usual	8	Before therapy After therapy	Depression
Wittenborn et al. (2019)	16 couples with one partner diagnosed with depression	Treatment as usual	15	Before therapy After each session	Relationship quality, depression
Ghochani et al. (2020)	28 couples dealing with infidelity	Waiting list, ACT + MBCT	8	Before therapy After therapy	Relational intimacy, trauma-related symptoms

Note. ACT, acceptance and commitment therapy; BPST, behavioral problem-solving therapy; CMT, cognitive marital therapy; CT, communication training; MBCT, Mindfulness-based cognitive therapy.

Table 6.2 for a summary of these studies' methods). In all of the studies, partners' reports of relationship quality at the end of EFT were higher than their pretherapy reports. In addition, three follow-up studies found that the posttherapy improvement in relationship quality was still observed 3 months and 2 and 3 years later (Halchuk et al., 2010; Johnson & Talitman, 1997; Wiebe, Johnson, Burgess Moser, et al., 2017, Wiebe et al., 2019). Wiebe et al. also documented posttherapy improvement in sexual satisfaction immediately after EFT and at a 2-year follow-up, and MacIntosh and Johnson (2008) found that PTSD symptoms dramatically decreased after 19 sessions of EFT in partners who had experienced childhood sexual abuse. Similar findings have been reported by Weissman et al. (2018) based on a study of seven couples in which one partner was a veteran diagnosed with PTSD and the couples completed 26 to 36 sessions of EFT.

Fortunately, some of these pre- and posttherapy assessment studies provide preliminary evidence concerning the hypothesized security-enhancing effects of EFT (see Table 6.2). Using Coan et al.'s (2006) "hand-holding" fMRI paradigm in a study of 32 married couples, Johnson et al. (2013) assessed the extent to which the women's brain responses indicated that their partner served as a safe haven before and after 21 EFT sessions. Specifically, female partners were informed of the possibility of receiving an electric shock while lying in an fMRI scanner, while holding a stranger's hand or their spouse's hand. Before therapy, fMRI recordings indicated that spousal hand-holding (as compared to the two other conditions) did not affect the way that participants' brains responded to the threat of electric shock. However, after EFT, holding a spouse's hand during the same procedure (versus no or stranger hand-holding) attenuated women's neural fear responses, as indicated by decreased activity in limbic areas and prefrontal cortex; and it also reduced their reports of pain when the shocks were administered. These findings imply that EFT can improve the ability of husbands to serve as a safe haven and that their affectionate touch can soothe their wife's fear and pain responses—a key example of security enhancement.

Burgess Moser et al. (2016) analyzed self-reports of attachment anxiety and avoidance (using the ECR scale) completed by Johnson et al.'s (2013) couples prior to therapy and immediately following each EFT session. They also analyzed independent coders' ratings of partners' attachment security (using Crowell et al.'s [2002] Secure Base Scoring System) during couple interactions before and after therapy. Findings indicated that self-reports of attachment insecurities decreased as EFT sessions progressed and that attachment anxiety showed the strongest decrease after sessions that included episodes of pursuer/blaming softening during couple interactions. In addition, there was significant pre- to posttherapy improvement in coders' ratings of partners' attachment security. Importantly, Wiebe, Johnson, Burgess Moser, et al. (2017) reported that couples in this sample continued to show decreases in attachment anxiety at a 2-year follow-up. In addition, there is evidence that decreases in attachment-related avoidance immediately after therapy (as compared to pretherapy levels) predicted greater relationship satisfaction (Wiebe, Johnson, Lafontaine, et al., 2017) and greater sexual satisfaction (Wiebe et al., 2019) 2 years later.

On the whole, these findings are quite supportive of Johnson's (2004) basic premise that EFT enhances partners' felt security, and that this enhancement contributes to improved relationship quality. However, the lack of a control group and small sample sizes are reasons to continue to view the findings as tentative. In addition, no data have been collected concerning EFT effects on two attachment-related variables that are crucial for security enhancement: partners' sensitive responsiveness and working models of self and others. Therefore, the field still needs large-scale RCTs testing the effectiveness of EFT in enhancing partners' sensitive responsiveness, promoting more positive working models of self and others, and enhancing felt security.

TABLE 6.2. Summary of Pre- and Posttherapy Assessment Studies on Effectiveness of EFT

Authors	Sample	Sessions	Timing of assessment	Assessed variables
Johnson & Greenberg (1985b)	14 distressed couples	8	Before therapy After therapy 2-month follow-up	Relationship quality, relational intimacy
Johnson & Talitman (1997)	32 distressed couples	12	Before therapy After therapy 3-month follow-up	Relationship quality, relational intimacy
MacIntosh & Johnson (2008)	10 couples in which woman experienced childhood sexual abuse	11–26 (M = 19)	Before therapy After therapy	Relationship quality, trauma-related symptoms
Johnson et al. (2013) Additional analyses of the data:	32 distressed couples	21	Before and after therapy	Brain responses in "hand-holding" paradigm
Dalgleish, Johnson, Burgess Moser, Lafontaine, et al. (2015)			Before and after therapy, and after each session	Relationship quality, relational trust
Burgess Moser et al. (2016)			Before and after therapy, and after each session	Relationship quality, within-relationship attachment orientations, attachment security
Wiebe, Johnson, Burgess Moser, et al. (2017); Wiebe, Johnson, Lafontaine, et al. (2017); Wiebe et al. (2019)			Before and after therapy, and at a 2-year follow-up	Relationship quality, within-relationship attachment orientations, attachment security, sexual satisfaction
N. Weissman et al. (2018)	7 couples in which one partner was a veteran diagnosed with PTSD	26–36	Before therapy After therapy	Relationship quality, PTSD, depression, quality of life; psychiatric symptoms

Research on Therapeutic Processes Contributing to EFT Effectiveness

Several studies have examined the specific in-session therapist interventions and couple reactions that contribute to the efficacy of EFT in improving relationship quality and enhancing attachment security (for reviews, see Brubacher & Wiebe, 2019; Greenman & Johnson, 2013). Based on these studies, Brubacher and Wiebe (2019) concluded that three key ingredients of therapeutic change within EFT sessions have been identified: (1) construction of a solid client–therapist working alliance, in general, and clients' agreement with the in-session tasks they are being asked to perform, in particular; (2) deepening of partners' emotional experiencing (i.e., increased awareness and expression of each partner's unmet attachment needs and primary emotions); (3) promotion of in-session affiliative, comforting interactions (episodes of blamer softening and withdrawer reengagement and enactments involving partners' self-disclosure and sensitive responsiveness).

Using the Couple Therapy Alliance Scale (Pinsof & Catherall, 1986) to assess partners' trust in their therapist and agreement with the therapy's goals and tasks, Johnson and Talitman (1997) found that task agreement was an important predictor of posttherapy improvement in relationship satisfaction. According to Brubacher and Wiebe (2019), "a strong therapeutic alliance requires that the couple agree with the use of therapist interventions and client tasks that are often new and uncomfortable. Therefore, it is important for EFT therapists to attune to whether the couple senses the relevance of the EFT interventions and tasks and experiences how they are ultimately helping them, in spite of momentary discomfort" (p. 295).

Brubacher (2018) proposed several therapeutic interventions that may contribute to task agreement, such as being genuinely transparent about the therapeutic tasks, creating a safe and accepting environment, reflecting and validating partners' discomfort with the therapeutic tasks, using evocative questions and conjectures to elicit clients' doubts and worries about these tasks, and repairing ruptures in task agreement as they occur within EFT sessions. Unfortunately, no systematic study has examined the contribution of each of these in-session interventions to enhancing partner's security and relationship quality.

Four studies indicate that partners' overt expression of emotions and attachment needs within EFT sessions is associated with positive therapeutic outcomes (Couture-Lalande et al., 2007; Johnson & Greenberg, 1988; Greenberg et al., 1993; Wiebe, Johnson, Lafontaine, et al., 2017). For example, in a study of six couples who completed eight sessions of EFT, Johnson and Greenberg (1988) found that couples who showed greater posttherapy increases in relationship quality were coded by raters as displaying higher levels of emotional experiencing and a greater number of proximity-seeking statements (i.e., statements that involve self-disclosure, sharing, or understanding) during the most productive sessions (as identified by both therapists and clients). Couture-Lalande et al. (2007) replicated these findings in a detailed analysis of verbatim transcripts of the fourth, seventh, 12th, and 16th EFT sessions of two couples (one who showed improvement in relationship satisfaction after EFT and one who did not show improvement).

There is also evidence that the occurrence of in-session pursuer/blamer softening events can contribute to positive therapeutic outcomes (Burgess Moser et al., 2016, 2018; Dalgleish, Johnson, Burgess Moser, Wiebe, et al., 2015). Burgess Moser et al. (2016) analyzed the best session (as rated by therapist and clients) of 32 couples who completed at least 10 EFT sessions and found that the occurrence of a pursuer/blamer softening event (as coded by independent raters) during the session was associated with improvement in relationship satisfaction immediately following the session and a reduction in attachment insecurities over time. Burgess Moser et al. (2018) also found that although self-reports of attachment anxiety increased immediately after the softening session, they showed a steep decrease during the following sessions and at the end of therapy. In addition, Dalgleish, Johnson, Burgess Moser, Wiebe, et al. (2015) found that the occurrence of in-session pursuer/blamer softening events was associated with improved relationship satisfaction following the session, but that this link was noted mainly among partners who scored low on avoidant attachment prior to therapy.

In a study of 24 couples identified as having suffered an attachment injury (e.g., extramarital affair, one partner withdrawing at a time of upheaval), Makinen and Johnson (2006) obtained preliminary evidence for the therapeutic benefits of in-session enactments that involved the offended partner's disclosure of primary emotions elicited by the injury and the other partner's empathic responding to this disclosure and expressing heartfelt remorse. Specifically, couples who successfully completed these in-session enactments (n = 15) reported greater relationship satisfaction after therapy than couples who did not complete these enactments (n = 9). Halchuk et al. (2010) followed up these couples 3 years later and found that couples who completed the in-session enactments appraised the attachment injury as less severe and reported higher relationship quality than those who did not complete the enactments. Similar findings were reported by Meneses and Greenberg (2011) in their study of eight couples undergoing EFT following infidelity on the part of the male partner.

In summary, the reviewed studies provide promising evidence concerning the therapeutic processes (task agreement, emotional experiencing, in-session softenings, and comforting enactments) hypothesized to create EFT's beneficial effects. However, some caution is still in order due to the small sample sizes in most of the studies and the lack of an integrative assessment of the various therapeutic processes in a single sample of couples. Moreover, with the exception of Burgess Moser et al. (2016, 2018), the reviewed studies have exclusively focused on posttherapy changes in relationship quality and have not examined the extent to which these therapeutic processes contribute to security enhancement—the key concept in attachment theory. More systematic research is needed using larger sample sizes, providing an integrative assessment of in-session processes, and examining their short-term and long-term effects on partners' felt security.

The Hold Me Tight Program

To facilitate implementation and dissemination of EFT in the wider community and to reach couples who are not necessarily distressed but want to improve the quality of their relationship, Johnson (2008) developed the HmT program, a couple relationship education program that provides a cheaper and less stigmatizing alternative to EFT. Like EFT, the HmT program is designed to increase partners' awareness of the attachment bases of relational tensions, help partners deescalate destructive patterns of interaction, and strengthen partners' sensitive responsiveness to each other's needs and feelings. Rather than having as its primary focus the improvement of communication skills, which is the focus of most other couple relationship education programs (e.g., Hawkins et al., 2008; Markman et al., 2008), the HmT program seeks to enhance partners' felt security, which can then support constructive communication patterns (Johnson, 2008). Of course, other relationship education programs, such as the Prevention and Relationship Enhancement Program (PREP; Markman et al., 1988), also attempt to create security and emotional connection, but this is not the main focus of such programs, which are not primarily grounded in attachment theory and research.

HmT is a group-based program for couples that includes a standardized 16-hour protocol. It can be delivered in either of two formats: (1) eight 2-hour weekly sessions, as outlined in the HmT guide (Johnson, 2010), or (2) a modified weekend retreat format. According to the HmT manual, groups can include between four and 30 couples, and two facilitators are recommended when the group is larger than six to eight couples, making it possible for facilitators to work with each couple during the in-session exercises (Johnson, 2010). In the first session, couples introduce themselves and talk about what they would like to gain from the program. Next, the facilitator presents educational material concerning attachment, couple relationships, and the importance of a secure emotional bond. The remaining seven sessions coincide with the seven "conversations for connection" presented in Johnson's (2008) book for the general public, *Hold Me Tight*.

In the first conversation, partners learn to identify their negative interaction patterns and the ways in which attachment worries, fears, and defenses shape these patterns. In the second conversation, partners learn to identify their primary emotions and feelings of vulnerability ("raw spots"), which might underlie anger, blame, and distancing during couple interactions. They are also encouraged to share these raw spots with each other. In the third conversation, partners revisit a moment of relational tension ("rocky moment") and learn to talk openly about the raw spots that emerged during the moment and to soften pursuer/blamer or withdrawal responses during the interaction. In the fourth conversation, partners learn how to be more accessible, emotionally responsive, and deeply engaged with each other.

In the fifth conversation, partners learn how to hear and respond in an empathically comforting manner to each other's pain. Specifically, each partner takes turns sharing a significant hurt he or she experienced in the relationship while the other partner is guided and encouraged to help soothe and heal the hurt. In the sixth conversation, couples learn how to improve their sex lives by creating a more secure emotional bond and how to improve emotional connection during sex. The last conversation focuses on how to maintain the gains made in the HmT program and sustain a security-enhanced emotional bond over time.

During these conversations, the HmT facilitator's main job is to create a secure base from which partners can disclose their raw spots and explore and learn new, security-enhancing patterns of couple interaction, and can do so in an accepting and nonjudgmental atmosphere. For each of the conversations, facilitators first teach the relevant attachment-related principles and then show video clips of couples talking in a responsive and comforting manner about the targeted topic. Each couple then engages in a back-and-forth dialogue on the session's topic while the facilitator moves between couples and coaches them in shaping a responsive and comforting interaction. Participants also receive relevant homework, which is discussed at the start of the following session. Unlike EFT therapists who focus on tracking, heightening, and structuring emotional and relational experiences as they unfold during a therapy session, HmT facilitators spend a great deal of time teaching, coaching couples, providing feedback during structured interactions, and responding to couples' homework.

HmT facilitators are not required to be licensed therapists. Anyone willing to purchase the required materials can facilitate an HmT group. While not required before applying the program, there are training seminars that facilitators can take. The program materials include the HmT book, the Facilitators' Guide, a DVD presenting couples completing the conversations, and a short DVD talk on attachment as a "guide to couple relationships for HmT facilitators." To date, several variants of the program have been developed, such as *Hold Me Tight/Let Me Go* for parents and teens, *Healing Hearts Together* for partners facing cardiac disease, and *Hold Me Tight Online* for couples who want to take the HmT program at home on their own schedule.

Research Evidence on HmT Effectiveness

Unfortunately, no RCT has been published examining the effects of the HmT program on partners' attachment security and relationship quality, as compared with a waiting-list control group or other couple relationship education programs. Evidence concerning HmT program effectiveness is based on six pre- to postassessment studies that did not include a control group. Three studies have been conducted with small samples of couples (*N*'s of 14, 15, and 23), showing that, as compared to a preintervention assessment, relationship satisfaction had increased by the end of the HmT program (Morgis et al., 2019; Stavrianopoulos, 2015; Wong et al., 2018). In addition, Morgis et al. (2019) reported a pre- to postintervention increase in sexual intimacy and satisfaction, and Wong et al. (2018) found that self-reports of avoidant attachment (but not attachment anxiety) decreased after the HmT program.

Using a larger sample of couples (*N* = 95) that participated in 16 HmT groups, Kennedy et al. (2019) measured partners' relationship quality on four occasions: baseline, preprogram, postprogram, and at 3- or 6-month follow-ups. As compared to preintervention measures, relationship quality had increased immediately following the HmT program but was not sustained at that level 3 or 6 months later; that is, improvements in relationship quality associated with the HmT program seemed to fade fairly quickly. According to Kennedy et al., because HmT is briefer and less intense than EFT, participants might not have reached the threshold of positive relational experiences and skills needed to sustain improved relationship satisfaction over time.

In another pre- to postassessment study, Conradi et al. (2018) studied 129 Dutch couples (79 self-referred and 50 therapist-referred) that participated in 22 HmT groups. These researchers collected self-reports of relationship satisfaction and relationship-specific attachment security (with the Accessibility, Responsiveness, Engagement Questionnaire; Johnson, 2008) before the program, immediately after the program, and 4 months later. As compared to their preprogram scores, self-referred couples showed improvements in both relationship satisfaction and attachment security after the HmT program, and these improvements were maintained 4 months later. Clinician-referred couples, who were more distressed and less securely attached before entering the program, also showed improvements in relationship satisfaction and attachment security immediately after the program but not at the 4-month follow-up. Thus, the psychological benefits of the HmT program seem to fade fairly quickly in highly distressed couples.

The sixth pre- to postassessment study was conducted in a sample of 39 couples in which one partner has had a cardiac vascular disease (Tulloch et al., 2021). In this study, patients and their partner underwent the Healing Hearts Together intervention—the variant of HmT for couples coping with cardiac diseases (Tulloch et al., 2017)—and both of them completed self-report scales tapping relationship quality, mental health, and quality of life before and after the intervention. Findings revealed significant pre- to postintervention changes in all of the assessed variables. As compared to their preintervention scores, both patients and their partners reported lower levels of relationship distress, depression, and anxiety, and better quality of life immediately after the intervention. It seems that this variant of the HmT program was beneficial for not only improving relationship quality but also alleviating psychological distress in both the ill partner and the healthy partner.

Overall, the six studies suggest that the HmT program has positive effects on partners' attachment security and relationship quality. However, because none of the studies included a control group, we can't be certain that the changes attributed to the intervention were not due to something other than the HmT program itself. Future studies should test the effectiveness of this promising attachment-based program using more rigorous random assignment designs and comparing its effects to other relationship education programs with alternative foci.

The studies conducted to date suggest that the positive effects of the HmT program fade within a few months, especially among distressed, clinically at-risk couples. For these couples, the intervention probably requires more direct consideration of each partner's specific attachment injuries, a task beyond the reach of a relatively brief, group-oriented educational intervention. Future studies should systematically examine the obstacles encountered by distressed couples during and following participation in the HmT program.

Strengthening the Effectiveness of Attachment-Based Interventions for Couples

Research on the effectiveness of EFT and the HmT program provides promising evidence that partners' felt security can be enhanced within the context of couple relationships (Wiebe & Johnson, 2016). These application-oriented studies complement the findings from the laboratory studies we reviewed earlier, which showed that comforting, supportive interactions with a responsive romantic partner can reduce attachment insecurities (Arriaga et al., 2018). However, although promising, the existing applied studies are only a first step in clarifying the role played by attachment-theoretical variables in improving couple relationships. Given this first step, more rigorous RCTs should now be conducted to examine the hypothesized effects of the interventions on partners' attachment orientations (anxiety and avoidance) and their working models of self and others. These studies should also examine the extent to which therapeutic changes are sustained over months and years without further intervention. Moreover, future studies should examine the extent to which postintervention security enhancement is associated with the key processes that, according to Johnson (2004, 2008), underlie the beneficial effects of EFT and the HmT program: partners' increased expression of attachment needs and their improved ability to soften destructive reactions while remaining sensitive and responsive to each other's needs.

EFT emphasizes the role of emotion in therapeutic change and security enhancement. Specifically, Johnson (2004) claims that powerful primary emotions (e.g., fear, hurt, despair) resulting from unmet attachment needs underlie rigid, destructive patterns of interacting (e.g., pursuit, withdrawal); that these emotions can be softened and restructured during in-session enactments; and that new emotions can be enlisted to create more constructive interactional patterns. Hence, the most effective way to enhance a person's felt security, according to Johnson (2004), is to access, express, comprehend, and reorganize primary vulnerability-related experiences.

However, we want to keep in mind that increased emotional awareness, regulation, and expression are not the only path to reshaping couple interactions and enhancing felt security. It can be complemented by other pathways reviewed in Chapter 2, using methods that have been implemented in attachment-based interventions designed to enhance felt security within parent–child relationships (see Chapter 4). One such path is increasing the capacity for *mentalization*, the tendency to represent and hold in mind one's own and a partner's needs, feelings, and thoughts (Fonagy et al., 2002). Increasing partners' accurate reflection on their own mental states can make them more aware of their unmet attachment needs and the feelings, expectations, and behavioral tendencies they experience and enact during couple interactions (Luyten et al., 2012). Moreover, increasing mentalization with respect to the other partner's mental states can make it easier to understand and empathize with the causes of the partner's formerly misunderstood or misinterpreted reactions (Fonagy & Target, 1997).

The potential therapeutic benefit of heightening partners' mentalization within EFT sessions has been emphasized by MacIntosh (2013), who identified partners' difficulties in mentalizing as a key impediment to fully engaging with therapeutic tasks. In his view, many of the core EFT interventions, such as affective heightening and enactments, require partners to simultaneously hold in mind their own and their partners' mental states, which is difficult for people with poor mentalizing skills. MacIntosh et al. (2019) pursued this idea in a qualitative analysis of mentalizing responses during EFT sessions of couples in which one or both partners were survivors of childhood sexual abuse.

EFT and the HmT program might be enriched by incorporating mentalization-enhancing practices and techniques that were originally developed for attachment-based parent–child interventions (e.g., Minding the Baby, child–parent psychotherapy; see Chapter 4) or individual psychotherapy (e.g., mentalization-based treatment; see Chapter 7). Future research could evaluate the extent to which this kind of expansion strengthens the effectiveness of EFT and the HmT program in enhancing attachment security within couple relationships.

Attachment-based interventions for couples could also benefit from incorporating practices and techniques derived from cognitive-behavioral therapies, which aim to change partners' insecure working models of self and others. But these interventions should not lose sight of the emotions associated with the mental representations targeted for change. According to attachment theory and research, insecure working models result from a history of frustrating, disappointing, or frightening interactions, and they tend to negatively bias the processing of social information in general, and relational events in particular (Dykas & Cassidy, 2011). These models cause insecure people to expect, attend to, and recall destructive couple interactions and to ignore, dismiss, reject, misinterpret, and forget disconfirming positive couple interactions. This is why Arriaga et al. (2018) claim that a partner's responsiveness can enhance felt security only if it challenges the validity of insecure working models. Without the creation of more positive mental representations, dominant insecure working models may negatively bias the processing of incoming information, including that provided by an EFT facilitator, thereby reducing the benefits of any security-enhancing relational experiences.

According to Johnson (2004, 2008), therapeutic processes within EFT and HmT sessions, such as the occurrence of softening events and responsive enactments, might by themselves instill more positive beliefs about oneself and a relationship partner (e.g., "I'm not a bad partner"; "My partner loves me") and facilitate the revision of insecure working models. However, the pervasive effects of these models on information processing can probably prevent partners from fully engaging in therapeutic tasks (e.g., by dismissing, rejecting, or misinterpreting therapist instructions) and thus interfere with the effectiveness of an intervention. Therefore, techniques that have been shown in cognitive-behavioral therapies to help people notice and change negative thought patterns (e.g., cognitive restructuring) or to soften the biasing effect of these patterns on information processing (e.g., attentional retraining) might facilitate engagement in therapeutic tasks and augment their effectiveness (Verhees et al., 2019).

Attachment-based interventions for couples might also benefit from contextually priming security-enhancing mental representations before and during an intervention (see Chapter 3 for a detailed description of security-priming techniques). There is evidence that security priming improves attitudes toward relational therapies, mainly among highly attachment-insecure clients who tend to be reluctant to seek professional help (Millings et al., 2019). Moreover, security-priming techniques can momentarily mitigate distress and help partners complete in-session enactments that require sensitive responsiveness to each other's needs. In fact, insecure partners are likely to have difficulty managing distress during softening exercises or supporting each other during in-session enactments, and security priming might momentarily reduce these difficulties and allow partners to engage more fully in the therapeutic tasks.

Johnson (2019a) explicitly noted that sensitive and responsive therapists can by themselves prime feelings of security and act as a secure base from which partners can fully engage in the challenging and sometimes demanding therapeutic tasks. However, therapists could also take advantage of other techniques (e.g., security-enhancing pictures in the therapy room, guided imagination exercises) that increase felt security and augment the beneficial effects of their interventions. Future studies should determine whether the incorporation of security-priming techniques can improve the effectiveness of EFT and the HmT program.

Concluding Remarks

Nearly 50 years after Bowlby (1979) stated that couple relationships, particularly marriages, are often adults' most important attachment relationships, we can be assured, based on extensive research, that these relationships have the power to endow partners with a sense of security. We also know that applications of attachment theory and research can contribute to the strengthening and healthy functioning of adult couple relationships, as they have to the quality of parent–child relationships. As seen throughout this chapter, numerous laboratory experiments and longitudinal studies of dating and married couples indicate that although attachment insecurities can interfere with relationship quality and satisfaction, the presence of a sensitive and responsive partner can enhance a person's sense of attachment security. Moreover, attachment theory and research are being successfully applied in a particular kind of couple therapy (EFT) and in a couple relationship education program (HmT) aimed at improving relationship quality. Research conducted to date, while still preliminary in certain respects, provides encouraging evidence for the broaden-and-build effects of these interventions.

CHAPTER 7

An Attachment-Informed Approach to Individual Psychotherapy

Bowlby had in mind a variety of clinical phenomena when writing his trilogy on attachment, and as an active clinician himself, he understood the importance of clinical applications of psychological research. Still, he didn't write much about such applications during most of his career, preferring to understand and explain how attachment works before telling clinicians how to treat and prevent its malfunctions. Only in 1988, near the end of his life, did Bowlby summarize his ideas about applying attachment theory clinically, in a book titled *A Secure Base*. (The title was a homage to Mary Ainsworth, who coined that term.) He conceptualized the client–therapist relationship as an attachment bond and the therapist as a safe haven and secure base. As such, the therapist can help move clients toward greater felt security, with all of its positive implications for emotion regulation, mentalization, and interpersonal functioning (see Chapter 2). In attachment theory's terms, these are the broad aims of psychotherapy.

Over the past three decades, since the publication of *A Secure Base*, there has been an explosion of research examining security-enhancement processes within psychotherapy. These studies have shown convincingly that a sensitive and responsive therapist can facilitate calm exploration of and reflection on painful attachment-related experiences and maladaptive beliefs, and can contribute to the construction of a more secure pattern of attachment. Importantly for clinicians, these security-enhancement processes have been found to contribute beneficially to therapeutic processes and the achievement of desired outcomes. This impressive body of evidence has encouraged several clinicians to apply attachment theory systematically to the domain of individual psychotherapy, with the aim of strengthening clients' felt security in relation to the therapist as a key part of therapeutic change. In this chapter, we review evidence concerning security-enhancement processes in psychotherapy and describe therapeutic practices and psychotherapy modalities informed by attachment theory and research.

Security-Enhancement Processes within the Therapist–Client Relationship

According to Bowlby (1988), just as a sensitive and responsive mother induces a sense of attachment security in her child—thus facilitating the child's exploration of the world by making it clear that support will be available if needed—a therapist can encourage and bolster a client's felt security, which facilitates inner exploration and therapeutic progress. (Bowlby used the term *exploration*, already well established with reference to a parent providing a child with a "secure base for exploration," to refer to a client's exploration of memories, feelings, behavior patterns, and self-identity.) A therapist can be an important source of safe-haven support, comforting and reassuring emotionally troubled clients, abetting their coping efforts, and helping them manage the distress associated with articulating and exploring painful memories, current conflicts, and sources of doubt and confusion. Moreover, the therapist can be a secure base, encouraging, validating, valuing, and applauding clients' inner exploration, their efforts to understand their accumulated, and often forgotten, suppressed or misunderstood attachment experiences, and their attempts to identify and revise negatively biased beliefs and maladaptive ways of coping and relating. As therapy continues, the therapist can provide a secure base for a client's exploration of new possibilities in life outside the therapy setting.

Of course, not every therapeutic relationship involves an attachment bond, which is something that evolves only gradually and under certain conditions over time. The extent to which a client–therapist relationship fulfills the definitional criteria for an attachment bond after, say, 6 months of therapeutic sessions may be different from what it was in the initial phases of treatment. According to Mallinckrodt (2010), many client–therapist dyads that finish their work and meet the definitional criteria of an attachment bond do not start out meeting all of them. Indeed, much of the effort of therapy can be considered an effort to transform a weak bond into a strong attachment that inspires felt security and serves as a secure base for exploration (Mallinckrodt, 2010). Bowlby (1988) believed that due to the central role played by attachment insecurities in the genesis of emotional and relational difficulties, the creation of a safe and secure client–therapist relationship should be a major therapeutic goal in itself and a crucial mechanism of therapeutic change.

Bowlby (1988) discussed five therapeutic tasks that contribute to security enhancement. The first is to create a warm and comforting safe haven to which clients can confidently return whenever they feel distressed or confused, either during or between therapeutic sessions. This task, best represented by the welcoming and holding hands in the circle-of-security diagram (see Chapter 4, Figure 4.1), is a precondition for the entire therapeutic process. Without such a safe haven, clients are likely to be afraid to explore and disclose thoughts and feelings, instead remaining closed, distrustful, or ambivalent about the therapist's intentions and interventions. Moreover, if a therapist is unable to provide clients with confidence that they can rely on him or her when needed, the therapist will not be able to create a relationship that clients experience as refreshingly and therapeutically different from previous ones, which were likely characterized by disinterest, rejection, or unpredictability. In Bowlby's words, "The therapist strives to be reliable, attentive, and sympathetically responsive to his patient's exploration, and so far as he can, to see and feel the world through his patient's eyes, namely to be empathic" (p. 152). (Unfortunately, writing in British English in the 1980s, Bowlby used the "general he" to refer to infants, therapists, and clients. We have chosen not to edit quotations to update this style.)

The other four tasks involve the therapist's provision of secure-base support: helping, encouraging, and empowering clients to delve deeply into fully or partially occluded memories and distorted wishes and feelings, resulting in expanded self-understanding. These tasks are best represented by the encouraging and celebrating hands in the circle-of-security diagram (see Chapter 4, Figure 4.1). The process of exploration in psychotherapy is bound to be frequently difficult and painful, because the client must confront long-forgotten or defensively distorted experiences and strong emotions, and explore perplexities that he or she has been unable to face, manage, or understand alone. Only when accompanied and empowered by a sensitive and engaged therapist can a client explore, uncover, and understand deep-seated fears, well-practiced defenses, and distorted perceptions. Allen (2012) aptly recalled that he "once remarked in a trauma-education group, 'The mind can be a scary place.' A patient quipped, 'Yes, and you wouldn't want to go in there alone!' "

These four therapeutic tasks include supporting and encouraging clients as they consider how their working models of self and others influence the way they think, feel, and act in relationships, including the therapeutic relationship. They also involve helping clients assess how current thoughts, feelings, and behaviors may have originated in childhood experiences with parents or other caregivers, or in subsequent relationships with important partners. Finally, therapists must help clients consider ways in which their historically influenced modes of thinking and behaving are poorly adapted to their current lives, and to imagine and practice alternative, healthier ways of coping and interacting.

Cobb and Davila (2009) noted that because attachment-related working models are at least partially unconscious, clients need a therapist's support, encouragement, and, sometimes, guidance if they are to become aware of previously unrecognized biases and failed relational strategies. Clients also need a therapist to provide reality-testing tools that reveal the dysfunctional nature and destructive consequences of misguided working models. In most cases, clients have a long history of self-destructively misinterpreting their own goals and actions, generating the opposite of the emotional outcomes intended, and hurting other people with whom they hoped to have mutually rewarding relationships (Cobb & Davila, 2009).

Bowlby (1988) stressed the importance of two kinds of exploratory ventures: delving into past relationship experiences and analyzing current behaviors and experiences, including with the therapist. Exploration of past attachment experiences helps clients become more aware of how they construe and distort current relationships, and exploring current relationships helps them reflect on earlier attachment experiences. However, for the most part, Bowlby recommended that therapists focus on interactions in present-day relationships as well as here-and-now therapist–client interactions, exploring the past "only for the light it throws on [the client's] current ways of feeling and dealing with life" (p. 141). (This was in contrast to the potentially endless, unfocused past recollections practiced by some of Bowlby's psychoanalytic predecessors and contemporary colleagues.) Bowlby also recommended approaching clients as knowledgeable partners, trusting them to engage in the work necessary for change, and being aware that clients' perceptions of a therapist are shaped not only by working models (i.e., by transference) but also by the way the therapist actually treats them.

Figure 7.1 summarizes the interpersonal and intrapersonal processes underlying security enhancement within psychotherapy. At the interpersonal level, a therapist's sensitive provision of safe-haven and secure-base forms of support and the resulting development of a client's secure attachment to the therapist can activate a broaden-and-build cycle of security that has positive repercussions for the therapist–client relationship, the therapeutic work, and eventual therapeutic outcomes. At the intrapersonal level, this broaden-and-build cycle, empowered by a caring and skillful therapist, can sustain a client's effective emotion regulation and inner exploration (see Chapter 2) and fortify a collaborative relationship with the therapist. It can also result in more accurate reflection on clients' own and others' feelings, thoughts, and intentions (increased *mentalization*) and the creation of more reality-attuned working models. The combination of these interrelated intrapersonal processes helps to shape and consolidate more secure patterns of attachment outside the therapy room, which in turn further strengthens broaden-and-build processes within the therapy relationship. Figure 7.1 also includes attachment-related factors, such as clients' and therapists' pretherapy attachment insecurities, which can interfere with security enhancement and therapeutic change.

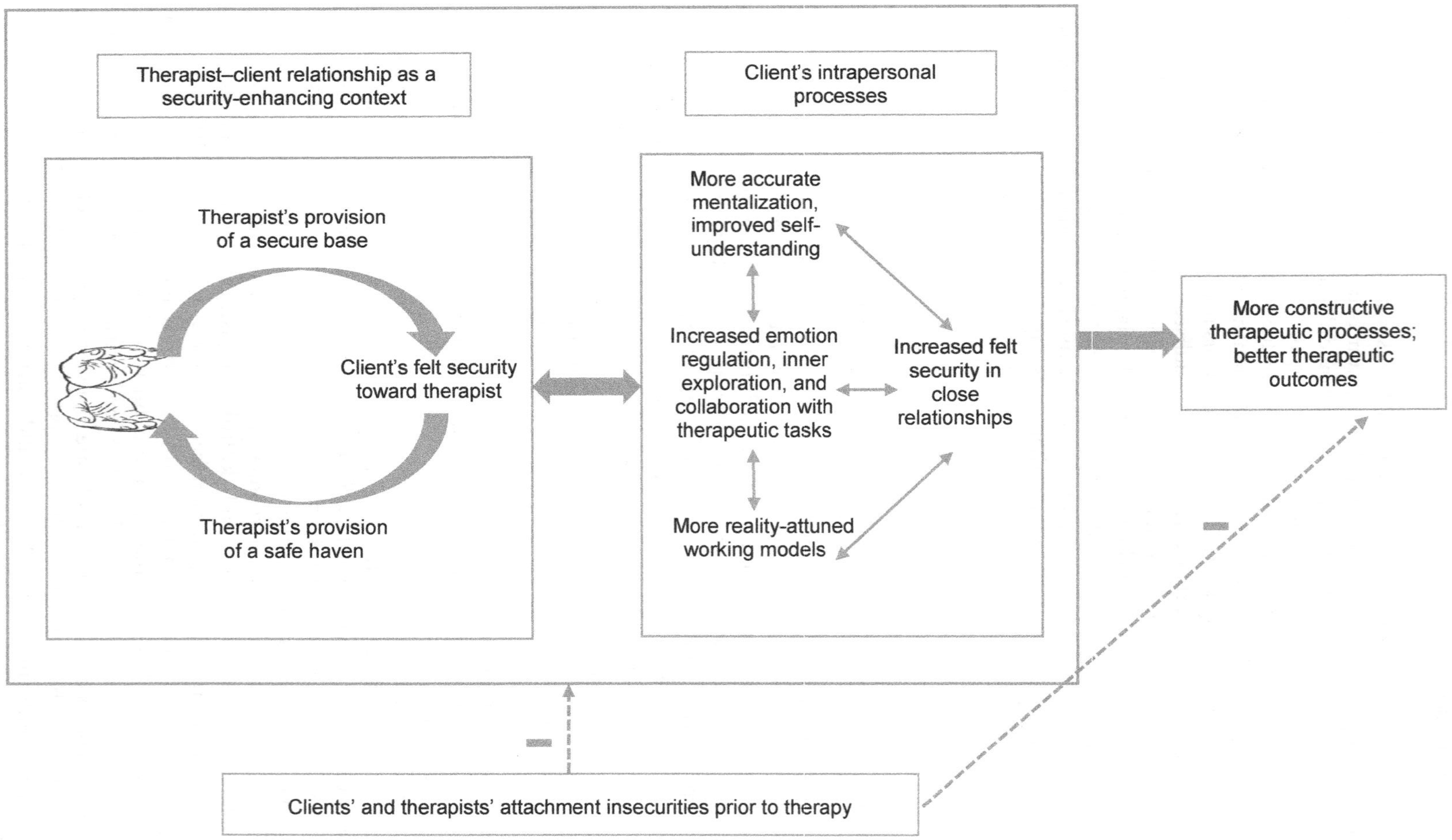

FIGURE 7.1. Security-enhancement processes within psychotherapy.

In the following sections, we review studies examining the processes summarized in Figure 7.1. We first review evidence that a certain kind of client–therapist relationship can be a security-enhancing context that contributes to beneficial therapeutic developments and outcomes. We then present data concerning intrapersonal changes in clients' mentalization and attachment security over the course of therapy and the implications of these changes for therapeutic outcomes. We also review evidence that the attachment insecurities that clients and therapists bring to therapy can interfere with the formation of a secure client–therapist bond and retard therapeutic change. For clinicians, this review provides an empirical basis for designing specific attachment-informed practices that increase the effectiveness of their therapeutic work, regardless of their theoretical orientation (e.g., psychodynamic, cognitive-behavioral, or humanistic).

The Therapist–Client Relationship as a Security-Enhancing Context

When considering the validity of Bowlby's (1988) claims about the security-enhancing qualities of the client–therapist relationship and their implications for therapeutic change, we need to answer two important questions:

1. Can a sensitive and responsive therapist increase a client's felt security?
2. Is the formation of a client's secure attachment to a therapist an important step in enhancing therapeutic change?

In the following sections, we review studies addressing these questions.

The Therapist's Responsiveness and Clients' Felt Security

Clients typically enter therapy in a state of frustration, anxiety, or demoralization, which naturally causes them to yearn for support and relief. Attachment needs are easily directed toward therapists, because therapists, at least when a client believes in their healing powers, are perceived as "stronger and wiser" caregivers, possessing the hallmarks of a good attachment figure. Therapists are expected to know better than their clients how to deal with the clients' problems, and they occupy the caregiving role in the relationship. Therefore, clients naturally seek their therapist's support, and a therapist's skilled performance as a sensitive and responsive caregiver is likely to have beneficial effects on clients' felt security (see Chapter 2).

To date, only a few studies have directly examined the idea that a therapist's sensitive responsiveness increases clients' felt security. Three studies involved coding behavioral markers of the therapist's responsiveness and attunement to clients' affects or nonverbal gestures (nonverbal synchrony) within therapeutic sessions. All three studies found that these markers are associated with a reduction in clients' attachment insecurities over the course of therapy (Håvås et al., 2015; Ramseyer & Tschacher, 2011; Schoenherr et al., 2021). For example, Håvås et al. (2015) video-recorded an early session of therapy with clients diagnosed with personality disorders and had trained observers rate the therapist's attunement to the client's affects. They found that a therapist's degree of nonverbal attunement to the client's affects during the early session predicted a decrease in the client's reports of attachment-related avoidance by the end of therapy (compared to the pretherapy level of avoidance). Moreover, nonverbal affect attunement and a therapist's nonverbal expressions of regard for a client's experiences during the early session predicted a decrease in attachment anxiety over the course of therapy. In other words, this aspect of a therapist's work increases a client's attachment security.

In another study, Watson et al. (2014) examined the security-enhancing effects of clients' perception of their therapist as an empathic, understanding, and caring figure. Clients who received a 15-session course of therapy for depression rated their therapist's sensitivity after the ninth and 12th therapeutic sessions. They also completed a self-report scale measuring attachment security before and after therapy. Clients who perceived their therapist as more sensitive were more likely to show pre- to posttherapy increases in attachment security. These findings parallel those of studies on parent–child relationships and couple relationships reviewed in Chapters 4–6, and they imply that the link between perceived caregiver responsiveness and subsequent felt attachment security is established within psychotherapy.

More extensive data have been collected on the positive implications of a therapist's sensitive responsiveness for therapeutic work and outcomes (for reviews and meta-analyses, see Elliott et al., 2018; Farber et al., 2018). For example, Zuroff and Blatt (2006) analyzed clients' ratings of their therapist's accurate empathy (e.g., "nearly always knows what I mean"), positive regard (e.g., "feels a true liking for me"), and genuineness (e.g., "is comfortable and at ease in our relationship") during therapy and found that these ratings predicted relief from depression at the end of therapy and 18 months later, regardless of the type of therapy employed (interpersonal therapy or CBT). These findings have been replicated and extended in several studies assessing therapists' expressions of positive regard, acceptance, and nonpossessive warmth, as rated by either clients or external observers (e.g., Barnicot et al., 2014; Bedics et al., 2012; Zuroff et al., 2010). Based on a recent meta-analysis of 64 studies (3,528 clients), Farber et al. (2018) reported a significant moderate association between therapists' expressions of positive regard and positive therapeutic outcomes.

A number of studies have indicated that a therapist's accuracy in identifying and addressing a client's emotions (empathic sensitivity) within a therapeutic session is associated with clients' positive evaluations of the session and with more therapeutic progress in the long run (e.g., Atzil-Slonim et al., 2018; Duan & Kivlighan, 2002; Kwon & Jo, 2012). Moreover, clients of a more sensitive and empathic therapist (as rated by clients or external observers) are more likely to form a trusting and cooperative relationship with the therapist (e.g., Malin & Pos, 2015; McClintock et al., 2018; Murphy & Cramer, 2014). In a meta-analysis of 82 studies (6,138 clients), Elliott et al. (2018) found a strong association between therapist's sensitivity and the quality of the therapeutic relationship.

There is also evidence that appraising a therapist as a responsive figure facilitates the successful resolution of in-session disagreements and conflicts (Ben David-Sela et al., 2021; Eubanks et al., 2021). In Ben David-Sela et al.'s (2021) study, for example, clients rated their therapist's supportiveness four times during therapy (Weeks 1, 3, 5, and 7), and judges watched videotapes of the next-week therapy session (Weeks 2, 4, 6, and 8) and coded behavioral markers of ruptures in the therapist–client relationship, as well as markers of successful resolution of the ruptures within the session. Perceiving the therapist as more supportive in a given session was associated with more successful resolution of relational ruptures during the next session. It seems that a therapist's supportiveness (at least as perceived by clients) sustains collaborative therapeutic work even during moments of emotional friction.

The Therapeutic Benefits of Clients' Felt Security in Relation to Their Therapist

In applying attachment theory to psychotherapy, Mallinckrodt et al. (1995) developed the Client Attachment to Therapist Scale (CATS), which assesses (1) secure attachment to the therapist (confidence in the therapist's availability and responsiveness when needed), (2) avoidant attachment to a therapist (distrust of the therapist, being reluctant to self-disclose in therapy), and (3) anxious attachment to a therapist (longing to be at one with the therapist and worrying about his or her approval and love). Importantly, although clients' CATS scores might have been thought merely to reflect their global attachment orientations prior to therapy, studies have consistently yielded only low to moderate correlations between those two constructs (e.g., Arbuckle et al., 2012; Wiseman & Tishby, 2014). In fact, a meta-analysis of nine studies examining this association yielded effects sizes ranging from only 0.12 to 0.18 (Mallinckrodt & Jeong, 2015). Hence, clients' felt security in relation to their therapist may, as hoped, be shaped by other factors, such as the therapist's responsiveness, rather than being a mere generalization (or projection) of pretherapy dominant working models.

There is mounting evidence that clients' felt security in relation to their therapist (as measured by the CATS) is associated with better therapeutic outcomes (e.g., Fuertes et al., 2007; Petrowski et al., 2019; Sauer et al., 2010). For example, Sauer et al. assessed attachment to therapist at the third therapy session and administered a standardized measure of distress at intake, the third session, and at therapy termination. Findings indicate that the CATS security score was associated with greater reduction in clients' distress over the course of therapy. In addition, clients who scored higher on the CATS Anxiety subscale (indicating anxious attachment to the therapist) were more likely to show increases in distress over the course of therapy.

Mallinckrodt et al. (2017) raised two important qualifications in their discussion of the therapeutic benefits of clients' felt security in relation to their therapist. First, these benefits are most likely to be observed when the clients' anxious attachment to the therapist is low (what Mallinckrodt et al. called *individuated-secure attachment*) but not when clients show signs of anxious hyperactivation within therapeutic sessions, such as demanding that the therapist disclose his or her personal feelings and thoughts or experiencing intense distress when the therapist is unavailable (*pseudo-secure attachment*). Second, the beneficial effects of secure attachment to the therapist are especially strong for clients who hold negative working models of others before therapy. According to Mallinckrodt et al., moving a client who is reluctant to rely on others in times of need to trust a therapist's benevolence and to comfortably approach him or her during a therapeutic session seems to be one of the strongest predictors of therapeutic change.

Clients' felt security with respect to their therapist (in the CATS) has also been found to contribute to the formation of what Bordin (1979) called a *therapist–client working alliance*—agreeing with the therapist about therapy's tasks and goals, and adopting a trusting and collaborative stance toward therapy (e.g., Bachelor et al., 2010; Mallinckrodt et al., 2015; Yotsidi et al., 2019). In their meta-analysis, Mallinckrodt and Jeong (2015) found a strong association between the CATS security score and the strength of the working alliance (as rated by clients, therapists, or observers). Moreover, research shows that clients' felt security with respect to a therapist facilitates the successful resolution of inevitable ruptures in the working alliance, which occur during moments when clients and therapists are out of sync. Using the Patient Attachment Coding System (PACS; Talia et al., 2014)—an observer-rated measure of in-session behavioral markers of a client's attachment to a therapist—Miller-Bottome et al. (2019) found that higher scores on a measure of secure attachment in a given session predicted successful repair of alliance ruptures during that session (as rated by the client or the therapist).

Developing a secure attachment to a therapist also helps clients explore and share personal issues (e.g., Mallinckrodt et al., 2005; Romano et al., 2008; Saypol & Farber, 2010). For example, Saypol and Farber found that clients who felt more secure in relation to their therapist were more likely to disclose personal issues during therapeutic sessions (as rated by observers) and to feel good after the disclosure. Similarly, Mallinckrodt et al. (2005) reported that clients who felt more secure in relation to their therapist were more likely to engage in in-session exploration of inner experiences and to perceive therapeutic sessions as smooth and deep. Notably, these associations could not be explained by ratings of the working alliance and seemed to be a unique reflection of the sense of security clients experienced in relation to their therapist.

Overall, the reviewed studies provide positive answers to the two questions we asked regarding the potential security-enhancing properties of the client–therapist relationship. First, a therapist's responsiveness can enhance a client's felt security with regard to the therapist. Second, a therapist's responsiveness and the resulting formation of a within-therapy secure attachment contribute to constructive therapeutic processes and positive therapeutic outcomes.

Intrapersonal Attachment-Related Changes over the Course of Psychotherapy

The observed positive effects of clients' secure attachment to their therapist on therapeutic processes (e.g., working alliance, self-disclosure, inner exploration) seem to reflect the underlying action of the broaden-and-build cycle of attachment security. As reviewed in Chapter 2, this cycle favors endorsement of pro-relational, collaborative attitudes and behaviors, and confident engagement in exploratory ventures, even if these involve perplexity and uncertainty. Within psychotherapy, this cycle can increase clients' mentalization of their own and others' internal states, which can broaden and improve their understanding of what happened to them in the past and what is happening to them "here and now" inside and outside the therapy room. Moreover, clients can become better able to revise insecure working models, because they now have the skills, knowledge, and strength necessary to understand that early models of negative attachment experiences are not accurate or adequate representations of current relational experiences. All of these intrapersonal processes can bolster clients' global sense of attachment security, which further allows and sustains inner exploration, accurate mentalization, and therapeutic change (see Figure 7.1).

In the following sections, we review evidence concerning these intrapersonal processes. Specifically, we show that psychotherapy can improve mentalization and promote more secure attachment patterns, and that these changes contribute to positive clinical outcomes.

Changes in Clients' Mentalization during the Course of Therapy

In a pioneering study, Levy et al. (2006) assessed markers of clients' mentalization in response to the AAI (using Fonagy et al.'s [1991] *reflective functioning score*) at the onset and after 12 months of transference-focused psychotherapy for borderline personality disorder. They found that clients' mentalization improved over the course of therapy. Moreover, this improvement was associated with enhanced attachment security by the end of therapy (as also assessed with the AAI).

Subsequent studies employed Levy et al.'s (2006) methodology and found that among clients with diverse mental disorders and across different therapeutic modalities, improvement in clients' mentalization over the course of therapy was associated with positive changes in symptom severity, global distress, and personality organization (e.g., Chiesa et al., 2021; Fischer-Kern et al., 2015; Katznelson et al., 2020). Importantly, this association was also observed using different methods of assessing changes in clients' mentalization over the course of therapy, such as the Reflective Functioning Questionnaire, the Metacognition

Assessment Interview, or markers of mentalization in transcripts of therapeutic sessions (e.g., Carcione et al., 2019; De Meulemeester et al., 2018; Maillard et al., 2020).

A related line of research has focused on self-understanding—"patients' understanding of associations between past and present experiences, typical relationship patterns, and the relation between interpersonal challenges, emotional experience, and psychological symptoms" (Jennissen et al., 2018, p. 966). Several studies have found that pre- to post-therapy improvement in self-understanding (as rated by clients or observers) is associated with more positive therapeutic outcomes (see Jennissen et al., 2018, for a meta-analysis). Moreover, increases in clients' self-understanding in a given session are followed by lower complaint ratings in the following session (Kivlighan et al., 2000). And when therapists reported having used more interventions aimed at increasing clients' self-understanding within a session (e.g., drawing clients' attention to knowledge they already possessed but viewing it in a new light), clients reported less symptomatic distress following that session (Fisher et al., 2020). Importantly, this association was mediated by clients' own reports of self-understanding during the session.

Changes in Clients' Attachment Patterns during Therapy

Although attachment states of mind (assessed with the AAI) or self-reports of attachment orientations in close relationships reflect relatively stable patterns of relating, psychotherapy can move clients away from insecure and toward secure patterns (Taylor et al., 2015). In two separate studies, Blatt et al. (1996) and Harpaz-Rotem and Blatt (2005) assessed the severity of psychopathology of seriously disturbed, hospitalized adolescents at the beginning and end of long-term intensive therapy. In addition, Blatt et al. (1996) assessed changes in the structure of the adolescents' descriptions of mother, father, self, and therapist across the course of therapy, whereas Harpaz-Rotem and Blatt (2005) assessed changes in the description of a significant other whom each patient elected to describe at the beginning and end of treatment. In both studies, there were increases in the coherence of attachment-related representations over the course of therapy—a definitional component of attachment security (Hesse, 2016)—and these differences were associated with symptom relief.

Several researchers have directly assessed clients' attachment states of mind or self-reports of attachment orientations before and after therapy, and have found positive changes in attachment security (but see Strauss et al., 2011, for an exception). Fonagy et al. (1996) reported that a significant proportion of psychiatric patients receiving psychodynamic psychotherapy changed to a secure attachment state of mind in the AAI over the course of treatment. And Travis et al. (2001) found an increase in clients' self-reports of secure attachment over the course of time-limited dynamic psychotherapy, and this increase was associated with decreases in the severity of symptoms. Similar findings have been reported in studies of clients receiving transference-focused psychotherapy for borderline personality disorder (Diamond et al., 2003; Levy et al., 2006; Tmej et al., 2021), clients receiving interpersonal psychotherapy for depression (Gunlicks-Stoessel et al., 2019; Ravitz et al., 2008; Y. Zhou et al., 2021), and clients receiving psychotherapy for PTSD or domestic violence (Lawson et al., 2006; Muller & Rosenkranz, 2009).

The Interfering Effects of Clients' and Therapists' Attachment Insecurities

Although the findings we have reviewed so far indicate that a sensitive and responsive therapist can augment felt security in his or her clients and cultivate a broaden-and-build cycle of security within therapeutic sessions, we are quick to acknowledge that security enhancement can be disrupted by attachment insecurities that some clients and therapists bring to therapy. These insecurities can prevent the formation of a secure client–therapist bond, interfere with constructive therapeutic work, and militate against therapeutic change. Of course, a skillful and responsive therapist can try to sensitively manage client's insecurities and move forward with in-session security-enhancement processes. Moreover, therapists may be able to understand and moderate their own insecurities (through mentalizing) and prevent them from negatively biasing their reactions to clients (*countertransference*). These issues have been empirically studied.

Clients' Pretherapy Attachment Insecurities

Clients' subjective construal of the therapist as an attachment figure can result not only in the therapist being a target of proximity seeking but also in the arousal of attachment-related worries, defenses, and hostile projections. For many attachment-insecure clients, the therapeutic relationship can reactivate core attachment-related fears and negative views of others, which in turn can create negative cognitive and emotional reactions to the therapist. Both psychoanalytic theorists and social-cognitive researchers refer to this process as *transference* (e.g., Greenson, 1967; Miranda & Andersen, 2010). This generalization (or projection) of pretherapy attachment insecurities can sometimes not only disrupt therapeutic work but it also may offer an opportunity for a skillful and sensitive therapist to make useful observations and interventions that provide clients with greater self-insight.

Clients' pretherapy attachment insecurities are likely to interfere with the formation and maintenance of a trusting working alliance with a therapist. Although anxious clients' desire for connection and intimacy may cause them to agree readily with their therapist about the goals and tasks of therapy, their relational ambivalence can create obstacles to therapeutic work. Moreover, their hunger for attention and care; misinterpretation of others' responses as signs of disapproval, rejection, or criticism; and unregulated outbursts of frustration or anger (Mikulincer & Shaver, 2016) can increase the frequency and intensity of ruptures in the therapeutic relationship. The working alliance can also be hindered by avoidant clients' distrust of others and reluctance to engage in intimate exchanges or to deepen interdependence with the therapist. Avoidant people's desire for self-reliance can work against accepting a therapist's suggestions regarding therapeutic goals and tasks, while their defensive privacy shield may prevent constructive discussions concerning client–therapist disagreements and resolution of ruptures in the working alliance.

As expected, clients' pretherapy attachment insecurities tend to impair the quality of in-session interactions with a therapist. For example, clients' reports of attachment anxiety prior to therapy are associated with observers' ratings of lower client in-session engagement in complementary interactions (e.g., friendliness followed by friendliness) and movement synchrony (e.g., changing sitting posture after a therapist underlines his or her speech with gestures) with a therapist (Maxwell et al., 2012; Schoenherr et al., 2021). In other in-session studies of clients in psychodynamic psychotherapy, trained observers rated avoidant clients (assessed with the AAI) as seeking less contact and proximity to the therapist, talking less during the session, and having shorter speaking turns (Daniel et al., 2018; Egozi et al., 2021; Talia et al., 2014). Attachment-anxious clients (per the AAI) were rated by trained observers as more likely to resist therapists' interventions, to seek more proximity to the therapist, and to show more in-session fluctuations in mood states (Egozi et al., 2021; Talia et al., 2014; Woodhouse & Gelso, 2008). Gupta et al. (2018) analyzed 814 clients' in-session occurrences of laughter and found that independent observers rated the laughter of more avoidant clients as less cheerful and more contemptuous and the laughter of more attachment-anxious clients as more nervous.

Clients' mental representations of a therapist tend to be biased by their attachment insecurities prior to therapy. For example, self-reports of attachment-related avoidance prior to therapy are associated with perceptions of the therapist as "too close" at the midpoint or termination of therapy, whereas self-reports of attachment anxiety are associated with perception of the therapist as "too distant" (Mallinckrodt et al., 2015). Using the Therapist Representation Inventory, Geller and Farber (2015) found that more insecure clients, either anxious or avoidant, expressed more doubts about the soothing abilities of the therapist. Among avoidant clients, these doubts were coupled with persecutory images of a malevolent and hostile therapist—a direct projection of their negative working models of others. But among attachment-anxious clients, these doubts about the therapist's competence were coupled with a strong desire for a personal relationship with him or her beyond the therapy room despite these doubts—an example of their relational ambivalence and intense proximity seeking.

On this basis, one can understand the frequently observed finding that clients' pretherapy attachment insecurities impair the quality of the therapeutic relationship, as evident in clients' or therapists' reports regarding the strength of their alliance or independent observers' ratings of behavioral markers of in-session alliance (e.g., Coyne et al., 2018; Eames & Roth, 2000; Folke et al., 2016). But three meta-analyses (Bernecker et al., 2014; Diener et al., 2009; Diener & Monroe, 2011) yielded only small, though significant, correlations between clients' attachment insecurities and working alliance (ranging between .12 and .17). It seems that although clients' attachment insecurities prior to therapy may interfere to some extent with the formation of a trusting therapeutic relationship, they do not seem to be a crucial factor, perhaps because of the compensatory effects of a sensitive and responsive therapist.

Attachment insecurities measured before therapy can also interfere with positive clinical outcomes at the end of therapy (e.g., Reiner et al., 2016; Smith et al., 2012; Wiseman & Tishby, 2014). For example, Byrd et al. (2010) used archival data from 66 psychotherapy clients treated at a university graduate program training clinic and found that self-reports of avoidant attachment prior to therapy were associated with poor psychotherapy outcomes, and that problems in the working alliance were a partial mediator of the association between avoidance and outcome. Sauer et al. (2020) evaluated session-by-session changes in distress from the beginning to the end of therapy and found that more attachment-anxious clients exhibited lower levels of improvement throughout the middle period of therapy. In two meta-analyses of 14 and 36 studies (1,467 and 3,158 clients), Levy et al. (2011, 2018) found a moderate to strong association between clients' pretherapy attachment insecurities and poorer clinical outcomes.

Therapists' Attachment Insecurities

Therapists' attachment insecurities can also interfere with therapeutic work. Whereas a secure therapist should generally find it easy to occupy the role of security provider and create a good working alliance, even with a difficult client, an insecure therapist is likely to complicate the therapeutic process. Whereas avoidant therapists may lack the skills needed to provide sensitive care and promote emotional bonds with clients, attachment-anxious therapists may experience a desire to merge or lose boundaries with clients and have difficulty regulating emotions, which can obviously interfere with objectivity and the creation of a calm and relaxed therapeutic climate. As a result, insecure therapists may be less able to remain open to their clients' needs and more susceptible to the negative countertransference reactions that insecure clients frequently evoke.

Research findings support these expectations. Clients of more attachment-insecure therapists are more likely to report a weak working alliance during therapy (e.g., Black et al., 2005; Dinger et al., 2009; Sauer et al., 2003). In addition, more attachment-insecure therapists are less likely to appraise their relationship with a client as a real and genuine interpersonal bond and tend to be less empathic with their client's feelings and more critical and rejecting, especially when paired with insecure clients (Fuertes et al., 2019; Mohr et al., 2005; Rubino et al., 2000). There is also evidence that more avoidant therapists are less able to reflect on their client's mental states and are less accurate in understanding clients' problems (Berry et al., 2008).

In a study of in-session ruptures in the therapist–client working alliance, Marmarosh et al. (2015) examined the contribution of therapists' self-reports of attachment insecurities to the way they react to these ruptures. Specifically, novice therapists completed a measure tapping perceptions of ruptures and repairs following the eighth session with their first clients. More attachment-anxious therapists reported more in-session ruptures, felt more tension during the rupture, and were more likely to expend effort in trying to heal the damaged bond. However, despite these increased efforts, anxious therapists were not more likely to report rupture repair.

Research Summary

In line with expectations based on attachment theory, there is evidence that clients' sense of attachment security, either therapist-specific or global, can be enhanced over the course of therapy and positively contribute to therapeutic processes and outcomes. Moreover, we reviewed findings that security enhancement within psychotherapy is closely associated with a therapist's sensitive responsiveness and a client's increasing in-session inner exploration and mentalization over the course of therapy. Research also highlights the importance of dealing with clients' and therapists' insecurities, because they can interfere with successful therapeutic outcomes.

Therapeutic Applications of Attachment Theory and Research

To date, partly based on the large body of research reviewed in the previous sections, many clinicians from different therapeutic orientations view attachment theory as an important framework for making sense of clients' histories, discourse and thought patterns, and relationship difficulties, and as a rich source of information concerning therapeutic processes and outcomes. However, whereas attachment theory and research have informed the practice of psychotherapy and provided a basis for the development of several therapeutic approaches, there is no distinct school of therapy for adult clients called "attachment therapy." Unlike Freud, Rogers, or Beck, Bowlby did not create a detailed clinical model for practice, only a rough outline of the therapeutic tasks involved in providing clients with a secure base for exploration. He believed that clinicians, regardless of their therapeutic orientation, could improve their therapeutic work by incorporating insights from attachment theory and research, such as the importance of clients' attachment needs, the ways in which these needs play out in the client–therapist relationship, and the therapeutic implications of a therapist's sensitive responsiveness (Costello, 2013; Eagle 2017; Wiseman, 2017).

With this kind of perspective in mind, Obegi and Berant (2009) identified two broad types of clinical applications of attachment theory. The first, which they called *attachment-informed psychotherapy* and we prefer to call *attachment-informed therapeutic practices*, refers to the use of attachment-related concepts and research findings to inform and supplement clinical practices based on some other established clinical approach (e.g., CBT). The second, which Obegi and Berant called *attachment-based psychotherapy* and Levy and Johnson (2019) called *attachment-based interventions,* refers to interventions that explicitly draw upon attachment theory in conceptualizing the client–therapist relationship and specific therapeutic tasks and goals (e.g., interpersonal therapy, accelerated experiential dynamic psychotherapy, mentalization-based treatment). As Obegi and Berant stated, "All of these therapies are related to attachment theory in the same way that cognitive-behavioral therapy (CBT), for example, is related to cognitive theory" (p. 3). In the following sections, we present the basics of attachment-informed therapeutic practices, followed by a brief review of some of the most important attachment-based interventions, as well as research findings regarding their effectiveness.

Attachment-Informed Therapeutic Practices

Attachment-informed therapeutic practices are mainly directed at enhancing clients' felt security rather than explicitly dealing with their poor self-esteem, dysfunctional obsessive thoughts and compulsions, or deficits in emotion regulation or interpersonal skills—problematic areas that can be tackled by other, already-existing therapeutic techniques. In fact, according to attachment theory and research, felt security can have positive effects in any of these areas and can facilitate therapeutic change (Cobb & Davila, 2009). There is little in attachment theory that elevates the importance of one of these problematic areas above the others or that privileges one set of therapeutic techniques over another. The single principle that attachment-informed clinicians follow is to fortify the broaden-and-build cycle of security by (1) creating an in-session climate of security that relieves stress, inspires hope, and increases trust and collaboration, and (2) supporting and encouraging inner exploration, accurate reflection on maladaptive working models, and experimentation with new ways of relating and coping.

Creating a Climate of Security

Above all, attachment-informed therapists endeavor to create an in-session *climate of security,* without which broaden-and-build processes cannot proceed. Such a climate requires certain therapeutic attitudes and practices, many of which overlap with those described by Rogers (1961) in his eloquent description of what it means to practice humanistic experiential psychotherapy. In attachment terms, these are defining features of security-enhancing attachment figures (see Chapter 2). Thus, adopting an attachment-informed approach means endeavoring to be consistently trustworthy, dependable, and emotionally available, responsive, and engaged during therapy sessions. It also means creating a permissive and sufficiently accepting setting where clients can disclose as freely as they are able. They should be able to feel confident that they will not be shamed or invalidated as they disclose their problems and concerns.

Creating a security-enhancing climate also requires assuaging clients' distress, at least to some degree (safe-haven support). This may come in the form of acceptance, reassurance, understanding, validation, positive regard, nonjudgmental listening, and an active focus early in treatment on symptom reduction. These and other practices communicate to clients that a wise, kind, reliable, and committed person is on their side. Over time, this should engender clients' confidence that help is available, that emotional balance and equanimity can be restored, and that crises can be weathered with the support and encouragement of a security-enhancing therapist. According to Slade and Holmes (2019), attachment-informed therapists "adopt a position of 'radical acceptance' of clients' adaptations and their necessity for survival, especially when patients are very disturbed. These capacities are crucial to diminishing the threat patients feel in addressing their pain and suffering, and allowing themselves to trust the therapist" (p. 154).

We should also mention a promising technique that may be worth adding to an attachment-informed toolbox for creating a climate of security: contextually priming security-enhancing mental representations during therapeutic sessions and between sessions (see Chapter 3). Therapists, for example, can ask clients to visualize a loving and kind relationship partner within the session or to reflect and write about particular comforting, supportive interactions with this figure at home between sessions. As reviewed in Chapter 3, a substantial amount of research suggests that these techniques jump-start broaden-and-build processes by momentarily instilling a sense of attachment security. Specifically, these techniques might facilitate distress regulation and increase curiosity, exploration, and endorsement of a pro-relational collaborative stance, all of which can facilitate therapeutic work and outcomes.

Handling Clients' Attachment Insecurities

Another component of attachment-informed therapeutic practices is to customize treatment based on each client's specific attachment dynamics. Attachment-informed clinicians conscientiously attend to in-session manifestations of clients' attachment needs, fears, and defenses, and tailor their responses to provide the most effective intervention for dealing with the observed attachment insecurities and softening their destructive consequences. For example, early in treatment, anxious and avoidant clients differ in what constitutes a comfortable therapeutic distance, and the levels of validation and reassurance desired by anxious clients might be perceived as noxious by avoidant clients, causing them to drop out before treatment makes much headway (Mallinckrodt et al., 2009). Therefore, with the aim of creating a secure bond early in therapy, attachment-informed therapists attempt to meet anxious clients' needs for reassurance and validation, while being empathic with, and respectful of, avoidant clients' need to feel self-reliant (see Chapter 6 for similar *safe/softening* strategies within couple relationships). However, once a fairly secure bond is established, therapists can gradually shift toward a more optimal therapeutic distance and gently challenge clients by responding "out of style" to their attachment dynamics (Mallinckrodt et al., 2009).

According to Mallinckrodt (2000), attachment-informed therapists need to be aware and sensitive when clients feel sufficiently safe and secure within therapy to accept and digest what he called *counter-complementary attachment proximity strategies*—interventions that challenge clients' habitual attachment-related expectations and inclinations. At these potential turning points, therapists' reactions can gently collide with clients' attachment-related demands and gradually disconfirm their expectations and maladaptive patterns of relating. This collision provides an opportunity for corrective emotional experiences, inner exploration, and revision of insecure working models.

For avoidant clients, who prefer interpersonal distance and tend to encourage others' emotional detachment from them, corrective emotional experiences can be provided by therapists slightly increasing proximity and insisting on deepening clients' disclosures. For attachment-anxious clients, who prefer to remain in a somewhat infantile, dependent position, corrective emotional experiences can be provided mainly by therapists encouraging them to take a more autonomous stance in dealing with their problems. The anxious client's tendency to get emotionally caught up in chaotic recounting of past injuries and current conflicts can be gently countered by the therapist easing the client back to a calmer, more focused, more constructive dialogue. These therapists' responses resemble the security-enhancing attitudes and responses of romantic partners and spouses prescribed by Arriaga et al.'s (2018) attachment security enhancement model (see Chapter 6).

Daly and Mallinckrodt (2009) interviewed 12 therapists about ways in which they deal with clients' attachment insecurities, finding that most of them relied on these counter-complementary attachment proximity strategies to challenge clients' working models and facilitate therapeutic change. Moreover, Tyrrell et al. (1999) reported that more avoidant clients found more helpful the therapists who increased relational closeness and deepened emotional experiencing over the course of therapy, whereas attachment-anxious clients found more helpful the therapists who supported their capacity for autonomy and self-reliance. According to Slade and Holmes (2019):

> The expression of negative emotions is helpful to clients with avoidant attachment styles, but less so with preoccupied [anxious] clients. Here, "dwelling in the negative" is a habitual stance, which can be reinforced by therapists' relentless emphasis on rage/anger/envy, and so on. Therapists' capacity to notice and encourage a "Dutchman's breeches" smidgeon of blue in an otherwise overcast emotional sky can be an important skill. Overall, with dismissing clients, the aim is "breaking" rigid, emotionless accounts; with the preoccupied [i.e., anxious] and disorganized, it is "making" coherent stories out of overwhelming, unbounded, and chaotic emotions. (p. 154)

Although these counter-complementary attachment proximity strategies are useful ways to foster therapeutic change, we should acknowledge that their enactment is a challenging task for therapists, one that involves direct confrontation with clients' habitual relational inclinations and their methods of pulling interaction partners into particular familiar positions. Dozier and Tyrell (1998) explained that therapists should themselves have a solid sense of security in order to be able to respond to a client in a counter-complementary manner. According to Mallinckrodt (2000), this approach requires considerable interpersonal sensitivity and responsiveness in understanding what clients may do to recreate familiar relational patterns in the therapeutic setting and how to break maladaptive patterns without overwhelming clients with anxiety.

Mallinckrodt (2000) used a creative analogy of control rods in a nuclear reactor to symbolize the extreme sensitivity needed for effective counter-complementary interventions: "If the rods are inserted too far, the energy source (client anxiety) is overcontrolled, all the reactions cease, and the reactor core cools. If the rods are withdrawn too far the energy source becomes uncontained and a 'melt down' ensues" (p. 251). This aptly characterizes ways in which attachment-insecure therapists can insensitively activate and actually strengthen clients' insecure attachment strategies (Dozier et al., 1994; Romano et al., 2009).

Attachment-informed clinicians try to choose interventions according to the specific deficits inherent in the attachment strategies of their insecure clients. Numerous interventions can address one or more of these deficits. To name just a few: Cognitive techniques can challenge distorted ways of thinking that perpetuate attachment insecurities; emotion-focused techniques can promote better emotion regulation and communication of relationship needs; behavioral experiments can undermine long-held beliefs and expectations; narrative techniques can loosen the grip of rigid personal accounts that artificially narrow response alternatives; and psychoeducation can redress skill deficits. (For a discussion of how different therapeutic approaches can be supplemented by attachment concepts, see Obegi & Berant, 2009.)

Attachment-Informed Assessment and Case Formulation

The need to customize treatment based on the attachment dynamics of a particular client highlights the importance of conducting an attachment-informed assessment before formulating a treatment plan, anticipating treatment obstacles, and identifying useful targets for change. Therefore, at intake, attachment-informed therapists assess clients' attachment-system functioning at both the intrapersonal level (e.g., social perceptions, affective experiences and capacities, representations of self and others, defenses, and mentalizing skills) and the interpersonal level (e.g., style of relating, ways of speaking about feelings, quality of relationships, availability and quality of support systems). Key components of this assessment include taking a client's history of attachment relationships and experiences, attending to their narrative style, and collecting data on attachment-related mental representations. The goal is not only to determine a client's attachment style, which may be somewhat different with different relationship partners, but to develop hypotheses about the idiosyncratic workings of a particular client's attachment system in different relational contexts, his or her reliance on specific attachment-related strategies, and the developmental origins of these strategies (Slade, 2004).

In order to assess a client's attachment history and narrative style, attachment-informed therapists can use a semistructured approach that takes cues from the AAI (see Hesse, 2016, for an overview). Answers to questions from this interview draw therapists' attention to the availability, responsiveness, and stability of attachment figures during childhood and adolescence; significant separations, losses, and attachment injuries; the coherence of a client's autobiographical narrative; and the ways in which he or she violates narrative coherence by what Holmes (2001) called "clinging to rigid stories" or "being overwhelmed by unstoried experience" (p. 88). Attachment-informed therapists also collect information on clients' secure-base scripts, working models of self and others, and relational beliefs and inclinations. They are particularly interested in how these mental representations manifest themselves in response to stressors such as hurt feelings, illnesses, separations, or losses. They are interested in questions such as the following: How do patients respond cognitively, affectively, and behaviorally to threats? Do they confidently turn to attachment figures, cling to such figures, or withdraw? In times of need, how do they perceive themselves and relationship partners' responses? How do they feel about intimacy and closeness? What are they likely to do during interpersonal conflicts?

Data collected on attachment history, narrative style, and attachment-related mental representations usually turns up at least one attachment-related issue that is salient and relevant to treatment (Hardy et al., 2004). Exposure to such an issue predictably evokes the maladaptive attachment strategies that have made a client vulnerable to current problems and that play a role in perpetuating these problems. Stated differently, the goal of case formulation is to delineate the circumstances and factors that block the broaden-and-build processes that would normally flow from attachment security. Once these blocks are identified, a dynamic formulation can be created, usually comprising four components: (1) the precipitating attachment-related events, (2) the typical cognitive–affective meanings ascribed to these events, (3) the strategies clients use to cope with these events, and (4) the ways these strategies leave patients susceptible to the problems that prompted seeking treatment (Obegi & Berant, 2009).

Broadening Clients' Perspectives and Self-Understanding

As summarized in Figure 7.1, security enhancement and therapeutic change are facilitated not only by establishing a secure client–therapist bond but also by the active and tailored methods therapists use to broaden clients' perspectives, improve their mentalization capacities, and facilitate the creation of more reality-attuned working models. Reliance on counter-complementary attachment proximity strategies is one method for challenging insecure working models. However, it needs to be supplemented with other therapeutic attitudes and practices that encourage exploration of and reflection on these models and help clients open themselves to more adaptive ways of thinking and feeling about self and others.

Attachment-informed therapists aim to foster openness and mentalization while being warm and compassionate, sensitive and empathic with a client's needs and feelings, and responsive to his or her bids for proximity and support. Therapists monitor a client's in-session attachment needs and emotional arousal while the client discloses and reflects on his or her past or current experiences, or responds to the therapist's interventions. The therapist has to provide just enough of a safe haven so that the client's inner exploration can be sustained without collapsing or generating unmanageable distress. In actively moving a client to explore memories and feelings, rework perspectives on self and others, and offer corrective remarks aimed at improving mentalization, attachment-informed therapists try to balance not being too directive and not damaging the client's secure feelings toward the therapist.

Attachment-Based Psychotherapies

In their examination of attachment theory and psychotherapy, Levy and Johnson (2019) noted that various therapeutic approaches have incorporated a few principles of attachment theory concerning the therapist's provision of support and a focus on relational experiences (e.g., supportive psychodynamic therapy, transference-focused psychotherapy). But there are four approaches in particular whose conceptualization of therapeutic tasks and goals is fully and coherently derived from attachment theory and research: interpersonal psychotherapy (IPT; Klerman et al., 1984), mentalization-based treatment (MBT; Bateman & Fonagy, 2004), accelerated experiential dynamic psychotherapy (AEDP; Fosha, 2000), and emotionally focused individual therapy (EFIT; Johnson & Campbell, 2022). All of these therapies emphasize the importance of instilling a secure in-session climate and revising insecure working models and patterns of relating for bringing about therapeutic change. But the four approaches diverge in their specific foci (interpersonal functioning, emotion regulation, mentalization) and in the techniques they use for moving clients toward greater security. For our purposes, the four approaches, considered as a set, illustrate well how attachment theory and research are being applied in psychotherapy.

Interpersonal Psychotherapy

IPT is a time-limited (12–16 sessions) and manualized individual therapy derived from a theoretical integration of Bowlby's writings with the work of interpersonally oriented neo-Freudian psychoanalysts such as Karen Horney and Harry Stack Sullivan. Despite being derived mainly from psychodynamic theories, IPT incorporates technical elements from CBT, such as formal assessments, psychoeducation, and homework assignments. It was originally developed to treat adults diagnosed with major depression (Klerman et al., 1984), but it has since been expanded and adapted to treat other disorders, such as postpartum depression, suicidal tendencies, social anxiety, eating disorders, and PTSD (e.g., Markowitz, 2010; Markowitz et al., 2014; Markowitz & Weissman, 2004). In addition, ITP has been adapted to treat depressed adolescents (Mufson et al., 1993).

In all of its versions, IPT is based on Bowlby's understanding that mental disorders emerge in the context of frustrating and painful interpersonal interactions, and that relational insecurities and maladaptive relational patterns sustain these disorders over time (Klerman & Weissman, 1994). Also, in line with attachment theory, IPT's founders believed that a safe and secure relationship with a sensitive and responsive therapist is a useful means for improving clients' interpersonal functioning and thus bringing about symptom alleviation (Klerman et al., 1984). The main goal of IPT is to move clients toward more security-based, adaptive ways of relating and to facilitate positive changes in interpersonal functioning, which can in turn contribute to improved mental health. The key mechanisms of therapeutic change are the creation of a secure in-session climate and the provision of a secure base from which clients can confidently explore and practice more adaptive patterns of relating (Klerman et al., 1984).

Unlike Bowlby's dual focus on current and past relational experiences, IPT therapists focus mainly on clients' "here and now" relational thoughts, feelings, and inclinations. Although IPT founders recognized the importance of early painful attachment experiences in the development of mental disorders (Klerman et al., 1984), the time-limited nature of IPT does not allow therapists and clients to delve into Bowlby's fourth therapeutic task of exploring the historical origins of clients' current relational problems. Instead, IPT therapists switch the focus from early experiences to clients' current interpersonal functioning, with the aim of encouraging a more adaptive pattern of relating (Markowitz & Weissman, 2012).

To instill a safe and secure in-session climate, IPT therapists are trained to be warm, supportive, and nonjudgmental; to express acceptance and positive regard for a client; to be attentive, emotionally engaged, and respectful concerning a client's disclosures; and to be able and willing to share their own personal experiences when this disclosure can advance a client's self-understanding. However, IPT therapists do not usually offer explicit suggestions regarding a client's change efforts; rather, the change should emerge organically from secure in-session interactions. Because of the time-limited nature of IPT, transference-related issues are not usually addressed during therapy unless a client's needs and feelings toward the therapist are clearly disrupting the formation of a secure therapeutic relationship (M. Weissman et al., 2000).

Therapists are trained to follow the IPT treatment manual (M. Weissman et al., 2000, 2007, 2018). It outlines three phases of treatment (assessment, active treatment, and termination) and the specific tasks and goals of each phase. In the assessment phase (Sessions 1–4), therapists and clients together define a core relational insecurity, crisis, or difficulty that becomes the primary focus of therapy (e.g., excessive dependence, fear of intimacy, inability to disengage emotionally from a lost relationship). This phase includes (1) evaluating clients' symptoms and patterns of relating; (2) providing a case formulation, which includes a diagnosis of clients' mental health problems and links this diagnosis to their core relational difficulty; and (3) agreeing on a treatment plan.

Therapists and clients explore the relational meaning of clients' symptoms. For example, they talk about how clients' maladaptive relational patterns might have contributed to their symptoms and how these symptoms are affecting current relationships. They also talk about clients' close relationship partners, clients' own relational needs and expectations, and the satisfying and unsatisfying aspects of their relationships. The therapist helps clients verbalize the changes they desire in these relationships, and the steps toward this relational change are formulated and built into the treatment plan. At the end of this phase, a core relational problem is identified, and resolving this problem is agreed upon as a major therapeutic goal.

The active treatment phase (Sessions 5–14) focuses on resolving the relational problem. During each session, the therapist supportively invites clients to talk about relational experiences they have had during the past week and how these experiences relate to the specific problem they identified in the assessment phase. The therapist then encourages clients to explore and reflect on these relational experiences and provides the comfort and reassurance needed to soothe any distress that might result from this exploration (secure-base support). As the therapy progresses, the therapist helps clients to use alternative, more effective ways of coping with their core relational problem, to explore and practice new patterns of relating to established relationship partners, and to develop interest in new relationships. According to Lipsitz and Markowitz (2013), "IPT attempts not to fix a problem in the patient, but to help the patient fix the problem in the interpersonal context and her relationship to this problem, thereby helping her to enhance her life situation and to recover from the psychiatric syndrome" (p. 1138). In the termination phase (Sessions 14–16), the focus is on reviewing and consolidating therapeutic changes, anticipating future problems, and working through the sadness of ending the therapeutic relationship.

The effectiveness of IPT was initially examined in an RCT for major depressive disorders conducted at Harvard and Yale Universities' mental health centers (Weissman et al., 1981). As compared to antidepressant drug therapy or an unscheduled treatment control condition (each participant was assigned to a psychiatrist and was told to call the psychiatrist whenever he or she needed to do so), IPT was more effective in alleviating depressive symptoms, improving work performance and interest, and decreasing suicidal ideation. IPT's effectiveness was also evident in an RCT conducted by the National Institute of Mental Health's Treatment of Depression Collaborative Research Program, which showed that IPT was as effective as CBT—the "gold-standard" depression treatment at the time—for alleviating depressive symptoms (Elkin et al., 1989).

Over the past 35 years, there have been hundreds of studies demonstrating the beneficial outcomes of IPT for a wide variety of mental disorders, and several meta-analyses have provided support for its effectiveness among adults and adolescents (Althobaiti et al., 2020; Cuijpers et al., 2008, 2011, 2016; Mychailyszyn & Elson, 2018; Pu et al., 2017; Sockol, 2018). For example, Cuijpers et al. (2016) meta-analyzed 90 studies (11,434 depressed clients) and found moderate-to-strong positive effects of IPT on depression, compared to control conditions. They concluded that IPT alleviates symptoms at the acute phase of depression and prevents the onset and relapse of depressive disorders. Overall, IPT is one of the best-examined therapies, and it seems to be effective in improving mental health among clinically diagnosed adolescents and adults.

Mentalization-Based Treatment

MBT is a manualized form of psychodynamic psychotherapy resulting from the integration of attachment theory, Kleinian object relations theory, and Fonagy et al.'s (1995) developmental theory of mentalizing (Bateman & Fonagy, 2004, 2012). MBT was originally developed to treat adolescents and adults diagnosed with borderline personality disorder (Bateman & Fonagy, 1999), but clinicians have used MBT in treating other mental disorders, such as eating disorders, depression, antisocial behavior, and suicidal tendencies (e.g., Rossouw & Fonagy, 2012; Jacobsen et al., 2015; Robinson et al., 2016) as well as problems encountered by troubled children and their parents (Midgley & Vrouva, 2012). MBT usually takes 18 months of weekly individual and group sessions. Whereas individual sessions allow clients to broaden their mentalizing and emotion regulation skills within a safe and secure relationship with the therapist, group sessions allow clients to practice these skills in a more complex, but still supportive and warm, social setting (Karterud, 2015).

MBT focuses on clients' security-based capacities for exploration and mentalization. As reviewed in Chapter 2, security-enhancing interactions with a responsive attachment figure encourage people to engage in exploratory ventures, including exploration of their own personal memories and experiences, and reflection on their own and others' needs and feelings (*mentalization*). These security-based capacities have been found to improve distress regulation, to underlie the formation of a coherent representation of self and others, and to contribute to mental health (see Chapter 2). In contrast, painful interactions with a neglectful or abusive attachment figure are likely to compromise mentalization, thereby interfering with self-understanding, impairing emotion regulation, and increasing the risk for mental disorders.

The main goal of MBT is to repair clients' mentalization deficits in the context of a safe and secure relationship with a sensitive and responsive therapist (Allen et al., 2008). However, before embarking on this challenging task, the initial goal of the therapist is to assist clients in stabilizing emotional arousal and soothing distress (i.e., providing a safe haven). In fact, clients' insecure attachment at the beginning of therapy, combined with intense, emotion-laden interactions with the therapist, can heighten distress and endanger the continuity of therapy. Following Bowlby's (1988) model of therapeutic change, an MBT therapist first provides effective safe-haven support, and only after distress is under control does the therapist provide a secure base to clients for exploring and reflecting on their subjective experience. During this exploration process, the MBT therapist supports and applauds clients' mentalization efforts, while at the same time clarifying and elaborating clients' reflections in a nonintrusive manner and gently challenging nonmentalizing stances (e.g., assuming that what is in one's mind accurately reflects reality). Moreover, the therapist continuously tracks and monitors clients' in-session level of distress and assists them in regulating any intrusion of negative feelings and thoughts that might destabilize the exploration and mentalization processes. In this way, clients become more accurate in understanding themselves and others with positive repercussions for mental health.

Bateman and Fonagy (2004) described the core components of a therapist's provision of a secure base that supports in-session exploration and mentalization. This therapeutic stance includes humility derived from a sense of "not knowing," genuine interest in exploring the mind, and constructing a partnership with the client rather than adopting an "expert" role. It also involves gently identifying clients' problems in mentalization, offering alternative ways of thinking about clients' experiences (e.g., "I can see how you get to that but when I think about it, I wonder whether Jimmie may have been preoccupied with something else rather than ignoring you"), and legitimizing and accepting different perspectives on external events and inner experiences. In addition, it includes actively asking clients for detailed descriptions of their experiences rather than asking for explanations (e.g., "What is it like?"; "What would make a difference?"; "How did you manage that?"), sensitively informing them when something they say is unclear, and inviting them to provide clarification or consider alternative perspectives.

In MBT, the therapist demonstrates appreciation of clients' exploratory efforts and respects the way they understand their inner experience. However, at the same time, he or she may sensitively provide alternative perspectives if they can improve clients' mentalization. These alternative perspectives are not provided in an overly challenging or confrontational manner but as possibilities residing along with a sense of not knowing and an authentic interest in understanding clients' experience (e.g., "I don't know, but if it were me, I might feel . . ."). Moreover, an MBT therapist avoids mentalizing *for* clients by providing interpretations or by instructing them on how to appraise their own or others' behavior. The main role of the MBT therapist is to encourage clients to open themselves to alternative perspectives and help them arrive at more autonomous and accurate self-understandings.

Another important component of the therapeutic process is the therapist's monitoring, recognition, and acceptance of his or her own empathic failures in mentalizing and understanding clients' experience (Bateman & Fonagy, 2004). These failures, which can shake clients' felt security and rupture the working alliance, are opportunities for exploring and reflecting on different alternatives of understanding inner experiences, and, if successfully resolved, can improve and deepen clients' mentalization. According to Bateman and Fonagy (2010), "In this collaborative patient–therapist relationship, the two partners involved have a joint responsibility to understand mental processes underpinning events within and without therapy" (p. 13).

In MBT, the therapist's task is to improve clients' mentalization by inviting them to be curious and inquire about their own and others' needs and feelings (e.g., "What is it that you feel about that?"), and especially about the mental states that emerge within the context of the therapist–client relationship. The focus is on current experiences, and the past is discussed only if it serves to elucidate clients' here-and-now experiences. When clients are able to reflect to some extent on their current experiences, the MBT therapist attempts to help them to identify, explore, and reflect on their affective responses to others, including the therapist. In this stage, clients are often asked to reflect on their relational feelings and think about what might have caused them, and how they might have affected their current feelings and behavior. The therapist also invites clients to explore and reflect on discrepancies between the way they are currently feeling and their nonverbal, subtle expressions of these feelings during in-session interactions. In this way, the therapist helps clients to attend to and make sense of less conscious sensations and feelings.

As the treatment progresses, the MBT therapist helps clients reflect on the way they feel in response to his or her comments and interventions. (Bateman & Fonagy, 2004, call this the *therapist's affect focus*). For example, imagine a client who describes a situation in which she failed to accomplish a task in the workplace and felt guilty about it. In the session, the client seems anxious and preoccupied after listening to the therapist's comments. An MBT therapist would ask the client to explore and reflect on her current anxiety and how it may be related to the way she thinks the therapist is responding to her disclosure of guilt feelings. In this way, the therapist helps clients understand not only their own affect but also their experience of talking about what is on their mind in the presence of another person. Moreover, the therapist encourages clients to express and work through their feelings while actually interacting with another person.

The effectiveness of MBT was first examined by Bateman and Fonagy (1999) in an RCT conducted with 44 partially hospitalized clients diagnosed with borderline personality disorder. As compared to clients who received standard psychiatric care, clients who received MBT showed more therapeutic gains across a range of outcomes: decreased self-reports of depression, anxiety, and global distress; fewer suicide attempts and self-harms; fewer and shorter inpatient admissions; decreased use of psychotropic medication; and improved interpersonal functioning and social adjustment. Importantly, follow-up studies conducted 18 months and 8 years later revealed that the gains of clients who received MBT were sustained; they exhibited continued improvement on most measures compared to the control group (Bateman & Fonagy, 2001, 2008). These findings were fully replicated in a larger RCT conducted with 134 outpatients diagnosed with borderline personality who were randomly allocated to 18-month MBT or structured clinical management (Bateman & Fonagy, 2009, 2016).

In 2019, Malda-Castillo et al. (2019) conducted a systematic review of other outcome studies on MBT effectiveness. They included seven additional RCTs that tested the effectiveness of MBT in treating adults and adolescents diagnosed with personality disorders, depression, suicidality, or eating disorders, and mothers struggling with addiction (Hertzmann et al., 2016; Laurenssen et al., 2018; Philips et al., 2018; Robinson et al., 2016;

Rossouw & Fonagy, 2012; Suchman et al., 2010, 2017). In addition, Malda-Castillo et al. (2019) reviewed seven studies that examined pre- to posttherapy changes in mental health in samples of adolescents and adults diagnosed with borderline personality disorder or eating disorders (Bales et al., 2012; 2015; Balestrieri et al., 2015; Bo et al., 2017; Hauber et al., 2017; Laurenssen et al., 2014; Thomsen et al., 2017). In the majority of these studies, clients who received MBT showed more improvement than those in treatment-as-usual or waiting-list control conditions and more posttherapy symptom alleviation compared to pretherapy levels (Malda-Castillo et al., 2019).

Only one RCT (Rossouw & Fonagy, 2012) tested MBT effects on clients' felt security, and found that, as compared to a treatment-as-usual condition, MBT led to a higher posttherapy reduction in self-reports of avoidant attachment among depressed adolescents. This is a promising finding, but more RCTs are needed to confirm MBT's effectiveness in fostering secure patterns of relating. Further research is also needed to examine the proposed mechanisms of change in MBT (secure client–therapist relationship, clients' in-session mentalization) and the effects of specific MBT interventions (e.g., therapist's affect focus). Despite these remaining research needs, the concept of mentalizing and its use in therapy sessions are important developments in the application of attachment theory and research to psychotherapy.

Accelerated Experiential Dynamic Psychotherapy

AEDP is a short-term, individual therapy based on an integration of attachment theory and psychodynamic and experiential practices (Fosha, 2000, 2021). Like Bowlby, Fosha (2000) highlighted the difficulties in emotion regulation that attachment injuries and insecurities create and their key role in the formation and maintenance of mental disorders. Moreover, she recognized the healing effects of explicitly creating a secure in-session climate so that clients can safely express and explore emotions that have been persistently warded off, and can experience more positive emotional states with an emotionally engaged and responsive therapist (Fosha, 2002, 2004).

The main goal of AEDP is to move clients toward more security-based, constructive ways of regulating distress and savoring positive emotional experiences (Fosha, 2002, 2004). From an attachment perspective, the focus of AEDP is the positive affectivity derived from the broaden-and-build cycle of attachment security. As we explained and documented in Chapter 2, comforting interactions with a responsive attachment figure facilitate distress regulation and sustain longer periods of positive feelings, which contribute to overall mental health. In the same way, supported and empowered by a responsive therapist, clients can feel safe and secure enough to explore, disclose, and actively deal with painful experiences, fully enjoy emergent positive feelings, and return to daily life with renewed confidence in their own strength and value and in others' love and benevolence. These are AEDP's key mechanisms of therapeutic change (Fosha, 2021). They are notable in including an emphasis on positive emotions.

In AEDP, the therapist attempts to provide a safe haven and secure base by not only being sensitive and responsive to clients' moment-to-moment needs and feelings but also being emotionally engaged and willing to self-disclose his or her own feelings and personal information in the service of the client. According to Fosha (2000), "AEDP's clinical stance demands at least as much from the therapist as from the patient: the patient cannot be expected to rapidly open up to a therapist who remains hidden and shielded. The emotional atmosphere should be one in which the patient feels safe and the therapist brave" (p. 213).

Fosha (2021) listed seven concepts that define therapists' tasks and therapeutic processes. The first is *undoing aloneness*. The therapist explicitly expresses to clients that they are working together in facing whatever experiences or memories the client finds difficult to bear or acknowledge alone. A therapist's self-disclosure can contribute to this task, particularly the use of phrases such as "Me, too," "I feel this way, too," or "We are all in the same boat" (Yalom, 1995, p. 6). As a result, clients become more confident in their therapist's emotional availability and responsiveness—the sine qua non of felt security.

The second concept is *transformance/privileging the positive*. The therapist attempts to create a secure in-session climate so that clients' natural strivings for growth and change can emerge. Like Bowlby, Fosha (2000) believed that the human mind is strongly inclined toward exploration, growth, and self-healing, and the therapist's main job is to provide the safe and secure conditions in which these growth-oriented processes can thrive. In addition, the AEDP therapist is trained not only to work through clients' painful memories but also to amplify and deepen clients' positive memories and capitalize on in-session moments of positive affectivity (e.g., laughing together). The therapist privileges in-session positive experiences that reflect client–therapist mutual appreciation and delight, which can solidify their emotional bond.

The third concept is *moment-to-moment tracking and making the implicit explicit and specific*. The therapist tracks momentary shifts in clients' needs and feelings (as manifested in both nonverbal and verbal channels) and reflects them back as a means of increasing clients' awareness of their "here and now" experience (e.g., "You feel embarrassed," "Now you feel comfortable"). The fourth concept is *true self/true other/responsiveness to need in the moment*. In performing this task, the therapist helps clients develop an inner sense that they are being met and responded to by an authentic, true other in a way that is just right for them. However, this does not mean that clients need to experience the therapist as a perfect, idealized figure, but rather as a responsive other in the "here and now"—one who at painful moments asks where he or she can help, gets things right or, after empathic failures, works to get it right (Fosha, 2005).

The fifth concept is *affirming, celebrating, delighting*. The therapist explicitly celebrates and affirms each sign of the client's progress, just as a responsive parent celebrates and applauds a child's first steps, first words, first examples of creative play (secure-base support). In this way, the therapist attempts to shift clients' attention from what is wrong to what is going well. The sixth concept is *meta-therapeutic processing*, by which the therapist helps and encourages clients to explore and reflect on their positive in-session experiences. As clients look back and review a successfully completed transformation, positive feelings, such as gratitude and pride, and a sense of achievement or satisfaction may arise. Reflection on these feelings can arouse still more positive emotions and a greater sense of personal strength and value, resulting in desired clinical outcomes.

The seventh concept is *the map of the transformational process*. AEDP work is guided by a four-state transformation model (Fosha et al., 2019). Therapy begins with clients in a distressed, defensive state, from which the therapist tries to gradually shift them to a position in which they are more connected with their core emotions and growth-oriented strivings. In State 1, the therapist attempts to create a secure in-session climate to minimize defensive tendencies and increase clients' awareness of their inner experience. In State 2, the therapist helps clients access, explore, and work through distressing emotional experiences and memories until positive affect emerges and adaptive action tendencies are observed. In State 3, the emergence of positive affect is itself processed (meta-therapeutic processing), which both consolidates the positive shift and generates its own set of growth-oriented phenomena. By eliciting positive affect, meta-therapeutic processing often stimulates additional rounds of positive shifts and meta-processing, which continue in succession until the client reaches a calm, peaceful state of mind (State 4). This final state is characterized by deep, genuine, reflective experiences and the consolidation of therapeutic gains. AEDP therapists are trained to attend to clients' nonverbal and verbal affective markers in order to detect whether the transformational process is on track and what can be done to move clients forward.

Unfortunately, to date, no RCT has been published examining the effectiveness of AEDP. In fact, there is only one study, which relied on a pre- to posttherapy design without a control condition, that has examined AEDP's effectiveness (Iwakabe et al., 2020, 2022). Sixty-two self-referred adults who underwent 16 AEDP sessions were assessed before therapy, immediately after the 16 sessions, and 6 or 12 months later. They completed self-report measures of psychiatric symptoms, psychological distress, self-esteem, self-compassion, and a variety of psychological hardships (e.g., interpersonal problems, difficulties in emotion regulation, automatic negative thoughts) before and after therapy and 6 or 12 months later. As compared to the pretherapy assessment, clients reported alleviation of distress and psychiatric symptoms, and improvement in all of the assessed domains following therapy. These positive effects were maintained at the 6- and 12-month follow-ups and were observed in both clients with severe pretherapy problems and clients with fewer and less severe problems.

These findings provide preliminary empirical support for AEDP. However, future studies should test AEDP's effectiveness using more rigorous random assignment designs, comparing its effects to other therapeutic modalities, examining the hypothesized mechanisms of change, and tracking maintenance of therapeutic gains over long follow-up periods. At present, we find this approach attractive because of its promising depth and breadth and its unusual focus on positive experiences and encouragement of a therapist's self-disclosures and shared therapist–client expressions of positive feelings.

Emotionally Focused Individual Therapy

In 2019, Sue Johnson proposed an individual-therapy version of EFT (see Chapter 6 for the original couple therapy version). (A primer for EFIT was published when we were in the last stages of writing this chapter; see Johnson & Campbell, 2022). As with AEDP, the main goal of this recently developed therapy is to move clients toward more open, mindful, and constructive ways of processing painful emotions (sadness, fear, shame) aroused by the frustration of attachment needs. Strong emphasis is placed on the exploration, regulation, and acceptance of difficult emotions that have been persistently warded off, doing so with the support and encouragement of a responsive and skillful therapist. In Johnson's (2019a) words, "EFIT seeks to give clients an integrative corrective emotional experience in which they explore new ways to engage with their own experience, with others, and the existential dilemmas of life" (p. 75).

Johnson and Campbell (2022) described four main therapeutic tasks. In the first task, the therapist provides clients with safe-haven forms of support (e.g., comfort, reassurance) and assists them in restoring emotional balance whenever they feel distressed and dysregulated during a therapeutic session (as a "surrogate attachment figure"; Johnson, 2019a). In this way, the therapist challenges clients' insecure working models of self (as unloved) and others (as unavailable and rejecting), strengthens their confidence in the therapist's support when needed, and provides a scaffold for maintaining emotional stability while exploring and processing painful, distressing emotions.

The other three tasks involve the therapist's provision of secure-base forms of support (e.g., encouragement, empowerment) that facilitate constructive processing of painful emotions and savoring of more positive emotional experiences. In the second task, the therapist encourages and assists clients in dealing with "in session transformative moments where vulnerability is encountered with emotional balance and difficult emotions are ordered and made specific and coherent" (Johnson & Campbell, 2022, p. 29). The therapist helps clients to identify, explore, reflect on, and accept vulnerability-related emotions that emerge during the therapeutic sessions while talking about themselves or close relationships. Moreover, the therapist coaches clients in exploring how these painful emotions shape insecure (anxious, avoidant, or both) patterns of relating and underlie emotional problems. The therapist also helps clients understand how insecure patterns of relating exacerbate their negative emotional experiences and prevent corrective emotional experiences.

In the third task, the therapist helps and coaches clients to be emotionally available, nonjudgmental, and fully engaged when reflecting on and talking about their unmet attachment needs and painful emotions, and when interacting with others. With the support and guidance of a responsive and skillful therapist, clients develop what Rogers (1961) called *existential living*—"openness to the flow of experience, trusting this experience, and being able to use it as a compass—a guide in life—actively choosing perspectives and responses while taking responsibility and being open to growth and ongoing development" (Johnson & Campbell, 2022, p. 29). In the fourth task, the therapist encourages and celebrates clients' exploration of and reflection on their own strengths, personal achievements, and positive relational experiences. In so doing, the therapist strengthens the client's sense of personal value and competence and teaches them to savor these resilience-promoting feelings.

Although EFIT views clients' emotional problems as results of a painful attachment history, the focus of therapy is on clients' "here-and-now" experiences. The therapist attempts to be empathically attuned to the client's in-session subjective experiences, and to the needs and feelings that emerge during in-session interactions. And then, by using evocative questions, repetitions, conjectures, imagery, and metaphors, the therapist helps clients to deepen and expand on their current emotional experience and make it more specific and easier to understand and digest. In this way, with the support and encouragement of a responsive therapist, clients can confidently and calmly process painful emotions, understand how they underlie their personal and interpersonal problems, and practice more adaptive ways of regulating emotions. Moreover, they can explore and reflect on how emotional reactions like these seen in therapy also emerge during frustrating interpersonal exchanges, while at the same experimenting and practicing more secure patterns of relating.

EFIT includes three stages. In the first stage, *stabilization*, the therapist attempts to create a solid working alliance and instill a secure in-session climate. The therapist supports and encourages clients to explore and reflect on how their current emotional problems relate to their attachment history and insecure patterns of relating. By adopting a nonjudgmental, validating, and compassionate stance, the therapist "shapes a safe haven and secure base in the session, distils the client's strengths and finds the logic in the client's stuck patterns of inner processing and interactions, and then gradually leads the client into new ways of constructing emotions, framing models of self and other, and shaping interactions with significant others" (Johnson, 2019a, p. 100).

In the second stage, *restructuring*, the therapist encourages clients to take greater risks in confronting difficult emotions when talking about disowned aspects of themselves or recalling or imagining distressing social interactions. The therapist then supports and sensitively guides clients in processing, deepening, and expanding the current emotional experience, until they reach a better understanding of its meaning and its personal and relational implications. (This is obviously closely related to Fonagy's notion of mentalization.) The therapist also assists clients in fully embracing the new insights they achieve concerning themselves and others.

According to Johnson and Campbell (2022), this deepening and restructuring of in-session emotions provides clients with corrective emotional experiences and an opportunity to develop more positive models of self and others. "As clients deeply engage in, claim, and congruently express previous unformulated or avoided experience in the presence of a trusted other, this expands the sense of self and the person's repertoire of interactional responses. Core definitions of the self and others become available and open to modification" (p. 140).

In the third and last stage, *consolidation*, the therapist supports and encourages clients to apply the newly acquired more secure working models in dealing with practical problems and close relationships. The therapist works with clients to construct a new narrative focused on an emerging sense of personal value, courage, competence, and strength. The therapist also joins clients in creating a vision of the future in which difficult emotions are well-regulated, allowing clients to engage fully in life tasks, approach relationship partners constructively, and make personal decisions in a secure and relaxed manner. "Confident that clients' felt sense of security will continue to evolve, the therapist also guides clients in continuing to shape this new narrative beyond the therapeutic process" (Johnson & Campbell, 2022, p. 160).

Unfortunately, no research findings have yet been published that examine the effects of EFIT on clients' working models, felt security, patterns of relating, or mental health. However, we are aware that relevant data are currently being collected and analyzed. Based on Johnson's previous development and evaluation of EFT for couples, we are optimistic about her new approach, EFIT, becoming another successful form of attachment-based individual psychotherapy.

Concluding Remarks

Although Bowlby created his theory within a clinical context and for the benefit of clinicians and their clients, developmental, personality, and social psychologists did much of the work of subjecting his ideas to empirical test. Nevertheless, over the past four decades, attachment theory has found its way into various approaches to psychotherapy—at first by playing a supporting role, then increasingly by providing parts of a core framework for new psychotherapies. These therapies leverage attachment theory's ability to connect early experiences to later emotion-regulation strategies and interpersonal behaviors; to conceptually integrate diverse methods of promoting positive change; to value actual interpersonal relationships as well as the intrapsychic realm; and to make sense of supportive, therapeutic relationships. Considerable work is still needed to explore and validate attachment theory's implications for psychotherapy. However, Bowlby's eclectic approach to theory construction, his theory's insights into intimate relationships, and attachment researchers' diligence in testing his ideas portend an exciting future for attachment-related psychotherapies.

CHAPTER 8

Other Therapeutic Applications of Attachment Theory and Research

Beyond applications of attachment theory in individual psychotherapy of fairly broad and conventional kinds, reviewed in Chapter 7, the theory is also relevant to more specialized kinds of therapy, three of which are considered in this chapter: grief therapy, spiritually integrated psychotherapy, and animal-assisted therapy. We should note from the beginning that although attachment theory offers a coherent and research-based framework for these three kinds of therapy, no systematic research has been conducted to test the contributions of the attachment-informed practices included in these therapies. We hope this chapter inspires scholars and practitioners to apply attachment-informed practices in grief therapy, spiritually integrated psychotherapy, and animal-assisted therapy, and to examine their effects on clinical outcomes.

Grief therapy helps bereaved clients emotionally process and adjust to the death of a loved one. Beginning with Bowlby's (1980) pioneering books on attachment and loss, attachment theory and research have provided important ideas and information concerning complicated grief and grief resolution that can contribute to the effectiveness of grief therapy. Spiritually integrated psychotherapy (SIP; Pargament, 2011) is an attempt to provide spiritual resources to troubled believers and help them cope with life stresses and adversities. An attachment perspective on religion and spirituality (the *religion-as-attachment model*; Granqvist, 2020) proposes that believers can form an attachment relationship with God, and that felt security with respect to God is an important psychological resource that can be strengthened or restored during spiritually integrated therapy. Animal-assisted therapy involves in-session interactions between a client, an animal (a "therapeutic pet"), and a therapist, with the pet being viewed as an integral part of the therapeutic work. From an attachment perspective, the pet serves as an additional in-session safe haven and secure base. Feeling safe and secure with regard to an affectionate, responsive pet can benefit therapeutic work and improve clinical outcomes.

An Attachment Perspective on Grief Therapy

The death of a loved one (e.g., spouse, parent, sibling, child) is one of the most painful and devastating experiences in most people's lives. It naturally triggers acute grief reactions:

intense psychological pain, unfocused anxiety, sleeplessness, and anger; desperate longing for the lost person; and lack of interest and engagement in everyday activities that would normally provide pleasure, such as working, gardening, reading, or going to a movie with friends (McCoyd et al., 2021; O'Connor, 2022). In most cases, these debilitating grief responses subside and disappear after some weeks or months, emotional balance is restored, and the bereaved person can return to daily activities with renewed energy. However, in around 7–10% of cases, there may be profound and prolonged mental sequelae, including what is now considered a clinical disorder, *complicated grief* (World Health Association, 2018). This disorder is characterized by overwhelming distress and yearning, emotional numbness, cognitive disorientation, loss of a sense of self, and loss of purpose or meaning in life (Maciejewski et al., 2016). Besides interfering with normal life activities, these extreme and prolonged grief reactions can increase the risk of cardiovascular, neuroendocrine, and immune dysregulation (Fagundes & Wu, 2020), which may be responsible for widows' and widowers' well-documented increased risk of premature death (Moon et al., 2014).

Grief therapy is intended to help bereaved individuals who suffer from prolonged and debilitating grief reactions and are unable to cope with, and adjust to, a loss on their own. The therapy can take different forms and include a variety of techniques, depending on the therapist's theoretical orientation and skills; the characteristics of the relationship with the deceased and the nature of the loss; the bereaved person's history, strengths, and emotional problems; and the setting in which the therapy is provided (Neimeyer & Jordan, 2013). However, the different modalities of grief therapy have in common the goal of helping clients manage their grief reactions, understand and deal with obstacles that prevent adjustment to their loss (e.g., unresolved conflicts in the relationship with the deceased, clients' worries about their capacity to deal with life's challenges without the deceased), and find ways to move forward (Neimeyer, 2012; Rubin et al., 2012).

In their book *Attachment-Informed Grief Therapy*, Kosminsky and Jordan (2016) offered the following definition of grief therapy:

> Grief therapy is a concentrated form of empathically attuned and skillfully applied social support, in which the therapist helps the bereaved person re-regulate after a significant loss by serving as a transitional attachment figure. This includes addressing deficits in affect regulation and mentalizing related to both the loss at hand, and early neglect or trauma, as needed. In an environment that encourages exploration and growth, the bereavement therapist supports the bereaved in experiencing and tolerating feelings relating to grief, integrating new information and skills, and developing a new self-narrative that incorporates the impact of the loss. The goal of grief therapy is integration of the loss on a psychological and neurological level. Successful grief therapy encourages a state of flexible attention to the loss, and to the relationships, roles and experiences that are still available to the bereaved individual, in order that they may re-engage in life, without relinquishing their attachment to the deceased. (p. 100)

Notice that this definition was written from an attachment perspective. It emphasizes the core elements of an attachment-informed approach to any kind of therapeutic change, as described in Chapter 7: the therapist as a sensitive and responsive attachment figure, the creation of a secure in-session climate, and the provision of a secure base for the client's inner exploration, mentalization, and processing of painful emotions and feelings of vulnerability. However, as Kosminsky and Jordan (2016) noted, although the definition directs attention to attachment-informed practices that can improve clinical outcomes, "it does not change the goal of grief therapy" (p. 101). No matter which theoretical orientation one adopts, the goal of grief therapy is to alleviate a client's suffering, make sense of the lost relationship and its personal importance, reorganize mental representations of the person as permanently gone, confidently reengage in life, and successfully establish new satisfying relationships (Neimeyer, 2012). Adopting the attachment-informed practices presented in Chapter 7 can facilitate the attainment of these goals.

Attachment theory provides a conceptual framework for understanding grief reactions and grief resolution, and for guiding therapeutic work with bereaved clients (Bowlby, 1980; Fraley & Shaver, 2016). First of all, attachment theory emphasizes the devastating disruption of one's deep, visceral sense of security and the resulting feelings of vulnerability, helplessness, abandonment, and loneliness that can follow the death of a loved one. Second, the theory characterizes successful grief resolution as resulting from a reorganization of one's network of security providers, which can restore felt security through both the symbolic activation of mental representations of the deceased and actual interactions with living security providers, old and new. Third, the theory suggests that insecure-attachment working models and styles can contribute to and maintain complicated grief reactions; that is, they can retard or obstruct grief resolution if not managed effectively during therapy. These theoretical ideas emphasize the main tasks of grief therapy: working through the disruption of felt security; reorganizing the network of security providers; and managing attachment insecurities, the softening of which can facilitate grief resolution and reengagement in normal life.

The Meaning of Grief Reactions

From an attachment perspective, grief reactions are due to the shattering of a sense of safety and security that had, perhaps only implicitly, been continuously supported by the now absent attachment figure (Weiss, 1993). These reactions mirror the fear, anger, and sadness that infants experience and display when separated from their attachment figure (Johnson's *primary emotions;* 2019a). The seemingly irrational anxiety and fear that follow a loss are reactions to the sudden deficit in the customary sense of safety and protection (the absence of a safe haven). The anger is what Bowlby (1969/1982) called "protest" against the undeserved and "unfair" deprivation of a safe haven and secure base. The sadness, sometimes morphing into depression, is what Bowlby called "despair" in the case of a child experiencing an extended separation from a parent.

Undoubtedly, we all know from painful experiences what this anxiety, anger, and sadness feel like. When we, as adults, are confronted with the loss of a principal security provider, it's as if we have suddenly had a familiar, trustworthy security blanket yanked away, and our vulnerability, uncertainty, and in some cases fear of injury or death, is brought home with a jolt. In fact, losing a loved one is processed by the brain in ways similar to the experience of painful physical injuries that remind us, consciously and unconsciously, of death (Gillath, Bunge, et al., 2005). In this sense, psychological "pain" and physical pain are not just analogous, as most writers probably assume; they are neurologically similar. And making the similarity between physical and emotional pain more literal, at least during early childhood, having one's attachment figure physically absent can in fact be a matter of life or death (e.g., from predation, injuries, illness, or starvation).

In line with this reasoning, the intensity of grief is a function of the place and importance of the deceased spouse in the bereaved person's network of security providers. Parkes and Weiss (1983) suggested that individuals who lose the person on whom they most depend to provide a safe haven and secure base are the most likely to experience intense and prolonged grief reactions. Indeed, more intense grief is observed among people who describe themselves as having been more strongly attached to a deceased spouse (Jerga et al., 2011). In addition, continued attachment to a former partner (meaning that the ex-partner is still appraised as a principal attachment figure) is a source of intense distress following the partner's loss (Borelli et al., 2019).

This attachment-oriented conceptualization of grief reactions calls attention to the importance of a therapist's in-session provision of a safe haven and secure base. When one is counseling the bereaved, the creation of a secure in-session climate and the formation of a secure attachment to the therapist can temporarily restore, at least during therapy, some of the sense of security that was shattered by the loss. As a result, clients may become more confident that a safe haven and secure base is still possible to obtain, and this will help them become more willing and able to collaborate with the therapist and engage in therapeutic work.

With this renewed in-session sense of security, a therapist can sensitively coach and encourage clients to explore, mentalize, and process their insistent attachment-related needs and their painful feelings of vulnerability and loneliness brought on by the loss. Using techniques from therapies reviewed in Chapter 7 (e.g., IPT, MBT, AEPT), a clinician can help clients reach a better understanding of the attachment-related meaning and significance of the loss, to view their grief as a normal response to the disruption of a visceral sense of security, and to recognize and accept their intense needs for connection and support. This improved mentalization and processing of primary emotions can soften intense grief reactions and allow a bereaved client to more calmly and confidently engage in the reorganization of the client's security network, both mentally (where a kind of attachment to the lost figure can continue productively to exist) and externally, in old and new relationships with living figures.

Attachment Reorganization and Grief Resolution

According to Bowlby (1980), grief resolution through therapy involves moving the bereaved person beyond the lost relationship and helping him or her reorganize the network of security providers and renew or find alternative sources of felt security. However, contrary to some critiques of attachment theory's approach to grief, reorganization does not require or imply a complete emotional or cognitive "detachment" from the deceased. Rather, an attachment-informed therapist supports and encourages bereaved clients to oscillate their attention between two somewhat antagonistic psychological tasks. At some moments during the therapeutic session, the therapist assists clients in attending to the lost relationship, maintaining a symbolic attachment to the lost partner, and integrating the lost relationship into a revised model of reality, including an updated self-narrative (Stroebe & Schut, 2010, called this focus a *loss orientation*). At other moments during the session, the therapist coaches the client to accept the loss, attend to changing roles and responsibilities brought about by the loss, engage in everyday activities, and rearrange or "edit" the attachment-figure network by forming new attachments or upgrading old ones (Stroebe & Schut, 2010, called this focus a *restoration orientation*).

In this way, an attachment-informed therapist "helps the bereaved client to stay present with painful emotions and to gain perspective about the changed self and world created by the death" (Kosminsky & Jordan, 2016, p. 115). The proposed oscillation within and across therapy sessions is expected and encouraged to occur in real life outside of the therapy sessions as well. The client gradually accepts that there will be moments of painfully experiencing the loss, but also periods of renewed strength and ability to focus on other matters and meaningful activities.

Because a long-lasting attachment is represented in the brain by thousands of neural circuits (O'Connor, 2022), it is natural for these circuits to be suddenly reactivated by expected or unexpected reminders in waking life and by free associations during sleep, which can cause the deceased attachment figure to appear in emotional dreams. One main therapeutic task is to help clients reflect on these memories and to edit or rewrite them in an updated form—as part of something that is past, not something that can be revived in real, waking life. It can take more than a lifetime to complete this editing process. But once its nature is understood and accepted, it does not need to be debilitating. It can be momentarily jolting but not devastating, and it can even become a source of fond, nostalgic reflections.

While paying attention in therapy to the loss, the therapist can help clients transform the psychological functions of the deceased person so that he or she becomes an internal, symbolic source of security rather than a flesh-and-blood, real-world source. Clients are encouraged to maintain a symbolic bond with the deceased (visualizing the person's face, retrieving memories of comforting interactions with him or her, reviving feelings of being loved and cared for by him or her) and to let go of illusions that the deceased individual is still alive and able to offer tangible care. At the same time, the therapist can encourage clients to form and solidify emotional bonds with available, real-world attachment figures.

While attending to changing roles and responsibilities brought about by the loss, an attachment-informed therapist can help clients develop emotion-regulation and interpersonal skills needed for building and sustaining mutually satisfying close relationships. Because bereaved clients are likely to be self-focused, as is chronically the case with insecurely attached people, it may help to orient clients toward ways to be concerned about and helpful to others. Once the intended reorganization of clients' internal and external attachment networks is accomplished, they may be able to feel more vital, optimistic, and secure most of the time.

Of theoretical interest, the reorganization process requires a degree of both attachment to and detachment from the lost figure (Mikulincer & Shaver, 2013). By reactivating memories of the lost figure and yearning for his or her proximity and love, bereaved clients can explore the meaning and importance of the lost relationship and find ways to maintain a symbolic bond with the lost figure. When this continuing attachment is properly regulated during the course of therapy with the help of a sensitive, responsive, and skillful therapist, a client can work to incorporate the past into the present without splitting off important elements of personal and social identity related to the lost attachment figure. Some degree of detachment from the deceased can also contribute to the reorganization process, because it enables down-regulation of painful feelings and allows clients to explore the new reality and realize that life presents new and attractive opportunities following a loss. If this degree of detachment is applied only to the lost figure and is not generalized to other real and potential attachment figures, it can facilitate the reorganization of the attachment network.

Without at least some periods of feeling still attached to the deceased, clients may not be fully capable of understanding the depth and meaning of their loss. But without a degree of detachment from this figure, clients may remain psychologically stuck and unable to move on and resolve their grief. An attachment-informed therapist is aware of the importance of both attachment and detachment moments and periods, and can sensitively coach clients to expect and accept alternation (or *oscillation,* a term used by Stroebe et al., 2005). According to Stroebe et al.,

> Oscillation occurs in the short term (transient fluctuations in the course of any particular day) as well as across the passage of time, because adaptation to bereavement is a matter of slowly and painfully exploring and discovering what has been lost and what remains: what must be avoided or relinquished versus what can be retained, created, and built upon. (p. 52)

Over the course of therapy and with the successful transfer of attachment functions to living partners, the need for this kind of oscillation is gradually reduced, and felt security is gradually restored by a combination of attachment to the therapist, the now understood symbolic attachment to the lost figure, and the discovery of new or renewed attachments (Newsom et al., 2017).

In line with these ideas, findings indicate that successful adjustment to the death of a spouse requires both the maintenance of symbolic bonds with the lost figure and the formation of close relationships with new partners (Sbarra & Borelli, 2019). These findings also indicate that the beneficial consequences of continuing bonds with a deceased partner depend on the extent to which people accept the irreversibility of the loss and regard the lost partner as a symbolic rather than an actual source of security. In fact, illusions and hallucinations of a deceased partner, in which the partner is located externally, alive, and in an unchanged form (e.g., "I felt her physical touch"; "I saw him standing directly before me"; "I saw him on the other side of a crowd") tend to increase rather than reduce distress (e.g., Field et al., 2013).

Attachment Insecurities and the Reorganization Process

From an attachment perspective, successful reorganization of a bereaved client's network of security providers depends on the extent to which (1) the lost partner was a major source of security and (2) new potential relationship partners are available, willing, and able to provide security and comfort. When the lost partner was important but unreliable and/or punishing in some respects, continuing attachment to this figure seems to constrain people to distress, confusion, and ambivalence (like a child returning ambivalently to an abusive parent when there is no alternative attachment figure available). Moreover, hurtful, rejecting experiences with a new relationship partner who is emotionally unavailable or unresponsive to the bereaved person's needs and feelings may interfere with his or her reengagement in life, and it may reactivate intense longing for the deceased. In such cases, an attachment-informed therapist can help bereaved clients understand and work through all of the reactions that occur while grieving and recovering from loss. This might include helping clients further detach from a lost abusive partner and, if warranted, also withdraw from a destructive new relationship.

A person's attachment insecurities, either anxious, avoidant, or some combination of the two, may also interfere with the reorganization process during therapy. Attachment-anxious people's overdependence on the lost figure and self-focused worries may reactivate a desperate need for protection and support from this figure and make it difficult to suppress or let go of feelings, thoughts, and memories related to him or her. This maintenance of intense emotional connection with the lost attachment figure may make successful reorganization impossible and interfere with the establishment of healthy new relationships. Avoidant individuals might seem to detach fairly quickly from a lost attachment figure (or the mental representation of the figure) and thus find it difficult to process and create meaning from the loss. And despite seeming to be able to get quickly past the loss, their chronic reluctance to rely on others for support may interfere with the formation of new attachments. Research indicates that attachment anxiety is associated with illusions of a deceased partner still being physically alive (e.g., Field & Filanosky, 2010) and that both forms of insecurity contribute to complicated grief reactions (e.g., Fraley & Bonanno, 2004; Jerga et al., 2011; Mancini et al., 2009).

In Chapter 7, we explained that one of the major tasks in attachment-informed therapies is to deal with clients' attachment insecurities and tailor treatment based on each client's specific attachment dynamics. In grief therapy, an attachment-informed therapist needs to be aware of clients' insecurities and how they interfere with the reorganization process. He or she should attempt to soften clients' insecurities (meeting anxious clients' needs for reassurance and validation; validating avoidant clients' needs for self-reliance and autonomy) while they explore the meaning of the lost relationship and the possibilities of reengaging in life.

Once a fairly secure bond between client and therapist is established, an attachment-informed therapist can sustain the reorganization process by introducing *counter-complementary attachment* interventions that challenge clients' habitual, chronic, dispositional attachment-related inclinations (see Chapter 7). For avoidant clients, who are not willing to reflect on the lost relationship or deeply process painful emotions, some kind of exposure therapy that confronts clients with the reality of the loss and its emotional implications may be useful (Boelen et al., 2007). For anxious clients, who tend to withdraw from social, occupational, and recreational activities while dwelling on and ruminating about the loss, the reorganization process can be facilitated by encouraging them to engage in personally relevant and meaningful activities (Papa et al., 2013). These clients are not likely to be helped by interventions whose main aim is to direct attention to the loss. Such clients are already immersed in rumination. They need help in reorganizing their attachment network and beginning to look outward toward the future.

Summary

Attachment theory and research can equip grief therapists with ideas and knowledge that facilitate their therapeutic work and improve clinical outcomes. This knowledge includes the attachment-related meaning and implications of separation and loss, the ways in which a bereaved person's network of attachment figures can be reorganized during therapy, and the ways in which some clients' insecure attachment working models, and in some cases their insecure relationship with the deceased before he or she died, can interfere with therapeutic work. However, although Kosminsky and Jordan (2016) eloquently described the core elements of attachment-informed grief therapy, no manualized intervention has been developed along these lines and tested in rigorous RCTs. We look forward to seeing this kind of intervention develop. We hope future studies can examine the feasibility and effectiveness of attachment-informed grief therapy and explore in greater depth the attachment-related mechanisms of change underlying grief resolution and adjustment to loss.

Spiritually Integrated Psychotherapy

SIP involves the incorporation of spirituality and religion into therapy as a means of enhancing therapeutic change and improving clinical outcomes for religious or spiritually oriented clients (Pargament, 2011). Beyond the common tasks of secular therapies (e.g., creating a secure in-session climate, processing painful emotions, revising dysfunctional beliefs), a major task of spiritually oriented therapy is to provide clients with spiritual resources that facilitate therapeutic work. This task can be accomplished in diverse ways depending on therapists' and clients' spiritual/religious beliefs and practices, and on the therapist's theoretical orientation and skills. For example, a therapist might help a client reconsider particular religious images or beliefs that are contributing to distress and replace them with healthier beliefs (religious or nonreligious, depending on other aspects of the person's situation). This kind of change could be accomplished, for example, through ordinary cognitive-behavioral techniques, engaging in or encouraging prayer or other spiritual exercises to reduce distress, or increasing awareness of aspects of spirituality and religion that might have beneficial effects on subjective well-being and mental health (e.g., Pearce et al., 2015; Post & Wade, 2009; Rosmarin, 2018).

A spiritually oriented therapist can help clients identify, recognize, and reflect on their concerns about spirituality or religion, especially if these concerns seem to be blocking therapeutic progress (Pargament & Exline, 2022, called this "working with spiritual struggles"). Several studies have tested the effectiveness of SIP, with findings that indicate it is as effective on the whole as secular therapies for a wide variety of emotional and behavioral problems (see Anderson et al., 2015; Captari et al., 2018; and Gonçalves et al., 2015, for meta-analyses, but see Rosmarin, 2018, for a discussion of methodological limitations of these studies).

To date, no attachment-informed spiritually integrated approach to therapy has been published, implemented, or tested. However, we suspect that attachment theory and research can equip spiritually oriented therapists with useful tools for providing spiritual resources to troubled clients and working through their spiritual struggles. Of course, this kind of therapy, like the various secular forms of therapy, can benefit from attachment theory's emphasis on the health-promoting effects of a therapist's sensitive responsiveness, the formation of a secure client–therapist attachment, and clients' mentalizing of insecure working models and attachment injuries. In addition, however, spiritually oriented therapists might improve their therapeutic work by taking into account the *religion-as-attachment* model (Kirkpatrick, 1994, 2005; Granqvist, 2020), which proposes that secure attachment to a loving God is a core spiritual resource that sustains believers' mental health, and that attachment insecurities (anxiety, avoidance, or both) with regard to God can contribute to spiritual struggles and distress.

Strengthening Reliance on a Responsive God and Secure Attachment to God

Using the religion-as-attachment framework, a spiritually oriented therapist might help religious or spiritually inclined clients not only to trust and rely on the responsiveness and support of their good human attachment figures, if they have any (parents, friends, spouse, or the therapist) but also to rely on the protection and support that a loving God can provide. This therapeutic task is based on the notion that believers tend to perceive God as an attachment figure who can either be sensitive and responsive or not (Granqvist, 2020). (Most likely, their perceptions of God as an attachment figure are affected by their experiences, good and bad, with human attachment figures.) On the good side, they might expect God to be a safe haven and secure base ("Yea, though I walk through the valley of the shadow of death, I will fear no evil, for thou art with me"; Psalm 23:4; "On the day I called, you answered me and made me bold with strength in my soul"; Psalm 138:3).

A believer who experiences God in this way can feel safe and secure in the presence of such a powerful and benevolent attachment figure. Therefore, therapeutically increasing clients' confidence in God's provision of a safe haven and secure base in times of need and strengthening a secure attachment to God might help clients work through their personal difficulties and acquire new strengths. Of course, if a client has a negative, insecurity-supporting conception of God, for whatever reasons, a religiously oriented therapist would have to work through that major barrier.

In the following titled sections we present theoretical ideas and empirical evidence supporting the therapeutic application of the religion-as-attachment model. Specifically, we consider the possibilities that (1) most believers perceive and regard God as a security provider, (2) they tend to seek God's protection and support in times of need, (3) they feel soothed and empowered by sensing God's loving and responsive presence, and (4) the formation of a secure attachment to God contributes to well-being and mental health. Given these facts, one main task of an attachment-informed spiritually oriented therapist is to strengthen clients' reliance on a loving and responsive God in times of need and to help them form a secure attachment to God. This strengthened felt security can sustain broaden-and-build processes, with benefits for mental health, personal development, interpersonal functioning, and relationship quality (see Chapter 2).

(Incidentally, we say these things without ourselves being conventionally religious. We are not attempting here to promote religion; we are only attempting to clarify how religious or spiritually oriented therapists and clients can make good use of their beliefs to improve mental health.)

Relying on God's Support in Times of Need

Like parents, God is perceived by believers to be a "stronger and wiser" figure who has created everything, has the power to solve any problem, and is capable of protecting and supporting them when they face threats and challenges (Granqvist, 2020). This idea is central to theological doctrines in which God is described as omnipotent (able to do anything), omniscient (knows everything), and omnipresent (is everywhere). In most theistic faith traditions, religious people also believe that when they are facing threats and difficulties, God will not only be able to help but will also want to help. In other words, God is expected to be omnibenevolent (all good)—a kind and loving figure who is willing to protect and support believers in times of need. This is the most common image of God that appears in religious texts (Wenegrat, 1989).

By tagging God as a potential source of a safe haven and secure base, believers are likely to seek "his" proximity, protection, and support when facing threats and challenges, just as they seek the protection of human attachment figures (Granqvist, 2020). There is extensive evidence that believers turn to God when distressed and tend to strengthen their emotional connection to this attachment-like figure through prayer, the most prototypical proximity-seeking behavior in relation to God (for reviews, see Koenig et al., 2012; Pargament, 2011). People also tend to strengthen their faith, endorsement of religious beliefs, and engagement in religious practices in times of need (e.g., Davis et al., 2019, Keefe et al., 2001; Sibley & Bulbulia, 2012). A strengthened emotional connection with God can also be observed following experimental inductions of existential threats, such as making salient one's lack of control over life events or one's mortality (e.g., Kay et al., 2008; Vail et al., 2012).

The Soothing and Empowering Effects of Confidence in God's Responsiveness

Believers may feel comforted and empowered by sensing the loving presence of a responsive and supportive God in the same way that the availability of responsive human attachment figures allows them to feel safe and secure (Granqvist, 2020). From an attachment perspective, these soothing and empowering effects of a spiritual relationship with God depend on the extent to which God is perceived as loving and responsive (Kirkpatrick, 2005). In fact, representing God as nonresponsive, punitive, or frightening can increase rather than decrease distress and fear whenever one feels a need for God's protection. This can explain the inconsistent, and even contradictory, associations that studies and meta-analyses have found over the years between a person's level of religious faith or engaging in religious practices (including prayer) and mental health (e.g., Bradshaw & Kent, 2018; Koenig et al., 2012; Hackney & Sanders, 2003).

Findings are more consistent when assessing aspects of religiosity that involve spiritual connection with a loving and responsive God. For example, research has shown that reliance on what Pargament (1997) called *positive religious coping*—relying on God's power and benevolence with confidence in "his" responsiveness—is associated with more effective emotion regulation and greater well-being among survivors of natural or man-made disasters and among people coping with a chronic illness or depression (for meta-analyses, see Ano & Vasconcelles, 2005; Smith et al., 2003). In addition, studies directly assessing believers' perceptions or images of God have found that perceiving "him" as a loving and kind figure is associated with greater well-being and lower levels of distress and negative emotions (see Stulp et al., 2019, for a meta-analysis). In addition, perceptions of God as a loving and kind figure have been associated with more constructive ways of coping and lower levels of distress among people dealing with adversities (e.g., Cook et al., 2013; Gall & Bilodeau, 2018; Gall et al., 2009).

Additional evidence for the soothing and empowering effects of relying on a loving and responsive God comes from studies that assess believers' attachment security with regard to God (i.e., the extent to which they are confident that God's support will be available when needed). These studies rely on self-report measures of attachment orientations toward God (Beck & McDonald's [2004] Attachment to God Inventory; Rowatt & Kirkpatrick's [2002] Attachment to God scale). As in dyadic relationships, believers who form a secure attachment to God tend to rely on more constructive ways of coping with adversities and stressors (e.g., Cassibba et al., 2014; Massengale et al., 2017; Parenteau et al., 2019).

Secure attachment to God also seems to shield believers from diagnosable emotional disorders and to increase their psychological well-being and mental health (e.g., Ellison et al., 2014; Knabb & Pelletier, 2014; Njus & Scharmer, 2020). Believers who feel secure with respect to God can maintain emotional composure when faced with difficulties and stressors, and can rapidly restore it when the stress subsides. Indeed, several studies have confirmed the distress-buffering function of secure attachment to God: The well-known association between exposure to stressful life events and feeling distressed is weakened by secure attachment to God (e.g., Ellison et al., 2019).

Strengthening a Secure Attachment to God

Based on these theoretical ideas and empirical findings, one main task of an attachment-informed spiritually oriented therapist is to strengthen or restore clients' secure attachment to God. This can be accomplished by engaging clients in types of prayer that deepen their relationship with God (e.g., Hood et al.'s [1996] contemplative or meditational prayers) while encouraging them to explore and reflect on the loving and comforting presence of God during prayer. (This is obviously a form of security priming, discussed in Chapter 3.) The therapist can also encourage clients to recognize, articulate, and endorse the various aspects of positive religious coping when dealing with their troubles, such as relying on God's power, working with God as a partner, and feeling confident that God will provide comfort and strength (Pargament, 1997). The therapist can also increase a client's awareness of the possibility that everything that exists, including oneself and God, is part of a unified whole (Diebels & Leary's [2019] "sense of oneness"), thereby allowing clients to incorporate the power of God into their self-concept and enjoy the protection offered by this spiritual resource. Clients can also enjoy the sense of meaning that comes from seeing themselves as part of an important cosmic process.

A secure attachment to God might also be strengthened during therapy by inviting clients to recall situations in which they sensed the presence of a loving, accepting, and supportive God, and to reflect on and articulate the positive feelings and thoughts they experienced in those situations. (This is another form of security priming.) A therapist can also support clients in exploring and mentalizing the positive attributes of God that appear in religious writings, especially the attributes that help them feel safer and more secure. In addition, clients can be encouraged to reflect on comforting interactions they have had with responsive religious leaders (e.g., priests, rabbis) and supportive fellow members of their faith community. (Often these communities are among a religious individual's major sources of security, social engagement, and meaning.) According to Davis et al. (2021), these comforting interactions can contribute to the formation of an image of a responsive God and strengthen a secure attachment to God.

But successfully encouraging a secure attachment to God may not be easy when treating clients who have a painful history of attachment relationships with parents or religious authorities, or who suffer from serious attachment insecurities (anxiety, avoidance, or both) with respect to close relationships. Research indicates that believers tend to generalize the insecure working models and orientations they developed in close relationships with human partners to the relationship they form with God. As a result, people who report attachment insecurities in close relationships are more likely than other people to have an insecure attachment to God (e.g., Beck & McDonald, 2004; Granqvist et al., 2012; Rowatt & Kirkpatrick, 2002). This generalization might work against a therapist's effort to strengthen clients' secure attachment to God. However, the correlations are only moderate in size, suggesting that an insecure attachment orientation in close relationships will not always correspond with an insecure attachment to God, and that effective therapeutic interventions might be able to foster a secure attachment to God even among attachment-insecure clients.

Davis et al. (2021) raised the possibility that some insecure believers can "earn" a certain degree of attachment security by reparative experiences within the context of psychospiritual interventions aimed at strengthening secure attachment to God. Two studies provided some support for this possibility. Monroe and Jankowski (2016) found that a single 2-hour session of receptive prayer (practicing openness, acceptance, and surrender to God; encouraging participants to ask God questions and then wait patiently and silently for a response) led to positive pre- to postintervention changes in felt security with respect to God. In another intervention study involving Iranian adolescents with conduct disorders, 14 sessions of spiritual psychotherapy (vs. a waiting-list condition) reduced avoidant attachment to God immediately after the intervention, and generated an increase in felt security that lasted at least a month (Salmanian et al., 2020). More research is needed to specify the religious/spiritual contexts that favor these adaptive changes and allow the development of felt security with respect to God among people who are generally insecure with respect to attachment.

Managing Attachment Insecurities with Respect to God

In Chapter 7, we noted that one major task for attachment-informed therapists is to assess and identify attachment-insecure clients' needs, fears, and defenses prior to therapy, attend to the in-session manifestations of these insecurities, and provide the most effective intervention for avoiding or overcoming their destructive effects on therapeutic work. Therapists also need to encourage and coach clients to be aware of these in-session manifestations, to think about (mentalize) the ways in which their insecurities contribute to suffering and interfere with therapeutic change, and to experiment and practice more secure methods of distress regulation and relating to others.

In SIP, therapists need to accomplish these challenging tasks while also assessing and dealing with clients' insecurities (anxiety, avoidance, or both) with respect to God and provide a secure base for mentalizing about these insecurities and their destructive consequences. Moreover, they need to direct clients' attention and mentalizing efforts to the ways in which both general and God-specific insecurities prevent comfortable reliance on God in times of need, exacerbate spiritual struggles and negative images of God, and aggravate spirituality-related distress. Finally, they should encourage clients to experiment with and practice more secure ways of relating to God.

There is evidence that attachment insecurities do interfere with the search for a secure spiritual connection with God in times of need. For example, believers who are avoidant with respect to attachment are less likely to engage in meditative prayer or to practice intimate forms of spiritual connection with God (Byrd & Boe, 2001; Jankowski & Sandage, 2011). Similarly, believers who are avoidant in their attachment to God are less likely to seek spiritual support in times of need, and those who are anxious in their attachment to God are more likely to be overwhelmed by doubts and worries about God's responsiveness (e.g., Ano & Pargament, 2013; Belavich & Pargament, 2002). More avoidant believers also tend to score lower on a self-report measure of the extent to which people turn to and maintain contact with God and religion as a means of obtaining felt security (e.g., Granqvist, 2002).

Two experimental studies also showed that attachment insecurities in close relationships reduce symbolic reliance on God following a laboratory-induced threat. Birgegard and Granqvist (2004) found that an implicit separation threat increased the wish to be close to God only among attachment-secure participants, not among anxious or avoidant participants. Similarly, Granqvist et al. (2012) found that implicit exposure to threat-related words, such as *failure* or *death* (as compared with neutral words), heightened mental activation of God-related concepts (indicated by shorter reaction times in a lexical decision task) only among secure participants, not among those with higher scores on the ECR anxiety or avoidance scales. Together, these findings imply that insecure people experience less automatic activation of positive God-related mental representations under threatening conditions than do secure people.

Similar interfering effects of attachment insecurities have been noted with respect to perceptions and images of God. In one of the earliest studies of attachment and religion, Kirkpatrick and Shaver (1992) found that people who experienced attachment insecurity in human relationships reported less positive perceptions of God as a loving and benevolent figure. Since then, numerous studies have replicated this finding in other countries, using different measures of God images, and across faith traditions (see Granqvist, 2020, for a review). This association has also been observed in a study using a less explicit measure of God images (Granqvist et al., 2012). More attachment-insecure participants (as assessed with the ECR scale) reacted to exposure to the word *God* (as compared to a neutral word) with faster reactions to negative traits (e.g., rejecting, distant) in a lexical decision task and slower reactions to positive traits (e.g., loving, caring). This suggests that attachment insecurities developed in human relationships do tend to interfere with the appraisal of God as a loving figure.

Attachment-insecure people also seem to miss the psychological benefits of feeling connected to God. In a laboratory experiment conducted with Israeli Jews, Granqvist et al. (2012) implicitly primed participants with a religion-related picture (a Torah scroll) or a neutral picture (a generic book) before exposing participants to a neutral stimulus (an unfamiliar Chinese ideograph) and found that exposure to the religious picture increased implicit positive mood (higher liking of the neutral ideograph). However, this effect was found only among secure believers, not among those scoring high on attachment anxiety or avoidance. In another line of experimentation with American and Swedish Christians, contextually priming the concept of God (compared with neutral material) increased interest in engaging in challenging, risky recreational behaviors, such as scuba-diving or wilderness camping, but only among secure participants (Gruneau-Brulin et al., 2018; Kupor et al., 2015). "God priming" failed to increase exploratory risk taking among less secure participants.

Studies that have assessed patterns of attachment to God reveal that believers who are less secure with respect to God are less likely to perceive God as a loving and supportive figure and more likely to miss the comforting effects of prayer (e.g., Bradshaw & Kent, 2018; Tung et al., 2018). Moreover, believers who are anxious in their attachment to God are more likely to feel disappointed by and angry toward God, to experience inner conflict and distress with respect to religious/spiritual beliefs and practices, and to hold ambivalent attitudes toward God (e.g., Cooper et al., 2009; Sandage et al., 2015; Trevino et al., 2019). Believers who are avoidant with respect to God tend to feel less indebtedness and gratitude to God for their positive life experiences (Knabb et al., 2021; Nelson et al., 2022). They are also less likely to engage in what Batson et al. (1993) called "religious quest"—exploration and questioning of religious beliefs and practices (e.g., Beck, 2006), which goes along with their reluctance to engage in activities that might arouse negative emotions.

All of these research findings highlight the importance of handling both general and God-specific attachment insecurities within the context of spiritually integrated psychotherapy. Without dealing with these insecurities skillfully, a therapist may fail to increase clients' comfortable reliance on God's support and fail to foster more positive images of God. In fact, insecure clients are likely to dismiss or reject a therapist's invitation to engage in prayer intended to deepen their relationship with God or to explore and reflect on the loving and comforting presence of God.

A therapist's work along the lines we've been discussing could be enhanced by assessment of a client's attachment history and working models prior to therapy and customizing treatment based on this assessment. Therapists could rely on cognitive and emotion-focused techniques proposed by MBT, AEPT, or EFIT to improve clients' self-understanding (see Chapter 7). The addition of religious and spiritual issues in the context of therapy relies on the same attachment-theoretical ideas and research findings found relevant in other kinds of therapy, but with the addition of considering religious and spiritual problems and resources in attachment terms.

Summary

In this section, we have shown that attachment theory and research in general, and the religion-as-attachment model in particular, are highly relevant to practicing and improving SIP. Unfortunately, as far as we can tell, no attachment-informed spiritually integrated approach to psychotherapy has been published, implemented, or tested, so our fairly loose ideas about the approach should be viewed as tentative. The two of us are far from being experts in developing the details of this kind of intervention (neither of us is religious, and we are not formally clinically trained), but we hope that clinical researchers and practitioners who are favorable toward religiously and spiritually oriented psychotherapy will consider incorporating the religion-as-attachment model into this kind of therapy.

Animal-Assisted Therapy

Animal-assisted therapy (AAT) is an umbrella term for therapies of diverse kinds (e.g., CBT, psychodynamic, experiential) used with children, adolescents, or adults in which an animal is an integral part of the treatment process (Chandler, 2012). AAT involves in-session interactions between a client, an animal (usually a dog), and a therapist. Although some clients are pet owners themselves, they interact with a new pet (i.e., the *therapy pet*) during the therapeutic session. The therapist might invite clients to explore and reflect on their experience during and after these interactions, and to comment on what they and the therapy pet wanted and felt during their interaction (Chandler, 2012). Some therapists present therapy pets as co-therapists or therapy facilitators; others present them as their own pets. Still others let their clients decide how they wish to refer to the therapy pets (Kruger & Serpell, 2006).

The use of AAT and the body of empirical research examining its effectiveness has increased substantially over the last several years. And several meta-analyses have found that AAT is an effective intervention for treating a wide variety of psychiatric and neurological disorders among children, youth, and elderly adults with disorders such as PTSD, behavioral problems, depression, and dementia (e.g., Chang et al., 2021; Hediger et al., 2021; Zafra-Tanaka et al., 2019). However, there are still many unanswered questions about the therapeutic processes underlying AAT's clinical outcomes. For example, it's unlikely that the mere presence of a therapy pet is sufficient to be helpful (Fredrickson & Howie, 2000), so we need to know more about the psychological functions of the therapy pet and how interactions with the pet facilitate therapeutic change. According to Fine (2000), AAT needs to be based on sound theory before it can gain widespread acceptance. In our view, attachment theory offers a useful framework for thinking about the psychological processes underlying AAT and its potential clinical benefits.

Although no attachment-informed AAT has been published, implemented, or tested, attachment theory and research can usefully inform AAT therapists in several ways. Of course, all of the attachment-informed practices we described in Chapter 7 are relevant for improving therapeutic work and AAT's clinical outcomes. However, more important in the present context, attachment theory and research provide relevant information about the therapeutic processes associated with in-session interactions with the therapy pet. Specifically, pets can accomplish attachment functions (safe haven, secure base), and children, adolescents, and adults can form a secure attachment to a pet (Zilcha-Mano et al., 2011a). For this reason, a therapy pet can function as an additional in-session attachment figure (beyond the therapist) that can contribute to a secure in-session climate and the mentalization processes needed for therapeutic change.

Human–Pet Attachment

Children, adolescents, and adults often view their pet as one of their best friends and as a potential source of a safe haven and secure base (Kurdek, 2008). Of course, a pet, unlike a human attachment figure, cannot provide advice and guidance in dealing with one's anxieties (although a pet might be imagined to do this: "Yes, I know, honey; you are sorry to see me so sad"). In addition, a pet is not usually "stronger and wiser" than its owner. Rather, like a child, the pet needs its owner's attention and care if it is to survive. However, pets tend to be naturally perceived as benevolent and kind, and as capable of providing comfort in times of need. Research shows that pet owners often describe their pets as loving, accepting, warm, helpful, trustworthy, authentic, and nonjudgmental (e.g., Hoffmann et al., 2018).

Therefore, even in human–pet relationships, people can feel close to their pets, seek and enjoy this closeness, and view these benevolent creatures as potential providers of felt security (Kurdek, 2008).

In applying attachment theory to human–pet relationships, Zilcha-Mano et al. (2011a) argued that a pet can serve as a safe haven and provide its owner with affection, support, comfort, and relief in times of need. They also argued that a pet can serve as a secure base from which its owner can more confidently pursue activities, take risks, and explore the world. In their view, people hold implicit beliefs about the pet's responsiveness to their needs for safety and security, which in turn may predispose them to be soothed and empowered by their pet's presence and affectionate gestures and behaviors.

Indeed, there is experimental evidence that, as compared to a control condition in which a participant's pet was absent, bringing their pet to the laboratory or being instructed to think about the pet reduced pet owners' physiological indicators of distress (e.g., blood pressure) during a difficult cognitive task (Zilcha-Mano et al., 2012, Study 1). Moreover, the physical or cognitive presence of a pet during a laboratory session (vs. a pet-absence condition) led to higher aspirations and greater feelings of self-efficacy when writing about personal goals (Zilcha-Mano et al., 2012, Study 2). These findings indicate that the actual or symbolic availability of a pet can soothe and empower its owner during threatening or challenging circumstances. However, as in other attachment relationships, it's not the mere presence of the pet that has soothing and empowering effects; it is the extent to which pet owners enjoy the presence of an affectionate and responsive pet. In support of this view, there is experimental evidence that pet owners have higher levels of oxytocin and opiates in their blood during comforting interactions with their dog in the laboratory (e.g., when gently scratching the dog; talking gently to the dog) than when simply reading a book in the presence of the dog (Odendaal & Meintjes, 2003).

In addition, just as people mourn when their principal attachment figure dies (e.g., a parent, close friend, or spouse), they also mourn the loss of a loved pet. According to Kwong and Bartholomew (2011), losing a loved pet may be akin to losing a loved human relationship partner. Indeed, there is evidence that pet owners who have lost their pet tend to report levels of grief and distress comparable to the grief experienced after the death of a close person (Rujoiu & Rujoiu, 2014). Moreover, as in human–human relationships, the strength of the emotional connection with the pet is positively associated with the intensity of grief reactions following the pet's death (Field et al., 2009).

Based on these findings, Zilcha-Mano et al. (2011a) concluded that a loved pet accomplishes the four definitional criteria of an attachment figure: It is a target of proximity seeking, it can provide both a safe haven and a secure base, and its loss causes separation distress and grief reactions. Hence, people's relationship with a pet can be viewed as an attachment bond and, as in other attachment relationships, they can feel secure or insecure with regard to their pet. On this basis, Zilcha-Mano et al. (2011a) constructed the 26-item Pet Attachment Questionnaire (PAQ) to assess pet owners' attachment to their pet. Thirteen items on the scale tap avoidant attachment to a pet (e.g., "I try to avoid getting too close to my pet") and 13 items tap anxious attachment to a pet (e.g., "I'm often worried about what I'll do if something bad happens to my pet"). The PAQ has been used in several studies, with statistical analyses corroborating its good psychometric properties and factor analyses validating its two-dimensional structure (e.g., Douglas et al., 2021; Kiss et al., 2020; Zilcha-Mano et al., 2011a).

As with other attachment relationships, attachment insecurities in relation to a pet tend to bias perceptions of the pet's responsiveness and reduce the psychological benefits of the presence of the pet when the owner is facing threats and challenges. Using the PAQ,

Zilcha-Mano et al. (2011a) found that pet owners who reported higher levels of pet attachment anxiety or avoidance held more negative expectations regarding their pet's responsiveness at both explicit (self-report) and implicit (reaction time in a cognitive task) levels. In addition, Zilcha-Mano et al. (2012) found that attachment-related avoidance toward a pet, as assessed with the PAQ, was associated with failure of a pet to be able to provide either a safe haven or a secure base. Specifically, for people scoring relatively high on the PAQ Avoidance subscale, the physical or cognitive presence of a pet (as compared to no pet presence) failed to reduce blood pressure during a distressing task or to produce more confident exploration of personal goals.

As one might expect, the quality of a person's attachment to a pet seems to be shaped by his or her attachment insecurities in close relationships with people (Zilcha-Mano et al., 2011a). However, the matching is far from perfect, implying that people who are insecure in the context of human–human relationships do not necessarily form insecure attachments to their pets. Moreover, due to a pet's authentic and natural ability both to give and to receive unconditional love, care, and affection, it may be able to circumvent some of the relational worries and defenses that characterize attachment-insecure people in their relation to other people and make them feel more secure in relation to the pet (Rockett & Carr, 2014).

As Cusack (1988) said, "Loving an animal can be easier than loving a person, and unlike a person, the love the pet has for its companion is generally without condition or judgment" (p. 9). With an affectionate and responsive pet, even insecure people may sometimes feel accepted and loved, and may not automatically project their maladaptive working models onto the pet. It's also possible that for children whose parents do not meet their attachment needs, animal companions might help to fill the gaps. According to Levinson (1972), "These children have experienced so much hurt at the hands of people in their environment. It is only after they have had a satisfactory relationship with an animal that they can make a start at developing a human relationship" (p. 35).

This compensatory function of relationships with pets has been documented in AAT contexts, where interacting with a loving and responsive pet in a therapy room has been shown to increase closeness and felt security to a therapist among children with a history of abuse or neglect (Parish-Plass, 2008). Balluerka et al. (2014) randomly assigned adolescents in residential care who had suffered traumatic childhood experiences to either AAT or treatment as usual and found that those who were given the opportunity to interact with a pet in the therapy room showed a steeper posttherapy increase in attachment security toward their parents. In subsequent studies with the same population, at-risk adolescents who interacted with a pet during therapy showed better relationship quality with parents and more positive attitudes toward teachers than at-risk adolescences who received treatment as usual (Balluerka et al., 2015; Muela et al., 2017).

Overall, the reviewed findings imply that a therapy pet might be particularly suitable for enhancing clients' felt security and empowering broaden-and-build processes and therapeutic change. At the same time, we should keep in mind that even if a therapy pet facilitates security enhancement, some clients might project their rigid insecure working models onto the pet and recreate previous insecure attachments with the pet. For those clients, we believe that the attachment-informed practices described in the next section can transform the relationship with the therapy pet into a valuable and efficacious therapeutic tool.

An Attachment Perspective on AAT Practices

In 2011, together with Zilcha-Mano, we proposed several therapeutic practices based on attachment theory and research that can be used within AAT to deal with a client's unmet relational needs and maladaptive working models (Zilcha-Mano et al., 2011b). During the intake process, an attachment-informed therapist should pay careful attention to projections the client directs at a pet and the feelings he or she expresses toward the pet (e.g., "She [the therapy pet] doesn't let me touch her; I think she doesn't like me"; "I can't stand it when someone gets so close to me the way she does; it's so annoying") as indicative of clients' attachment anxiety or avoidance. The therapist should also notice clients' spontaneous gestures and behavior within the therapy triangle (i.e., clients' responses to the therapist, the therapy pet, and the therapist–pet interactions) and to understand them as reflections of the client's attachment-related working models. For example, noticing that a client is jealous and angry when the pet clings to the therapist could reflect clients' anxious working models and suggest potential targets for therapeutic work.

During the first stages of therapy, a pet's warmth, acceptance, and uninhibited affection may contribute to the development of a secure in-session climate. According to Zilcha-Mano et al. (2011b), the comforting quality of therapist–pet interactions may help clients view the therapist as an attentive and caring person. Clients who observe a therapist relating to a pet in a nurturing way may think, "The therapist may be kind to me, too" (Reichert, 1998). Moreover, the therapist–pet relationship may help the client experience the therapy session as a safe haven. Clients may feel that the therapist will accept them even if they act in a regressive or negative way, because the therapist accepts the pet even when it acts unpredictably or unfavorably. The client may identify with the pet's wishes and fears, and feel unconditionally accepted by the therapist.

When a secure attachment develops with the therapy pet, the pet may become a relied-upon provider of security. During difficult sessions, the pet can help the client feel more comfortable in taking risks while exploring and reflecting on attachment injuries and other past traumas. The pet can display signs of affection and reassurance during these difficult moments, and clients can touch, stroke, and hug the pet while talking about painful experiences—comforting behaviors in which they cannot engage with the therapist. Moreover, according to Zilcha-Mano et al. (2011b), the therapy pet may sustain feelings of stability and continuity of the therapeutic bond despite temporary ruptures in the working alliance with the therapist. In addition, feeling secure in the presence of the therapy pet might facilitate clients' exploration and mentalization. This might render clients more responsive to their therapist's invitations to explore and reflect on the way they relate to the therapy pet, to see how this relationship differs from the troubled relationships they have with human partners, and to consider what they learn from interactions with the therapy pet to improve their interpersonal relationships. In this way, the therapy pet can facilitate the revision of clients' attachment working models.

According to Zilcha-Mano et al. (2011b), the therapy pet may symbolize different and even contradictory parts of the client's self or some feared or hated part of the self or parts about which they feel ashamed. In this way, a pet can provide an outlet for unpleasant traits, such as intimacy avoidance or inability to grant autonomy to others. For example, an anxious client may comment on the therapy pet's behavior: "She begs for attention. She won't let you proceed with anything until you pet her. She wants to know that you really do love her. . . ." On these occasions, the therapist can invite clients to explore and reflect on their thoughts and consider which parts belong to the pet and which belong to themselves. Such therapeutic work may foster the formation of more differentiated working models of self and others (Lasher, 1998).

Having a pet in the therapy room might also soften in-session manifestations of avoidant and anxious attachment, and allow the therapist to challenge insecure working models in a less threatening manner (Zilcha-Mano et al., 2011b). Often, in conventional therapy (without animals), anxious clients frustrate a therapist's attempts to encourage autonomy and self-reliance, and avoidant clients frustrate the therapist's attempts to encourage relational closeness and intimacy. In contrast, as detailed below, comforting interactions with the therapy pet may enable clients to experience these therapeutic efforts in a more open and less defensive manner.

Avoidant tendencies may be gradually softened during in-session interactions with a pet, because clients may feel that the pet accepts, validates, and respects their needs for self-reliance and autonomy, and that they can optimally regulate proximity to a pet without being criticized or punished. In this way, clients may enjoy interacting with the pet, savor the psychological benefits of relational closeness and interdependence, and even accept the pet's expressions of attention and love. As a result, the therapy pet might help avoidant clients feel more comfortable with interdependence, and they might be less defensive and more accepting of the therapist's attempts to increase relational closeness and invitations to explore and reflect on relational experiences.

For attachment-anxious clients, comforting interactions with the therapy pet might signal safety in the relationship (Arriaga et al.'s [2018] *safe strategies*) and allay attachment-related worries, because the pet provides unwavering reassurance, love, and attention. According to Zilcha-Mano et al. (2011b), attachment-anxious clients "know that the therapy pet will be there waiting for them in the therapy room the next session (as part of the therapeutic contract)" (p. 548). They may therefore experience the relationship with the pet as more predictable, stable, and secure than the relationships they have with human relationship partners. As a result, they may be more relaxed and receptive to their therapist's invitation to engage in autonomy-promoting activities and to explore and reflect on ways of becoming more independent and dealing with life circumstances on their own.

In some cases, clients' insecure working models may block the opportunity to form a refreshing, rewarding, secure relationship with a pet. According to Zilcha-Mano et al. (2011b), the therapist should view these occasions as opportunities for therapeutic work. He or she should encourage and coach clients to explore and reflect on their attitudes and feelings toward the pet and consider how their insecure working models and patterns of relating contribute to their troubled interactions with the pet: "Consistent with Bowlby's (1988) claim that therapists should offer occasional guidance, the client–pet relationship may serve as a simpler sphere for re-evaluating a client's insecure working models and the resulting maladaptive perceptions, expectations, and interpretations of social interactions" (Zilcha-Mano et al., 2011b, p. 553).

Therapists can also assist clients in exploring and learning about the maladaptive consequences of their troubled interactions with the therapy pet. For example, an attachment-anxious client may be generally favorable toward the therapy pet but become upset or angry when the pet leaves the client to get a drink of water. The therapist can take advantage of these moments to help the client reflect on his or her attachment needs and fears, which underlie the negative reaction to the pet, and to understand how he or she can manage and deescalate this kind of maladaptive response. According to Zilcha-Mano et al. (2011b), "This unique relational microcosm can help to broaden and build a client's relational skills. Because pets tend to be more forgiving than human beings when mistakes are made, they allow clients to work on 'interpersonal' skills in the absence of an unappreciative human interaction partner" (p. 553).

In summary, in this section we have focused on the usefulness of attachment theory and research as a conceptual framework for understanding human–pet relationships and AAT. We reviewed Zilcha-Mano et al.'s (2011b) suggestions concerning how insights derived from attachment theory and research can inform and improve AAT's therapeutic practices. However, we wish to reiterate Zilcha-Mano et al.'s (2011b) conclusion that "much still remains to be understood about the theoretical and practical implications of conjoining AAT and attachment theory" (pp. 554–555). This is a worthy area for future research.

Concluding Remarks

In this chapter we have considered three specialized kinds of psychotherapy that incorporate or could benefit from the use of attachment theory and research: grief therapy, SIP, and AAT. These kinds of therapy are quite different from each other, but in some ways our accounts of them reverberate among each other. Pet-assisted therapy, for example, might be a useful contributor to grief therapy, because a bereaved client might be able to obtain comfort and consolation from a loving animal in a way that might not yet be possible with a person. Therapy that includes religious issues, especially the nature of God as a security provider, offers additional attachment-related paths for grief resolution and adjustment to loss. All three kinds of therapy exemplify diverse ways in which attachment issues, concepts, and research findings can be and are being applied.

CHAPTER 9

Attachment-Informed Practices in Working with Therapeutic Groups and Work Teams

In the first volume of his trilogy on attachment, Bowlby (1969/1982) raised the possibility that adolescents and adults seek a safe haven and secure base from not only relationship partners but also informal and formal groups: "During adolescence and adult life a measure of attachment behavior is commonly directed not only towards persons outside the family but also towards groups and institutions other than the family. A school or college, a work group, a religious group or a political group can come to constitute for many people a subordinate attachment figure, and for some people a principal attachment figure" (p. 207). This inclusionary view of attachment figures has inspired theorists and researchers concerned with group processes and group psychotherapy to study attachment system functioning within group contexts and to determine whether a responsive and supportive group is capable of increasing members' felt security (for reviews, see Marmarosh et al., 2013; Tasca & Maxwell, 2021).

The attachment-related processes that characterize close dyadic relationships (see Chapter 6) do seem also to occur in people's relationships with the groups to which they belong (i.e., *in-groups*, Mayseless & Popper, 2007). For example, when facing threats and challenges during group and intergroup interactions, people tend to rely on their in-group for protection and support. Moreover, people often construe a group that is responsive to their needs and feelings as a symbolic source of a safe haven and secure base. They can potentially form a secure attachment to this kind of group and benefit from the broaden-and-build processes it makes possible. Unfortunately, as with close relationships, the psychological benefits of group membership can be interfered with by members' attachment insecurities (Smith et al., 1999). But actual supportive group interactions can move even dispositionally insecure members toward greater felt security (Rom & Mikulincer, 2003). In other words, supportive group interactions can provide one among several foundations for both beneficial psychological and, as we will discuss, organizational transformations and development.

In this chapter, we focus on the important possibility that social groups can have security-enhancing effects, and we review applications of adult attachment theory and research to group therapy and other kinds of groups (e.g., work teams, sports teams, elderly communities). We first consider evidence concerning attachment-related processes in group relationships and focus on the possible safe-haven and secure-base effects of a responsive social group. We then consider how this growing body of evidence is being applied in what Marmarosh et al. (2013) call *attachment-informed group therapy*. We also offer tentative ideas and proposals for developing attachment-informed interventions in other kinds of groups, suggestions aimed at contributing to improved functioning of both individual group members and their groups as wholes.

Security-Enhancement Processes in Group Relationships

The groups to which people belong and with which they identify (*in-groups*), such as their peer group, sports team, political party, ethnic group, nation, or culture, offer possibilities for safety and security in times of need (Brewer, 2007). From an attachment perspective, in-groups possess the two characteristics that define a potential attachment figure—benevolence and competence (Mayseless & Popper, 2007). People tend to perceive in-groups as a benevolent context (in which something beneficial and nothing harmful might happen). In-group members tend to have similar personal characteristics, share common values and goals, and feel a sense of solidarity or community of interests (Tajfel & Turner, 1979). As a result, they naturally tend to perceive each other as cooperative, helpful, and trustworthy (e.g., Tracy et al., 2020), and they may perceive their group as a benevolent social entity (my group, my team, my church, etc.).

Moreover, in many situations, groups are perceived as more resourceful and powerful than single, individual members in coping with threats and challenges. According to the *defensive aggregation* principle (Hamilton, 1971), tight clustering of conspecifics (e.g., flocking in birds, schooling in fish, huddling in mammals) reduces the probability of predation and diminishes the adverse psychological effects of stressors. For these reasons, people may rely on their in-groups for protection and support in times of need. Of course, they can also turn to in-groups for nonattachment reasons (e.g., accomplishing group tasks, having fun), but during times of need, such groups may be perceived mainly as possible sources of a safe haven and secure base.

Several social psychologists have proposed that groups can provide important emotional and instrumental resources for dealing with threats and challenges (see Jetten et al., 2012, for a review). For example, group membership can protect against existential threats (injury and mortality; Castano & Dechesne, 2005); sustain self-esteem (Abrams & Hogg, 1988); restore a sense of personal control (Fritsche et al., 2008); and reduce uncertainty (Hogg, 2007). In our view, personal strength in the face of vulnerability and mortality, a heightened sense of agency and control, and reduced uncertainty-related threats are inherent aspects of the safe haven and secure base functions that a competent and benevolent group can provide. As reviewed in Chapter 2, these provisions enhance felt security and support broaden-and-build processes that increase self-esteem and improve emotion regulation and goal pursuit. Hence, we agree with Haslam et al.'s (2009) proposal that a group has the capacity to act as a "social cure" for its members.

Seeking Proximity to a Group in Times of Need

From an attachment perspective, proximity and support seeking in times of need can be directed to not only close relationship partners but also social groups. However, we're not saying that dyadic and group relationships possess identical characteristics or serve exactly the same functions. Whereas a close relationship partner can provide personalized support that is tailored to one's specific emotional needs, groups are better equipped to encourage all of their members to cooperate with each other to satisfy their needs and stick together to cope with threats and challenges (Brewer, 2007). Moreover, whereas in a dyadic relationship there is an identifiable unique person (e.g., friend, spouse) to whom one can turn in times of need, no personified attachment figure exists in many cases of attachment to a group.

The expansion of proximity seeking beyond intimate dyadic relationships to groups is possible due to a developmental move from seeking physical proximity to seeking psychological closeness as the primary attachment strategy. Whereas infants need to be physically close to their attachment figure in order to feel safe and secure, older children, adolescents, and adults can sustain felt security by relying on feelings of emotional connection with a supportive attachment figure. They can also feel comforted by calling upon accessible mental images, thoughts, or memories of a security provider, even if that figure is not physically present at the moment (Mikulincer & Shaver, 2007).

Once this developmental shift has occurred, attachment needs can be directed to an image of a security provider rather than to a concrete person, although often there is a particular concrete figure associated with the image. Just as an image of the mother may comfort a child suffering from a stomachache, the image of a cohesive and dependable community may comfort a person facing the disaster of a tornado or flood. Therefore, even though people do not always have a concrete, corporeal person available to whom they can direct their attachment behavior, it is worthwhile to study their seeking of proximity to groups.

Proximity seeking in the context of group relationships takes a variety of forms. First, people can attempt to maintain physical proximity to group members by doing things together and *huddling* with them (the term used for this kind of behavior among nonhuman animals) during periods of danger. People can also directly or indirectly ask for guidance, instrumental support, or emotional reassurance from their group, including asking for what Cutrona and Russell (1990) called *social network support* (messages from group members that promote feelings of inclusion, acceptance, and appreciation). One can also make efforts to feel closer and more connected to the group and to share the group's strengths and resources. These attempts often result in heightened *group identification*, the sense that group membership is personally valuable and central for self-definition (e.g., Doosje et al., 1995)—and the inclusion of the group within the self (*group-based social identity*; Brewer, 2001).

Evidence That Proximity-Seeking Bids in Times of Need Are Directed to Groups

There are everyday observations as well as research studies indicating that people are prone to rely on in-groups for protection and support in times of need (Butler et al., 2019). For example, people are more likely to perceive support to be available from an in-group than from an out-group (e.g., Haslam & Reicher, 2006) and to interpret support from in-group members (vs. out-group members) in the manner in which it is intended (e.g., Haslam et al., 2004). People also tend to "huddle" with group members when facing natural or man-made disasters (Mawson, 2005). Indeed, studies of behavior during major fires show that people tend to converge and cluster and to evacuate only as a group, steadfastly maintaining proximity with conspecifics (e.g., Sime, 1985).

People also tend to heighten identification with their in-group in threatening times. In a series of surveys, a dramatic increase in patriotism (love of country, in-group solidarity) and identification with national symbols (e.g., flag, anthem) was found among

American adults immediately after the 9/11 terrorist attacks (e.g., Li & Brewer, 2004). A similar increase in patriotism was reported recently by Sibley et al. (2020) among New Zealanders immediately following the COVID-19 outbreak (compared to a matched pre-pandemic group).

Heightened in-group identification has also been noted following exposure to physical threats (e.g., potential virus contagion; Bélanger et al., 2013), economic and ecological threats (e.g., Barth et al., 2018; Uhl et al., 2018), and threats to feelings of personal control and self-worth (e.g., Fritsche et al., 2013; Greenaway & Aknin, 2018; Stollberg et al., 2017). For example, participants who read an article about the threat of climate change showed greater adherence to in-group norms than those who read a neutral article (Barth et al., 2018). Interestingly, as compared with participants whose performance on an exam was not publicly evaluated, those who were informed that a research assistant would grade the exam and therefore would know how they performed were more likely to wear or use items (e.g., clothing, pens) that were visible reminders of their group membership (Greenaway & Aknin, 2018).

Terror management studies examining the psychological effects of experimentally making mortality salient provide some of the best evidence for attachment system activation in relation to a group. For example, Castano et al. (2002) found that, as compared to Italian participants in a control condition, Italians exposed to death reminders displayed stronger identification with Italians, perceived themselves to share more common characteristics with Italians, and held more positive attitudes toward Italians (vs. Germans). Moreover, mortality salience increases self-group overlap, causing people to overestimate their consensus with in-group members' opinions (e.g., Pyszczynski et al., 1996) and to hold positive attitudes toward in-group members (e.g., Florian & Mikulincer, 1998; Greenberg et al., 1990; Harmon-Jones et al., 1996). In summary, numerous studies support the hypothesis that people seek to be emotionally close and connected to their social group in times of need.

The Calming and Empowering Effects of Responsive Groups

Being part of a group and sharing its strengths and resources can help members feel less vulnerable and more confident when facing threats and challenges. As in relationships with close relationship partners, the actual or symbolic availability of a group (e.g., doing things together, retrieving fond memories of comforting group interactions) can alleviate stress and distress, because members feel they are not alone and unprotected. Rather, they can rely on the reassurance and support provided by a benevolent and powerful social entity.

However, group membership is not sufficient to produce these positive psychological effects, just as the mere presence of a friend or romantic partner does not necessarily have calming and empowering effects (see Chapter 6). From an attachment perspective, these effects depend on two factors. First, they are a function of members' emotional connection to, and reliance upon, the group for protection and support; that is, the group must be appraised as a "figure" that can be comfortably approached when one is facing threats and challenges. To the extent that members do not use the group as a safe haven and secure base, the extent of its calming and empowering effects is reduced.

Second, these positive effects depend on members' appraisal of the group as accepting, validating, and supporting their needs and aspirations. Members who experience lack of group support, reassurance, or encouragement when needed; exclusion from group meetings or tasks; minor incivilities (e.g., disrespectful comments, gossiping, disapproving looks); or severe aggressive and abusive behaviors (e.g., physical intimidation, bullying, sexual harassment) may not feel calmed or empowered by being part of such a group. Rather, the group itself might become a source of frustration, pain, and distress—multiplying rather than reducing insecurity.

A group may have calming and empowering effects when members are sensitive and responsive to each other's needs, empathically attending to each other, sharing personal experiences, and offering comfort and relief in times of need (safe-haven support). Moreover, to be a source of solid security, group members must try to understand and validate each other's interests, feelings, and beliefs. They also need to encourage each other to believe that they are capable and skillful in solving problems and managing distress (secure-base support).

In such a responsive group, members provide constructive help and advice to each other when things go wrong, while maintaining an accepting and nonjudgmental attitude in cases of setbacks or failures ("Everyone makes mistakes; it's unrealistic to expect us to be perfect all the time"). They cooperate with each other and work together to find the best way to deal with threats and challenges. They also value and respect each other as autonomous human beings who have their own personal needs, beliefs, and preferences. All of these constructive relational tendencies contribute to members' confidence in the group as a safe haven to which they can turn when feeling distressed or confused, and as a secure base for exploration and thriving.

In the research field of group processes, these relational tendencies converge in one of the most researched group-level constructs—*group cohesion* ("the tendency for a group to stick together and remain united in the pursuit of its instrumental objectives and/or for the satisfaction of member affective needs"; Carron et al., 1998, p. 213). From an attachment perspective, *group cohesion* refers to the extent to which a group as a whole is appraised as a responsive social entity. The greater the group's cohesiveness, the more its members feel understood, validated, and cared for by the group, and the more they feel they are in the same boat with other members when dealing with threats and challenges. Therefore, members of cohesive groups might feel secure with regard to their group and perform at their best during group activities.

Evidence That Responsive Groups Have Calming and Empowering Effects

Research confirms that being part of a group contributes to a person's ability to cope with and thrive in the context of life's inevitable threats and challenges (Jetten et al., 2012, 2017). But findings also indicate that people who have a stronger emotional connection to a group (*group identification*) are more likely to benefit from being part of the group (see Postmes et al., 2019, for a meta-analysis). For example, in seven studies based on a diverse range of participant samples (e.g., former residents of a homeless shelter, schoolchildren, older adults), group membership predicted enhanced self-esteem mainly when people felt strongly connected to their group (Jetten et al., 2015).

The positive psychological effects of group membership are also amplified by members' perceptions of group responsiveness. Studies of emotional responses to natural disasters, losses, and traumas provide the most dramatic evidence for the calming effects of perceived group responsiveness (Kaniasty, 2020). For example, survivors of Hurricane Ike who reported having received more emotional support from their community immediately after the disaster exhibited lower levels of posttraumatic stress 12 months later (Platt et al., 2016). Also, Shang et al. (2019) followed up survivors of the 2013 Lushan earthquake in China and found that survivors' appraisal of the quality of group-based support (the extent to which it fit their needs and was provided in a timely and sensitive manner) was predictive of less distress 2 years later.

In the workplace, genuine expressions of affection, reassurance, and acceptance between team members tend to promote job satisfaction, alleviate emotional burnout, and foster positive attitudes toward novelty and change (e.g., Bastian et al., 2018; Ng & Sorensen, 2008; Poortvliet et al., 2015). In a meta-analysis of 142 studies ($N = 68{,}354$) and a two-wave prospective study, Mathieu et al. (2019) found that perceptions of emotional and instrumental support from work teams have positive effects on employees' well-being and reduce negative emotional effects of job-related stressors (e.g., job insecurity, abusive supervision). Research has also shown that members who feel safe about being included and accepted by a team (which Edmondson, 1999, called *team psychological safety*) are more likely to be creative within the team and to feel confident in dealing with demanding tasks (Abror & Patrisia, 2020).

Research on group cohesion in the workplace has shown that although the relative strength of effects varies depending on the type of group and task assessed, members whose group is rated as more cohesive (by members or external observers) are more likely to feel and perform better during group tasks (for meta-analyses, see Beal et al., 2003; Evans & Dion, 1991; Gully et al., 1995). In group therapy, the cohesiveness of the therapeutic group, as rated by clients, therapists, or external observers during therapy, has been found to be associated with pre- to posttherapy increases in clients' self-esteem, well-being, and mental health (see Burlingame et al., 2018, for a meta-analysis).

There is also evidence that citizens' perceptions of *community cohesion* (the extent to which neighbors get together to deal with local problems and provide support to each other) have positive psychological effects. In a seminal study, Cutrona et al. (2000) found that an aggregate-level cohesion index for a neighborhood predicted lower levels of psychological distress among Black women living in poor neighborhoods. Subsequent studies have also found that highly cohesive neighborhoods have lower rates of mental disorder (e.g., Stockdale et al., 2007). Moreover, community cohesion has been found to buffer the negative mental health effects of physical and emotional abuse during childhood (e.g., Greenfield & Marks, 2010).

Although cohesive groups can have calming and empowering effects, it's important to note that some cohesive groups might still fail to attend to, accept, or support members' personal quests and expressions of their unique personal identity and autonomy. For example, there are some religious or terrorist sects that, despite being highly cohesive, reject any attempt of members to question the validity of the group's dominant beliefs or goals and vigorously (sometimes brutally) suppress any attempt to develop independent thinking. These groups thwart members' desire for secure-base support and reduce the likelihood of their autonomous growth and thriving.

In our view, the most desirable cohesive group is one that is responsive to the full spectrum of group members' needs, including their desire to be protected and comforted when distressed and to affirm their autonomy and unique voice within the group. As yet, however, we don't know whether the reviewed calming and empowering effects of group cohesion result from groups' responsiveness to attachment needs or exploration needs, or both. Unfortunately, with the exception of two studies linking autonomy support from peers in the workplace with job satisfaction, work engagement, and mental health (Liu et al., 2011; Moreau & Mageau, 2012), we have located no research assessing secure-base forms of support from a group and examining their calming and empowering effects. We need further research that involves the development of reliable and valid measures of secure-base support within groups and that addresses the unresolved theoretical and applied issues.

The Interfering Effects of Attachment Insecurities

As in the case of dyadic relationships, the positive effects of responsive and supportive groups on members' well-being, needs satisfaction, and thriving might be obstructed by attachment insecurities that members bring from relationships with their principal attachment figures or past groups into their experiences with current groups. For attachment-insecure members, targeting a group as a potential security provider can reactivate their typical fear of rejection and negative working models of self and others. As a result, they may hold negative expectations of a group's responsiveness and find it difficult to engage constructively and confidently in group activities. They may therefore remain distressed and defensive when interacting with the group.

Attachment insecurities are likely to interfere with the formation of a cohesive group. Although anxious people's desperate need for love and attention may cause them to readily identify with a group, their rejection sensitivity may prevent them from making a leap of faith and taking interpersonal risks (e.g., disclosing their feelings, expressing their beliefs) during group interactions. And their tendency to become distressed in a self-focused, ruminative way may prevent them from empathically listening and properly responding to other group members' disclosures.

The formation of a cohesive group can also be hindered by avoidant members' distrust of others' goodwill and their own reluctance to engage in activities that increase psychological connection to, and dependence on, others. In fact, making the group a definitional component of their identity is at odds with avoidant people's compulsive self-reliance and their desire to view themselves as unique and separate from others (Mikulincer et al., 1998).

Attachment-related worries and defenses might also negatively bias appraisals of group interactions, preventing attachment-insecure individuals from enjoying, savoring, and capitalizing on calming and empowering group interactions. We suspect, however, that a clearly cohesive group in which members feel accepted, understood, valued, and cared for might be appraised as a safe haven and secure base even by attachment-insecure people. The emerging positive appraisal might allow them to take more interpersonal risks during group interactions, find that they can trust others' goodwill, and thus take a first small step toward increasing their sense of felt security. We return to this possibility in the next section of this chapter.

Evidence on Attachment-Related Individual Differences in Group Processes

In the first systematic study of attachment to groups, Smith et al. (1999) constructed the Group Attachment Scale (GAS) to assess anxious attachment to groups (e.g., "I often worry my group will not always want me as a member") and avoidant attachment to groups (e.g., "I prefer not to depend on my group"). Findings revealed that attachment insecurities in close relationships (as measured with the ECR) tend to be projected onto groups. People who are attachment-anxious in close dyadic relationships are also more likely to experience attachment anxiety with respect to groups, and people who are more avoidant in close dyadic relationships are more likely to develop avoidant attachment to a group. But the correlations are only moderate in size, indicating that although group attachment insecurities may be special cases of global insecurities, they are also influenced by other factors, such as past and current experiences in groups.

Additional findings from Smith et al.'s (1999) studies indicated that higher scores on group attachment anxiety or avoidance predicted lower engagement in group activities, more negative evaluations of social groups (e.g., fraternities, sororities), and lower perceived support from groups. In addition, whereas group attachment anxiety was associated with stronger negative emotions toward groups, group avoidant attachment was associated with lower levels of positive affect toward, and identification with, social groups. These early findings have been conceptually replicated in subsequent studies (e.g., DeMarco & Newheiser, 2019).

There is also evidence that attachment insecurities in close relationships can negatively bias group-related beliefs, feelings, and behaviors. Across four studies, Rom and Mikulincer (2003) found that ratings of attachment anxiety or avoidance in close relationships (assessed with the ECR) were associated with more negative views of social groups, more negative memories of group interactions, and more intense negative emotions and poorer instrumental functioning during actual group tasks (as assessed by both self-reports and observers' ratings). Subsequent studies have also found that attachment insecurities in close relationships are associated with lower identification with in-groups, lower perceptions of group cohesion, and less loyalty to groups (e.g., Ames et al., 2011; Ronen & Mikulincer, 2009; Rosenthal et al., 2014).

In an experimental investigation of insecurity-based negative biases in perceived group responsiveness, Santascoy et al. (2018) manipulated the benevolence/warmth of a social group and examined attachment-related differences in positive evaluations of the group. In the warm condition, participants read about a fictitious group (the Kaonians) whose members are renowned for their hospitality and interpersonal warmth and were presented with testimonials praising the warmth of Kaonians. In the cold condition, participants read that Kaonians are notorious for their inhospitable and cold nature and were presented with testimonials criticizing their coldness. Whereas no attachment-related differences in the evaluation of Kaonians were found in the cold condition, more attachment-avoidant participants evaluated Kaonians less positively when they were presented as benevolent and kind.

Attachment insecurities in close relationships also seem to negatively bias relational attitudes and behavior during group therapy. For example, clients with higher levels of attachment anxiety or avoidance (assessed before therapy) are more likely to provide negative appraisals of group climate and cohesion during and after therapy (e.g., Gallagher et al., 2014; Lo Coco et al., 2016; Marmarosh et al., 2009) and to perceive lower levels of support from other group members during therapy (Harel et al., 2011). In addition, more attachment-avoidant clients tend to be less attracted to their therapeutic group and less accurate in appraising other group members' traits (Chen & Mallinckrodt, 2002; Mallinckrodt & Chen, 2004).

In another study of socioemotional functioning during group therapy, Shechtman and Rybko (2004) found that more attachment-insecure clients were rated by external observers as sharing less intimate personal information during the first group session. In addition, whereas more avoidant clients scored lower on self-disclosure at the end of the counseling process, therapists rated attachment-anxious clients as working less constructively during group sessions. There is also evidence that more avoidant clients are more likely to devalue other group members' disclosures during therapeutic sessions (Shechtman & Dvir, 2006) and to reject requests to share intimate feelings with the group (Illing et al., 2011).

All of these processes can interfere with the formation of a cohesive group, especially if many of the group members are insecure with respect to attachment (Kivlighan et al., 2012). Moreover, these processes can interfere with the effectiveness of group therapy. Indeed, research indicates that attachment insecurities in close relationships, assessed before group therapy, are associated with lower chances of completing therapy (e.g., Tasca, Ritchie, et al., 2006) and poorer therapeutic outcomes (e.g., Leitemo et al., 2020).

Can a Responsive Group Move Attachment-Insecure Members toward Greater Security?

Happily, the answer to this question appears to be yes. Despite the initial projection of previously established negative working models onto a group one has just entered, repeated interactions with a responsive group can gradually soften the negative relational attitudes of attachment-insecure members and move them toward greater security with respect to the group.

Managing Attachment Insecurities during Group Interactions

According to McCluskey (2002), a responsive group can soften the dysfunctional effects of attachment insecurities during group interactions: "Failures in early attachment relationships can be revisited within the context of therapeutic groups and groups can provide the context for supporting authentic connection with one's own affect and encourage resonance with the affect of other people" (p. 140).

Pursuing this idea, Rom and Mikulincer (2003) conducted two studies of new recruits in the Israel Defense Forces (IDF) whose performance in combat units was evaluated in a 2-day screening session. On the first day, participants completed the ECR measure of attachment anxiety and avoidance in close relationships. On the second day, they were randomly divided into small groups of five to eight members that each performed three group missions. Following each mission, they rated their emotional state and instrumental functioning during the mission, and the cohesiveness of their group. External observers also provided ratings of each participant's emotional state and instrumental functioning during the three group missions, and participants completed the GAS (Smith et al., 1999) at the end of the second screening day to register their anxiety and avoidance with respect to their group.

In both studies, Rom and Mikulincer (2003) found that group cohesion (operationalized as a group-level variable created by averaging the appraisals of all group members) reduced the detrimental effects of attachment anxiety on instrumental functioning during group missions. Although recruits scoring higher on the ECR Anxiety subscale were less likely to contribute effectively to their group's task performance (as rated by themselves or external observers) in low cohesive groups, they showed improved instrumental functioning in highly cohesive groups. Moreover, Rom and Mikulincer found that group cohesion significantly attenuated group-level attachment insecurities, whether anxiety or avoidance, and weakened the projection of dyadic attachment anxiety onto the group.

These findings imply that attachment-anxious people can feel appreciated, valued, and cared for by a cohesive group. This kind of benevolent and responsive group may meet their needs for closeness, protection, and support, and allow them to feel more secure with regard to a group and to engage more comfortably in group activities. Conceptually similar findings have been reported by Ames et al. (2011) and Reizer et al. (2022) studying other kinds of groups (e.g., therapeutic groups, work teams).

Sadly, group cohesion failed to improve the functioning of avoidant military recruits (Rom & Mikulincer, 2003). Some of the findings even suggested that a cohesive group exacerbated avoidant people's poor instrumental functioning. As reviewed earlier, avoidant people attempt to deal alone with threats and challenges, and resist relying on attachment figures for protection and support. This "compulsive self-reliance" (Bowlby's term) seems to be sustained even during interactions with a cohesive group. Perhaps a cohesive group, which involves a high level of interdependence among group members, is so uncomfortable for avoidant people that it exacerbates rather than calms their attachment-related fears and defenses.

Research also indicates that group cohesion is beneficial in improving the mental health of attachment-anxious people undergoing group therapy (Gallagher et al., 2014; Tasca, Balfour, et al., 2006). For example, Gallagher et al. (2014) examined the potentially beneficial effects of group cohesion in a 16-week psychodynamic therapy group for women with binge-eating disorder and found that increases in cohesiveness of the therapeutic group (measured weekly) over the course of therapy were associated with a reduction in binge eating among attachment-anxious clients. Although attachment anxiety (assessed with a self-report scale) was associated with more severe binge-eating symptoms before therapy, this association was weakened after 16 weeks of therapy in groups that became more cohesive during the therapeutic process.

Group cohesion also seems to strengthen the positive contributions of attachment-insecure people to group performance. According to Ein-Dor (2015), groups can benefit from having attachment-insecure members. Whereas attachment-anxious members are good "threat detectors" who rapidly inform other members about approaching dangers or imminent problems (e.g., Ein-Dor & Orgad, 2012), avoidant members are the quickest to act and react to threats and dangers, perhaps acting quickly to save themselves but inadvertently showing other group members how to save themselves (Ein-Dor et al., 2011a, 2011b). However, Lavy et al. (2015) found that the benefits of including attachment-insecure people in a group were observed only among highly cohesive groups. In other words, when a group is able to understand, validate, and care for all group members regardless of their attachment-related predispositions, attachment-insecure members seem to contribute positively to group performance, perhaps in unique ways.

Fostering Felt Security within a Group

As in dyadic relationships, the steady experience of comfort and support during group interactions may, over time, increase attachment-insecure group members' sense of lovability and worth ("I feel accepted, loved, and valued by group members") and their confidence that group support will be available when needed. As a result, they can rely on the if–then expectations prescribed by the secure-base script (e.g., "If I face a threat or challenge, I can approach other group members and they will be supportive"), and enjoy being part of a responsive group. All of these within-group positive beliefs and feelings foster broaden-and-build processes that are beneficial to both individual group members and the group as a whole. Moreover, when group membership is an important aspect of a person's identity, the psychological benefits might extend to other relational contexts and contribute to moving an insecure person toward greater felt security in general.

To date, there is only one published study examining the potential effects of a cohesive group on felt security. As mentioned earlier, Rom and Mikulincer (2003) found that people scoring relatively high on attachment anxiety in close relationships felt less anxious and avoidant in relation to a cohesive (vs. noncohesive) group immediately after performing group missions. However, we have no evidence concerning the extent to which this short-term positive effect of a cohesive group would be maintained over longer periods of time.

In the context of group therapy, 11 studies have examined pre-to-post therapy changes in a client's global attachment orientation and have consistently found security-enhancing effects of being a member of a therapeutic group (see Table 9.1 for a summary of these studies' methods and findings). Samples have included women with binge-eating disorder, attachment-insecure women, violent men, and psychiatric inpatients and outpatients.

TABLE 9.1. Summary of Studies Examining Changes in Attachment Orientations or States of Mind Following Group Therapy

Authors	Sample	Type of therapy	Attachment measure	Timing of assessment	Major findings
Kilmann et al. (1999)	23 attachment-insecure women	AFGI vs. no therapy	RSQ	Before therapy After therapy 6-month follow-up	Pre- to posttherapy reduction in attachment anxiety after AFGI (but not in control condition), which was maintained 6 months later.
Lawson et al. (2006)	33 violent men	Group therapy vs. no therapy	AAS	Before therapy After therapy	Pre- to posttherapy higher increase in the number of securely attached participants after group therapy than control condition. Means of the attachment dimensions did not show any significant change.
Tasca, Balfour, et al. (2007)	66 women with binge-eating disorder	GPIP, GCBT	ASQ	Before therapy After therapy	Pre- to posttherapy reductions in attachment anxiety and avoidance after either GPIP or GCBT.
Kirchmann et al. (2012)	265 inpatients in psychiatric hospitals	Group psychotherapy in routine care	RSQ	Before therapy After therapy 1-year follow-up	Pre- to posttherapy reductions in attachment anxiety and avoidance, which were maintained 1 year later.
Kinley & Reyno (2013)	145 psychiatric outpatients in day treatment program	Short, intensive group therapy	RSQ	Before therapy After therapy	Pre- to posttherapy reduction in attachment anxiety.
Keating et al. (2014)	87 women with binge-eating disorder	GPIP	GAS ASQ	GAS: Weeks 4, 8, 12, and at end of therapy	Attachment anxiety and avoidance to therapeutic group (GAS scores) decreased during therapy.

				ASQ: Before and after therapy, and 6 and 12 months later	Pre- to posttherapy reductions in global attachment avoidance and anxiety (ASQ scores), which were maintained 6 and 12 months later.
Maxwell et al. (2014)	102 women with binge-eating disorder	GPIP	ASQ	Before therapy After therapy 6-month follow up 12-month follow-up	Pre- to posttherapy reductions in attachment avoidance and anxiety, which were maintained 6 and 12 months later.
Maxwell et al. (2017)	63 women with binge-eating disorder	GPIP	AAI	Before therapy 6 months after therapy	60% of women classified as insecure before therapy showed clinically relevant changes to a secure state of mind after therapy.
Compare et al. (2018); Maxwell, Compare, et al. (2018)	118 women with binge-eating disorder	Emotion-focused group therapy	AAI	Before therapy 6 months after therapy	Pre- to posttherapy increases in coherence of mind (attachment security) and reflective functioning (mentalization).
Maxwell, Tasca, et al. (2018)	63 women with binge-eating disorder	GPIP	AAI	Before therapy 6 months after therapy	Pre- to posttherapy increase in reflective functioning but not in coherence of mind.
Tasca et al. (2019)	85 women with binge-eating disorder	GPIP vs. no therapy	ECR	Before therapy After therapy 6-month follow-up 12-month follow-up	Pre- to posttherapy reduction in attachment avoidance (but not in control condition), which were maintained 3 and 6 months later.

Note. AAI, Adult Attachment Interview; AAS, Adult Attachment Scale; ASQ, Attachment Styles Questionnaire; AFGI, attachment-focused group intervention; GAS, Group Attachment Scale; GCBT, group cognitive-behavioral therapy; GPIP, group psychodynamic interpersonal psychotherapy; RSQ, Relationship Style Questionnaire.

Therapeutic modalities were diverse, including group CBT, emotion-focused group therapy, and group psychodynamic interpersonal psychotherapy. Eight of the 11 studies relied on a pre- and posttherapy design without a control condition, and the three studies that included a control condition compared the effects of group therapy to a no-therapy condition. Changes in attachment orientations were assessed with self-report scales and the AAI, and most of the studies followed up these changes 6 and 12 months after the end of therapy.

In the eight studies that assessed pre- to posttherapy changes in self-reports of attachment insecurities, six found a significant reduction in attachment anxiety, and five found a significant reduction in attachment-related avoidance (see Table 9.1). In the three studies that assessed pre- to posttherapy changes in AAI scores, two of them reported increases in a secure state of mind and in reflective functioning. Importantly, all of these positive changes were sustained 6 and 12 months after the end of therapy. Only one study (Keating et al., 2014) also assessed attachment to the therapeutic group during therapy (Weeks 4, 8, 12, and 16 of therapy) and found that group attachment anxiety and avoidance decreased significantly during therapy. Moreover, reductions in group-specific attachment insecurities during therapy predicted decreases in global attachment insecurities 1 year later. Overall, it seems that therapeutic groups have an enduring positive effect on clients' attachment orientations.

Beyond methodological problems concerning the omission of a control condition and lack of uniformity in therapeutic modality, the studies we've reviewed here fail to provide evidence concerning the mechanisms of change underlying the effects of group therapy on attachment orientations. For example, none of the 11 studies examined whether changes in the cohesion of the therapeutic group over the course of therapy drove the observed pre- to posttherapy changes in felt security. Future studies should address these deficiencies by examining the effects of being a member of a cohesive therapeutic group on group-specific and global attachment orientations (i.e., including dyadic attachment orientations), and extending this line of research to work teams and social groups.

Research Summary

Research on attachment-related processes within groups indicates that a responsive group contributes to members' well-being and goal pursuit, but members' attachment insecurities can interfere with these calming and empowering group-level effects. In addition, there is initial evidence that being part of a responsive group can enhance felt security, but we need more systematic research testing the validity and generalizability of these findings. Nevertheless, enough has been learned so far to inspire applications. In the remainder of this chapter, we show how research is being applied in group therapy (e.g., Marmarosh et al., 2013) and how these applications can be extended to other kinds of group work.

Applications of Attachment Theory to Group Therapy

In a clinically oriented book dealing with group therapy informed by attachment theory and research, Marmarosh et al. (2013) showed that many modalities of group therapy, ranging from psychoanalytically oriented group therapy to cognitive-behavioral group therapy, have incorporated core attachment-theoretical concepts. For example, psychoanalytically oriented group therapists acknowledge that maladaptive mental representations of self and others that were formed in earlier relationships (i.e., attachment working models) might bias the ways in which group members respond to each other (Schermer & Pines, 1994).

These biases can be explored and better understood through observations and discussions in therapeutic groups.

In their interpersonal process theory of group therapy, Yalom and Leszcz (2005) emphasized the importance of group members' sensitivity and responsiveness to each other's feelings and needs during group interactions. In line with Bowlby's (1988) emphasis on a secure base for exploration, Yalom and Leszcz (2005) stated that feeling understood, validated, and cared for by a group, members are more willing and able to reflect on current group experiences and understand their unmet emotional needs and maladaptive beliefs. Even cognitive-behavioral group therapists emphasize the importance of fostering members' empathy for and acceptance of each other as a means of revising maladaptive beliefs (White & Freeman, 2000).

According to Marmarosh et al. (2013), although psychoanalytic, interpersonal, and cognitive-behavioral modes of group therapy differ in their focus (transference of inner representations, current interpersonal experiences, maladaptive cognitions and behaviors), all of them highlight the importance of attachment-related processes for therapeutic change. According to Marmarosh et al. (2013),

> The emotional experience in the here and now, the presence of a responsive group that allows for a corrective emotional experience, and the ability to reflect on oneself and others are all important aspects of group therapy, regardless of the group leader orientation, because they revise internal representations of self and other. . . . In group treatment, not only do members experience current relationships in the group, they also revisit the internal representations of previous attachments and injuries, implicitly and explicitly, that have left them struggling to maintain intimacy and coping with challenging symptoms. The members are able to reengage each other in a process of restructuring automatic implicit relational processes, bringing emotion, insight, and a narrative into current relational experiences. All group therapies emphasize the importance of addressing maladaptive cognitions of self and other, addressing over- or under-regulation of emotion, and facilitating genuine interpersonal interactions that foster the capacity for intimacy. (pp. 34–35)

Based on this analysis, Marmarosh et al. (2013) proposed a road map and clinical guide for applying attachment-informed practices in group therapy. As in individual therapy (see Chapter 7), these practices inform and supplement the clinical work of therapists across all forms of group therapy. However, beyond these practices, some clinicians have developed attachment-based group therapies that explicitly draw upon attachment theory in conceptualizing therapeutic tasks and goals (e.g., attachment-focused group intervention, group psychodynamic interpersonal therapy, group mentalization-based treatment). In the following sections, we summarize Marmarosh et al.'s conceptualization of attachment-informed practices in group therapy and then briefly review the most notable attachment-based group therapies.

Attachment-Informed Practices in Group Therapy

Attachment-informed practices in group therapy are based on Bowlby's (1988) therapeutic tasks, which we described in Chapter 7: creating a warm and comforting safe haven; supporting and encouraging clients' exploration, reflection on, and revision of, their insecure working models; and providing opportunities to practice new ways of relating and coping. They are also based on research findings that insecure working models tend to emerge during group interactions and interfere with security-enhancement processes (discussed earlier in this chapter). These practices deal specifically with (1) creating a safe and secure group, so that members can confidently share painful memories and feelings, and remain open to the therapist's and other group members' comments and feedback; (2) broadening members' self-understanding; and (3) addressing members' attachment insecurities during group interactions.

Creating a Safe and Secure Group

In group therapy, the initial task of creating a safe and secure therapeutic climate is twofold. As in individual therapy, an attachment-informed group therapist endeavors to become a reliable safe haven and secure base for clients, increasing their confidence that they can count on his or her support when needed and that problems arising during group interactions can be addressed and at least attenuated with the therapist's guidance. For this purpose, an attachment-informed group therapist adopts all of the therapeutic attitudes of a responsive caregiver described in Chapter 7.

However, unlike the situation in individual therapy, the creation of a secure therapeutic climate in group therapy also involves helping the group to become a source of comfort and reassurance for distressed members and a secure base for improving their mentalization and self-understanding. In other words, clients in attachment-informed group therapy are encouraged to explore, uncover, and understand what is bothering them while being accompanied and empowered by two security providers: a responsive and supportive therapist and an accepting, understanding, and caring group.

In attempting to promote members' secure attachment to the group, a group therapist endeavors to create a highly cohesive group, to which members feel strongly connected (Yalom & Leszcz's [2005] feeling of "we-ness") and which they can approach for reassurance, comfort, support, and encouragement when needed. As members courageously share their painful memories and feelings, and begin to feel accepted, understood, and valued by the group, they gradually come to construe the group as a reliable source of felt security and therapeutic support. With the recurrence of these comforting group experiences over time, the group gradually becomes a more important secure base than the therapist, who can then relinquish the position of primary caregiver and manage group interactions more as a partner (Pistole, 1997).

How does one facilitate the creation of a cohesive group? According to Pistole (1997) and Burlingame et al. (2001), the process begins in pregroup preparation and early group sessions. During pregroup preparation, an attachment-informed group therapist defines group rules of acceptance, support, and positive regard for other members, and informs clients about the importance of working together in a cooperative and trustworthy manner for the sake of meeting all members' needs. The therapist also instructs clients regarding the appropriate attitudes and skills needed for group participation, such as empathic listening, responsiveness, and nonjudgmental responses.

During early group sessions, the therapist takes an active role in assuaging clients' discomfort, while sharing personal experiences, because the group is not yet appraised as a secure base. Moreover, the therapist can introduce highly structured group activities that reduce ambiguity and encourage members' self-disclosure and empathic listening (Bednar et al., 1974). As a result, members can gradually increase their confidence in the availability of the group's support when needed. The therapist can then begin to introduce less structured group activities and place more responsibility on the group as a security provider (Burlingame et al., 2001).

In the early group sessions, an attachment-informed therapist can also "model emotional accessibility through his or her psychological presence, sensitive listening, responsiveness, respect for others, and interest in members' and the group's welfare" (Pistole, 1997,

p. 12). In this way, the therapist not only fosters clients' secure attachment to him or her but also encourages group cohesion as members vicariously learn to behave within the group in a more accepting, responsive, and collaborative manner. The therapist endeavors to be well-regulated and relaxed in his or her interventions, and to use comforting and encouraging words and prosody in comments and feedback. This provides a model for the climate of group interactions, the quality of member-to-member exchanges, and the ways in which members provide feedback to each other (Marmarosh et al., 2013).

Broadening Group Members' Self-Understanding

When members begin to feel safe and secure during group interactions, an attachment-informed therapist moves a step forward and invites group members to explore and reflect on their unmet needs, painful emotions, and maladaptive relational beliefs. Specifically, the therapist encourages members to identify and reflect on ways in which these needs, emotions, and beliefs distort both their perception of what is happening in the group and their responses to other members' disclosures. The therapist also offers members opportunities to understand that these distortions are a source of pain and suffering in their lives and impair the quality of their relationships.

As in individual therapy, this step fosters increased mentalization and the creation of more reality-attuned working models. In attachment-informed group therapy, however, these processes are based mainly on the disclosures, comments, and feedback provided by other group members. A sensitive and skillful therapist only refines and amplifies the personal and constructive insights group members provided to each other (Marmarosh et al., 2013).

According to Marmarosh et al. (2013), unlike in individual therapy, the group context provides multiple sources of corrective interpersonal feedback that can improve members' mentalization. In group therapy, powerful working models built on past experiences can be challenged through a process of *consensual validation,* in which the therapist and multiple group members offer the same feedback from which an individual member can learn about the inaccuracy of his or her current feeling and beliefs (Yalom & Leszcz, 2005). When receiving consensual feedback from multiple trustworthy, accepting, and supportive others, group members may find it harder than usual to deny or dismiss the feedback. Instead, they begin to share with the group some doubts about the validity of their beliefs and try to understand the source, meaning, and implications of their attachment-related distortions.

Here is how Marmarosh et al. (2013) described the group processes that contribute to heightened mentalization:

> When the group members start to share their perspectives, they begin to observe that what they imagined to be true is not accurate. They are projections. . . . The members learn that what looks like disinterest on the outside may have deeper, more complicated roots on the inside. The members also learn to be curious about their immediate reactions and how they avoid conflict and intimacy. They come to realize that to know what is going on within another person's mind, they need to ask and then listen. They also learn that what is going on within them may be hidden from view and that what they see in others may be more indicative of their own personal feelings and interpersonal histories. Through the real relationships in the group and the reflective process, group members gain insight into who they are, why they feel and behave the way they do, and how previous experiences influence them. (p. 111)

An attachment-informed therapist can take advantage of two unique features of group therapy for strengthening members' self-understanding. According to Yalom and Leszcz (2005), clients in group therapy can see in other members the same issues with which they personally are coping. Therefore, an attachment-informed group therapist can use this *hall of mirrors* (Yalom & Leszcz, 2005, p. 1162) to encourage members to share with others their common attachment-related issues and to learn about the ways each one is coping with them.

In addition, group therapy offers the opportunity to encounter and confront a wide range of attachment-related issues, because different members bring different attachment working models and problems to the group. An attachment-informed group therapist can invite members to explore and reflect on how they perceive and react to members with different working models and practice more adaptive ways of interacting with each of them. In this way, the group context can greatly contribute to the broadening of members' relational skills.

Handling Group Members' Attachment Insecurities

Working with groups from an attachment perspective, a therapist needs to be familiar with each group member's attachment history, working models, and style. This knowledge is paramount, because it allows the therapist to understand each member's needs and feelings within the therapeutic group, as well as the member's reactions to others' disclosures and feedback. According to Wallin (2007), "Such knowledge can also strengthen our ability to imagine, understand, and empathically resonate with the subjective experience, as well as the childhood histories, of our patients" (p. 85).

Hence, during pregroup preparation, an attachment-informed group therapist assesses members' attachment histories and current working models, as well as their group-related attitudes and habitual style of interacting within groups. As in individual therapy, this assessment not only provides information about each group member's attachment style, but it also enables the therapist to tentatively hypothesize about how each group member's working models and pattern of relating might facilitate or disrupt the development of a cohesive group.

When assessing the attachment histories and working models of group members, the therapist also considers the composition of the group in terms of attachment styles. In this way, he or she can develop hypotheses about how group members sharing or differing in attachment needs, fears, and defenses can positively relate or potentially collide with each other (e.g., how two group members anxiously seeking reassurance, love, and attention from the group might relate to each other during group activities). Moreover, the therapist can use information about the attachment-related composition of the group to customize treatment and choose the best strategy for working with a particular group.

When the group as a whole is high on attachment anxiety, or when working with group members who experience intense fears of rejection and doubts about their value and lovability, an attachment-informed group therapist attempts to allay these concerns early in therapy by providing unwavering signs of availability, responsiveness, and care. He or she can also explicitly ask group members to be accepting, empathic, and kind to each other. Moreover, the therapist can introduce highly structured group activities that direct members to express affection and positive regard to each other, signaling that the group is reassuring and safe (Arriaga et al.'s [2018] *safe* strategies; see Chapter 6).

When the group as a whole is high in attachment-related avoidance, or when working with group members who distrust others' intentions and feel uncomfortable with emotional closeness and interdependence, an attachment-informed group therapist can soften these concerns early in therapy by unconditionally accepting members' need for independence and self-reliance. Moreover, the therapist can encourage group members to respect and reinforce each other's uniqueness and autonomy. Therapists can also introduce highly structured group activities that do not demand highly intimate, emotion-laden disclosures, thereby making it feel less dangerous for avoidant members to engage actively in group activities (Arriaga et al.'s [2018] *softening* strategies; see Chapter 6).

Pregroup assessment of clients' attachment histories and working models can also help therapists decide about the composition of a particular group. Kivlighan et al. (2017), for example, found that if a group comprises mainly attachment-anxious members, adding members who are low on this dimension may contribute to group cohesion. However, when the group as a whole is high in attachment-related avoidance, adding a low-avoidant member may be dissonant with the group's tendency to maintain social distance and may actually reduce group cohesion. Kivlighan et al. say that avoidant individuals function best in groups that accept and respect their needs for self-reliance and autonomy.

As noted earlier, in the early stages of therapy, an attachment-informed group therapist attempts to meet the relational needs of both attachment-anxious and attachment-avoidant members (e.g., to feel loved and protected, to feel self-reliant) during group activities. In this way, he or she endeavors to create a cohesive group in which all of the members can feel safe and secure. However, with the consolidation of group cohesion, the therapist can begin to sensitively challenge members' insecure working models by using counter-complementary attachment proximity strategies (Mallinckrodt, 2000; see Chapter 7), stimulating members to question and revise their maladaptive beliefs and expectations (i.e., attachment-anxious members' negative representations of the self; attachment-avoidant members' negative representations of others).

Attachment-Based Group Psychotherapies

Several group therapeutic approaches have been built explicitly on the foundation of attachment theory and research. However, with the exception of group psychodynamic interpersonal psychotherapy (Tasca et al., 2005) and the Connection Project (Allen et al., 2021), systematic attempts to test the effectiveness of these approaches have been lacking. Therefore, after briefly presenting some of these insufficiently researched approaches, we devote most of this section to two approaches, group psychodynamic interpersonal psychotherapy (GPIP) and the Connection Project, the effectiveness of which has been examined in rigorous RCTs.

Based upon Bateman and Fonagy's (2004) mentalization-based treatment (MBT; see Chapter 7), Karterud (2015) developed a group therapy version of this attachment-based intervention (MBT-G). This approach adheres fully to the goals, tasks, and techniques of MBT, while attempting to create a group that supports and encourages members' exploration of and reflection on their emotional experiences and patterns of relating. Unfortunately, the single RCT that tested the effectiveness of MBT-G did not find it superior to treatment as usual in reducing psychiatric symptoms immediately after therapy in a sample of 113 adolescents with borderline personality disorder (Beck et al., 2020). Similarly disappointing findings were obtained when clinical outcomes were assessed 3 and 12 months after therapy (Jørgensen et al., 2021). Moreover, no data have been collected to determine the extent to which MBT-G improves clients' mentalization or enhances felt security. We hope that more RCTs will be conducted on this group therapy version of what is an effective attachment-based therapy for individuals (see Chapter 7 for a review of supportive findings regarding MBT's effectiveness).

In 1999, Kilmann et al. developed a 17-hour manualized group therapy (*attachment-focused group intervention*) for attachment-insecure people that focuses on exploration and revision of dysfunctional attachment dynamics. The therapy includes four segments. In the *relationship belief* segment (3 hours), group members are encouraged to explore and revise unrealistic relationship beliefs. In the *attachment issues* segment (10 hours), group members are encouraged to explore their insecure patterns of relating and the ways in which early experiences with parents shaped these patterns. In the last two segments, *relationships skills training* and *relationship strategies* (2 hours each), group members are encouraged to identify and discuss skills and attitudes that contribute to mutually satisfying relationships.

The effectiveness of this attachment-focused group intervention was examined in a single study. Kilmann et al. (1999) applied the intervention in a group of 13 attachment-insecure women and found that, as compared to a no-intervention group, the intervention reduced group members' dysfunctional relational beliefs and attachment anxiety. However, the small sample size, problems in the randomization process, and lack of comparison to other kinds of intervention raise doubts about the value of these findings. Moreover, no attempt to implement this intervention in other samples or to replicate the findings in larger samples has been made during the last 20 years. Therefore, we don't feel confident in evaluating the effectiveness of this attachment-focused group intervention.

The Connection Project

Based on principles from attachment theory and techniques from experiential therapies, Allen et al. (2021) created the Connection Project—a group-based intervention aimed at strengthening adolescents' feelings of social belongingness, improving the quality of their peer relationships, and fostering reliance on peers and friends as safe havens and secure bases. The program consists of nine to 12 sessions (around 60–75 minutes each) with small groups (around five to 15 members) of adolescents led by two trained facilitators. Facilitators are trained to create a secure in-session climate, while encouraging and coaching members to disclose personal experiences and challenges, to respond empathically and supportively to others' disclosures, and to enjoy moments of shared experience and togetherness. "The program used an experiential process to teach and model the formation of deep, supportive, and authentic relationships such that its effects would ultimately extend outward to group members' social interactions beyond the group" (Costello et al., 2022, p. 4).

The sessions are organized into three phases: (1) establishing a safe and supportive group context, (2) developing and enhancing a sense of social belonging, and (3) consolidating relationship gains. In the first phase, group activities are designed to increase members' felt security with respect to the group through repeated experiences of acceptance, positive regard, validation, and support within the group. In the second phase, the facilitators introduce group activities aimed at enhancing feelings of belongingness and togetherness within the group. These activities enable members to think about and savor shared experiences with their group and to realize that they are not alone in the ways they experience and deal with threats and challenges.

In the third phase, each member is invited and encouraged to talk about a challenge that he or she has faced and to reflect on what was learned from this difficult experience. Other group members are coached to respond in a sensitive and supportive way. "In the atmosphere of safety, belonging, and support that has been created by the final sessions, students often choose to reflect upon and share profound experiences in moving ways, which in turn evoke strong, spontaneous expressions of support from peers. Teens find that they truly are not alone and that others can really get to know and support them in a deep way" (Allen et al., 2021, p. 650). In the final session (a *strengths bombardment* session), members talk about the positive qualities and strengths of each member of the group, thereby strengthening members' positive working models of self and their confidence in others' benevolence.

The effectiveness of the Connection Project was examined in two RCTs—one with 610 high school students from economically and racially/ethnically marginalized groups (Allen et al., 2021) and the other with 438 first-year college students (Costello et al., 2022). In both studies, the youth were randomly assigned to either the Connection Project or a no-intervention (waiting-list) condition. In Allen et al.'s (2021) study, students in the Connection Project reported better peer relationships, more reliance on social support for coping with stress, more academic engagement, and less depression after the intervention than controls, and these gains were maintained 4 months later. Similar findings were reported by Costello et al. (2022): As compared to the no-intervention condition, the Connection Project resulted in reports of greater social belongingness and lower scores on loneliness and depression.

Overall, the two RCTs attest to the promise of the Connection Project, but more research is needed comparing this attachment-based intervention with other kinds of group-based programs and examining its effects in samples of more troubled youth. Future studies should also examine the extent to which the Connection Project is effective in fostering positive models of self and others, and moving attachment-insecure youth toward heightened felt security.

Group Psychodynamic Interpersonal Psychotherapy

Attachment theory is one of the conceptual pillars of GPIP (Tasca et al., 2005, 2021), a time-limited treatment (16 weekly 90-minute sessions) that combines principles from interpersonal, psychodynamic, and group psychotherapy theories. Tasca et al. (2005) borrowed from attachment theory the idea that frustration of attachment needs during interactions with a nonresponsive relationship partner elicits anger, anxiety, and sadness, and fosters reliance on maladaptive defenses that can create relational and emotional problems. In their view, these problems reflect the underlying action of *cyclical maladaptive interpersonal patterns* (CMIPs) that resemble Johnson's (2004) maladaptive dyadic cycles (see Chapter 6). These patterns include unmet attachment needs, resultant painful emotional experiences, defensive reactions, maladaptive beliefs about self and others, and destructive patterns of relating.

During treatment, the therapist focuses on members' "here-and-now" interactions with the group as a way of helping them identify, explore, and revise their CMIPs. Group members are encouraged to talk, elaborate, and provide comments and feedback to each other concerning their needs, feelings, maladaptive beliefs (what they expect from others, how others react to them, how they perceive themselves in the group), and relational problems (e.g., hostility, coldness, intrusiveness). These group-based explorations facilitate CMIP-related mentalization, which in turn can reduce relational difficulties and facilitate the revision of group members' insecure working models.

GPIP includes a pregroup preparation process during which therapists assess each group member's CMIPs (i.e., attachment needs, emotions, defenses, working models, relational problems) and their potential consequences for group interactions. In the early stage of therapy, the therapist focuses on developing a cohesive group in which members can feel safe and secure. At the same time, he or she encourages members to explore and reflect on their needs, feelings, beliefs, and relational problems in an open and constructive manner during group interactions.

In the middle stage, the therapist attempts to gently challenge group members' CMIPs during group interactions, with the intent of modifying their interactions with the group and the ways in which they relate to others outside the group. During the later therapy sessions, the therapist encourages group members to talk about past experiences of separation and loss, and link them to the end of therapy. Moreover, revised working models and adaptive relational patterns are reinforced and practiced.

The effectiveness of GPIP was first examined by Tasca, Ritchie, et al. (2006) in an RCT involving a sample of 135 women with binge-eating disorder randomly assigned to GPIP, group cognitive-behavioral therapy (GCBT), or a waiting-list condition. As compared to the waiting-list condition, GPIP reduced binge-eating symptoms, depressive feelings, and interpersonal problems up to 12 months posttreatment. However, GPIP did not outperform GCBT on these measures. In a second RCT, Tasca et al. (2019) provided unguided self-help to 135 women with binge-eating disorder, then randomly assigned those who remained in the study (n = 85) to either GPIP or a no-therapy condition. The self-help intervention was effective in reducing binge-eating symptoms, and GPIP did not result in further improvement in these symptoms. However, as compared to the no-therapy condition, GPIP reduced self-reports of relational problems and attachment avoidance over and above the effects of the self-help intervention.

Overall, GPIP seems to be a useful group therapy for women with binge-eating disorder. But we don't yet know whether it is effective in treating other psychological disorders. Future RCTs should evaluate the applicability and validity of GPIP as an effective transdiagnostic group therapy. It will also be important to discover the beneficial parts (effectiveness mediators) of GPIP—and of GCBT for that matter, the effectiveness of which may be due to attachment-related, not simply cognitive, processes.

Applications of Attachment Theory to Work Teams and Social Groups

Attachment theory and its extension to group processes can contribute to interventions in other areas of group work, such as work teams, sports and exercise teams, military units, support groups in health-related settings (e.g., oncology wards, rehabilitation units, community centers for elderly adults), and neighborhood communities. However, unlike the attachment-informed practices and attachment-based interventions in the field of group therapy, consciously applied attachment-related practices and interventions are rare and underdeveloped in most areas of group work. In this section, we want to remedy what we see as a deficiency by offering suggestions and recommendations gleaned from attachment theory and research. We hope that this will benefit coaches and group leaders who want to promote the functioning and thriving of both individual group members and their teams.

Before moving into specific details concerning attachment-informed practices in group work, we should make clear that attachment theory is relevant for both groups whose purpose is to foster the well-being and performance of individual group members (e.g., therapeutic groups, exercise groups, support groups) and groups whose purpose is to effect positive outcomes for an organization (e.g., work teams, military units, sports teams). When presenting attachment theory to military officers or managers of business organizations, we find that many of them react in a somewhat hostile and demeaning way. They believe that their teams need to focus on the task at hand and not divert precious resources to caring for each member's emotional needs ("Our teams are not support or therapeutic groups"). However, growing evidence for the broaden-and-build effects of cohesive groups tends to convince them that making members feel included, accepted, and supported by the group and construing the group as a secure base for exploration might be preconditions for improving group members' productivity and creativity. From an attachment perspective, developing a "support group" is a goal in itself in therapeutic/health settings and a necessary means of improving the performance of task-oriented groups and increasing their contribution to the organization.

In applying attachment theory to group settings, we must consider that groups develop gradually, beginning with a collection of individuals with their own interests and ambitions, and ending up, when all goes well, with a well-integrated group of collaborators with a common focus and shared goals. In 1965, Tuckman proposed, poetically, that groups develop through four stages: *forming*, *storming*, *norming*, and *performing*. In later writings, Tuckman and Jensen (1977) added a fifth stage (*adjourning*) for groups that have an endpoint.

From an attachment perspective, we view group development through the lens of Bowlby's (1982) stages of attachment-bond formation. This process begins with the perception of a group as a potential attachment figure and goes through the gradually increasing construal of this group as a secure base (a process that Bowlby, 1969/1982, called *attachment-in-the-making*) until group members feel safe and secure in the group (*full-blown attachment*). It ends in the formation of a mutually satisfying and highly committed partnership among group members (*goal-corrected partnership*) for the benefit of the group as whole.

Following Alexandre Dumas's immortal phrase in *The Three Musketeers*, we can say that group development involves consolidating first the sense of "All for one" (secure attachment to the group), which may launch a broaden-and-build process and foster the prosocial sense of "One for all." Attachment-informed practices are relevant both for encouraging the construal of the group as a secure base during the forming and storming stages, and facilitating effective group performance in the norming and performing stages.

Forming Stage

During the forming stage of group development, group members are often excited to be part of a new group, eager to begin working together, and tending to be polite and deferential to one another during group interactions. However, at the same time, they harbor questions and doubts about their place in the group, their contribution to the group, and the extent to which the group will meet their needs and expectations. Moreover, each member sees the group tasks and goals primarily from his or her own perspective and views the "group" as somewhat of a fiction. The main group work during the forming stage is to consolidate a working alliance between group members, defined by a sense of "groupness," a trusting comfortable group climate, and agreement about group task and goals.

During the forming stage, an attachment-informed coach or group leader attempts to portray the group as a safe haven and secure base in which all members can feel confident that their unique needs, feelings, beliefs, and behaviors will be accepted, understood, valued, and respected. In other words, much of the energy of an attachment-informed group leader during this initial stage is focused on fostering group members' sense of psychological connection to the group (including the increasing inclusion of the group within each member's self-identity), so that they can begin to rely on the group as a potential source of protection and support. The group leader also places strong emphasis on facilitating group members' responsiveness and supportiveness toward one another and gradually fostering a solid sense of group cohesion.

There are several well-established practices that an attachment-informed coach or group leader can use to foster members' emotional connection to a group. For example, group members can be encouraged to jointly explore, deliberate, and make decisions about core aspects of the group's life (e.g., C. Haslam, Haslam, Knight, et al., 2014) or to jointly reflect on group experiences that are important to individual members or the group as a whole (e.g., C. Haslam, Haslam, Ysseldyk, et al., 2014). They can also be encouraged to engage in joint activities (e.g., Morris et al., 2012), including those in which group members simultaneously perform the same task (e.g., individual painting) and those in which they perform interdependent tasks (e.g., group problem solving). Steffens et al. (2021) meta-analyzed 27 studies (N = 2,230) that applied one of these group practices and found that, as compared to control conditions, these practices enhanced group identification and made a moderate-to-strong contribution to members' quality of life, self-esteem, well-being, and mental health. And the practices had greater psychological benefits for members who identified strongly with the group.

In building group cohesion, an attachment-informed coach or group leader can use practices borrowed from group therapy. For example, the group leader can endorse the cohesion-building norms that Tasca et al. (2021) emphasize in GPIP, encouraging and reinforcing members for doing the following:

1. Openly disclosing their personal feelings and expressing their own beliefs and opinions without being afraid of being rejected or criticized.
2. Maintaining a positive and calm emotional tone.
3. Being attentive and genuinely interested in what other members are saying and accepting, valuing, and respecting their disclosures.
4. Providing kind and constructive feedback to other members aimed at improving both their own understanding and capacities and the climate and functioning of the group as a whole.
5. Taking into consideration the feedback provided by other members, since it is given from an accepting and respectful attitude.
6. Sticking together and remaining united in the pursuit of group goals despite disagreements and tensions.

An attachment-informed coach or group leader can also draw upon the Circle of Security (COS) intervention, which was originally developed to improve the quality of parent–child relationships (see Chapter 4). Specifically, the leader can expose group members to the COS vocabulary and graphics (see Figure 4.1) and represent the group as the *hands on the circle*—the secure base from which members explore and broaden their perspectives and the safe haven to which they can return for comfort and reassurance. Using COS graphics, group members can learn about their needs for attachment and exploration, the specific hardships they may experience during group activities, and the ways a group can make them feel safe and secure.

An attachment-informed coach or group leader can also video-record the initial sessions and invite members to view and review fragments of positive interaction moments during which group members were responsive and supportive to one another. In this way, the coach can highlight and reinforce members' responsiveness and supportiveness while making them more attentive and sensitive to other members' unique ways of being responsive and supportive. This experiential learning can be an effective means for fostering group cohesion.

Storming Stage

During the storming stage of group development, conflicts between group members, as well as concerns about losing personal freedom and worries about being rejected or unable to meet the group's goals, begin to surface. Members may become critical and express frustration about group goals, roles, and tasks, while noticing how the group responds to nonconsensual arguments and how it handles disagreements and conflicts. According to Tuckman (1965), "Group members become hostile toward one another and toward a therapist or trainer as a means of expressing their individuality and resisting the formation of group structure" (p. 386). These negative emotional responses are likely to interfere with group cohesion and members' felt security in relation to the group, thereby compromising effective group functioning.

This critical stage calls for group members to reappraise disagreements and conflicts as necessary evils in the formation of an effective group, confront these issues in a constructive manner, and come to a consensus about how to move forward as a group. Group leaders can help the group remain flexible and develop effective strategies for managing conflicts and pacifying members' worries about their value to the group or their potential loss of autonomy. In this way, group cohesion and a climate of security can be restored, and group members can refocus on group tasks and goals.

From an attachment perspective, the storming stage is dominated by the enactment of members' attachment worries and defenses within the group. For example, group members with predominantly avoidant defenses may be concerned with losing their uniqueness and autonomy during group interactions and may vigorously attempt to distinguish themselves and wall themselves off from other members. They may withdraw from activities that increase interdependence and uniformity within the group and may react with contempt, criticism, or hostility toward other members' disclosures or feedback.

Attachment-anxious group members may express frustration that their needs for affection and attention are not being met by the group and may insist, sometimes even in an intrusive or coercive manner, that the group attend to and care for them. They may misinterpret other members' comments as signs of rejection and react with accusations and anger. They may also demoralize the group by presenting themselves as unable to accomplish group tasks.

An attachment-informed coach or group leader considers the group members' attachment worries and help them to reflect on how these worries shape angry, demanding responses or emotional withdrawal and stonewalling. In addition, the leader can encourage and coach group members to use more constructive ways of communicating their needs for attention or autonomy. This makes it easier for other members to understand and empathize with an attachment-insecure member's feelings and responses, which can open the door to more supportive group interactions.

Using Johnson's (2004) terminology, these attachment-informed practices can help a group leader to *soften* group members' enactments of attachment insecurities. An attachment-avoidant person might be helped to feel understood and valued by the group, and then be able to remain constructively engaged during group activities (a process that Johnson called *withdrawer re-engagement*). Group members might also accept and understand an attachment-anxious member's neediness and vulnerability, and he or she might learn to express demands for attention and care in more constructive and easy-to-accept ways (*pursuer/blamer softening)*. Through these softenings, the storming group interactions might become less intense and less frequent, group members might again feel safe and secure in the group, and they might be able to focus on, and genuinely feel motivated to contribute to, the accomplishment of group tasks and goals.

Norming and Performing Stages

During the norming stage, intragroup conflicts occur less frequently, and group members take pleasure in the increased group cohesion and are able to work together harmoniously despite differences (Tuckman, 1965). This desirable group harmony pays off in the performing stage. Members become committed to the group's mission and are willing to invest time and energy in improving their individual performance and contributing fully to group creativity and productivity. In this way, the boundaries between individual performance and group success blur as group members become engaged in and highly committed to group tasks and goals.

Theoretically, we view the consolidation of members' secure attachment to a group to be what underlies the transition of a group to the norming and performing stages. In these stages, members feel confident in the responsiveness and supportiveness of the group and can move from an egoistic, self-protective focus to a more prosocial focus. They can appreciate the good qualities of other group members and the benefits of being in a highly cohesive group, making it easier for them to cooperate with others, confidently accommodate to the group's rules and norms, integrate these with their own self-interests, and genuinely commit themselves to the group's mission. As a result, they are more inclined to engage actively in progroup behavior, make conscious efforts to improve group performance, and help the group achieve its goals.

During the norming and performing stages, an attachment-informed coach or group leader should wait, watch, and intervene only when group members' attachment insecurities temporarily reemerge during group activities, and the group seems unable to deal with them by itself. The leader can also assist the group in developing suitable goal-related plans and strategies, while responding empathically and nonjudgmentally when the group encounters unexpected difficulties. In this way, the group leader reinforces members' natural broaden-and-build tendencies, hence heightening both their individual performance and progroup behavior.

Adjourning

Tuckman and Jensen (1977) recognized that termination of group activities and separation from group members are important issues throughout the life of a group and often arouse bittersweet feelings. Whereas group members can celebrate their individual performance and the achievements of the group as a whole, their strong emotional connection to the group and their close working relationships with other group members may cause them to feel anxious and sad about the group coming to an end. As with other close relationship losses, they may grieve the loss of the group. Their grief reactions can be manifested in apathy, lack of motivation and enthusiasm for new activities, and reluctance to join new groups. This natural process is worth discussing with the group before it ends.

Theoretically, the termination of group activities arouses anxiety and sadness related to the loss of a secure base. It may amplify attachment insecurities for some group members who have experienced painful, perhaps even traumatic separations and losses in the past. In these cases, an attachment-informed coach or group leader can help members reorganize their hierarchy of attachment figures by encouraging them to integrate the lost group into their self-identity and, at the same time, accept the loss and move on to membership in new groups.

During the adjourning stage, an attachment-informed coach or group leader can encourage members to use the group as an internal source of felt security. The leader can invite group members to bring to mind fond memories of group interactions and to reflect on the gifts and skills the group provided them. Group members can also be encouraged to stay in touch with one another and continue to provide safe-haven and secure-base support for one another even if they become parts of new groups. In this way, they can enter new groups with increased confidence in their value and competence and other members' likely goodwill and strengths.

Summary

Although we have provided some suggestions and recommendations rooted in attachment theory or extrapolated from attachment-informed practices in other domains (parent–child relationships, marital relationships, individual psychotherapy) for developing security-enhancing groups and facilitating group functioning, we know of no group development program based specifically on attachment-theory principles and evaluated empirically. However, some attachment-theory principles can be found in the work of coaches and group leaders that focus on group cohesion as a vehicle for improving group effectiveness. In fact, organizational scientists and professionals are becoming more aware of attachment theory and the benefits of cultivating emotionally safe groups (e.g., Ehrhardt & Ragins, 2019; Grady et al., 2020; Yip et al., 2018). We look forward to seeing this trend develop.

Concluding Remarks

We began this chapter with a seminal passage in which Bowlby (1969/1982) said that "a school or college, a work group, a religious group or a political group can come to constitute for many people a subordinate attachment figure, and for some people a principal attachment figure" (p. 207). For researchers, theorists, and clinicians working in Bowlby's shadow, this passage is a license to extend research findings from the study of close dyadic relationships, and from clinical applications in individual and couple therapy, to the study and improvement of groups of various kinds, from therapy groups to sports teams and work groups. Bowlby was correct that people can become attached to groups, and often to their leaders as well, via mechanisms similar to those in dyadic relationships, and with similar effects. This happens when a person views a group as a safe haven and secure base for exploration and personal development. Also, as expected based on attachment theory, achieving security in relation to a group provides a foundation for a broaden-and-build process of exploration, learning, and individual accomplishment, often while benefiting the group to which the individual member is attached.

A great deal is known about what a group therapist, coach, or leader can do to foster secure attachment to a group. A bit is also known about how individual differences in attachment, along the dimensions of attachment-related anxiety and avoidance, influence how a person perceives group members and group processes, and hinders (or in some cases helps) group goal attainment. There are still many openings and challenges for researchers and intervention designers who wish to explore the realm of attachment to groups in greater detail and to discover how to apply attachment-related insights more effectively.

CHAPTER 10

Attachment-Based Applications in School and Educational Settings

The broaden-and-build cycle of attachment security is critical to school success. As explained in Chapter 2, felt security sustains positive affectivity, optimism, self-esteem, and self-efficacy. It also promotes compliance and cooperation with reasonable social rules and trustworthy authorities. And it supports children's confident engagement and persistence when encountering opportunities to learn and master challenging tasks. This means that students—from preschoolers to university students—work and learn best when they are confident that support is available when needed.

As we've seen, felt security is initially developed within safe and secure interactions with responsive parents during infancy and childhood. However, positive interactions with an approachable and kind teacher during school hours can also create felt security within the classroom and launch broaden-and-build processes. This within-classroom felt security can even reduce the negative effects that insecure attachment to parents have on socio-emotional adjustment and academic performance (Sabol & Pianta, 2012; Verschueren & Koomen, 2012).

These possibilities have inspired researchers in educational psychology to study student–teacher relationships from an attachment perspective (Pianta, 1999). These researchers have suggested that teachers can offer a safe haven for alleviation of school-related distress and a secure base for exploration and learning. Since parents are not physically available during school hours, preschool or school-age children tend to rely on their teacher to fulfill safety and security needs in the classroom, and to use the teacher as an *ad hoc attachment figure* (Zajac & Kobak, 2006, p. 380). Children feel reassured and empowered when their teacher understands, validates, and cares for them when facing school-related threats and challenges. And this helps the children function optimally at school (Williford et al., 2016).

Over the past 30 years, evidence has been accruing in support of an attachment perspective on the student–teacher relationship. This research has encouraged the development of interventions that strengthen teacher responsiveness and improve the quality of student–teacher interactions as a way of contributing to students' felt security and school success (e.g., Cooper et al., 2017; Driscoll & Pianta, 2010; Spilt et al., 2012). In this chapter, we review research concerning security-enhancement processes in student–teacher relationships and describe some of the professional development programs for teachers that are informed by this line of research.

Security-Enhancement Processes in Student–Teacher Relationships

We begin by discussing the empirical basis for applying attachment theory to student–teacher relationships. We first review studies showing that children often direct attachment-like behaviors to their homeroom teacher when faced with threats and challenges. We then review studies involving preschoolers, school-age children, and adolescents that document the positive effects of comforting and supportive student–teacher relationships on students' socioemotional adjustment and academic achievement. We also review evidence that although the psychological benefits of supportive student–teacher relationships can be reduced by children's attachment insecurities carried over from relationships with parents, a responsive and supportive teacher can work through this interference and move even attachment-insecure children toward greater felt security, at least with respect to that teacher. For educational psychologists and counselors, the research findings we review can provide a road map for enhancing students' within-classroom felt security and their well-being and academic functioning at school.

Teachers as Ad Hoc Attachment Figures

An attachment-theoretical perspective on student–teacher relationships was pioneered by Robert Pianta (1992, 1999), who was interested in exploring the teachers' role in promoting children's well-being and academic functioning. Based on his pioneering work, many educational psychology researchers have become interested in understanding the attachment-like nature of the student–teacher relationship and the possibility that teachers can legitimately be viewed as attachment figures. These researchers were particularly curious about whether students rely on a teacher as a safe haven and secure base in times of need.

Within the school context, the search for a safe haven involves students' turning to a teacher when they are distressed or feel a need to be protected, comforted, or reassured. Students can also use the teacher as a secure base for exploration (to use Ainsworth's [1991] phrase), which includes relying on the teacher for encouragement and guidance when attempting to master new knowledge and skills. Whenever these attachment behaviors are directed to a teacher, we can infer that the student regards the teacher as an attachment figure, at least in the school context, and may form either a secure or insecure attachment to him or her (Howes & Ritchie, 1999).

In attempting to understand the attachment-like nature of the student–teacher relationship, researchers have focused on the notion that a child's network of attachment figures naturally expands during childhood (Kerns et al., 2006). As growing children begin to spend more time away from parents and engage in more diverse and complex social and academic activities, roles, and relationships, they can no longer rely on immediate protection and support from their physically absent parents. This doesn't mean that the bond with parents becomes weaker (Cassidy, 2016), but that the growing child may direct attachment-like behaviors to nonparental figures when feeling distressed at school or in other out-of-home settings (Mayseless, 2005). As a result, a child's network of attachment figures becomes more differentiated and diversified as the child comes to rely on different figures in different contexts (Mayseless, 2005).

When attending school and being physically separated from parents, children may naturally, and quite automatically, perceive their teacher as a potential security provider. A teacher, by being an expert in the academic domain, a person who is better emotionally regulated than anxious and puzzled fellow students, and who is trained to promote students' welfare, is likely to be perceived as a competent and benevolent figure. Thus, students expect a teacher to serve as a safe haven when one is sick, distressed, or afraid during school hours and as a secure base for learning and for acquiring knowledge and skills (Verschueren & Koomen, 2012).

Imagine, for example, a 6-year-old boy meeting his teacher for the first time. He will monitor the teacher for cues relevant to warmth and competence. If the teacher appears to have benevolent intentions and the skills needed to provide a secure base for learning within the classroom, the child will begin to trust the teacher and regard him or her as a potential attachment figure. Days later, when encountering a problem with a reading assignment, the child will optimistically, but perhaps still cautiously, approach the teacher and ask for assistance. The child's confidence in the teacher's warmth and competence will, of course, be strengthened if the teacher once again proves to be warmly supportive and skillful in solving the problem.

According to Hamre and Pianta (2001), a teacher's role in early childhood is quite similar to a parent's role: Teachers may provide a safe and calm environment for learning (safe-haven support) and may serve as a scaffold for children's development of important adaptive skills (secure-base support). At this early stage of development, children need to acquire foundational cognitive, social, and self-regulatory skills that will be needed, among other purposes, for success in school. Although most prominent during early childhood and among vulnerable and at-risk children (Sabol & Pianta, 2012), reliance on a teacher as an attachment figure can also occur later in life when adolescents and young adults face demanding academic challenges (Mayseless, 2016). They may, like young children, still seek the support, guidance, and encouragement of a teacher (or mentor, coach, or supervisor) when they step outside their comfort zone and tackle new and difficult academic tasks.

There is research evidence, in addition to informal observations, that children and adolescents sometimes direct attachment behaviors to teachers. For example, preschoolers turn to their kindergarten teacher for support when distressed by physical pain, fear-eliciting situations, or hurtful rejection by peers, or when confronting challenging academic tasks (Koomen & Hoeksma, 2003). In one study, Seibert and Kerns (2009) conducted open-ended interviews with children 7–12 years of age to identify attachment figures and found that children often direct attachment-like behaviors to teachers.

In several other studies, adolescents were found to describe teachers as supportive figures (e.g., Reid et al., 1989) but only as secondary sources of protection and support relative to parents and peers (Furman & Buhrmester, 1992). In fact, teachers are rarely mentioned by adolescents as having a significant or important influence on their lives (e.g., Reid et al., 1989). However, social support studies have shown that perceived support from teachers is a significant predictor of adolescents' motivation and academic achievement (e.g., Wentzel & Asher, 1995). And Wentzel (1998) found that perceived support from teachers makes a stronger contribution to students' school engagement than perceived support from parents or peers.

We are unaware of retrospective studies in which adults are asked to remember any teachers who played a special role in supporting them during difficult times or in scaffolding their academic advancement. But certainly, both of us can remember such special, sometimes life changing, teachers, professors, and mentors in our own lives.

Research also indicates that students can form secure or insecure attachments to a teacher. In a large sample of preschoolers (N = 3,062), Howes and Ritchie (1999) trained observers to watch interactions between a teacher and a specific child for 2 hours and to code the quality of the child's attachment to the teacher using the Attachment Q-Set (Waters & Deane, 1985). (The Q-set was designed for naturalistic observations of parent–child interactions.) They observed four major patterns of attachment that partially parallel the typology of child–parent attachments: secure, near-secure, avoidant, and resistant.

Secure children use the teacher as a secure base, accept his or her comfort and reassurance, share their activities with the teacher, and ask for help when needed. Near-secure children (a category used by Howes and Ritchie [1999]) react positively to their teacher's emotional and instructional support but do not voluntarily seek proximity to the teacher. Avoidant children avoid proximity to the teacher and reject his or her support and guidance. Resistant children (ones whom we would call anxious or anxious/ambivalent) are often upset and irritable with the teacher and tend to be demanding and angry toward him or her. As compared with less secure preschoolers, those with a secure attachment to their teacher engage in more cooperative play with peers and in more competent exploration of their environment. They also display more signs of school readiness, including linguistic, attentional, and metacognitive skills (e.g., Commodari, 2013; Howes & Ritchie, 1999; Howes & Smith, 1995a).

Of course, although children may seek protection and support from their teacher and may feel secure or insecure with regard to him or her, this doesn't mean that the children have a "full-fledged" attachment bond with their teacher similar to the one they have with their parents (Sabol & Pianta, 2012). The teacher–student relationship is less durable than the parent–child relationship, because children change teachers every school year in most educational systems. Also, the teacher–student relationship is less exclusive than the parent–child relationship, because children usually know that teachers must be shared with many other students (Lamb, 2005). Furthermore, especially in high school, students interact with multiple teachers throughout the day. But despite these important differences, children can still benefit greatly from comforting and supportive interactions with a teacher.

The Calming and Empowering Effects of Supportive Student–Teacher Relationships

Conceptual and Methodological Considerations

In applying attachment theory to educational settings, Pianta (1999) argued that a high-quality student–teacher relationship often involves a warm and kind teacher who is willing and able to be emotionally available and closely attentive when needed; to assist students in alleviating their distress; and to encourage and empower students to develop new interests, knowledge, and skills. In this positive relational context, students can feel calm and well-regulated, and more willing to cooperate with the teacher. Moreover, they can confidently engage in learning activities provided by the teacher and persist in challenging academic tasks with the confidence that the teacher's support is available if needed.

These positive outcomes may be attributable to comforting and empowering one-on-one interactions students have with the teacher. However, their improved well-being and academic functioning may also be derived from classroom-level interactions in which the teacher creates a climate of acceptance, positive regard, support, and empowerment for students (Hamre & Pianta, 2001). In both cases, students may be able to use a teacher as a secure base and as a developmental asset (a secure base) for learning and personal growth.

Based on an attachment-theoretical conceptualization of high-quality student–teacher relationships, Pianta and colleagues (e.g., Pianta, 1993; Pianta & Steinberg, 1992) developed the Student–Teacher Relationship Scale (STRS). Using this scale, teachers rate the extent to which they have a warm and close relationship with an individual student. The STRS identifies three distinct dimensions of a child–teacher relationship: closeness, conflict, and dependency. *Closeness* refers to the degree of warmth, positive affect, and supportiveness in the relationship and to students' use of the teacher as a secure base (e.g., "I share a warm relationship with this child"; "If upset, this child will seek comfort from me"). *Conflict* refers to the negativity or lack of rapport between this student and the teacher (e.g., "This child and I always seem to be struggling with each other"); *dependency* refers to the extent to which teachers complain about a child's clinginess or possessiveness (e.g., "This child is overly dependent on me").

The three STRS dimensions map conceptually onto parent–child attachment relationships by focusing on teachers' provision of a safe haven and secure base. According to Hamre and Pianta (2001), closeness is indicative of a teachers' responsiveness to an individual child; teachers may be kinder and more loving to children with whom they naturally have a close and affectionate relationship. Moreover, when teachers feel emotionally close to a student, they are likely to offer him or her reassurance, guidance, and instructional support, and to provide the student with scaffolding for the development of socioemotional and self-regulation skills. These positive relationships with teachers can then increase students' felt security and promote their natural inclinations to explore and learn (Pianta, 1999).

In contrast, a low-quality relationship characterized by conflict or overdependence may cause teachers to become frustrated and distressed when interacting with the child and may interfere with the provision of a safe haven and secure base for the child. A teacher's lack of responsiveness may result either from his or her own attachment insecurities and negative attitudes toward closeness or from a child's unfavorable behavior or rejection of support (see next section). In either case, such a negative climate may impair children's socioemotional adjustment to school and interfere with their engagement in academic tasks.

Originally, the STRS was administered to teachers rather than students, because studies were conducted with preschoolers or first graders who couldn't respond meaningfully to complex self-report scales. However, in subsequent studies conducted with older children and adolescents, students rated their own relationship with a teacher. In these studies, students either completed the STRS (e.g., Spilt et al., 2010) or directly rated (1) a teacher's provision of emotional support, reassurance, and guidance in times of need; (2) the teacher's respect for, and support of, the students' autonomy; or (3) feelings of being understood, validated, and cared for by the teacher (e.g., Davis, 2001; Gurland & Grolnick, 2003; Lynch & Cicchetti, 1997). Other researchers have relied on behavioral observations of student–teacher interactions and have had trained observers code the extent to which a teacher is responsive to a student's proximity-seeking bids and supports the student's autonomy (e.g., Spilt et al., 2018).

Still other researchers have assessed (through observational methods) the extent to which the teacher is capable of creating an emotionally supportive and empowering climate for the class as a whole (e.g., Cash et al., 2019). The Classroom Assessment Scoring System (CLASS; Pianta et al., 2007) is the most frequently used instrument for assessing the quality of teachers' interactions with students in the classroom. This instrument assesses three broad domains of teacher behavior: *classroom organization, emotional support,* and *instructional support.* Classroom organization involves a teacher's clear expression and consistent enforcement of behavioral expectations, as well as intentional efforts to provide children with learning opportunities, prevent unnecessary distractions in the classroom, and facilitate their engagement with learning materials. Emotional support is indicative of a teacher's overt expression of warmth and affection and his or her sensitivity and responsiveness to students' needs and feelings. Instructional support refers to a teacher's provision of a solid scaffold for children's development of higher-order thinking and problem skills, opportunities to generate new ideas, and constructive feedback that expands children's understanding and sustains task persistence.

Although classroom organization and instructional support can be seen as effective ways of sustaining students' exploration and learning, the emotional support domain naturally maps onto the construct of teacher's sensitive responsiveness. This domain includes three dimensions—positive climate, teacher sensitivity, and regard for students' individuality and autonomy, which converge to create comforting and supportive within-classroom interactions. *Positive climate* refers to the teacher's encouragement of affection and cooperation within the classroom. *Teacher sensitivity* includes noticing students' difficulties, acknowledging their emotions, being responsive to their problems, and providing them with support and guidance when needed (safe-haven support). *Regard for students' individuality and autonomy* involves teachers' encouragement of students' personal ideas and opinions, and respect for students' own voices during the learning process (secure-base support).

Research Evidence

The hypothesized calming and empowering effects of warm and supportive student–teacher relationships have been observed as early as preschool. Preschoolers with closer and more supportive relationships with their teacher are more likely to be happy and well-regulated in kindergarten and to show greater classroom engagement and greater school readiness (e.g., Hatfield & Williford, 2017; Nguyen et al., 2020; Pianta et al., 2020). Moreover, student–teacher closeness during preschool has been found to predict positive outcomes in first grade, such as better academic performance, lower mothers' ratings of students' depression and anxiety, and higher observers' ratings of students' social competence (Pianta & Stuhlman, 2004). Following children from kindergarten through eighth grade, Hamre and Pianta (2001) found that preschoolers with closer relationships with their teacher showed greater classroom engagement and fewer behavioral problems over the study period.

Similar calming and empowering effects have been found in studies assessing the quality of student–teacher relationships among school-age children and adolescents. Students who had a closer and more supportive relationship with a teacher (as rated by students, teachers, or external observers) also reported greater well-being and had a lower risk of emotional and behavioral problems (e.g., O'Connor et al., 2012). Moreover, first graders with a more responsive teacher were more likely to have diurnal patterns of salivary cortisol indicative of effective stress regulation (Ahnert et al., 2012). And more supportive student–teacher interactions recorded via diary assessments of adolescents at age 14 predicted less engagement in risky sexual behavior at age 15 (Kobak et al., 2012).

Importantly, the soothing effects of high-quality student–teacher relationships occur for students with and without learning or behavioral problems (Murray & Greenberg, 2001). Although children with behavioral or learning problems are at risk of developing a conflictual relationship with their teachers, a responsive and supportive teacher can soften this tendency and promote the students' well-being and socioemotional adjustment to school (e.g., Al-Yagon & Mikulincer, 2004). In this way, a comforting student–teacher relationship can protect at-risk children from the emergence and exacerbation of behavioral and emotional problems at school.

The quality of student–teacher relationships is also associated with students' academic motivation, self-esteem, and performance (O'Connor & McCartney, 2007). For example, Pianta, Belsky, et al. (2008) followed children from first to fifth grade and found that those who had a closer and more supportive relationship with their teacher exhibited greater growth in math and reading ability over the study period. This association was also found in a laboratory experiment in which a supportive teacher's message (vs. a neutral teacher's message) increased elementary schoolchildren's performance on a working memory task (Vandenbroucke et al., 2017). In two meta-analyses—one of 61 studies conducted with elementary school students (N = 88,417) and the other of 105 studies with elementary school students (N = 79,925) and 74 studies with high-school students (N = 107,473), Roorda et al. (2011, 2017) found that ratings of close and supportive student–teacher relationships were associated with greater school engagement and better grades.

Students' perceptions of a teacher's autonomy support also contribute to the students' well-being, school engagement, and academic achievement (e.g., Hospel & Galand, 2016; Jungert & Koestner, 2015). In a meta-analysis of 56 studies, Vanconcellos et al. (2020) found that physical education teachers' provision of autonomy support to their students had a moderate-to-strong association with students' better socioemotional adjustment within their classrooms. Teachers can improve students' well-being and performance not only by offering protection and comfort in times of stress and distress (i.e., safe-haven support) but also by respecting and encouraging their exploration and autonomy (i.e., providing a secure base).

The Interfering Effects of Attachment Insecurities

Children tend to use the working models formed during early interactions with parents as information-processing heuristics to guide their expectations and behaviors in relationships with other adults who are perceived as playing caregiving and growth-supporting roles, such as teachers, counselors, and coaches (e.g., Bretherton, 1995). As a result, whenever attachment-insecure children direct their unmet needs for a safe haven and secure base to a teacher, their negative working models of parental figures may be generalized to the teacher and negatively bias their expectations, feelings, and behavior toward the teacher. In other words, insecure attachment to parents can negatively bias the quality of the relationships a child forms with teachers in the early school years (O'Connor & McCartney, 2006).

These negative biases tend to be generalized to several different domains of student–teacher relationships. For example, the negative and pessimistic expectations that attachment-insecure children import from unsatisfying relationships with parents can foster doubts about the trustworthiness and kindness of a teacher and contribute to devaluing appraisals and memories of the teacher's behavior (Hamre & Pianta, 2001). Indeed, children who have more conflictual relationships with parents are less likely to perceive their teacher as supportive (e.g., Barber & Olsen, 2004). As well, attachment-insecure college students are likely to form negative impressions of their instructors' teaching effectiveness and supportiveness, and to decline instructors' offers of support (e.g., Reid & Scharfe, 2019). The associations are only moderate in size, however, suggesting that clear-cut, explicit, and reliable expressions of a teacher's support over time might be able to weaken the association.

In addition, children with a history of frustrating or disappointing interactions with cold and rejecting or unreliably responsive parents may have learned that relying on others is not a productive way to reduce fear, pain, and suffering. As a result, they may have difficulty in seeking comforting proximity to a teacher and asking for the teacher's support in times of need. Moreover, they may miss opportunities to learn about their teacher's responsiveness and to feel protected, valued, and supported by the teacher. Indeed, Sroufe et al. (1983) found that preschool children with insecure attachment to parents were less likely than securely attached children to approach their teacher and ask for support when injured, ill, or distressed. Similarly, more attachment-insecure adolescents and young adults are less prone to seek help and guidance from teachers or college counselors (e.g., Cheng et al., 2015; Larose et al., 2005).

Beyond negatively biasing children's appraisal of teachers' behavior and interfering with the seeking of support from teachers, an insecure parent–child relationship can result in the formation of a corresponding insecure attachment to teachers. For example, Booth-LaForce et al. (2003) used the Attachment Q-Set at 24 months to rate the quality of toddlers' attachment to both mothers and caregivers in day care centers and found a significant correlation between the safe-haven/secure-base composite score of child–mother and child–caregiver observed interactions. In a meta-analysis of 40 studies (N = 2,867 children), Ahnert et al. (2006) found a significant, albeit modest, association between preschoolers' attachment (secure–insecure) to parents and their attachment to a teacher or care provider. Because the findings are correlational, however, we can't rule out alternative interpretations (e.g., responsive mothers selecting responsive caregivers) of the observed concordance between attachment to mother and attachment to caregiver–teacher.

Insecure attachment to parents can also encourage more conflictual relationships with teachers. Longitudinal data from the NICHD Study of Early Child Care and Youth Development revealed that insecure attachment to the mother in early childhood significantly predicted more conflictual relationships with teachers at 54 months, kindergarten, first grade, and fifth grade (O'Connor & McCartney, 2006; O'Connor et al., 2012). Similarly, 5-year-old children who, in a narrative task, conveyed more negative (insecure) representations of their parents (as being indifferent and unavailable) experienced greater conflict with their teacher at age 6 (Rydell et al., 2005).

Magro et al. (2020) used prospective longitudinal data from the NICHD Study of Early Child Care and Youth Development (N = 1,306) to investigate whether the association between early attachment experiences with mothers and subsequent student–teacher relationship quality remains stable or diminishes over time. The contribution of lack of maternal responsiveness in infancy to lower levels of student–teacher closeness was reduced between kindergarten and grade 6. However, the contribution of lack of early maternal responsiveness to teacher–student conflict endured over the study period and was partially accounted for by child behavioral problems. These findings support the idea that when early negative attachment experiences contribute to a child's behavioral problems, they may also contribute to conflictual student–teacher relationships over time. However, the findings also suggest that as a child grows, his or her emotional closeness to a teacher becomes less dependent on early negative attachment experiences with parents, perhaps because some children have cumulative positive experiences with warm and kind teachers.

In analyzing the interfering effects of children's attachment insecurities, we should keep in mind that some teachers might actually be less responsive and supportive to an insecure child than teachers of an attachment-secure child. For example, interactions with children who are regularly rejecting and distant (avoidant children) or who exhibit overly demanding and clinging behavior (anxious children) might provoke a teacher's annoyance, frustration, and distress, which may hinder his or her ability to provide a safe haven and secure base (Belsky, 2005). However, if a teacher is secure and resilient enough to resist an insecure child's rejection or complaints, the teacher may still be able to provide clear-cut signs of warmth and care, which can gradually move an insecure child toward greater felt security.

This possibility is nicely illustrated in Lifshin et al.'s (2020) prospective longitudinal study of first graders. In that study, a teacher's attachment security (indicated mainly by relatively low scores on the avoidance dimension), as measured at the beginning of first grade, prospectively predicted the formation of closer and less conflictual relationships with children over the course of the academic year (as rated by the children). More important, this positive effect of the teacher's felt security was observed even among children who were attachment-insecure in relation to their mother.

Increasing Attachment-Insecure Children's Felt Security

Can a responsive teacher provide corrective experiences for children or adolescents who have had a history of frustrating and painful attachment experiences with parents? And can such a teacher buffer the deleterious effects of an insecure familial environment on students' well-being and academic functioning at school? We suspect that whenever a teacher becomes a target of children's attachment behaviors, comforting and empowering interactions with a responsive teacher can help the children feel safer and more secure at school, even if they are insecure with regard to parents (Sabol & Pianta, 2012).

Of course, this doesn't mean that children's working models of parental attachment figures will be totally reshaped by a responsive teacher. We are saying only that a new secure representation of an adult attachment figure can be added to a child's network of attachment figures. This addition can positively affect the child's expectations regarding other teachers and other extrafamilial sources of a safe haven and secure base (e.g., mentors, coaches, supervisors), and thus expand the child's mental *islands of security*.

The modest association between children's attachment to parents and their attachment to a teacher (see previous section), and the fact that some studies have failed to find a significant association between these two constructs (e.g., Howes & Hamilton, 1992, Cassibba et al., 2000) suggest that teacher responsiveness might have an important corrective effect on an already-in-process insecure trajectory. Indeed, Ahnert et al.'s (2006) meta-analysis indicated that children's felt security increased as their care provider or teacher created a more supportive climate in a child care center or school setting. Findings also suggest that responsive teachers can be successful in providing beneficial relational experiences that are different in quality from the early negative relationships that insecure children experienced with their parents (e.g., van IJzendoorn et al., 1992; Howes & Ritchie, 1998; Howes & Smith, 1995b).

In an examination of the effects of teacher responsiveness on the quality of the relationships that attachment-insecure preschoolers form with a teacher, Buyse et al. (2011) conducted behavioral observations of the quality of child–mother attachment at home and teacher's responsiveness in the kindergarten classroom. Child–teacher closeness was rated by the teacher. Findings indicated that children with less secure attachments to parents had less close and comforting relationships with teachers, unless the teacher was rated by external observers as highly responsive and supportive. In this latter case, attachment-insecure children were no longer at risk for developing poor relationships with teachers.

Comforting and empowering interactions with responsive teachers can also reduce the deleterious effects of negative early experiences with parents and resulting attachment insecurities on students' socioemotional and academic functioning at school. For instance, Burchinal et al. (2002) followed children in child care centers from preschool to second grade and found that among children whose parents used less sensitive and responsive parenting practices, the children who had close relationships with a teacher exhibited more gains in reading scores compared to children without such close relationships. Similarly, O'Connor et al. (2012) reported that a closer child–teacher relationship weakened the link between a child's insecure attachment to mother at age 3 and behavioral problems in fifth grade.

Ben-Gal Dahan and Mikulincer (2021) conducted two studies with adolescents to examine the extent to which perceived teacher responsiveness reduced the association between attachment insecurities and lack of persistence in academic tasks (self-reports of persistence in schoolwork, actual persistence in a cognitive task). In the second study, Ben-Gal Dahan and Mikulincer manipulated the symbolic presence of participants' teacher during task performance (teacher priming). Across the two studies, attachment anxiety (as assessed by the ECR) was associated with decreased task persistence. But the perception of the teacher as a responsive figure contributed to greater persistence and reduced the detrimental effects of attachment anxiety. Findings from the second study also showed that the protective effect of perceived teacher responsiveness on task persistence was found only when the teacher was made contextually salient, not when the teacher's imagined presence was not primed.

These findings indicate that perceived teacher responsiveness is a contextual source of security and has beneficial effects on task persistence, but only when the teacher is symbolically present (through experimental priming). This is relevant to the classroom setting in which the teacher is actually present while students engage in academic tasks under the teacher's supervision and guidance. However, outside of school, it seems that mental representations of the teacher's responsiveness are less relevant for determining students' task persistence. In those situations, their behavior is likely to be influenced more by global attachment orientations or other sources of attachment security, such as support provided by parents or close friends.

Longitudinal studies provide preliminary evidence that high-quality student–teacher relationships not only reduce the detrimental effects of poor parenting but also sustain and reinforce the broaden-and-build effects of parental responsiveness. For example, Ansari and Pianta (2018) used data from the NICHD Study of Early Child Care and Youth Development ($N = 1{,}307$) to examine the effects of maternal sensitivity (measured at child ages 6, 15, 24, 36, and 54 months) and the quality of student–teacher relationships (measured during first, third, and fifth grades) on academic achievement from 54 months to ninth grade. They found that maternal sensitivity had the strongest positive effect on academic achievement from the end of preschool through age 15 when coupled with both close student–teacher relationships and a supportive classroom climate during elementary school. In contrast, the benefits of maternal sensitivity were absent when children experienced lack of teacher support during elementary school. These findings highlight the role of teachers as a potential source of felt security and broaden-and-build processes within classrooms.

Research Summary

The research we have reviewed here indicates that teachers can accomplish attachment functions at school, and that children who have a warm and comforting relationship with a responsive teacher feel and function optimally in classroom. Moreover, a responsive teacher who deals constructively with students' insecurities and meets their socioemotional needs can move them toward greater felt security and improve their school success. This means that responsive teachers can provide a revitalizing, corrective relational experience for insecure students, helping them to revise negative views of relationships and supporting their efforts to explore and learn at school. And this points to the importance of attachment-based interventions aimed at improving teachers' responsiveness and supportiveness, which might well be effective in supporting students' security, well-being, and academic functioning.

Attachment-Based Interventions to Improve Student–Teacher Relationships

In the past 20 years, partly based on the research reviewed in the previous sections, several scholars have employed interventions originally focused on parent–child relationships (e.g., VIPP-SD, ABC; see Chapter 4) to improve the responsiveness and supportiveness of child care providers in child care centers (e.g., Werner et al., 2018). Moreover, intervention programs have been developed for student–teacher relationships within classrooms, focusing on students' socioemotional adjustment and academic performance. Some of these programs, such as the teacher module of the Incredible Years program (Webster-Stratton, 2005), are part of a multicomponent intervention that targets parents, teachers, and children, and aims at improving not only teachers' responsiveness but also their use of effective behavioral methods.

Other programs target only teachers, are informed by attachment theory and research, and are focused mainly on enhancing teachers' responsiveness, their mentalizing abilities, or their functioning as a secure base within the classroom. In this section, we focus on these attachment-based professional development programs for teachers. For each of the programs, we describe key features of the intervention and review research regarding its effectiveness in improving the quality of student–teacher relationships and improving students' school success.

Enhancing Teacher Responsiveness and the Quality of Student–Teacher Relationships

Following evidence highlighting the security-enhancing effects and broaden-and-build implications of close and warm student–teacher relationships, Pianta and colleagues developed three process-oriented professional development programs to promote teachers' responsiveness and supportiveness within the classroom. In all three of these programs, "rather than providing teachers with general knowledge unconnected to teachers' classrooms, process inputs focus on providing teachers knowledge, skills, and support within individual classroom contexts and experiences in order to change teaching practices" (Sabol & Pianta, 2012, p. 222). However, the three programs differ in the techniques used: web-based coaching, face-to-face consultation, or academic instruction. They also differ in the focus of the intervention: teachers' responses during classroom interactions with their students or teachers' responses during a dyadic interaction with a specific student.

My Teaching Partner

My Teaching Partner (MTP) is an individualized, web-based coaching program for teachers aimed at enhancing their ability to form warm and supportive relationships with their students (Pianta, Mashburn, et al., 2008). The MTP program helps teachers identify their own destructive and constructive responses to students' needs and feelings, and improve their responsiveness and supportiveness in the classroom. For this purpose, an MTP coach provides ongoing feedback to teachers through a standardized protocol focused on specific aspects of teaching practices observed during video-recorded classroom interactions. The coach uses the CLASS (described earlier in this chapter) as a foundation for analyzing teachers' classroom behaviors and providing feedback with respect to teachers' provision of emotional and instructional support and classroom organization.

Teachers are assigned for an entire academic year to one trained MTP coach. Every two weeks, teachers video-record interactions with their students during a specific classroom activity (e.g., a math lesson, a small-group discussion) and mail the recording to their coach. The coach then edits the recording into a series of 1- to 2-minute segments, each focusing on a specific teaching skill (e.g., supporting students' autonomy) explained in the MTP manual. For each edited segment, the coach prepares specific written feedback that explicitly focuses on the targeted skill and raises questions that call the teacher's attention to aspects of his or her behavior in the classroom. The feedback focuses on both positive and less-positive teacher behaviors, while maintaining a constructive, problem-solving focus and a nonjudgmental tone.

The coach posts these materials on a private website so the teacher can view the edited video segments and read and respond to the feedback and questions. Teachers and coaches then meet online in a video-chat format to discuss the feedback, questions, and the teacher's responses and reflections. The MTP coach and teacher also co-construct an action plan for the teacher to follow when working to improve his or her teaching practices. Each coaching cycle spans 2 weeks, and its form is repeated throughout the academic year (12 cycles).

Teachers are also given an opportunity to consult with the MTP coach by phone concerning problematic interactions with students. In addition, they have on-demand access to video-clip exemplars of high-quality teacher–student interactions (from a video library of over 200 clips). Thus, teachers can watch, at will, exemplars of other teachers' constructive responses in the form of 1- to 2-minute video clips focusing on a specific CLASS-related skill. The clips are accompanied by a written description of the teacher's behavior, using concepts drawn from the CLASS manual and tailored to the clip. Teachers can also chat with the MTP coach through the website and discuss the effective teacher responses portrayed in the video clip. Through these means, the MTP coach helps teachers become more sensitive and reflective (i.e., mentalizing) observers of their own teaching practices and learn to deal in a more constructive manner with students' needs, demands, and responses.

The effectiveness of the MTP program has been examined in five published RCTs (see Table 10.1 for a summary of these studies' methods). Four of the RCTs were conducted with PreK and preschool teachers, and one RCT was conducted with teachers in middle and high schools. In PreK and preschool settings, the MTP program includes a module aimed at improving teachers' instruction of language and literacy skills, and teacher–student interactions were videotaped mainly during language/literacy-related activities. As can be seen in Table 10.1, the MTP program was compared to well-matched control conditions, such as professional development as usual (with no attachment-based program), access to instructional materials and detailed lesson guides, or access to a website with video clips of effective teacher–student interactions.

The contribution of the MTP program to changes in the quality of teacher–student interactions (using behavioral observations and the CLASS coding manual) has been examined in four of the five RCTs (see Table 10.1). In all four, as compared to teachers in the control conditions, teachers in the MTP program were rated by trained observers (based on classroom video recordings) as exhibiting greater improvement over the course of the program in classroom organization and provision of emotional and instructional support.

TABLE 10.1. Summary of Studies Examining the Effectiveness of the MTP Program

				Pre- and postintervention assessments	
Authors	Sample	Intervention group	Control group	Teacher	Student
Pianta, Mashburn, et al. (2008); Hamre et al. (2010); Mashburn et al. (2010); Ansari & Pianta (2018)*	113/134 teachers in a PreK program and 1,165 children in their classrooms	One-year MTP combined with a language/literacy and socioemotional curriculum	Access to website with video clips of teacher–students interactions	Quality of teacher–student interactions (CLASS) during the program	Children's language/literacy skills and executive functions before and after the program
Allen et al. (2011); Mikami et al. (2011); Gregory et al. (2014*)	78/88 teachers in middle and high school and 1,493/2,237 students in their classrooms	One-year MTP program tailored for teachers in secondary classrooms	Professional development as usual	Quality of teacher–student interactions (CLASS) during the program	Quality of peer interactions and classroom engagement before and after the program Test grades before and 1 year after the program
Downer et al. (2011)*	161 teachers in a PreK program and 1,338 students in their classrooms	One-year MTP program	Access to instructional materials and detailed lesson guides	—	Children's language/literacy skills before and after the program
Pianta et al. (2014)	177 preschool teachers (subsample of Pianta et al.'s [2017] RCT)	One-year MTP program	—	Quality of teacher–student interactions (CLASS) before and after the program	—
Early et al. (2017)*	311 teachers in a PreK program	One-year MTP program	Access to website with video clips of teacher–student interactions	Quality of teacher–student interactions (CLASS) before and after the program	—
Pianta et al. (2017); Downer et al. (2014)*	325 preschool teachers and 1,407 students in their classroom	One-year MTP program	Professional development as usual	Quality of teacher–student interactions (CLASS) during the program	Children's language/literacy skills and executive functions before and after the program and 1 year later
Pianta et al. (2021)	393 preschool teachers and 1,570 students in their classrooms (sample taken from Pianta et al.'s [2017] RCT)	One-year MTP program	—	Quality of teacher–student interactions (CLASS) during the program	Children's language/literacy skills and executive functions before and after the program

Note. An asterisk (*) indicates an RCT.

These positive effects were found in samples of both preschool teachers and teachers in middle and high schools.

Unfortunately, none of the five RCTs collected data on students' attachment working models or orientations (degree of attachment anxiety and avoidance) toward parents or teachers. However, four of the five RCTs collected data on other child outcomes (see Table 10.1). As compared to control conditions, toddlers and preschool children of teachers in the MTP program made greater pre- to postintervention gains in language and literacy skills, as well as in executive functions (e.g., inhibitory control, working memory). In the RCT conducted in middle and high schools, the MTP program, as compared to a control condition, resulted in greater improvement in students' peer interactions, classroom engagement, and academic achievement.

Findings from RCTs conducted in preschool also indicated that some of the children's gains were maintained at a 1-year follow up (Pianta et al., 2017). Moreover, these gains were larger when teachers completed more MTP coaching cycles during the program (Pianta et al., 2017). In addition, RCTs conducted with either preschoolers or children in middle and high schools revealed that MTP's positive effects on students' school outcomes were explained by improvement in the quality of student–teacher interactions (Gregory et al., 2014; Pianta et al., 2021).

Overall, there is good evidence that the MTP program is an effective coaching intervention for heightening teachers' responsiveness and supportiveness within their classrooms and improving students' school success. However, we still need research that identifies the mediating and moderating factors such as students' felt security and attachment patterns. In addition, more research is needed to identify the specific intervention elements that contribute to MTP's effectiveness at different ages, from toddlerhood to adolescence.

Banking Time

Banking Time (Driscoll & Pianta, 2010; Pianta & Hamre, 2001) is an attachment-based dyadic intervention intended to improve a teacher's responsiveness to a specific child with whom he or she has trouble serving as a secure base. The name of the intervention, Banking Time, derives from the idea that when teachers invest time and energy in being responsive and supportive to a child, the student–teacher relationship becomes a resource for the child in the classroom in times of need (e.g., when the child is asked to complete a difficult academic task). In this way, Banking Time can strengthen a child's felt security with regard to a teacher, allowing the child to feel and work at his or her best at school.

The principles of Banking Time are based on teacher–child interaction therapy (TCIT, McIntosh et al., 2000). In the first part of TCIT, a teacher interacts with a particular child in a nondirective fashion guided by attachment-theory principles. These sessions are aimed at developing and consolidating positive teacher-child interactions and strengthening the child's appraisal of the teacher as a responsive and supportive figure. TCIT also includes a second component, based on learning theory, aimed at improving the teacher's management of a child's behavioral problems (McIntosh et al., 2000). Both parts of the intervention continue for 6 weeks. A number of studies have shown that TCIT is an effective intervention for decreasing children's externalizing problem behaviors (e.g., Lyon et al., 2009). However, these studies were small in scale and did not use a randomized controlled design.

In Banking Time, a teacher and a child engage in a set of time-limited (10- to 15-minute), one-on-one playful interactions two to three times a week in a quiet area of the school. The teachers are coached to use specific techniques for effectively meeting the child's needs and for interpreting his or her gestures and actions in a constructive manner. These sessions can be repeated for an entire academic year and provide the child with regular opportunities to feel comforted and empowered by the teacher.

The aim of the brief sessions is to help the child develop more positive expectations about the teacher's kindness and benevolence, and to feel more confident about the teacher's availability and support in times of need. In this way, the comforting teacher's responses can gradually counteract a child's negative working models of adults (especially parents) that tend to lead to conflictual interactions with teachers. For this purpose, teachers are trained to convey acceptance, sensitivity, and responsiveness in their nonverbal gestures (e.g., tone of voice), verbal messages, and interactive behaviors; to provide safe-haven support when the child is showing signs of distress; and to support and encourage the child's exploration and autonomy.

Banking Time sessions occur when the teacher is available to provide full attention to the child and are not contingent on the child's behavior. During each session, the teacher and child engage in an activity chosen by the child. The meeting is led by the child, and the teacher only watches, listens, and conveys acceptance, understanding, and validation. The teacher is instructed not to ask questions, give commands, or teach a lesson, but rather to (1) observe the child's actions, (2) narrate the child's actions, and (3) label the child's feelings and emotions. (All three are aspects of mentalization; see Chapters 4 and 7.)

The teacher carefully watches and takes note of the child's behavior, words, and feelings, as well as the teacher's own thoughts and feelings. The teacher also describes aloud what the child is doing in an interested tone of voice and overtly communicates that the teacher is able to read and understand the child's emotional states. In this way, the child learns that the teacher is attending, accepting, and validating his or her feelings and behaviors, thereby increasing confidence in the teacher's responsiveness and support. In addition, the teacher chooses a specific theme that conveys a message to the child about comforting aspects of their relationship (e.g., "I'm here to help if you need me"), so the child can increase the use of the teacher as a secure base within the context of the classroom.

Teachers work with a Banking Time coach throughout the entire program. In the beginning, a coach meets a teacher for about 1½ hours to describe the intervention goals and techniques and to provide a copy of the Banking Time teacher's manual. Following this initial session, teachers and coaches have a face-to-face meeting once every 2 weeks and a phone meeting on the alternate weeks. The focus of these meetings is to ensure that teachers fully follow the Banking Time guidelines during teacher–student interactions. Throughout the program, teachers video-record an individual Banking Time session once a week and send this footage to their coach. The coach uses short clips from this footage in the next face-to-face meeting to improve the teacher's responsiveness and address any questions or concerns.

The effectiveness of Banking Time has been examined in three RCTs and one quasi-experimental study conducted with preschool teachers and with students with whom teachers had relational difficulties. In the first RCT conducted with only 29 preschool teachers, Driscoll and Pianta (2010) found that Banking Time (vs. a typical classroom routine) led to larger pre- to postintervention improvements in teachers' reports of relationship closeness to the targeted students and in students' classroom behavior (improved frustration tolerance and task orientation, as well as reduced conduct problems). Similar gains in teachers' reported relationship closeness to problematic students have been observed in Driscoll et al.'s (2011) nonexperimental study. Specifically, teachers who voluntarily chose to participate in Banking Time sessions reported greater pre- to postintervention increases in relationship closeness than teachers who chose not to participate in Banking Time.

More recently, Vancraeyveldt et al. (2015) conducted an RCT with Flemish preschool teachers, examining the effectiveness of an adapted version of Banking Time that included teacher training in behavior modification techniques. Findings indicated that teachers in the dual-intervention condition (compared with teachers in a control condition) reported greater pre- to postintervention increases in relationship closeness with the targeted students and larger decreases in student inattention/hyperactivity and behavioral problems. Importantly, follow-up analyses indicated that these positive effects were already present after Banking Time was implemented alone, without any behavior modification training.

In the most recent and largest RCT (Williford et al., 2017), Banking Time, as compared to two control conditions (teachers met with a child without any coaching; business as usual), led to greater increases in the observed quality of student–teacher interactions over the course of the program. Moreover, Banking Time led to larger decreases in students' behavioral problems (as rated by parents or teachers) and greater improvement in students' emotion regulation (as indicated by a decline in cortisol release during the morning). Using data from this RCT, subsequent studies revealed that teachers who displayed more fidelity to Banking Time coaching or reported a more positive relationship with the coach showed greater improvements in observed student–teacher interactions (Alamos et al., 2018; Partee et al., 2022).

Overall, the findings are encouraging and attest to the effectiveness of Banking Time for improving both teachers' responsiveness to a particular problematic student and students' behavioral problems and classroom behavior. However, it is important to note that all of the studies were conducted with preschoolers. So far, no study has applied Banking Time in elementary, middle, or high schools. More important, from our attachment perspective, although teachers in the Banking Time program reported increases in relationship closeness, no information was collected concerning students' attachment working models or attachment orientations with respect to parents or teachers. Moreover, none of the studies assessed students' well-being and engagement with and performance on academic tasks. Therefore, we do not know whether Banking Time supports students' broaden-and-build processes at school.

Semester-Long Academic Course on Student–Teacher Relationships

Hamre et al. (2012) developed a semester-long academic course, entitled *Support of Language and Literacy Development in Preschool Classrooms through Effective Teacher–Child Interactions and Relationships*. This course was aimed at improving preschool teachers' responsiveness and preschoolers' language and literacy skills. It was specifically designed (1) to increase teachers' knowledge concerning the vital role that teacher responsiveness and support play in facilitating children's learning and (2) to train teachers to observe and label their constructive and destructive responses within the classroom.

The course is delivered to a small group of preschool teachers (between five and 15) in fourteen 3-hour sessions. Instructors have experience in early childhood education and attend a weeklong training focused on attachment theory principles, the importance of student–teacher relationships, and the ongoing implementation of the course. The instructors are also provided with an instructor's manual as well as PowerPoint presentations, videos, and written assignments for each course session. LoCasale-Crouch et al. (2011) video-recorded these sessions and found that instructors showed high levels of implementation fidelity.

In the first three sessions, teachers reflect on and discuss the importance of preschool experiences for child development and the importance of comforting child–teacher interactions and relationships for promoting children's socioemotional well-being and school readiness. Teachers are also introduced to the three broad domains of the CLASS: emotional support, classroom organization, and instructional support. The fourth and fifth sessions focus on teachers' provision of emotional support; the sixth session on classroom organization; and the seventh and eighth sessions on providing instructional guidance and support. Within each of these sessions, teachers are introduced to the ingredients of high-quality teacher–student interactions and exposed to videos in which they analyze the extent to which these ingredients are present in the video clip. Homework includes readings plus watching and analyzing additional videos online.

The next three sessions (Sessions 9–11) focus on language development and instruction. Teachers watch videos dealing with effective language instruction, are provided with language-instruction activities, and are instructed to use them in their classrooms. Sessions 12 and 13 focus on literacy development and instruction. In the final session, teachers are asked to film themselves delivering a literacy and language activity, to share their video with fellow teachers, and to reflect on and discuss examples of effective or ineffective interactions with students during the video-recorded activity.

Hamre et al. (2012) examined the effectiveness of this course in an RCT with 440 preschool teachers who were randomly assigned to the course or to business as usual (though they may have been taking other courses at the time of the study). As compared to teachers in the control condition, the teachers who took the course reported having more knowledge about effective interactions, better observation skills, and more supportive classroom interactions after the study period (relative to a preintervention assessment). Furthermore, teachers who took the course were rated by external observers as being more supportive during video-recorded classroom interactions than controls. This positive effect was found immediately after the end of the course and in observations conducted approximately 9–12 months later.

Using the same sample, Pianta et al. (2017) examined the effectiveness of the course on children's outcomes. In this study, data were collected on children's language and literacy skills and executive functions (e.g., inhibitory control) before and immediately after the course and at a 1-year follow-up. Findings indicated that the course had important benefits for children's development. Students of teachers who took the course made greater gains in language/literacy skills and inhibitory control than children in the control condition. Importantly, these gains were maintained 1 year later.

Unfortunately, as with studies conducted on the MTP and Banking Time programs, no data were collected on changes in students' felt security with respect to parents or teachers. Therefore, it is still premature to say that these attachment-based interventions aimed at improving the quality of student–teacher relationships accomplish their hypothesized security-enhancing mission. We also don't know whether the intervention works equally well for children with different attachment orientations. More RCTs are needed to provide this theoretically important information.

Enhancing Teachers' Mentalization of Children's Needs and Feelings

In Chapter 4, we reviewed the positive effects that mentalization-based interventions with parents (e.g., Minding the Baby, child–parent psychotherapy) have on their child's felt security and socioemotional development. In recent years, inspired by the success of these parenting interventions, several scholars have designed similar mentalization-based professional development programs for teachers. All of these programs, although differing in techniques and the targeted children's specific problems, share in common the belief that increasing a teacher's ability to accurately reflect on his or her students' needs and feelings can improve student–teacher relationships and improve students' well-being and academic functioning at school.

Peaceful Schools

The Peaceful Schools program (Twemlow et al., 2001, 2018) is a whole-school approach designed to enhance both teachers' and students' mentalizing capacities, with the aim of creating more comforting teacher–student and peer relationships and reducing violence and bullying at school. According to Twemlow and Sacco (2012), violent individuals and communities have difficulty accurately reflecting on others' needs and feelings. If so, increasing community members' mentalizing capacities should reduce violence and contribute to more harmonious relationships.

Peaceful Schools is a teacher-implemented, manualized program with four components (Twemlow et al., 2018). The first component is a positive climate campaign using learning methods and materials aimed at supporting and encouraging teachers' and students' reflection on mental states. This component also includes increasing teachers' and students' awareness of the important role that certain kinds of mental states play in violent and peaceful relationships. The second component is a classroom management plan that helps teachers stop using coercive discipline and encourages them to reflect on, understand, and constructively deal with students' conduct problems and aggressive behavior. Teachers are coached to rely on their mentalizing capacities in managing conflictual and violent interactions within classroom.

The third component is a physical education program—Gentle Warriors—that helps students self-regulate their anger and adopt nonaggressive physical and cognitive strategies when faced with interpersonal offenses and bullying episodes at school. The last component is a mentorship program that trains teachers to assist students in mastering the needed skills for reacting in a mentalistic, nonaggressive way to violent interactions outside the classroom. The program also introduces reflection periods (around 10 minutes) in the classroom at the end of each day devoted to talking, reflecting, and understanding what happened that day at school, including especially any violent episodes.

The effectiveness of the Peaceful Schools program was evaluated in a single published RCT conducted with nine middle and high schools (Fonagy et al., 2009). The schools were randomly assigned to either the program or two control conditions: (1) school psychiatric consultation (a child psychiatrist meeting with school's mental health teams once a week and providing consultation to teachers when needed) and (2) no intervention. In this RCT, the program was implemented over a 2-year period. Throughout the 2 years, the Peaceful Schools team held monthly consultations with teachers. In the first year, teachers also received a 1-day group training, and students received nine sessions of the Gentle Warriors program. In the second year, teachers received a half-day refresher group training and students received three sessions of the Gentle Warriors program.

As compared to the two control conditions, the Peaceful Schools program reduced students' aggressiveness and bullying and promoted greater empathy over the 2-year study period. Moreover, the positive effects were maintained a year after the end of the program. However, no data were collected on hypothesized changes in teachers' and students' mentalizing capacities, and no information was provided about the relevance of the program for students' felt security and attachment-related broaden-and-build processes at school. Therefore, there is no evidence to support Twemlow et al.'s (2018) claim that the goal of the program "is to create in the school (and in the community) a family in which secure attachments predominate" (p. 365). Future RCTs should assess students' felt security before and after the program in order to examine whether the Peaceful Schools program accomplishes its attachment-related mission.

Relationship-Focused Reflection

Spilt et al. (2012) developed the Relationship-Focused Reflection (RFR) program to help teachers think about their relationship with individual students. The program is aimed at enhancing teachers' ability to reflect on, understand, and narrate the conflictual interactions they have with a student, with special attention on the positive and negative emotions they experience during these interactions.

The intervention includes two sessions (45–60 minutes each) of a teacher with an RFR consultant focusing on a specific student. (The two sessions can be repeated with regard to the relationship of the teacher with another student.) In the first session, a teacher's narrative about the relationship with the targeted student is elicited with the Teacher Relationship Interview (TRI; Pianta, 1999). The teacher is asked to describe concrete classroom interactions with the student, and the thoughts and feelings elicited by these interactions.

In the second session, the RFR consultant helps the teacher link up the narrative to actual interactions with the student using segments of video recordings of these interactions. In addition, the consultant presents the teacher with a unique profile describing the teacher's strengths and difficulties in his or her relationship with the student. This relational profile, based on the TRI coding manual, includes feedback about (1) the teacher's capacity to empathize with and understand the student's feelings and needs, (2) the teacher's ability to provide an effective safe haven and secure base when needed, (3) his or her perceived self-efficacy in dealing with the student's behavior, and (4) his or her feelings (positive, negative) toward the student. The consultant and teacher discuss and reflect on the profile together and construct a plan for improving the teacher's sensitivity and responsiveness, making the student feel safer and more secure within the classroom, and supporting his or her academic performance.

Spilt et al. (2012) examined the effectiveness of the RFR program in an RCT with 32 Dutch preschool teachers who were assigned to the program or to a comparison intervention aimed at improving a teacher's interpersonal skills. For each teacher, two students were selected with above-median levels of behavioral problems, and pre- to postintervention changes were assessed in teacher reports of closeness and conflict with the targeted students and in behavioral observations of teacher sensitivity during video-recorded interactions with each of these students (i.e., the extent a teacher provided support tailored to the student's needs). Compared to the control condition, the RFR program yielded more positive changes in teacher-rated relationship closeness and observers' ratings of teacher sensitivity to the students. Similar findings were reported in a recent RCT conducted with 78 Dutch elementary school teachers who were randomly assigned to the RFR program or a no-intervention group (Bosman et al., 2021).

Although these findings are encouraging, no information was provided about the potential effects of the RFR program on teachers' mentalizing capacities or on targeted children's felt security or their behavioral problems. We therefore can't draw firm conclusions about teacher's mentalizing capacities as the mechanism of change underlying the effects of the RFR program. We also can't determine whether the RFR program actually makes the targeted children more safe and secure with respect to their teacher.

Key2Teach

The Key2Teach program (Hoogendijk et al., 2018) is an extension of the RFR program for improving teachers' mentalization of conflictual interactions with an individual student. Key2Teach consists of 12 meetings (each around 45–60 minutes) of a teacher with a trained coach focusing on a targeted student with whom the teacher has a conflictual relationship.

The first phase of the program consists of four meetings designed to enhance the teacher's awareness and understanding of his or her own mental representation of the relationship with the student and how it influences his or her feelings and behaviors during interactions with the student. This phase incorporates two building blocks. The first two sessions are identical to the RFR program sessions, in which the teacher describes his or her relationship with the targeted student, receives a unique relationship profile based on the narrative, and reflects on the relational difficulties with the student and how to improve the relationship. The third and fourth sessions are designed to increase the teacher's awareness and understanding of the relation between his or her mental representations and behavior toward the student. During these sessions, the teacher and coach discuss mental states (needs, motives, feelings, thoughts) and overt behaviors of both the teacher and the student based on a video clip of a classroom interaction prepared by the coach. At the end of the first phase, the teacher and coach articulate a temporary working hypothesis about the mental states underlying the conflictual relationship.

The second phase includes eight sessions designed to reduce dysfunctional interactions by providing the teacher opportunities to practice more constructive patterns of interaction. For this purpose, the coach makes use of video interaction guidance and synchronous coaching. Using video clips of the teacher's interactions with the student, the coach and the teacher reflect on the observed interaction patterns in relation to the formulated working hypothesis. Then, coach and teacher select appropriate keywords, which are short, specific, and representative of constructive patterns of interaction (e.g., support provision) to be used during synchronous coaching sessions. In these sessions, the coach is situated at the back of the classroom during a lesson. Using bug-in-ear technology, the coach provides the teacher with a relevant keyword when there is an opportunity to practice a constructive pattern of interaction, and the teacher is asked to follow the coach's instructions. These lessons are video-recorded, and the teacher and coach watch the video clip together, reflect on the teacher's mental states during the lesson, and consider what further steps he or she might take to improve the relationship with the student.

Hoogendijk, Holland, et al. (2020) conducted an RCT with 103 Dutch elementary school teachers who were randomly assigned to the Key2Teach program or educational support as usual and were then followed for an academic year. Teachers' reports of the quality of the student–teacher relationship were collected before the intervention, immediately after the intervention, and at the end of the academic year. As compared to the control condition, the Key2Teach program produced greater pre- to postintervention increases in teachers' reports of relationship closeness with the targeted students and larger decreases in teachers' reports of relationship conflict. Using the data from this RCT, Hoogendijk, Tick, et al. (2020) found that Key2Teach led to greater improvement in students' behavioral problems (as rated by teachers) than the control condition. Unfortunately, however, as with the other programs we've reviewed, no data were collected regarding changes in teachers' mentalizing capacities and students' felt security.

Expanding the COS to the Teacher–Student Relationship

Following the conceptualization of teachers as attachment figures, Cooper et al. (2017) expanded the use of the COS intervention (see Chapter 4), first to care providers in child care centers, then to teachers in PreK, preschool, and elementary school settings (COS-Classroom [COS-C]). In all of these settings, the COS-C program is based on the language, concepts, graphs, and techniques used in the COS-Parenting protocol (see Chapter 4 for a description), but with teachers rather than parents as the intervention's target.

The main focus of the COS-C program is enhancing teachers' responsiveness and improving their capacity to repair inevitable rapport ruptures that occur during teacher–student interactions. Teachers are also assisted in developing a better understanding of students' needs and feelings, recognizing how their responses to these needs and feelings affect student behavior, and using more effective strategies to regulate their own emotions during teacher–student interactions. In this way, the COS-C is aimed at improving teachers' functioning as a safe haven and secure base and thereby increasing students' felt security and likelihood of school success.

The COS-C curriculum includes 12 group sessions (with small groups of around eight teachers) and four individual classroom visits for each teacher over a period of approximately 6 months. During the first 2 months, the group meets with a COS-C facilitator each week for a 90-minute workshop session (a total of eight "collaborative learning workshops"). In each of these eight sessions, teachers view and discuss video clips taken from the COS-P video library. Based on the intervention manual, the facilitator stops the video clip at particular junctures, introduces COS basic concepts and graphics, and helps teachers apply these concepts when reflecting on their own and students' behavior in the classroom. In these sessions, teachers are engaged as experts in their own learning, and the facilitator's role is to serve as a secure base for teachers to reflect on their strengths and struggles, to guide teachers' discussion of student needs, and to foster an accepting and supportive group climate where teachers can feel safe to explore and share their personal feelings and thoughts without fear of being rejected or criticized.

In the eight collaborative learning workshops, teachers learn about children's safety and exploration needs, the way they express these needs, the role of teachers as providers of a safe haven and secure base, and how teachers' failure to accomplish this role might result in students' attachment insecurities and less constructive responses to teachers (e.g., being demanding, controlling, or withdrawing). Teachers also learn how to identify and empathically respond to a student's expressions of safety needs and to encourage the student's exploration and autonomy bids. In addition, teachers learn how to manage their own attachment-related fears and defenses during interactions with their students.

During the next 4 months, the group meets once a month with the facilitator for a 90-minute "collaborative consultation session" (a total of four sessions). The focus of these sessions is the relationship of each teacher with a student with whom the teacher is having trouble relating. To this end, the COS-S facilitator invites each teacher to choose a problematic student, describe his or her behaviors during typical interactions with the student, and characterize the feelings these interactions evoked.

In each of the four collaborative consultation sessions, two teachers (the focal teachers) separately reflect on and discuss their problematic teacher–student relationship, and the other teachers are encouraged to support the focal teacher and learn from his or her observations and insights. The COS-C facilitator then helps the focal teachers to reflect on what they are doing and what they can do better to meet the targeted student's needs and enhance his or her felt security. Through this reflection process, teachers move from attempting to control a student's misbehavior to trying to understand what unmet needs and painful feelings the student is trying to communicate through the behavior. On this basis, teachers attempt to develop an action plan for improving their responsiveness during interactions with the difficult student.

Beyond the four collaborative consultation sessions, the COS-C facilitator visits each teacher's classroom once a month during the last 4 months of the program (four visits). During these visits, the facilitator observes the teacher's and targeted student's behaviors, then coaches the teacher about specific steps that can be taken to improve his or her functioning as a safe haven and secure base for the student. In this way, teachers can apply the knowledge they acquired from the program to reflect on, understand, and improve the quality of the problematic relationship.

Throughout the program, the COS-C facilitator helps teachers create a supportive climate in their classrooms and offers teachers classroom routines that support the formation of secure student–teacher relationships. For example, the COS-C facilitator might propose the creation of small, stable groups of students that meet throughout the day with a specific teacher. Cooper et al. (2017) noted that teachers in this small-group arrangement "report shifting from thinking, 'Someone needs to attend to that child' to 'That is one of my children.' By virtue of focusing on a smaller number of children, teachers report developing a greater knowledge, acceptance, and commitment plus a greater appreciation of their influence on the children" (p. 33).

Unfortunately, no RCT or even pre- and postintervention assessments have been made to assess the effectiveness of the COS-C program. We suspect that this program is a valuable way to improve teachers' responsiveness in the same way that the original COS program and COS-P protocols are effective in promoting secure parent–child relationships. However, we need systematically collected empirical data attesting to COS-C's effectiveness.

Conclusions and Future Directions in Research, Translation, and Policy

Overall, professional development programs that support teachers' awareness and understanding of students' needs and feelings, and strengthen teachers' ability to provide a safe haven and secure base for students within their classrooms, appear to have positive effects on the quality of student–teacher interactions and relationships. Moreover, they have been found effective in producing positive changes in students' psychological well-being and engagement, and academic performance at school. The findings are in line with the attachment theory premise that humans function best when they have confidence in the availability of a trusted, supportive, "stronger and wiser" other who serves as a secure base in times of need. By increasing a teacher's responsiveness and supportiveness, the professional development programs reviewed here probably make students feel safer and more secure with regard to the teacher and sustain their natural broaden-and-build tendencies.

However, this encouraging conclusion remains speculative, because the reviewed studies did not include data on changes in students' attachment working models and felt security with regard to teachers over the course of an intervention program. Although reports of increased closeness can be seen as a proxy for a secure student–teacher relationship (Hamre & Pianta, 2001), we do not yet know whether the professional development programs we've reviewed are effective in counteracting the detrimental effects of an insecure child–parent relationship on the quality of child–teacher relationships and children's well-being and academic functioning at school. Future studies should examine whether attachment-based professional development programs allow attachment-insecure students to feel more secure at school.

Future studies should also examine potential differences in the effectiveness of attachment-based professional development programs as a function of the kinds of insecurity (anxiety, avoidance, disorganization) that characterize a student's attachment to parents. In addition, they should delineate the specific components of each program that are most important for heightening felt security in each kind of insecure student. For example, students scoring high on attachment-related avoidance may benefit most from a teacher who is trained to respect these students' self-reliance and gently engages them in structured, enjoyable classroom interactions. In contrast, attachment-anxious students may be most likely to form a secure attachment to a teacher when he or she is trained to show the students that they are important to the teacher (e.g., "I was thinking about you when . . .") and to help the students strengthen their feelings of self-worth and self-efficacy. These examples are derived from research findings in parent–child relationships and romantic/marital couple relationships (see Chapters 4–6), and their validity needs to be carefully examined in future studies of student–teacher relationships.

In addition, no study has examined whether and how the effectiveness of attachment-based interventions is moderated by teachers' own attachment orientations (degrees of attachment anxiety and avoidance). Assessment of these orientations could be important for improving the effectiveness of interventions and tailoring them to individual teachers. Although teachers' attachment orientations may not be easy to change, and interventions may not be able to reduce teachers' attachment-related insecurities directly, strategic interventions could nevertheless assist insecure teachers to improve their responses to students' needs for safety and security. For example, avoidant teachers might feel more comfortable with, and be more accepting of, interventions that explicitly emphasize that the adoption of a caring and empathic attitude toward students increases their autonomy and independence rather than encouraging dependence and neediness.

Of course, our ability to worry about these details is made possible by how much has already been done and learned by the researchers whose work we've discussed in this chapter. Conducting large-scale intervention studies with the cooperation of parents and school authorities is extremely difficult, yet many talented, ambitious scholars have been doing it.

Attachment-based professional development programs could be extended to mentors, mental health counselors, and academic supervisors in colleges and universities. All of these people can serve as security providers, and the formation of a secure relationship with one or more of them could help undergraduate and graduate students cope with distressing academic demands, assignments, and exams. In fact, from our personal experiences as students at all levels and long histories of mentoring doctoral students and supervising their research, we know they perform best when feeling protected and supported by an accepting, validating, and caring professor. University authorities need to understand that students are more likely to digest new material, think broadly and creatively, articulate their ideas effectively, and devote time and energy to academic tasks when they feel confident that their mentor or supervisor will be responsive and supportive.

With the exception of the Peaceful Schools program, the programs we reviewed train teachers without targeting other school personnel (e.g., counselors, coaches, librarians, administrators). However, some students undoubtedly feel closely involved with some of these figures and rely on their protection and support in times of need. Therefore, attachment-based interventions might target other school personnel in addition to teachers and train them to be more responsive to students' safety and security needs. This reasoning inspired Anderson et al. (2004) to develop the school-based Check & Connect program for elementary and middle school students at risk for dropping out of school. The program was aimed at improving students' school engagement by training a member of the school staff ("the interventionist"), not necessarily a teacher, to connect with a student, provide persistent and continuous support to him or her, and conduct an ongoing evaluation of the student's engagement. Results indicated that students of interventionists who reported a closer relationship with the student showed greater increases in school attendance and engagement over the course of the program. But this is only a preliminary study, and more systematic RCTs are needed to test the effectiveness of attachment-based interventions involving whichever adult person a student targets as an attachment-like figure at school.

Another characteristic of the attachment-based programs reviewed in this chapter is that they target teachers who are currently working in schools (i.e., they involve in-service training), not those who are studying to become teachers. Improving within-classroom responsiveness of education students (teachers in training) might be difficult before they have actual classroom experiences. However, implementation of attachment-based interventions in university teacher-training programs could be an important step in socializing teachers-to-be for their role as security-enhancing attachment figures for students.

Introducing teachers-in-training early on to basic attachment concepts and to the premise that an effective teacher is, first of all, a kind and responsive caregiver could be very useful. It could help students create what might be called an *attachment-based professional identity* ("One basic goal of a teacher is to serve as a safe haven and secure base for students"). This initial socialization phase could be followed up with (1) workshops that involve watching and reflecting on video clips of security-enhancing teacher–student interactions, (2) studying relevant portions of the academic course developed by Hamre et al. (2012, see previous section), and (3) using an adapted version of the MTP coaching or COS-C programs when student teachers actually begin to work with students in schools.

There is preliminary evidence that preservice attachment-related training for teachers-to-be can in fact improve student–teacher relationships (e.g., Rimm-Kaufman et al., 2003). For example, Fukkink et al. (2019) developed a training program for Dutch students in early childhood education programs (Caregiver Interaction Profile for Pre-Service [CIP-PS]), in which preservice teachers learned about the importance of a teacher's sensitive responsiveness and support of students' autonomy needs. They watched and reflected on video clips of their own behavior during classroom interactions. Findings indicated that preservice teachers with relatively low scores on sensitive responsiveness, support for autonomy, limit setting, and positive verbal communication during classroom interactions (as rated by trained observers) before the training displayed significant improvement in these interaction skills after the training.

However, overall comparisons between the CIP-PS group (not just the initially poor performers) and a no-intervention group failed to show a significant benefit of the CIP-PS program. These findings are very preliminary, and we need more systematic RCTs examining the validity of Sabol and Pianta's (2012) conclusion that "there may be potential to train teachers on relational practices before they enter the teaching profession" (p. 225).

Attachment-based professional programs are designed to provide teachers with the interaction skills needed to form security-enhancing relationships with their students. However, being sensitive, responsive, and supportive is a demanding, effortful task in general, and it can be particularly stressful when one is interacting with problematic students. In fact, like students who learn better when feeling safer and more secure, teachers need to feel safe, secure, supported, connected, valued, heard, and competent in order to serve as effective secure bases for students. In all of the reviewed programs, the trained coach or consultant is instructed to help the teachers restore emotional balance when distressed and to support and encourage them as they attempt to master new interaction skills. Moreover, in the COS-C program, the collaborative learning groups are meant to provide a secure base for their members. Unfortunately, we lack empirical data showing that the coach/consultant or the training group in the reviewed programs did indeed help teachers feel safer and more secure. Future studies should address this issue.

In this respect, attachment-based professional development programs for teachers could benefit greatly by incorporating techniques from group counseling and therapy (see Chapter 9) to increase the cohesiveness of a teachers' group and strengthen the support this group provides to its members. Moreover, attachment-based interventionists could enhance teachers' felt security by incorporating techniques from leadership development programs aimed at training a school's principal to create a security-enhancing organizational climate and culture at school. All of these group and organizational interventions could strengthen the effectiveness of attachment-based professional development programs for teachers, because teachers are likely to work best when feeling supported by their peers and school principal.

This reasoning highlights the notion of a *chain of security* for security providers: Teachers can act as a secure base for their students mainly when they feel secure in relation to their teacher peer group and school principal. Students' felt security and school success are affected not only by a teacher's responsiveness but also indirectly by the extent to which the school's principal creates a comforting and supportive school climate and provides a secure base for teachers. Students' felt security may even be indirectly affected by the extent to which educational authorities and policymakers in the school district, state, or nation place emphasis on, and provide the needed resources for, fostering warm and supportive relationships within a school so that teachers can perform optimally and children can learn and grow optimally. It is difficult to think of a more important goal for a healthy society.

During the last decade, scholars have begun to design systematic attachment-based interventions aimed at transforming an entire school into a security-enhancing organization (e.g., *Attachment Aware Schools*; Rose et al., 2019), but so far, we don't have much evidence concerning the feasibility and effectiveness of such programs. Moreover, there hasn't yet been an attempt to work at the district, state, or national level to enact policies, regulations, and guidelines that support security-enhancing schoolwide and in-classroom practices. A fully systemic approach calls for district, state, and national policies that place the formation of secure student–teacher relationships alongside academic performance as the core of teaching and education. This is a challenging agenda for the future but one worthy of our aspirations.

CHAPTER 11

Applying Attachment-Theoretical Principles in Medical Settings

Attachment theory was born in a medical context. John Bowlby was a physician (a psychiatrist), and many of his early ideas about anxiety, attachment, and separation were spurred by observations of young children who were separated from their parents during hospitalization. Together with a talented social worker, James Robertson, who made powerfully moving films of children who were hospitalized for medical treatment and whose parents were not allowed to visit them, Bowlby concluded that this kind of separation can put a child at risk for depression, physical ailments, and even death (Robertson & Bowlby, 1952). Besides contributing to Bowlby's early theorizing, these early research ventures and filming experiences helped to change visitation policies in British hospitals, as well as, eventually, hospitals around the world. Today it's not unusual for a loved one to sleep overnight in a patient's hospital room to provide comfort and support.

In the first volume of his attachment trilogy, Bowlby (1969/1982) emphasized the relevance of attachment theory for medical settings, noting that the desire for proximity to and protection and support from a loving and responsive attachment figure can be aroused, at all ages, by physical pain and health- and injury-related threats and concerns, including death. In his view, illness and medical treatments are often sources of distress and suffering, and people attempt to cope with them by relying on an attachment figure's provision of a safe haven and secure base. Hence, patients' perceptions of attachment-figure responsiveness, felt security, and attachment-related fears and defenses can shape the way they experience and manage medical treatments, with dramatic effects on health deterioration or restoration (Maunder & Hunter, 2015). Moreover, as explained in Chapter 2, attachment-related psychological processes are inextricably involved in distress management, subjective well-being, self-efficacy, and social behavior, which can have long-term effects on physical health and illness (Pietromonaco et al., 2015).

In this chapter, we consider the relevance of attachment theory for health and health care. We begin by reviewing adult attachment research on the implications of felt security and attachment insecurities (anxiety and avoidance) for health maintenance and illness management. We then discuss ways of applying attachment-theoretical principles in medical settings to improve patients' felt security, psychological well-being, and health restoration. In particular, we focus on the attachment-related functions and beneficial health-related effects of supportive informal caregivers (family members, friends) and professional health care providers (physicians, nurses) when a person is coping with illness. We view these professionals as attachment figures in a medical context, and we offer an attachment-informed approach for enhancing their responsiveness as a way to promote good medical outcomes (Maunder & Hunter, 2015).

This application of attachment theory and research is fairly new and still developing. We hope this chapter provides ideas and research evidence useful for designing effective attachment-informed training programs and interventions that not only improve patients' outcomes but also help, more generally, to create a caring and humane health care system.

Attachment and Health

Despite the impact that Robertson and Bowlby's (1952) observations had on hospital policies, Bowlby himself and most attachment researchers, including ourselves, have devoted more attention to mental health than to physical health, studying attachment processes in psychotherapeutic rather than medical settings. In recent years, however, the theory has been extended into the domain of physical health and has proven useful for understanding the ways in which psychological and social-relational processes are involved in the etiology and treatment of acute and chronic health problems. As in the mental health domain, felt security seems to promote physical health, protect individuals from injuries and ailments, and facilitate illness management (Meredith & Strong, 2019). Moreover, perceptions of being understood, validated, and cared for by others (key components of felt security) have been shown to predict better health outcomes in medical settings (Maunder & Hunter, 2015). In contrast, attachment insecurities, either attachment anxiety or avoidance, have been found to be associated with poorer physical health and poorer medical-treatment outcomes (Pietromonaco & Collins, 2017).

In a pioneering early literature review, Maunder and Hunter (2001) proposed three attachment-related mechanisms that increase the risk of physical illness among people who are insecure with respect to attachment. First, their negative appraisals of stressful life events, difficulties in regulating emotions, and less effective utilization of social support can increase the likelihood of dysregulated, health-damaging physiological responses. Second, insecure people's tendency to rely on external means of distress regulation, such as smoking, alcohol/drug consumption, emotional eating, and risky sex, can endanger or damage health. Third, attachment-insecure people are less willing and able to seek medical assistance and may not adhere to medical regimens, increasing the severity of physical ailments and interfering with recovery and healing.

This attachment-theoretical analysis has now received attention from several adult attachment researchers, who have probed the relevance of the theory for understanding the psychological and relational mechanisms underlying health maintenance and deterioration (Pietromonaco et al., 2015). These researchers have examined attachment-related differences in somatic complaints and physical disorders, biological responses to stress, health-promoting behavior, responses to physical pain, and the quality of relationships between patients and health care providers. In the following sections, we consider studies on each of these topics.

Health Status, Somatic Complaints, and Physical Disorders

Supporting an attachment-theoretical analysis of physical health, several researchers have found that self-reports of attachment anxiety and avoidance are linked with lower subjective ratings of health, even after controlling for other personality and mental health variables (e.g., Feeney, 1995; Kealy et al., 2021; Sadava et al., 2009). There is also evidence that attachment insecurities are associated with a wide variety of physical health problems. For example, in a nationally representative sample of over 5,600 participants, McWilliams and Bailey (2010) found that self-reports of attachment anxiety were associated with greater likelihood of stroke, heart attack, and high blood pressure, even after controlling for psychiatric disorders. In addition, Davis et al. (2014) found that attachment insecurities assessed with the AAI were associated with increased risk of metabolic syndromes, such as elevated fasting glucose and high triglycerides.

Additional studies indicate that attachment insecurities are associated with the severity of medically diagnosed physical diseases. In a sample of clinical tinnitus patients (who experienced a ringing or buzzing in their ears in the absence of external sounds), Granqvist et al. (2001) found that both attachment anxiety and avoidance were associated with more severe tinnitus. In addition, self-reports of attachment insecurities have been associated with greater disease severity among patients with Crohn's disease, ulcerative colitis, or fibromyalgia (Agostini et al., 2010; Gick & Sirois, 2010; Oliveira & Costa, 2009).

Despite the volume and diversity of theory-supporting evidence, it's worth noting that most of the findings we've mentioned so far are derived from cross-sectional correlational research designs that cannot determine the direction of causality. We have to consider that although attachment insecurities might indeed contribute to the emergence and severity of a physical disorder, the existence of a disease might by itself disrupt the quality of patients' close relationships, causing the patients to feel less secure. Another problem with most of the existing studies is that they have failed to consider other ("third") factors that might contribute to both the attachment insecurities and the occurrence or severity of diseases, such as genetic predispositions or low SES.

Fortunately, a few longitudinal studies have been conducted on the attachment–health relationship and have examined the long-term contributions of attachment insecurities to physical disorders. Using data from the Minnesota Longitudinal Study of Risk and Adaptation (MLSRA), Puig et al. (2013) explored whether attachment in infancy is associated with health outcomes 30 years later. After controlling for health-related confounds at age 32, participants who were insecurely attached (anxious or avoidant) in the Strange Situation at ages 12 and 18 months were more likely than their secure counterparts to report inflammation-based illnesses in adulthood. In addition, participants classified as attachment-anxious during infancy reported more nonspecific physical symptoms at age 32 than those classified as secure.

There is also evidence for the long-term health-related effects of maternal sensitivity during early childhood. For example, Farrell et al. (2019) reported that lower levels of maternal sensitivity across the first 3 years of life predicted greater risk for cardiovascular diseases at ages 37 and 39, and this link was mediated by lack of secure-base-script representations (as coded from AAIs conducted at ages 19 and 26 years). A similar pattern of findings was reported in a 5-year longitudinal study of young children: Lack of maternal sensitivity at 18 months predicted greater likelihood of somatization at age 5 (Maunder et al., 2017). These findings increase our confidence in the hypothesized contribution of insecure attachment to the emergence of physical ailments.

Our confidence is reinforced by research showing that attachment insecurities are associated with more severe symptoms among patients whose physical disorders lack an organic explanation, even after controlling for mental health (e.g., Riem et al., 2018). In one such study, Maunder et al. (2000) found higher average avoidance scores among patients with ulcerative colitis (UC) who had no genetic marker for developing the disorder than among patients with a UC genetic marker. This implies that avoidant attachment is involved in developing the disorder rather than being a mere consequence of the disorder, because it would be difficult to explain why genetically unexplained UC produced more avoidance than genetically caused UC.

Biological Responses to Stress

It's clearly the case that prolonged, intense, and dysregulated physiological responses to threats and life adversities have negative effects on health (Uchino et al., 1996). From an attachment perspective, we view these physiological responses as shaped in part by attachment-related experiences and working models, with felt security fostering the development of better emotion- and self-regulation strategies and attachment insecurities exacerbating and perpetuating physiological dysregulation (Pietromonaco et al., 2015). As reviewed in Chapter 2, people who are secure with respect to attachment make more optimistic appraisals of threatening events, believe in their ability to cope with them, and tend to rely on the adaptive coping strategies prescribed by the secure-base script, such as support seeking and problem solving. As a result, secure individuals tend to be well regulated and less prone to experience intense stress-related physiological responses when coping with potentially threatening events.

In contrast, attachment-insecure people hold less optimistic appraisals of threats and rely on less adaptive strategies for coping with them, such as emotion suppression, cognitive distancing, exaggerated stress responses, and negative rumination (Mikulincer & Shaver, 2016). As a result, insecure individuals tend to react to threats with prolonged and intense physiological responses that can damage physical health. In this section, we consider four biological responses to stress that have been linked to attachment insecurities and have negative effects on health: cardiovascular reactivity to stress, hypothalamic–pituitary–adrenal (HPA) axis activation and cortisol release, dysregulated immune function, and accelerated cellular aging.

Stress-Related Cardiovascular Reactivity

People who habitually exhibit heightened cardiovascular reactivity to threats (e.g., raised blood pressure, decreased heart-rate variability, accelerated pulse rate) tend to be at increased risk for heart-related diseases, such as myocardial infarction, stroke, or hypertension (see Chida & Steptoe, 2010, for a review and meta-analysis). This is the case for attachment-insecure people whose emotion regulation deficiencies contribute to dysregulated cardiovascular responses. For example, self-reported attachment insecurities have been related to decreased heart-rate variability and increased blood pressure in response to various laboratory stressors, such as recalling a stressful situation, performing a demanding task, or discussing a relationship problem with a romantic partner (Kim, 2006; Maunder, Lancee, et al., 2006). In addition, attachment-anxious adults (assessed with the AAI or self-report scales) tend to exhibit increased heart rate while discussing a relationship conflict with their romantic partner (Ben-Naim et al., 2013; Roisman, 2007).

Diamond and Hicks (2005) exposed young men to two anger-provoking situations (math tasks accompanied by discouraging feedback from the experimenter; recollection of a recent anger-eliciting event) and recorded participants' vagal tone (indexed by resting levels of respiration-related variability in heart rate), a common index of parasympathetic down-regulation of negative emotions. Diamond and Hicks found that participants who scored higher on attachment anxiety (as assessed with the ECR) had lower vagal tone. This indicates that the parasympathetic nervous system responded less quickly and flexibly to the stressful tasks, and that attachment-anxious individuals recovered poorly from frustration and anger.

In expanding the study of attachment-related differences in cardiovascular reactivity beyond the laboratory, Gallo and Matthews (2006) monitored adolescents' blood pressure and heart rate for 36 hours while they reported on their current or most recent interpersonal interactions. In line with laboratory findings, attachment anxiety was associated with raised blood pressure during interactions with friends. Similarly, avoidance was associated with higher ambulatory blood pressure during conflictual interactions. In short, attachment insecurities amplify dysfunctional cardiovascular reactions to daily interpersonal interactions.

There is also evidence that insecure individuals' heightened cardiovascular reactivity is impervious to the expected calming presence of a romantic partner or the experience of being loved and supported. For example, Feeney and Kirkpatrick (1996) found that attachment-anxious and avoidant women reacted to the presence of their romantic partner (as compared to a no-partner condition) while performing a stressful arithmetic task with increased rather than reduced cardiovascular reactivity (heart rate and blood pressure). Similarly, Rockliff et al. (2008) found that self-reports of attachment anxiety were related to increased cardiovascular reactivity (lower levels of heart rate variability) in response to compassion-focused imagery (imagining being loved and cared for by another person). In an observational laboratory study, Kordahji et al. (2015) video-recorded dating couples while one partner (the "care seeker") disclosed a personal problem to the other (the "caregiver") and found that more avoidant care seekers experienced less reduction in cardiovascular reactivity when they received a partner's support during the interaction. However, attachment-anxious men (but not women) showed reduced cardiovascular reactivity when they received more support.

Cortisol Release

Cortisol, a steroid hormone released as part of activation of the HPA axis, prepares the body to respond adaptively to threats and challenges. However, heightened cortisol release that persists even after the stressful event ends (a chronic cortisol response) can disrupt normal functioning of the metabolic and immune systems, exhaust bodily resources, and lead to long-term health problems (e.g., Steptoe et al., 2016). Several studies have assessed attachment-related differences in salivary cortisol levels during and following laboratory-induced stressors (e.g., aversive noise, the Trier Social Stress Test), and found that heightened cortisol release is related to attachment insecurities (e.g., Kidd et al., 2011; Monteleone et al., 2019; Smyth et al., 2015). However, other studies have found no significant attachment–cortisol link (e.g., Ditzen et al., 2008; Smeets, 2010). These inconsistencies could be due, in part, to variations in the stressors and participants' ages (young adults, midlife adults).

Attachment-related differences in cortisol release have also been found in response to a relationship conflict in the lab. Specifically, attachment insecurities (assessed with the ECR) are associated with higher levels of salivary cortisol following a conflict discussion with a romantic partner (e.g., Hertz et al., 2015; Laurent & Powers, 2007; Powers et al., 2006). The same thing has been noted even following days of couple conflict outside the lab (Hicks & Diamond, 2011). However, Brooks et al. (2011) failed to replicate these findings; in their study, only women with avoidant partners exhibited increased cortisol responses to a conflict discussion. Laurent and Powers (2007) also observed this avoidant-partner effect, noting that it was strongest when both partners scored relatively high on avoidance. In a couple-level analysis of cortisol responses during conflictual marital interactions, Beck et al. (2013) found that couples in which anxious wives were paired with avoidant husbands had the strongest cortisol responses.

Research also indicates that attachment-insecure people react to other relationship threats (partner's rejection, separation) with heightened cortisol release. Dewitte et al. (2010) manipulated indicators of a romantic partner's rejection in the lab and found that more attachment-anxious individuals reacted to these signs with higher cortisol release. In a diary study conducted across 12 consecutive days, Diamond et al. (2008) found that attachment anxiety was associated with more severe physical symptoms and higher levels of salivary cortisol during and following days of physical separation from a romantic partner who was absent because of work-related travel. Rifkin-Graboi (2008) found that attachment-avoidant people (assessed with the AAI), as compared with secure people, showed greater cortisol reactivity during and after tasks that involved thinking about separation and loss experiences.

Other studies that have gone beyond examining acute cortisol responses to stress indicate that more attachment-anxious people tend to show higher daily cortisol levels over several days (e.g., Jaremka et al., 2013). In addition, attachment anxiety is associated with raised bedtime cortisol levels (Kidd et al., 2013), which suggests that anxious attachment not only elevates cortisol levels during waking hours but also interferes with the ability to reduce arousal when preparing to sleep. These findings suggest that attachment-related worries and doubts are related to chronic cortisol release even when no direct threat is present.

Dysregulated Immune Functioning: Pro-Inflammatory Responses

Research in the field of psychoneuroimmunology has shown that exposure to stressors early in life can create a *pro-inflammatory phenotype* in the immune system, fostering the release of hormone-like messengers (e.g., cykotines) and predisposing a person to chronic, low-grade inflammation (Miller et al., 2011). This kind of inflammatory response underlies a wide array of maladies, including cardiovascular diseases, diabetes, cancer, and autoimmune disorders (e.g., Danesh et al., 1998). According to Ehrlich et al. (2016), frustrating and stressful interactions with nonresponsive caregivers during early childhood, and the resulting attachment insecurities, may contribute to formation of the pro-inflammatory phenotype. To us this suggests that attachment-insecure people may be at risk for dysregulated immune functioning, chronic low-grade inflammation, and related diseases.

In a pioneering study conducted with a small sample of Italian women nurses, Picardi et al. (2007) found that self-reports of attachment-related avoidance were associated with lower natural killer cell cytotoxicity, which can result in impaired responses to viruses. This association was replicated in a follow-up study in which immune measures were collected 4, 8, and 12 months after the assessment of attachment insecurities (Picardi et al., 2013). Other researchers have found that self-reports of attachment anxiety are associated with lower numbers of T cells and greater Epstein–Barr virus titers (Fagundes et al., 2014; Jaremka et al., 2013)—two well-known indicators of immune dysregulation (Miller et al., 2011).

More recently, Ehrlich et al. (2019) found that self-reports of attachment anxiety were associated with a common marker of inflammatory activity—high levels of C-reactive protein (CRP)—in a sample of young African American adults. Heightened CRP levels have also been found in toddlers and school-age children classified as insecure or disorganized in the Strange Situation during infancy (Bernard et al., 2019; Nelson et al., 2020) and in adolescents who perceived lack of secure-base support from their parents (Jones et al., 2017).

Overall, these diverse research findings strongly suggest that attachment-insecure individuals have a diminished ability to mount a cellular defense against pathogens and a heightened proclivity for inflammation.

Attachment insecurities also increase the risk of inflammatory responses to distressing events. For example, self-reports of attachment-related avoidance have been associated with increased production of interleukin-6 (IL-6, an index of inflammatory activity) among romantic partners following a relationship conflict discussion in the laboratory (Gouin et al., 2009) and among patients following coronary artery bypass graft surgery (Kidd et al., 2014). In a prospective longitudinal study, Gouin and MacNeil (2019) assessed inflammation responses of international students migrating to a new country immediately after their arrival and again 2 and 5 months later. Findings indicated that self-reports of attachment anxiety assessed upon arrival to the host country predicted larger increases in CRP over the 5-month study period. Similarly, attachment anxiety has been associated with an increase in cellular markers of inflammation (i.e., increased stimulated monocyte IL-6 production) among bereaved individuals who had recently lost a spouse (LeRoy et al., 2020).

Robles et al. (2013) provided an additional intriguing piece of evidence regarding attachment-insecure people's dysregulated immune responses. They focused on the role that attachment security and insecurities play in recovery from injuries to skin barrier function. Dating couples completed the revised ECR scale, and during two separate laboratory visits, normal skin barrier function was disrupted using a tape-stripping procedure (rapidly removing a small piece of adhesive tape from the skin to remove part of its protective outer layer). This procedure was followed by a discussion of personal concerns in one visit and relationship problems in the other. Skin barrier recovery was assessed by measuring transepidermal water loss up to 2 hours after skin disruption. Attachment-related avoidance predicted slower skin barrier recovery among women, and attachment anxiety predicted slower skin barrier recovery among men. The observed effects remained significant after controlling for transepidermal water loss in undisturbed skin, suggesting that the observed findings could not be explained by other skin-related factors such as sweating.

Stress-Induced Cellular Aging: Shortened Telomere Length

One well-known indicator of cellular aging is leukocyte telomere length. Telomeres are repetitive TTAGGG sequences located at the ends of chromosomes, which confer genomic stability (de Lange, 2002). At each cell division, telomeres progressively shorten, creating a negative correlation between telomere length and biological age. Apart from normal aging, there is evidence that early life stressors and traumatic events can shorten telomere length and thus increase the risk of premature aging and aging-related diseases (e.g., Price et al., 2013; Solomon et al., 2017).

This biological response to stress might be expected to occur mainly among attachment-insecure people. They tend to amplify and perpetuate distress (in the case of anxious people) or pay a metabolic price for coping with the stress alone, without others' support (in the case of avoidant people). People who are secure with respect to attachment have more internal and external coping resources and thus may be less likely to show signs of accelerated cellular aging in response to life stressors (Ein-Dor et al., 2020).

Five studies support the hypothesis that insecure attachment strengthens the link between stress and cellular aging. In an assessment of cellular aging among young adults, Dagan et al. (2018) found that retrospective accounts of adverse childhood experiences were associated with shorter telomere length only among avoidant participants (assessed with the AAI). Ein-Dor et al. (2020) assessed cellular aging in a sample of former Israeli prisoners of war 40 years after the experience of captivity and found that self-reports of avoidant attachment (on the ECR, assessed 30, 35, and 40 years after captivity) predicted shorter telomere length. Ehrlich et al. (2021) also found that avoidant attachment at age 20 accelerated negative changes in telomere length from ages 20–27 among African American women exposed to neighborhood poverty. Murdock, Seiler, et al. (2018) collected young adults' retrospective accounts of social rejection during childhood and found that these accounts were associated with shorter telomere length only among participants who scored relatively high on the ECR Anxiety scale. In this sample, avoidant attachment was not related to telomere length. In another correlational study, Murdock, Zilioli, et al. (2018) found that self-reports of both attachment anxiety and avoidance were associated with shorter telomere length, and this association was mediated by insecure participants' heightened perceived stress.

Ein-Dor et al. (2020) found that wives' reports of attachment anxiety were associated with shorter telomeres among former prisoners of war. According to these researchers, attachment-anxious wives tend to be overly dependent, often demand attention and care, and react with overwhelming distress to relational discord, which may be taxing for the traumatized veteran and hence accelerate his cellular aging. Wives' attachment-related avoidance was unexpectedly found to be beneficial: It was associated with longer telomeres among former prisoners of war. According to Ein-Dor et al., former prisoners of war often struggle with myriad physical and mental problems, and with horrific memories of captivity. Under these conditions, a wife's somewhat distant, nonprobing stance may help her husband gain perspective and maintain emotional stability. Of course, we must regard these dyadic findings with caution; they may be unique to couples coping with the trauma of war captivity.

Health-Related Behaviors

Beyond underlying maladaptive physiological responses to stress, attachment insecurities may increase the likelihood of physical disorders by interfering with health-promoting behaviors and fostering behaviors that increase health risks. People who score relatively high on measures of attachment-related avoidance habitually distrust others' intentions, are reluctant to rely on their assistance and support, and tend to suppress negative emotions and feelings (Mikulincer & Shaver, 2016). Therefore, we might expect them to be less aware of physical problems and less willing to seek the help of health care providers and adhere to these professionals' prescriptions and advice. More avoidant people might also be more likely to smoke, consume alcohol and drugs, or engage in activities that can create a self-induced positive mood at the price of endangering health (e.g., promiscuous sex, gambling, risky driving) as a means of distracting and calming themselves and avoiding painful self-awareness.

People who score relatively high on measures of attachment anxiety, who have problems with distress regulation, might also use alcohol, drugs, or food to calm themselves and reduce the flow of distressing thoughts and memories. In addition, their sensitivity to threat-related cues, chronic hyperarousal, and tendency to ruminate (Mikulincer & Shaver, 2016) might deplete self-regulatory resources that are necessary for maintaining health and coping effectively with illness. As a result, attachment-anxious individuals might find it hard to calmly explore and learn about symptoms and treatments and to exert self-discipline (e.g., exercising, dieting, taking prescribed medicines). Their anxious hypervigilance might also impair sleep quality, which could add to resource depletion and difficulties in engaging in focused, effortful health-promoting behaviors.

Health-Promoting Behaviors

In the first comprehensive study of attachment and health-promoting behaviors, Feeney and Ryan (1994) found that avoidant attachment was related to fewer self-reported health care visits over a 10-week period, even after controlling for the severity of physical symptoms. They also found that attachment-anxious individuals expressed greater concern about their weight (even after controlling for body mass), but failed to take the necessary steps (e.g., physical exercise) to lose weight.

These findings have been replicated and extended in subsequent studies. For example, attachment insecurities are associated with less engagement in physical activity, poorer diet, and less regular use of seat belts (e.g., Ahrens et al., 2012; Davis et al., 2014; Li, Bunke, et al., 2016). In addition, insecure individuals are less likely to take preventive medical tests. For example, more avoidant and anxious women are less likely to report receiving cervical cancer screening and mammograms, and to conduct breast self-examinations (Hill & Gick, 2013; Tuck & Consedine, 2015). Another example: More avoidant men are less likely to undergo prostate-specific antigen testing and digital rectal examination (Consedine et al., 2013).

Research also indicates that attachment insecurities reduce adherence to medical regimens. For example, attachment insecurities among diabetics are associated with less faithful glucose monitoring and higher levels of HbA1c, a physiological indicator of poor glucose control (e.g., Bazzarian & Besharat, 2012; Ciechanowski et al., 2001; Rosenberg & Shields, 2009). In addition, Ciechanowski et al. (2004) found that more avoidant individuals with diabetes engaged in less exercise and foot care, maintained a poorer diet, and took their medication less regularly. Similar findings linking attachment insecurities with poorer adherence to medical regimens have been reported in samples of people living with HIV (Blake Helms et al., 2017), patients diagnosed with lupus (Bennett et al., 2011), and obese individuals (Aarts et al., 2013).

Health-Endangering Behaviors

Several studies indicate that attachment anxiety interferes with safe sex. For example, more anxious individuals have more negative beliefs about condom use (e.g., "Condoms are boring"; "They reduce intimacy"), are less likely to use condoms, and are less willing to change their risky sexual practices (e.g., Bogaert & Sadava, 2002; Feeney et al., 1999, 2000). In a 14-day diary study of daily condom use among college students, Strachman and Impett (2009) found that attachment-anxious participants were less likely to use condoms on days in which they had more conflictual interactions with their romantic partner, which suggests that their reluctance to use condoms is related to their relationship worries. It seems likely that anxious people's desire to get psychologically close to their sexual partners while hoping not to "turn them off," causes them to put their own and their partners' health at risk.

People scoring higher on attachment-related avoidance hold more positive attitudes toward condom use and are more likely to use them (Feeney et al., 2000)—one circumstance in which willingness to forgo intimacy may be health promoting. However, avoidant people's openness to having casual sex with relative strangers, without talking about their own and their partner's sexual histories (e.g., Bogaert & Sadava, 2002), can sometimes result in unsafe sex. This possibility is reinforced by avoidant men's tendency to use alcohol and drugs before sex, perhaps to reduce doubts about intimacy or their sexual performance (Tracy et al., 2003).

Attachment insecurities are associated with obesity (as indexed by body mass index and waist-to-hip ratio), a major health problem in many countries, in samples of adolescents and young adults (e.g., Diener et al., 2016), suggesting that attachment-insecure people have nonoptimal eating habits. Indeed, a meta-analysis of 70 studies (with 19,470 participants) yielded moderate but significant correlations between self-reports of attachment anxiety and avoidance and less healthy eating behaviors, such as binge eating, emotional eating, and high-caloric food consumption (Faber et al., 2018). Adding to these correlational findings, Wilkinson et al. (2013) found that normal-weight participants who were asked to think about and visualize a relationship in which they felt anxious (using Hazan & Shaver's [1987] prototypes) ate more high-caloric snacks that those asked to think about a secure condition.

Adult attachment studies have also turned up associations between self-reports of attachment anxiety and avoidance and higher levels of cigarette smoking, alcohol consumption, and drug use in community samples of adolescents and young adults (e.g., Cooper et al., 1998; Murase et al., 2021; Olsson et al., 2013). Importantly, although most of these studies have relied on one-time cross-sectional research designs, longitudinal studies have also consistently shown that insecure attachment prospectively predicts substance abuse at a later time (e.g., Burge et al., 1997). In a recent meta-analysis of 34 longitudinal studies (with 56,721 participants and time frames ranging from 1 month to 20 years), Fairbairn et al. (2018) found that attachment insecurity temporally preceded increases in substance abuse, and that the pathway from earlier insecure attachment to later substance abuse was significantly stronger than that from earlier substance abuse to later insecure attachment.

Another health hazard associated with attachment insecurity is poor sleep quality. From an evolutionary perspective, security-related beliefs that the world is a safe place in which other people are benevolent and supportive are conducive to healthy sleep, which involves being unattuned to imagined dangers in the environment and being, while asleep, unable to defend against them (Dahl & El-Sheikh, 2007). Indeed, several studies have found that lack of felt security (as indexed by higher scores on attachment anxiety and avoidance scales) is associated with reports of sleep disturbances, including difficulties in initiating and maintaining sleep during the night, early morning awakenings, and daytime sleepiness (e.g., Adams & McWilliams, 2015; Elsey et al., 2019; Kent de Grey et al., 2019).

Attachment insecurities are also associated with electrophysiological markers of poor sleep (particular electroencephalographic patterns of brain activity during sleep), such as elevated levels of alpha waves and reduced lengths of "deep-sleep" Stages 3 and 4 (e.g., Sloan et al., 2007; Troxel et al., 2007; Troxel & Germain, 2011). In a 4-day study, Gur-Yaish et al. (2020) monitored bodily activity (using an actigraph) during nighttime sleep and found that more attachment-insecure participants had more troubled sleep (e.g., more waking episodes during the night) and that these patterns were mainly evident on days when they reported having negative interactions with their spouse. Overall, research suggests that attachment insecurities are associated with heightened vigilance or arousal during sleep (metaphorically, "sleeping with one eye open").

Responses to Physical Pain

Attachment-insecure people's health can be damaged by their maladaptive responses to physical pain. These responses can intensify and perpetuate dysregulated biological responses and reluctance to undergo prescribed but painful medical treatments (Mikail et al., 1994). There is evidence that self-reports of attachment insecurities are associated with greater reported pain intensity and pain-related suffering among individuals with chronic pain (e.g., Forsythe et al., 2012). Attachment insecurities also prospectively predict more intense pain during labor and delivery (Quinn et al., 2015), heightened pain-related suffering and physical disability after a whiplash injury (Andersen et al., 2013, 2019), and more severe headache after performing a distressing task (Berry & Drummond, 2014).

In addition, attachment insecurities can interfere with the potentially beneficial effects of others' supportive presence on the experience of pain (e.g., Krahé et al., 2015). Wilson and Simpson (2016) found that greater spousal support during childbirth predicted lowered reports of pain intensity among attachment-secure women but not among attachment-insecure women. In fact, avoidant women actually reported greater childbirth-related pain when their spouse provided more support.

Other research has shown that attachment anxiety is associated with pain catastrophizing (i.e., the tendency to magnify the threat intensity of a pain stimulus and to feel helpless in the presence of pain), lower perceived efficacy in dealing with pain, more worrying about pain, and more engagement in physical activities that exacerbate rather than mitigate pain (e.g., Andrews et al., 2014; Kratz et al., 2012; McWilliams & Holmberg, 2010; Meredith et al., 2006, 2008). These findings have been replicated in laboratory studies in which pain is experimentally induced by applying a noxious thermal or ischemic stimulus (e.g., Andersen et al., 2018; Sambo et al., 2010; Wilson & Ruben, 2011). Interestingly, Frias and Shaver (2014) found that attachment anxiety was associated with greater physical pain sensitivity in a cold-pressor task mainly following episodes of social exclusion in a Cyberball task, implying that anxious people's pain sensitivity is affected by attachment-related injuries and worries.

Attachment-anxious people's negative appraisals of pain might be generalized to the way they perceive physical disorders, which in turn might interfere with psychological well-being. Vilchinsky et al. (2013) examined this possibility in a 6-month prospective study of midlife men who were recovering from a heart attack. In that study, attachment anxiety was associated with more pessimistic, hopeless appraisals of recovering from the attack during hospitalization, which in turn predicted increased depression and anxiety 6 months later.

The Quality of Patients' Relationships with Health Care Providers

In their attachment-informed model of health-related behavior, Hunter and Maunder (2001) proposed that patients' attachment insecurities can impair the quality of the relationships they form with health care providers (physicians, nurses), thereby negatively affecting the medical services they receive. According to Hunter and Maunder, individuals scoring high on measures of attachment anxiety have little confidence in the availability and responsiveness of health care providers in times of need and so use various means to keep their medical team close by and engaged (e.g., repeatedly complaining about physical problems, exaggerating their helplessness and need). These anxious, controlling, and sometimes coercive proximity-seeking behaviors may discourage and "burn out" health care providers and make them reluctant to approach the patient. Hunter and Maunder also suggested that avoidant individuals' negative models of others might cause them to distrust the intentions, knowledge, and skills of health care providers and show disdain and contempt for them. This could then frustrate the medical team members and cause them to back away from avoidant patients.

These ideas have been tested and supported in studies conducted in medical settings. For example, Holwerda et al. (2013) followed up cancer patients 3 and 9 months after their diagnosis and found that more attachment-insecure patients reported less trust in and satisfaction with their doctors. Hillen et al. (2014) showed video clips of consultations of oncologists with cancer patients and found that more avoidant patients appraised the videotaped oncologists as less trustworthy. Other studies have found that patients' attachment insecurities are associated with self-reports of poorer working alliances with physicians, more conflictual patterns of communication with them, and less satisfaction with medical care (e.g., Harding et al., 2015; McWilliams, 2018; Zaporowska-Stachowiak et al., 2019).

In an attempt to overcome methodological problems associated with patient self-reports, Maunder, Panzer, et al. (2006) asked physicians (who were blind to patients' attachment scores) to rate the difficulty of their relationships with particular patients. The results indicated that physicians had more troubled relationships with insecure than with secure patients. It seems that insecure patients' relational problems, which have been studied mainly in the domain of close personal relationships (e.g., marriages), are also evident in doctor–patient relationships.

As in other attachment relationships (e.g., infant–parent, client–therapist), physicians' own attachment insecurities might also influence the quality of the patient–physician relationship. Attachment-avoidant physicians might find it difficult to provide emotional support and reassurance to a distressed patient. Attachment-anxious physicians might be so focused on their own worries and so concerned about their own stress levels that they find it difficult to attend empathically to their patients' feelings and needs.

In support of this theoretical reasoning, there is evidence that more attachment-insecure physicians have more communication difficulties in primary care consultations (Cherry et al., 2018). Moreover, their patients are less satisfied with the medical care these insecure physicians provide (Kafetsios et al., 2016). In a study conducted with undergraduate medical students undergoing their qualifying Objective Structured Clinical Examination, Fletcher et al. (2016) found that self-reports of attachment insecurities predicted worse communication and clinical skills during a consultation with a simulated patient (as rated by examiners and the patient).

Research Summary

Overall, research indicates that people who are relatively insecure with respect to attachment have poorer health and are at greater risk of suffering from physical disorders. The research conducted to date fits well with Maunder and Hunter's (2001) model concerning the psychological and biological processes underlying the connections between attachment and health. Attachment insecurities are associated with dysregulated biological responses to stress, maladaptive psychological responses to pain, engagement in health-endangering behaviors, and difficulty trusting health care providers and complying with their recommendations, all of which contribute to poorer heath.

Findings from studies of dyads (e.g., marital couples) call our attention to the association between one relationship partner's insecure attachment and the other partner's impaired heath. These findings fit well with Pietromonaco et al.'s (2015) claim that the health of one partner in a dyadic relationship can be damaged by both his or her own attachment insecurities and those of the other partner. These findings are relevant for understanding dyadic processes in medical settings that can either facilitate or interfere with patients' illness management (e.g., adherence to treatment, engagement in health-promoting behavior) and recovery of health.

The research we've discussed here has practical implications for designing attachment-informed approaches to health care. Health professionals and patients' informal caregivers (family members, friends) can be informed about the negative implications for health of insecure attachment and about the broaden-and-build processes that flow from felt security. Moreover, medical professionals can be encouraged and trained to enhance patients' felt security by being more responsive to their needs and feelings, and providing more effective support and care, which may reduce the dysfunctional manifestations of patients' attachment insecurities and facilitate the healing process. For understandable reasons, the training of doctors and nurses focuses primarily on physiological and technical matters, which are difficult enough to master. But it would also be very beneficial if these professionals also learned how to be effective context-specific attachment figures.

Applying Attachment-Theoretical Principles to Improve Health and Health Care

As stated in Chapter 2, interactions with a responsive attachment figure who effectively provides a safe haven and secure base in a given social context can momentarily instill felt security and foster broaden-and-build processes, with benefits for well-being and health. Therefore, an attachment-informed approach to improving the effectiveness of health care services should (1) identify figures who are likely to be viewed by a patient as potential providers of a safe haven and secure base, and (2) encourage and instruct these potential security providers to adopt a more responsive and supportive attitude toward patients in general, and attachment-insecure patients in particular. Usually, patients appraise and relate to informal caregivers (family members, close friends) and their medical team (physicians, nurses) as potential security providers, so interventions aimed at increasing these people's responsiveness should have beneficial effects on patients' health and well-being.

The Safe-Haven and Secure-Base Functions of Informal Caregivers in Health Care Settings

Attachment research has shown that children, adolescents, and adults often direct proximity- and support-seeking bids to close relationship partners (e.g., parents during infancy and childhood; siblings, friends, romantic partners, and spouses during adolescence and adulthood; adult children during old age) when facing threats and challenges (Zeifman & Hazan, 2016). These close relationship partners are a person's most important sources of a safe haven and secure base, crucial for managing emotions and maintaining mental health and interpersonal functioning throughout life. In health care settings, the attachment functions served by family members and close friends become critical, because a patient often urgently needs support, care, and encouragement in order to cope effectively with, and recover from, illness.

In this section, we review evidence showing that responsive and supportive family members and friends help patients not only to feel safer and more secure but also to be healthier in general and more resilient in the face of illness or injury. We also review evidence concerning the psychological factors that can interfere with informal caregivers' responsiveness (e.g., caregiver burden, attachment insecurities) and attachment-based approaches for overcoming these obstacles and sustaining informal caregivers' effective support. In so doing, we hope to encourage health care professionals to pay more attention to the attachment functions served by informal caregivers, to take them into account when planning medical treatments, and to view them as critical therapeutic agents during the healing process.

Beneficial Health-Related Effects of Informal Caregivers' Responsiveness

In Chapter 6, we reviewed evidence from studies of romantic and marital relationships that the responsiveness and supportiveness of one partner can enhance the other partner's felt security, with beneficial implications for psychological well-being and relationship quality. Here we want to briefly review evidence showing that partner responsiveness is also beneficial for physical health.

Experimental findings indicate that the physical or mental presence of a responsive close relationship partner while a person undergoes a laboratory-induced stressor dramatically reduces cardiac dysregulation (e.g., Bourassa et al., 2019). Daily diary studies indicate that feeling supported by a close relationship partner is associated with healthier daily cortisol release patterns, less susceptibility to infections following stressful days, and fewer self-reported physical symptoms (e.g., Cohen et al., 2015; Ditzen et al., 2008; Lun et al., 2008). In a prospective longitudinal study, Slatcher et al. (2015) found that perceived partner responsiveness at the beginning of the study predicted healthier diurnal cortisol release patterns 10 years later. Overall, a responsive and supportive close relationship partner seems to make people not only happier and more secure but also healthier and less susceptible to physical illness.

Although the reviewed studies support the hypothesized role of close relationship partners in sustaining physical health, they were all conducted in healthy samples of young adults who were not currently ill. Therefore, their findings can only hint that a responsive relationship partner reduces the risk of health problems. However, no conclusion can be drawn concerning the role a responsive partner plays in facilitating healing from an already present illness. Moreover, the specific provisions people seek from a close relationship partner when facing a chronic illness or painful medical procedure (e.g., going together to medical treatments, sharing responsibility for managing the illness) differ dramatically from the regular care a partner is asked to provide in daily life or during laboratory-induced stress.

In conceptualizing relationships partners' responsiveness and supportiveness in medical settings, Bodenmann (1997) and Lyons et al. (1998) introduced the concept of *dyadic/communal coping*, a process in which a partner joins forces and collaborates with a patient to cope with an illness. Specifically, family members and friends might help the person appraise and address the illness (e.g., "This is 'our' problem rather than 'your' problem"), share responsibilities for managing the illness, provide instrumental support and emotional reassurance when needed, and engage in comforting and autonomy-respecting interactions (see Cutrona et al., 2018; Helgeson et al., 2018, for reviews). They might also assist the patient in executing complex self-management tasks and adhering to medical regimens, and help the patient sustain an optimistic outlook and broaden his or her understanding of the nature and implications of the illness. As a result, patients can feel understood, validated, and cared for by their family members or close friends and realize that they do not have to cope alone with the illness.

Numerous cross-sectional and prospective longitudinal studies conducted with patients in health care settings indicate that their perceptions of being supported, respected, and appreciated by family members and friends are associated with greater adherence to medical guidelines, enhanced well-being, and healthier physiological markers (e.g., Haviland et al., 2017; Lee et al., 2019; Maki, 2020). In a 24-day diary study of patients with type 2 diabetes, for example, Stephens et al. (2013) found that participants adhered better to a diabetic diet on days when their spouses provided more support for proper dietary choices. Similarly, patients with knee arthritis engaged in healthier physical activity and took more steps on days when their spouses encouraged them to exercise (Martire et al., 2013).

Studies assessing informal caregiver reports of dyadic coping have shown that appraising the illness as shared with the patient and acting in a collaborative and supportive manner contribute to a patient's well-being and physical health, better adherence to treatments, and faster recovery from illness (e.g., Berg et al., 2020; Zajdel et al., 2018, 2021). In addition, observational studies of illness-related discussions between a patient and his or her spouse have confirmed that more supportive and comforting interactions and more collaboration during the discussion are positively associated with the patient's well-being and physical health (e.g., Helgeson et al., 2022; Kuhn et al., 2017; Lau et al., 2019). In a review of 30 studies, Rosland et al. (2012) concluded that family members' responsiveness to patients' needs and feelings, as well as their provision of secure-base (autonomy) forms of support, predict better illness management and improved patient survival.

Overall, the findings fit well with Helgeson et al.'s (2018) model of the health-related benefits of dyadic/communal coping. The process begins when informal caregivers make a shared illness appraisal ("our problem") and share responsibility with the patient for coping with the illness. This appraisal then leads informal caregivers to collaborate with the patient ("work together") in sustaining his or her well-being and adhering to medical treatments. Both shared appraisal and a collaborative attitude converge in (1) informal support providers' greater responsiveness to patients' needs and feelings and improved provision of safe-haven and secure-base support, and (2) patients' trust and reliance on informal caregivers for managing the illness. This in turn has beneficial effects on the patient's health. In line with attachment-theoretical reasoning, patients' perceptions of partner responsiveness and enhanced felt security are the most direct predictors of health restoration.

Obstacles to Informal Caregivers' Responsiveness

Engagement in dyadic/communal coping requires effort, and it may not occur if informal caregivers lack motivation, ability, or mental resources to share responsibility and collaborate with the patient. Some family members or friends might be unwilling to engage in dyadic/communal coping, might reject a patient's bids for protection and support, or emotionally detach or behaviorally withdraw from him or her. Others might have a positive attitude toward caregiving but be unable to engage in dyadic/communal coping because they lack the emotion-regulatory skills needed to maintain a calm, well-regulated state of mind when interacting with the patient or spending prolonged periods of time in a hospital. Still others might overidentify with the patient's suffering and neglect their own need for care, which could result in emotional burnout and depression (a condition that Figley [2002] called *compassion fatigue*) and less effective care.

In all of these cases, informal caregivers may fail to support and empower the patient. Instead, they may engage in behavior that undermines the patient's felt security and well-being, such as criticizing his or her illness management, distracting him or her from adhering to prescribed treatment, hiding information about the illness, or adopting an overcontrolling stance that underestimates the patient's capabilities and disrespects his or her autonomy.

These motivational, regulatory, and affective obstacles to dyadic/communal coping can be aggravated by informal caregivers' attachment insecurities. Avoidant family members or friends who habitually have a negative, cynical view of others and are reluctant to engage in interdependent relations may be less willing to share responsibility with the patient and actively collaborate in managing the illness. Attachment-anxious informal caregivers who typically have difficulty managing their own distress or tend to neglect their own needs when attending to the needs of others may be less capable than more secure individuals of effectively supporting and empowering a patient's efforts to manage an illness, and they may be more susceptible to compassion fatigue.

These hypothesized negative effects of caregivers' attachment-related insecurities on dyadic/communal coping have received initial support from an observational study in which participants were video-recorded while interacting with a confederate of the experimenter, whom they thought had recently been diagnosed with cancer (Westmaas & Silver, 2001). As expected, avoidant participants were rated by observers as less verbally and nonverbally supportive, and as making less eye contact during the interaction. Attachment anxiety was not associated with supportiveness, but more anxious participants reported greater discomfort while interacting with the confederate and were more likely to report self-critical thoughts after the interaction. Although the findings are certainly interesting, it is important to note that the participants had no relationship with the confederate, so we cannot be sure that the same attachment-related deficiencies in dyadic/communal coping would be observed when a close relationship partner is actually injured or ill.

Subsequent studies conducted in medical settings have overcome this limitation and have shown that informal caregivers' attachment insecurities do in fact interfere with care provision. For example, higher scores on attachment anxiety or avoidance scales are associated with less frequent provision of emotional support to a spouse who is coping with cancer, less engagement in dyadic/communal coping with him or her, and less respect for the spouse's autonomy (e.g., Crangle et al., 2020; Kim & Carver, 2007; Kim et al., 2008). In addition, whereas avoidant attachment was associated with less responsive caregiving to a spouse with cancer, anxious attachment was associated with more intrusive caregiving (Braun et al., 2012). Anxious attachment was also associated with the adoption of a more overprotective stance when offering support to a spouse who had suffered a heart attack (O'Bertos et al., 2020), and more frequent harmful caregiver behavior (i.e., psychological or physical mistreatment) when caring for a cognitively or physically impaired spouse (Morse et al., 2012).

There is also evidence that attachment-anxious caregivers of patients with cancer or dementia report higher levels of personal distress, caregiver burden, burnout, and depression (e.g., Ávila et al., 2016; Perren et al., 2007; Rodin et al., 2007). Moreover, self-reported attachment anxiety has been found to strengthen the link between caregiving burden and depression among spouses of patients suffering from acute coronary syndrome (Vilchinsky et al., 2015). More caregiving burden was related to more depression only among anxiously attached spouses, not among more secure spouses.

Patients' attachment insecurities can also interfere with a partner's dyadic/communal coping and its beneficial effects on health. Attachment-avoidant patients, who are typically reluctant to acknowledge and share their problems with others, may make it difficult for partners to appraise the illness as a shared issue and engage in collaborative coping. Moreover, avoidant patients may appraise their partners' caregiving attempts as intrusive, because they prefer self-reliance and hence reject their partner's invitation to engage in dyadic/communal coping. Attachment-anxious patients' typical clinging and demanding stance toward partners, and their tendency to ruminate on self-focused worries and exaggerate expressions of distress, might demoralize their partner and perhaps increase caregiver burden and compassion fatigue. As a result, informal caregivers might provide less effective support to attachment-anxious patients.

To date, only two published studies have examined these possibilities. Van Vleet and Helgeson (2019) conducted a study of patients with type 2 diabetes and found that dyadic/communal coping (as coded from video-recorded patient–spouse interactions in which partners discussed difficulties managing diabetes) was beneficial only among patients who scored relatively low on the ECR Avoidance scale. However, when avoidance was high, dyadic/communal coping was associated with lower relationship quality and greater patient distress. In another study of patients recovering from a first heart attack, spouses' sensitive caregiving (as assessed by a self-report scale) predicted lower levels of patients' disease-related anxiety 6 months later, but only among patients who scored relatively low on the ECR Anxiety scale (George-Levi et al., 2020).

Enhancing Informal Caregivers' Responsiveness

Based on the kinds of research reviewed here, several dyadic interventions have been developed for increasing informal caregivers' involvement in their partners' medical treatment and healing process (for reviews, see Kedia et al., 2020; Martire & Helgeson, 2017). Some of these approaches attempt to create a more secure relational climate by (1) enhancing a patient's confidence in an informal caregiver's health-related suggestions and guidance, and (2) coaching the caregiver to maintain constructive, nonconflictual patterns of communication related to the illness and treatment. Other approaches attempt to sustain and enhance the provision of secure-base support by fostering an informal caregiver's acceptance, support, encouragement, and respect for a patient's illness-management efforts. Although these interventions have not been explicitly based on attachment theory (see some exceptions below), most of them implicitly follow the core attachment-theoretical principle that fostering more sensitive and supportive patterns of dyadic interactions can improve a patient's mental and physical health.

In the field of childhood illness, Martire and Helgeson (2017) reviewed two evidence-based interventions that target a child's parents and have been shown to improve the child's ability to manage his or her diabetes. One approach, Family Teamwork (Anderson et al., 1999), is explicitly designed to increase parents' involvement and collaborative management of their child's illness while maintaining a supportive, respectful, encouraging, and nonintrusive attitude toward the child's own coping attempts. The second approach, behavioral family systems therapy (Wysocki et al., 2008), focuses on improving the quality of parent–child relationships and fostering constructive patterns of communication regarding illness-related issues. These approaches can be tailored to other childhood diseases (e.g., asthma) and can foster more comforting parent–child interactions and more constructive patterns of dyadic coping.

Unfortunately, none of the attachment-based interventions that we reviewed in Chapter 4, which are aimed at improving parents' responsiveness more generally (VIPP, ABC, COS, MTB, CPP), have been implemented in medical settings or tailored to illness management. In our opinion, such implementation would be worthwhile. Attachment-based interventions demonstrably improve children's emotion regulation, self-regulatory skills, and overall well-being (see Chapter 4), which could benefit children's health and illness management.

In addition, attachment-based interventions focus on two parental qualities that are not addressed by other parent–child interventions but might be critical for improving children's health. First, attachment-based interventions put strong emphasis on increasing parents' mentalizing capacity when thinking about their child's needs and feelings. This might help parents sensitively and respectfully adjust their care to what their child really wants and needs. Second, attachment-based interventions address parents' own attachment fears and defenses, and the ways in which they can disrupt the parent–child relationship. This enhanced self-understanding could remove obstacles to the parents' provision of care to an ill child.

In attempting to improve illness management in adulthood, several interventions have targeted a patient's romantic partner or spouse as the main informal caregiver and have engaged the two partners in a kind of illness-relevant couple counseling. Some of these interventions teach partners about the optimal ways of helping patients manage their illness (e.g., Baucom et al., 2012). Other interventions place stronger emphasis on the quality of the relationship, by fostering positive couple interactions, enhancing constructive patterns of couple conflict resolution, and encouraging the well spouse to support and empower the ill spouse's illness-management efforts (e.g., Remien et al., 2005; Sorkin et al., 2014; Trief et al., 2011). All of these interventions have been found to produce positive changes in patients' adherence to treatment guidelines and engagement in health-promoting behaviors. However, they have only small effects on patients' subjective well-being and marital functioning (Martire & Helgeson, 2017).

The two attachment-based couple interventions reviewed in Chapter 6, emotionally focused therapy (EFT) and the Hold me Tight (HmT) couple relationship education program, have been implemented in medical settings and tailored to help couples who are coping with a chronic illness. McLean et al. (2013) adapted EFT for treating couples in which one partner was diagnosed with advanced cancer ($N = 42$). They found that, as compared to standard care, eight EFT sessions increased both partners' reports of marital satisfaction and patients' perceptions of their spouses' empathic care immediately after the intervention and 2 months later. No significant EFT effect was found on patients' depression or spouses' reported caregiver burden.

Tulloch et al. (2021) adapted the HmT relationship education program for counseling couples in which one partner has a cardiovascular disease (*Healing Hearts Together* intervention). As reviewed in Chapter 6, findings from 39 couples indicated that the pre- to postintervention produced increases in both partners' marital satisfaction, well-being, and quality of life. Although these finding are promising, RCTs should also examine the effects of these couple interventions on patients' illness management and health.

The Safe-Haven and Secure-Base Functions of Health Care Providers

In this section, we consider health care providers as context-specific attachment-like figures that, beyond providing effective medical treatment, can also provide a safe haven and secure base for patients and facilitate illness management and healing. We begin by elaborating on the idea that health care providers can serve attachment-like functions in medical settings, and that patients often direct attachment behaviors to physicians and nurses while coping with illness. We then review studies of patient-centered care, documenting the positive effects of health care providers' sensitive responsiveness on patients' recovery and health. Finally, we elaborate on the ways in which attachment theory and research can inform patient-centered care and help health care professionals deal with attachment-insecure patients.

We hope this section contributes to the integration of attachment theory and patient-centered medicine. We also hope it encourages medical and nursing schools to incorporate attachment theory into the academic curriculum and train students as not only technically oriented doctors and nurses but also responsive caregivers who can provide patients a secure base for illness management.

Do Patients Construe Health Care Providers as Fulfilling Attachment Functions?

According to Maunder and Hunter (2001), patients naturally tend to perceive health care providers (physicians, nurses) as more competent and informed than themselves and their informal caregivers in treating injuries and illnesses. It therefore makes sense that patients often construe health care providers as *stronger and wiser* caregivers and expect them to accomplish the attachment-like functions of providing a safe haven and secure base. Moreover, patients may direct proximity- and support-seeking bids to health care providers, and feel safe and secure when being understood, validated, and cared for by these professional caregivers.

Based on this reasoning, Maunder and Hunter (2016) constructed a self-report scale to assess whether a health care provider is viewed as a safe haven (e.g., "In some circumstances, I might count on this person to help me feel better") and a secure base (e.g., "This person makes me feel more confident about my health"). Patients were asked to nominate health care providers "who matter to you more than others" and to complete the scale for each of the identified providers. The scale showed adequate internal consistency, and 91% of the participants were able to identify at least one health care provider who mattered most. And the majority appraised these health care providers as fulfilling safe-haven and secure-base functions.

Patients' construal of health care providers as attachment-like figures is also evident in qualitative studies that have assessed patients' needs, preferences, and expectations in medical settings. For example, Frederiksen et al. (2010) identified three core components of an attachment bond in patients' accounts of their relationship with general practitioners. First, patients explicitly expressed a need to form a long-term, stable relationship with their doctor. Second, this need became stronger in times when patients were ill or anxious. Third, patients stated that it was difficult to change their doctor even if they were dissatisfied with the relationship and the care provided. In addition, meta-analyses of studies examining older people's needs and preferences with regard to medical and nursing care revealed both safe-haven needs (e.g., to feel safe) and secure-base needs (e.g., to feel competent and autonomous). In other words, older people hope doctors and nurses, like benevolent attachment figures, will care for them and empower their sense of self-worth and personal autonomy (e.g., Herrler et al., 2021).

Does Health Care Providers' Responsiveness Have Soothing and Empowering Effects?

Patients' construal of a health care provider as an attachment-like figure implies that the provider's responsiveness to patients' needs and feelings can enhance patients' felt security and thereby improve illness management and health restoration. This attachment-informed reasoning is evident in the *Learning Objectives for Medical Student Education* of the Association of American Medical Colleges, which states that "physicians must be compassionate and empathetic in caring for patients." Similarly, the American Medical Association's first principle of medical ethics says that "a physician shall be dedicated to providing competent medical care, with compassion and respect for human dignity and rights." These statements, although not explicitly informed by attachment theory, illustrate the importance that medical associations attach to physicians' empathic and caring attitudes and behaviors as components of high-quality health care. In other words, caring for patients' health involves not only the provision of effective medical treatment but also a compassionate, responsive attitude toward distressed patients.

Health care providers' responsiveness to patients' needs and feelings seems to be a core aspect of *patient-centered care* (Stewart et al., 1995). Although "patient-centered care" is a multifaceted construct that has been conceptualized and operationalized in various ways, compassionate care and shared decision making are integral to most definitions (Epstein & Street, 2007). Compassionate care includes health care professionals' efforts to attend to, understand, validate, and care for a patient's needs and subjective experiences and to convey warmth and support as part of creating a trusting relationship (Hojat et al., 2002). This construct resembles Reis's (2014) construct of "responsiveness" and involves understanding, validation, and compassion. Shared decision making requires health care professionals' respect for a patient's preferences and beliefs, empathic attention to his or her perspectives and judgments when making treatment decisions, and working collaboratively to reach mutually agreeable actions (Barry & Edgman-Levitan, 2012). This construct resembles Feeney's (2004) concept of secure-base support, which involves empowerment of patient autonomy.

There is considerable research linking physicians' compassionate care and shared decision making (as rated by physicians, patients, or external observers) to positive patient outcomes. For example, patients of physicians who score higher on measures of compassionate care and shared decision making are more likely to adhere to prescribed therapies and to comply with physicians' recommendations (e.g., Haas et al., 2022; Mercer et al., 2016; Moss et al., 2019). Moreover, studies show that physicians' provision of compassionate care and engagement in shared decision making are associated with patients' improved physical heath and greater satisfaction with care (e.g., Cuevas et al., 2019; Georgopoulou et al., 2018; Hojat et al., 2011).

Although an exhaustive review of relevant studies on the effects of patient-centered care on patients' outcomes is beyond the scope of this chapter, we will provide three examples. In a survey conducted in the United Kingdom, the United States, and Canada, Reis et al. (2008) found that the extent to which patients felt that their primary care physician was responsive to their needs and feelings and was genuinely interested in their thoughts and concerns was associated with self-reports of better physical health. Importantly, this association was significant even after the researchers controlled for general satisfaction with the physician. Relatedly, Sultan et al. (2011) found that physicians' accurate understanding of the beliefs of patients with diabetes concerning their illness was associated with better patient self-care (e.g., improved diet, increased blood glucose self-testing). In another study, patients with a common cold who appraised their physician as more empathically responsive had shorter and less severe cold symptoms and better immune functioning (Rakel et al., 2009).

Following this line of reasoning and research, a variety of psychoeducational programs have been developed over the years to enhance medical students' and physicians' sensitive responsiveness to patients' psychological needs (for reviews, see Kelm et al., 2014; Patel et al., 2019). Unfortunately, these programs have not been informed by attachment theory and research, dramatically differ in the skills and behaviors each of them tries to improve, and yield no information concerning the hypothesized effects of cultivation of physicians' responsiveness on patients' health and quality of life. Moreover, many of the evaluation studies of these programs suffer from poor research designs (e.g., small samples, nonrandom assignment), lack of standardized intervention protocols, and poor or absent assessment of patients' perceptions of physicians' responsiveness before and after the program (Kelm et al., 2014).

Despite these shortcomings, a review by Patel et al. (2019) of 52 studies revealed that most of the studies (75%) found that the program improved medical students' or physicians' empathy or compassion for patients (as rated by physicians, patients, and observers). They also found that the most effective programs for improving patients' perceptions of a physician's empathy and compassion included teaching trainees to detect patients' emotions, to recognize and respond to opportunities for compassion, and to express nonverbal signs of warmth and affection, as well as verbal messages of acceptance, validation, and support. We hope that future studies will thoroughly examine the extent to which these programs are effective in enhancing patients' felt security and improving their physical health.

Can Attachment Theory Inform Patient-Centered Care and Improve Its Positive Effects on Patients' Health?

In our view, attachment theory and research could be useful for training physicians and nurses to become more attuned to patients' needs and feelings, helping them deal with troubled, attachment-insecure patients, and designing more effective medical treatments. Unfortunately, no evidence-based training program has been informed by attachment principles, but some attachment scholars have provided recommendations regarding applications of attachment theory to medical settings (e.g., Jimenez, 2017; Maunder & Hunter, 2015; Thompson & Ciechanowski, 2003).

Patient-centered education programs for physicians and nurses highlight the importance of cultivating empathic responsiveness to patients' needs and feelings. Attachment theory can benefit these programs by making explicit that patients coping with illness are sometimes asking physicians and nurses for safe-haven support and at other times for secure-base support (see Figure 4.1, Chapter 4, depicting the Circle of Security). The theory can help health care professionals identify which need is dominant at a given moment and how to flexibly and empathically respond to what a patient currently needs.

Physicians and nurses can be trained to respond to a patient's need for a safe haven by emphasizing the safety of medical procedures, articulating comforting and soothing verbal and nonverbal messages, and providing emotional reassurance that everything is likely to go well. Safe-haven concerns can be addressed by explicit and genuine messages that medical professionals are currently available and fully engaged with the patient. In addition, medical professionals can be trained to respond to patients' need for a secure base by engaging patients in shared decision making and empowering their sense of self-efficacy and coping ability. Patients' sense of having a reliable secure base can also be reinforced by training medical professionals to trust in patients' strengths and skills, applaud and celebrate patients' illness-management efforts, and reassure patients that support will be available if physical health worsens or treatment becomes excessively painful.

Attachment theory can be important in informing health care professionals about patients' possible attachment-related fears and defenses, and how these states can impair physical health and disrupt adherence to medical treatment. Physicians and nurses can then better understand why a patient is responding negatively to a medical treatment, why their interactions with the patient are so troubled and frustrating, and how to tailor their responses to lessen the patient's insecurities and provide better clinical care. For this purpose, screening of a patient's attachment history, working models, and orientations might be integrated into clinical protocols (Jimenez, 2017), and physicians and nurses might be trained to use this kind of screening when planning treatment and interacting with patients.

Thompson and Ciechanowski (2003) offered some examples of how such screening can be a valuable tool for health care professionals:

> Realizing that the patient with a fearful attachment style [a combination of anxiety and avoidance] can be simultaneously desperate for care and yet unable to trust any care might help the physician be less defensive and take the role of caring for such patients less personally. Similarly, it helps to know that a patient with a dismissing [avoidant] attachment style has unknowingly learned to reject attachment needs as a paradoxical strategy to receive any care at all. Likewise, when experiencing the helplessness engendered by a clinging [anxious] patient, the physician can attend more objectively to the patient's underlying needs, rather than respond to the most apparent problems, by recognizing the patient's preoccupied attachment patterns. (p. 223)

By becoming aware of, and learning about, the specific needs, fears, defenses, and interpersonal complexities that characterize attachment anxiety and avoidance, physicians and nurses can improve their ability to respond effectively to each kind of insecure patient (either anxious, dismissingly avoidant, or fearfully avoidant). Although all insecure people lack a basic sense of attachment security, they differ in what they need from physicians and nurses (e.g., protection and support vs. self-reliance and autonomy). Moreover, they differ in the ways they cope with health-related distress (e.g., distress amplification vs. distress suppression). Therefore, if physicians and nurses wish to provide effective patient-centered care, they need to know what is driving and bothering a patient, so that they can tailor clinical interventions to address the patient's dominant form of attachment insecurity.

In their 2015 book, *Love, Fear, and Health*, Maunder and Hunter (2015) offered practical recommendations about how to tailor clinical interventions to a patient's main form of attachment insecurity. Interestingly, these recommendations fit well with Arriaga et al.'s (2018) model of attachment security enhancement in couple relationships (see Chapter 6). This similarity is not surprising, because both romantic partners in couple relationships and health care professionals in medical settings can potentially function as safe havens and secure bases.

With regard to attachment-anxious patients, Maunder and Hunter (2015) made four recommendations. First, health care providers should attempt to soothe the patient and prevent his or her habitual tendency to hyperactivate distressing thoughts and feelings. Specifically, they can approach patients in a calm and competent manner, use specific therapeutic tools to reduce anxiety and catastrophic ideation (e.g., cognitive-behavioral techniques, mindfulness training), show genuine interest in patients' concerns, and support and encourage them to approach and rely on loved others (family members, close friends) to feel more comfortable.

Second, they need to provide unwavering reassurance and support even before patients request this, thereby softening anxious patients' tendency to exaggerate distress expressions in order to receive care. Third, health care providers should attempt to soften the incoherent speech and angry responses that characterize attachment-anxious patients by helping them to be less fearful, and clearer and more precise when speaking about their illness. Fourth, health care providers need to provide opportunities for anxious patients to learn about their own competence and self-efficacy in coping with their illness, and to support and empower patients' assertiveness and autonomy. In this way, physicians and nurses can provide a secure base from which anxious patients can develop greater fortitude and self-efficacy (Maunder & Hunter, 2015).

In the case of avoidant patients, who feel uncomfortable with dependence, Maunder and Hunter (2015) proposed that health care providers soften these concerns by validating patients' need for self-reliance and conveying a sense that it is possible and beneficial to retain a sense of autonomy and self-efficacy while adhering to medical treatments. These softening techniques include expressing respect for a patient's autonomy, allowing the patient to set the desired level of self-disclosure and interpersonal distance, and letting the patient speak first and then respond and elaborate on what he or she said (called *following*). In addition, health care providers can soften an avoidant patient's underutilization of care (lack of reports of pain, nonadherence to medical treatments) by scheduling medical checkups rather than waiting for the patient to call. They can also negotiate adherence to treatment through less threatening techniques (e.g., humor, anecdotes, metaphors) and rely on principles and techniques of motivational interviewing (Rollnick et al., 2008) that involve respect and support of patient autonomy.

A richer understanding of the health benefits of mentalization is another valuable attachment-informed adjunct for patient-centered care. Physicians and nurses might be trained to cultivate genuine interest in what is happening in a patient's mind and adopt what Bateman and Fonagy (2004) called a *mentalizing stance* (see Chapter 7). In medical settings, this stance includes encouraging different perspectives on a patient's illness-related concerns, actively asking patients for detailed descriptions of what is happening to them, and sensitively inviting them to provide clarification when something they say is unclear.

Attachment theory and research can also inform health care professionals regarding their own attachment insecurities and how these mental states can negatively bias their responses to some patients and interfere with the healing process. As a result, physicians and nurses can be more aware of their own attachment fears and defenses. They can also better understand which kind of patient or kind of interpersonal interaction activates or aggravates their attachment insecurities and arouses their characteristic defenses. They may then be more capable of offering effective patient-centered care despite negative biases imposed by their insecure working models.

For example, avoidant health care providers might react more negatively to a clinging, overdependent patient, because his or her demands for proximity and support elicit discomfort with relational closeness and interdependence. In contrast, more attachment-anxious health care providers might react more negatively to a cool, rejecting patient, because the patient's detached attitude arouses the provider's own fears of rejection and worries about lack of respect and acceptance. Of course, providing physicians and nurses with a secure base for exploration and reflection on their own insecure working models might buffer these negative reactions and foster the formation of more empathic and caring relationships with patients.

As noted in previous chapters, being a sensitive, responsive, and supportive attachment figure is a demanding, sometimes tiring task, and a person needs to feel safe, secure, supported, respected, valued, and appreciated in order to serve as an effective secure base for needy others. In health care settings, fully taking the role of a responsive caregiver can increase the likelihood of emotional burnout and compassion fatigue on the part of physicians and nurses, particularly when they are caring for troubled, attachment-insecure patients. Therefore, an attachment-informed approach to health care should include an organizational or leadership development module aimed at training authorities in health care settings (e.g., head physicians, chief nursing officers, hospital administrators) to be security-providing leaders (Moriano et al., 2021) and to create an organizational climate and culture that sustains a chain of security flowing from authorities to physicians and nurses and from them to patients.

Concluding Remarks

Medical settings are the epitome of attachment theory's main focus: one person relying on another, at least temporarily viewed as stronger and wiser, to provide safety and support. Medical professionals have all undergone extensive training in science and their specialty's technology, often leaving little time and energy for education concerning interpersonal relationships and their own and their patients' attachment-related needs. Perhaps those needs could be ignored if they were irrelevant to the main goal of treating illness and injuries and returning patients to good health. But as we have shown in this chapter, the attachment needs and defenses of informal and formal care providers and patients affect the treatment process and the health outcomes of interactions between medical professionals and their patients.

Further work is needed to create and evaluate attachment-informed training programs for medical and nursing students, as well as treatment protocols based on an attachment perspective. So far, there is only one RCT providing supportive evidence concerning the effectiveness of collaborative care for patients with diabetes and coronary artery disease, which although not being an explicitly attachment-informed treatment, used attachment-theory concepts for training and supervising nurses who coordinated patients' care (Katon et al., 2010). We hope the ideas and findings in this chapter encourage both researchers and practitioners to use attachment theory's concepts and principles to improve the psychosocial aspects of medical treatment.

CHAPTER 12

Applying Attachment-Theoretical Principles in Organizations

As explained in previous chapters, the broaden-and-build cycle of adult attachment security is sustained by not only responsive close relationship partners (e.g., family members, a spouse) but also responsive therapists, teachers, and health workers, as well as supportive social groups. In recent years, evidence has been growing that broaden-and-build processes can also occur in large organizations (e.g., the workplace, the military) and can be shaped by the quality of the relationships that organization members have with their leaders and with the organization as a whole. Following the early lead of Hazan and Shaver's (1990) pioneering study of attachment-related differences in orientations toward one's workplace and the expansion of attachment theory to organizational settings (Mayseless & Popper, 2007), attachment researchers have begun to study the security-enhancing effects of responsive organizational leaders (e.g., managers, military officers) and a supportive organizational climate.

We begin this chapter by reviewing empirical evidence regarding the ability of social organizations and leaders to function as security-enhancing figures. We then evaluate the important possibility that attachment theory and research can be used to create organizational interventions that improve the performance of both individual members and an entire organization. We must admit at the outset, however, that although research already shows that responsive leaders and supportive organizations can enhance members' well-being and job performance, no attachment-informed intervention has yet been designed and implemented with the aim of advancing security-enhancing leadership and organizational climate. We hope the chapter inspires and encourages scholars and practitioners to apply the knowledge gained by attachment researchers when designing evidence-based, effective organizational interventions.

Security-Enhancement Processes within Organizations

In applying attachment theory to organizational settings, researchers have examined attachment-related processes connected with three potential providers of security: (1) fellow organization members, (2) organizational leaders, and (3) the organization as a whole.

In Chapter 9, we focused on a person's relationship with other organization members (e.g., coworkers, work team members, members of a military unit) and the security-enhancing effects of comforting and empowering group interactions with these members. In this chapter, we focus on the attachment functions served by organizational leaders and organizations as wholes.

Attachment and Leadership

In an elaboration and extension of Freud's (1930/1961) metaphor of the leader as a father, Popper and Mayseless (2003) applied attachment theory to leader–follower relationships, and proposed that there is a notable correspondence between the features of leaders and those of other attachment figures: "Leaders, like parents, are figures whose role includes guiding, directing, taking charge, and taking care of others less powerful than they and whose fate is highly dependent on them" (p. 42). Like security-enhancing attachment figures, effective leaders are likely to be sensitive and responsive to the needs of organization members (e.g., employees, citizens); provide advice, guidance, and emotional reassurance to members; assist them in building their sense of self-worth, competence, and autonomy; support them in taking on new challenges and acquiring new skills; and encourage their personal growth (Haslam et al., 2015).

Therefore, it's reasonable to expect that people may view leaders as competent and benevolent figures who can provide both a safe haven and a secure base (Mayseless & Popper, 2007, 2019). Indeed, studies of people's implicit leadership theories indicate that leaders are prototypically characterized by traits signaling competence (intelligence, strength, charisma) and benevolence (sensitivity, dedication) (e.g., Epitropaki & Martin, 2005). And Nichols and Cottrell (2014) found that people portray the ideal leader as highly intelligent and trustworthy.

Relying on Leaders for Protection and Support in Times of Need

Just as proximity and support seeking from parents, friends, and romantic partners is activated by threats and challenges, a desire for a stronger and wiser leader tends to arise especially in times of personal or collective crisis, trauma, or uncertainty (Mayseless & Popper, 2007). During such times, people tend to adopt the role of a vulnerable, dependent, and needy "child," and wish to feel close to a leader who can protect them and provide useful guidance. In such cases, the search for proximity to a competent and benevolent leader is a predictable attachment behavior and implies a willingness to become increasingly dependent on the leader for promoting felt security. As happens with dyadic-relationship attachment figures, distressed followers may approach a leader in hopes that he or she will assist them in managing distress and taking on new challenges.

This desire for a stronger and wiser leader need not be viewed as infantile or regressive. In fact, reliance on a leader for support can result in a secure base for personal growth toward mature autonomy. Just as students with caring teachers become increasingly independent learners, and just as well-parented children tend to become high-functioning adults, people can become better, stronger, and wiser adults, and in some cases become leaders in their own right, under the guidance and good judgment of an effective leader.

The tendency to seek proximity to a leader in times of need is illustrated in the *rally behind the leader* phenomenon—increasing trust in and reliance on a leader during a collective crisis. This phenomenon was first documented in 1970 by John Mueller, a political scientist who found that sudden international crises during the Cold War led Americans to rally behind their leaders and increase their trust in American presidents. In a subsequent review, Baker and Oneal (2001) suggested that military crises, mainly when they are sudden, dramatic, and international in scope, can, in and of themselves, arouse increased support for a president. Indeed, dramatic increases in support for American presidents were found following the attack on Pearl Harbor in 1941, the Bay of Pigs crisis in 1962, the entry of the United States into the Gulf War in 1991, the 9/11 terrorist attacks in 2001, and the invasion of Iraq in 2003 (Lambert et al., 2011). This tendency has also been noted in laboratory studies: As compared to a control group, American participants who were reminded of the 9/11 attacks (by watching a short video clip) expressed more favorable attitudes toward then-President George W. Bush (Lambert et al., 2011).

The Calming and Empowering Effects of Responsive Leaders

On the one hand, responsive and supportive leaders, like other security-enhancing figures, can support broaden-and-build processes in subordinates. According to Popper and Mayseless (2003), sustaining felt security in subordinates is an effective leader's method of empowering them and increasing their competence, autonomy, and well-being. Moreover, providing a safe haven and secure base is the key to the corrective, therapeutic changes a good leader can sometimes induce in maladjusted or troubled followers. Like a therapist who provides a secure base for exploring personal and interpersonal problems (see Chapter 7), a leader (e.g., a manager, military officer, rabbi, or president) can provide a secure base for initiating and sustaining adaptive changes in working models of self and relationships and in personal and social behavior.

On the other hand, as in other cases of attachment-figure nonresponsiveness, a leader's unwillingness or inability to meet others' needs for safety and security can exacerbate followers' worries and demoralization. Moreover, this kind of rejecting and frustrating leader can increase either followers' childish, anxious dependence on the destructive figure (in the case of attachment-anxious followers) or their tendency to emotionally detach from the leader and reject the leader's guidance (in the case of attachment-avoidant followers). In both cases, these responses can radically alter the relationship between leader and subordinates and transform what began as a hoped-for safe haven and secure base into a destructive, conflicted, hostile relationship that is self-defeating for both leader and subordinates.

The general idea that a leader who is sensitive and responsive to followers' needs has positive effects on their well-being, instrumental behavior, and goal pursuit recurs in several major leadership theories. In fact, a leader's sensitive responsiveness is a core feature of several researched styles of effective leadership. For example, Howell (1988) defined *socialized leadership* as a leader's use of his or her strength and resources to serve and empower others' needs and aspirations, while respecting their rights and feelings. In his definition of *servant leadership,* Greenleaf (1977) emphasized a leader's prioritizing of others' needs and interests, and investing efforts to meet these needs and empower others. As can be seen in the Servant Leadership Scale (Liden et al., 2008), items refer to a leader's provision of both safe-haven and secure-base forms of support (e.g., "My manager cares about my personal well-being," "My manager encourages me to handle important work decisions on my own").

A leader's responsiveness is also a central issue in Conger and Kanungo's (1988) theory of *empowering leadership*—supporting others' motivation and development, and promoting their psychological empowerment and capability. This is illustrated in the items used to assess this style (e.g., "My leader listens to me"; "My leader advises me to look for the opportunities in the problem"; Amundsen & Martinsen, 2014). The leader as a secure base (in our terms) is also a core theme in Bass's (1985) conception of *transformational leadership*—inspiring trust in others while empowering them to "do more than they originally expected to do" (p. 20).

Hundreds of studies and several narrative reviews and meta-analyses have shown that styles of leadership that emphasize a leader's responsiveness to subordinates' needs (socialized, servant, empowering, transformational) are positively associated with subordinates' well-being, feelings of self-worth and self-efficacy, and task performance in a wide variety of organizational contexts (for meta-analyses, see Lee et al., 2018, 2020; Montano et al., 2017). In addition, there is strong evidence that dyadic supervisor-employee relationships in the workplace characterized by trust, responsiveness, respect, and support are associated with employees' well-being, job satisfaction, improved job performance, and reduced job-related stress and emotional burnout (for meta-analyses, see Legood et al., 2021; Montano et al., 2017).

Working specifically from an attachment perspective, Davidovitz et al. (2007) examined the calming and empowering effects of leaders' responsiveness in two studies conducted in a military setting. In one study, officers' own reports of providing support to soldiers during demanding and challenging assignments were positively associated with their soldiers' ratings of morale and instrumental functioning within their units. In a second study, Davidovitz et al. assessed soldiers' ratings of the responsiveness of their direct officer during an intensive period of combat training and found that these ratings were associated with improved mental health 2 months later (relative to their mental health before the training period).

In extending these findings to the workplace, studies have shown that employees who appraise their manager as more responsive and supportive tend to report higher levels of job satisfaction and lower levels of emotional burnout (e.g., Lavy, 2014; Molero et al., 2019; Moriano et al., 2021). Similarly, workers who perceive their manager as more available, encouraging, and noninterfering have been found to expend more effort at work and to suggest new ideas that can improve work-related procedures (Wu & Parker, 2017). Interestingly, these beneficial effects of a manager's provision of a secure base were most prominent among attachment-insecure employees, implying that a leader's responsiveness can compensate to some extent for followers' dispositional attachment insecurities.

Research also indicates that employees whose manager is responsive to their autonomy needs feel calmer and more confident than employees of a leader who protects them in times of need but disrespects their autonomous motivation and aspirations. (In our terms, a security-enhancing leader provides both a safe haven in times of distress and a secure base for personal exploration and growth.) In a seminal study, Deci et al. (1989) observed that employees in a Fortune 500 firm who perceived their manager as supporting their autonomy reported greater job satisfaction. Since then, research has shown that managers who are more autonomy supportive contribute positively to employees' well-being, work engagement, and job performance (see Slemp et al., 2018, for a meta-analysis).

The Interfering Effects of Subordinates' Attachment Insecurities

Although the findings reviewed so far indicate that a responsive and supportive leader can have reassuring and empowering effects on subordinates, attachment insecurities that subordinates bring to their relationship with a leader can interfere with these broaden-and-build processes. Attachment-insecure people, either anxious or avoidant, can be reluctant to seek support and comfort from leaders and be unable or unwilling to cultivate supportive relationships with leaders and benefit from their support during periods of stress.

Fortunately, like attachment figures in other kinds of relationships, a skillful and responsive leader may be able to manage subordinates' insecurities and move them toward greater felt security.

In support of this view, research indicates that soldiers or employees with more anxious or avoidant attachment orientations are less likely to appraise their military officer or manager as a supportive, visionary, and effective leader (e.g., Davidovitz et al., 2007; Molero et al., 2013; Moss, 2009). Also, more avoidant employees tend to have lower trust in their manager (Harms et al., 2016), and employees scoring higher on measures of attachment anxiety or avoidance tend to report less satisfying relationships with their managers (see Fein et al., 2020, for a review). These associations are only moderate in size, however, suggesting that actual signs of a leader's responsiveness or other positive attitudes toward subordinates can reduce the destructive relational effects of attachment insecurities.

Similar attachment-related differences have been found in the quality of mentoring relationships in academic settings and workplaces. Mentees scoring higher on attachment anxiety or avoidance are less likely to seek support from a mentor, to perceive their mentor as supportive, and to feel satisfied with the mentorship relationship (e.g., Georgiou et al., 2008; Larose et al., 2005; Poteat et al., 2015). In addition, mentees' attachment anxiety is associated with less feedback seeking from mentors and lower acceptance of a mentor's feedback (Allen et al., 2010). Using data from mentors' logbooks (at nine time points during a yearlong mentoring program), Larose et al. (2019) reported that mentees' avoidant attachment uniquely predicted lower satisfaction with their mentoring relationships, mainly during times when the mentor addressed a mentee's personal issues.

The Interfering Effects of Leaders' Attachment Insecurities

Leaders' attachment insecurities can also compromise the quality of leader–follower relationships and prevent leaders from functioning as effective providers of a safe haven and secure base. As in other relationships (parent–child, teacher–student, therapist–client), felt security is crucial for being a responsive leader and successfully fulfilling the role of a security-enhancing figure. Without feeling safe and secure, a leader tends to be preoccupied with his or her own needs for self-protection instead of being concerned with meeting followers' needs and promoting their welfare. (This is the well-documented negative relationship between attachment insecurity and ability to function effectively as a caregiver; see Chapter 2.) In contrast, secure leaders can genuinely enjoy being a caregiver and confidently engage in the process of bolstering followers' sense of self-efficacy and movement toward personal and organizational goals.

Studies conducted in military contexts provide support for these ideas. More attachment-insecure officers score lower on socialized and transformational styles of leadership, report less sensitivity and responsiveness to their soldiers' needs, and are rated by the soldiers as less supportive and reassuring (Davidovitz et al., 2007; Popper et al., 2000). In addition, recruits working under more attachment-avoidant officers are less likely to report being understood and cared for by their officers (Thompson et al., 2021).

Davidovitz et al. (2007) found that leaders' attachment insecurities go hand in hand with self-focused motives to lead rather than other-focused (prosocial) motives and with lower expectations of self-efficacy in dealing with leadership-related tasks. In addition, soldiers of more avoidant officers were more likely to experience negative changes in their mental health during a 4-month intensive combat training program (Davidovitz et al., 2007). At the beginning of training, mental health was exclusively associated with soldiers' own attachment insecurities. However, by the end of training, soldiers' deterioration in mental health was a function of their officer's attachment-related avoidance, and this effect was mediated by soldiers' appraisal of their officer's lack of responsiveness.

As for business or religious rather than military organizations, research also indicates that attachment-insecure managers are less likely to adopt socialized and transformational styles of leadership (Rom & Benatov, 2018; Shalit et al., 2010) and more likely to hold negative views of employees (Thompson et al., 2018). In a recent study of religious leaders, Foulkes-Bert et al. (2019) found that attachment insecurities in close relationships and with regard to God were associated with weaker endorsement of transformational leadership. In addition, attachment-insecure managers are less likely than secure ones to delegate responsibility and power to subordinates, and more likely to create centralized authority structures (Johnston, 2000). Managers' attachment insecurities are also associated with employees' emotional burnout and job dissatisfaction, and these links appear to be mediated by managers' discomfort with caregiving and problems in working with groups (Kafetsios et al., 2014; Ronen & Mikulincer, 2012; Ronen & Zuroff, 2017).

In a creative but speculative theoretical article, Keller (2003) claimed that combinations of an avoidant leader and anxious subordinates, or an anxious leader and avoidant subordinates, are the most problematic. As in marital relationships, these configurations can create destructive demand–withdrawal patterns of interdependent behavior (see Chapter 6). Interestingly, Keller suggested that a combination of avoidant leader and avoidant follower might be more benign: "The avoidant follower may be grateful to be left alone without intrusions from the leader, while the avoidant leader may admire the follower's independence" (p. 152). Keller's interesting ideas await empirical examination, however. To date, research has focused on leaders' or followers' attachment styles but not on the ways in which various configurations of attachment styles affect the quality of leader–follower relations.

Moving Subordinates toward Greater Felt Security

Can a responsive leader provide corrective experiences for people who have a history of troubled attachment experiences with parents, friends, or romantic partners? And can such a leader increase felt security among insecure subordinates? Based on studies of other kinds of attachment relationships, we suspect that although subordinates' insecure working models may at first be generalized to (i.e., projected onto) the leader and negatively bias their expectations, feelings, and behaviors toward him or her (see previous section), comforting and empowering interactions with a responsive and supportive leader may counter the generalized insecure models and promote greater security.

As in other attachment relationships, these security-enhancing interactions may expand followers' mental *islands of security* in their network of attachment-figure representations. Unfortunately, no study has yet tested the validity of these ideas. In fact, no study has assessed changes in a person' felt security after repeatedly interacting with a responsive organizational leader or following interventions aimed at increasing a leader's responsiveness.

Research Summary

Attachment research on leadership shows that people do seek a leader's protection and support in times of need, and that a responsive and supportive leader can contribute to their well-being and performance. However, as in other dyadic relationships, attachment insecurities on the part of followers or leaders can interfere with a leader's provision of a safe haven and secure base, and therefore prevent a follower's formation of a secure attachment to the leader. Practically speaking, this means that responsive leaders should be aware of, and attempt to manage, their own and their subordinates' insecurities if they wish to encourage broaden-and-build processes in individual followers and bring about positive organizational outcomes. Unfortunately, there are not yet any good evaluation studies on this topic, so we can't be sure of the details concerning our central idea that supportive interactions with a responsive leader can move insecure subordinates toward greater security.

The Attachment-Like Functions of Organizations

The organizations to which most adults belong (e.g., workplaces, social clubs, churches) and the social institutions with which they interact (e.g., government, police, social service agencies), although often being somewhat impersonal, can also be a source of perceived safety and felt security. These social entities often have the power and resources to provide protection and support, and people usually expect to be well treated by them as valued and respected organization members or citizens (Granqvist, 2020; Mayseless & Popper, 2007). In fact, people are typically dependent on these organizations for safety and security. For example, people may rely on a workplace for economic security, social identity, and a sense of worth; they may depend on police for physical protection; and they may seek a material safety net provided by welfare agencies in cases of economic strain or crisis. Moreover, hospitals and courts are expected to be attentive and responsive when dealing with personal or relational problems (e.g., physical illness, divorce), and the government is expected to provide guidance and helpful information for confronting collective threats (e.g., a novel virus pandemic, an earthquake, climate change) and to set regulations that guarantee citizens' rights, autonomy, and well-being.

Relying on Social Organizations for Protection and Support in Times of Need

From an attachment perspective, collective threats and stressors might increase people's reliance on organizational sources of safety and security. Indeed, longitudinal surveys conducted in the United States and Switzerland revealed that people expressed greater trust in government and public health agencies during the H1N1 (swine flu) pandemic than in a prepandemic assessment (Bangerter et al., 2012; Quinn et al., 2013). Similar findings were reported by Sibley et al. (2020), who examined the effects of a nationwide lockdown in response to the COVID-19 outbreak by comparing matched samples of New Zealanders assessed before and during the first 18 days of lockdown. People in the pandemic/lockdown group reported more trust in the government and in the police, and they expressed more positive attitudes toward them than was the case before the pandemic.

There is also evidence that experimentally induced threats increase reliance on governmental services and foster more positive attitudes toward the workplace. For example, as compared with a control condition, a threat to personal control (created by a memory task that required participants to recall uncontrollable events) was found to increase explicit requests for help from the government (Kay et al., 2008). And a mortality salience manipulation caused Russian students to give government more responsibility and control over their lives (Prusova & Gulevich, 2019). The same kind of experimental death reminder led employees to endorse more aspects of their workplace culture than employees in a control condition (Jonas et al., 2011). Beyond these experimental findings, a cross-national survey conducted in 67 countries found that people who felt less control over their lives were more likely to turn to their government in times of need (Kay et al., 2008).

The Calming and Empowering Effects of Responsive Organizations

As with smaller group relationships, social organizations can also provide their members a collective sense of safety and security. In the workplace, employees facing work-related threats and challenges can feel safe and secure by knowing about the availability of institutional processes aimed at supporting their well-being and health, such as grievance systems, help lines, and human resources services. Similarly, welfare institutions, either governmental or nongovernmental, can be active providers of felt security for citizens of all ages. They can increase citizens' confidence in the availability of education, health care, housing, and social services when needed throughout childhood, adolescence, and adulthood; guarantee high-quality care to elderly adults; and even provide security beyond death by taking care of burials.

According to Gruneau Brulin (2021), "These services create a social safety net which liberates the individual from the dependency of personal bonds determined by one's cultural and socioeconomic background. Instead, the individuals are free to have relationships of their own choice" (p. 19). In other words, a social organization that is sensitive and responsive to its members' needs can provide a secure base from which they are able to autonomously pursue their goals with confidence that support is available when needed. However, if the organization is not responsive to its members' needs for safety and security and does not concern itself with their welfare, being a member of such an uncaring organization can have negative rather than positive psychological effects. Only when being part of a social organization results in increased support, acceptance, and validation of their needs do people feel safe, composed, and confident in dealing with challenging and demanding tasks within (and perhaps also outside) the organization.

The idea that responsiveness is a key for understanding the positive psychological effects of social organizations was originally addressed by Eisenberger et al. (1986), who conceptualized and operationalized the construct of *organizational support*—the extent to which people perceive that an organization meets their needs, supports their personal aspirations, and cares about their well-being. Interestingly, Eisenberger et al.'s premises are similar to the arguments Bowlby (1969/1982) offered when analyzing the attachment-like functions of social groups and organizations. People tend to anthropomorphize organizations, assign human-like qualities to them (e.g., reliable, supportive, benevolent, rejecting, harsh), and then emotionally react to organizational gestures and actions in the same way they react to human relationship partners (e.g., feeling pleased when appreciated or supported and hurt or angry when mistreated or excluded).

According to Eisenberger et al. (1986), people also tend to develop organization-specific beliefs regarding the extent to which an organization cares about their needs, goals, and feelings. In our estimation, these organization-specific beliefs can contribute positively to a member's felt security in relation to the organization or, instead, arouse attachment-related fears and defenses. As a result, positive beliefs about an organization's concern for and responsiveness toward members can be expected to contribute to members' broaden-and-build cycle of attachment security and allow them to feel and function at their best within the organization.

During the past 30 years, hundreds of studies and several meta-analyses have provided strong evidence of the positive effects of employees' perceptions of organizational support within a workplace. For example, in a meta-analysis of 167 studies, Riggle et al. (2009) found that perceived support from the workplace had a moderate-to-strong positive association with employees' job engagement and satisfaction and the quality of their job performance. A more recent meta-analysis of 558 studies replicated these findings and also concluded that perceived support from the workplace is associated with lower levels of distress and job-related burnout (Kurtessis et al., 2017). Perceived organizational support in the workplace also seems to provide a secure base for exploration: Employees who are more confident in their workplace's support are more likely to propose novel exploratory ideas and deliver creative solutions while working on job-related tasks (e.g., Yu & Frenkel, 2013).

There is also evidence that perceived support from their workplace can protect employees' health and well-being from the detrimental effects of job-related stressors and traumas (see Baran et al., 2012, for a review). For example, perceived workplace support was found to weaken the association between daily task setbacks and next-day increases in emotional exhaustion among employees who were teleworking full-time during the COVID-19 lockdown (Chong et al., 2020). Similarly, T. Zhou et al. (2021) assessed psychological responses of Chinese medical staff members who worked in Wuhan during the COVID-19 outbreak and found that perceived support from their workplace measured in March 2020 predicted stronger self-efficacy beliefs, greater reliance on problem-focused strategies for coping with work demands, and lower levels of PTSD a month later.

The positive psychological effects of perceived organizational responsiveness can also be observed in studies assessing citizens' appraisals of the support provided by governmental institutions in times of need. For example, studies conducted in China and Thailand after a natural disaster (e.g., earthquake or tsunami) revealed that survivors' perceptions of postdisaster governmental support were associated with greater well-being and lower levels of depression and PTSD (Huang et al., 2016; Tang, 2007). Similarly, survivors of the Fort McMurray wildfire in Canada who perceived more postdisaster governmental support were less likely to suffer from generalized anxiety disorders 6 months after the wildfire (Agyapong et al., 2018). In a recent study of the impact of COVID-19-related lockdowns and quarantines on psychological distress in a national sample of Chinese citizens, perceptions of government support prospectively predicted smaller increases in quarantine-related distress over a 2-month period (Gan et al., 2022). Overall, these findings indicate that people coping with collective threats do seem to benefit from feeling protected and supported by responsive governmental agencies.

The Interfering Effects of Attachment Insecurities

As in other attachment relationships, attachment insecurities that organization members carry with them from painful past experiences with close relationship partners or other social organizations can be generalized to the ways in which they mentally represent their current organization and negatively bias their perception of organizational support. As a result, attachment-insecure people may have pessimistic expectations about their organization. Moreover, they may be reluctant to rely on this social entity in times of need, rejecting or dismissing its supportive efforts.

There is some evidence that organization members' attachment insecurities negatively bias perceptions of organizational support. For example, Hazan and Shaver (1990), in their early study of attachment and work, found that attachment-insecure people, compared with secure coworkers, reported stronger feelings of being misunderstood and underappreciated at their workplace. Moreover, three subsequent studies found that attachment-related avoidance is associated with lower appraisals of organizational support, fairness, and psychological safety in the workplace (Byrne et al., 2017; Chopik, 2015; Ronen & Mikulincer, 2009).

Research also indicates that attachment insecurities can interfere with the safe-haven and secure-base effects of a supportive organization. In a cross-sectional study, Littman-Ovadia et al. (2013) found that perceptions of an organization as supporting workers' personal goals (autonomy support) were associated with greater well-being in the workplace (less emotional burnout, more job engagement) only among workers who scored relatively low on avoidant attachment. Avoidant workers missed the emotional benefits of being part of an organization that could provide a secure base for autonomous growth.

Attachment insecurities can also reduce pro-organizational tendencies and behavior; that is, attachment-insecure members may be less likely to be committed to their organization and invest efforts in behalf of the organization. They also might be reluctant to endorse what Organ (1997) called *organizational citizenship behaviors*, such as being cooperative with other organization members, respecting their needs and rights, and inhibiting proclivities and behaviors that might reduce organizational effectiveness (e.g., tardiness, theft, sabotage). Indeed, using either self-report scales or the AAI to measure adult attachment security and insecurities, a host of correlational studies have found that dispositional attachment insecurities are associated with lower levels of organizational commitment and organizational citizenship behaviors (e.g., Reizer, 2019; Schmidt, 2016; Scrima et al., 2015).

There is preliminary evidence that attachment insecurities can disrupt compliance with an organization's expectations, rules, and demands. In a recent study assessing Swedish adults' compliance with governmental guidelines for stopping the spread of COVID-19, Gruneau Brulin et al. (2022) found that more attachment-anxious or -avoidant participants reported lower adherence to these guidelines. Findings also indicated that lack of trust in governmental institutions mediated this association. Specifically, less secure participants reported less trust in government (indicating less security), which in turn contributed to lower compliance with governmental guidelines.

Moving Organization Members toward Greater Felt Security

After showing that a supportive organization can improve members' well-being and instrumental functioning, and that members' attachment insecurities can interfere with these positive effects, a question arises as to whether organizational support can override these insecurities and move insecure people toward greater felt security with respect to an organization and perhaps contribute to an improved generalized sense of attachment security. Unfortunately, there is as yet no research evidence to answer this question.

Up until 2020, self-report measures of individual differences in attachment to a social organization were atheoretical and focused on the strength of the attachment bond rather than attachment security and the various kinds of insecurity (anxiety, avoidance, disorganization) associated with it (e.g., Venkataramani et al., 2013). In 2020, Feeney et al. (2020) constructed the seven-item Organizational Attachment Scale (OAS) to measure individual differences in attachment anxiety and avoidance with respect to a specific organization. However, they collected data only concerning the intended two-factor structure of the scale and the construct validity of the Anxiety and Avoidance scores. They did not provide information about the extent to which organizational support affects these scores.

Future studies should examine both generalization of attachment insecurities in close relationships to insecurities in relation to organizations and reductions in these insecurities created by supportive and empowering organizational experiences. Specifically, researchers should test the extent to which positive organizational experiences encourage the formation of a more secure attachment to this social entity. It will be important to study the specific kinds of organizational experiences that heighten both the perception of organizational support and members' felt security.

Research Summary

Research clearly shows that people increase their symbolic proximity to organizations to which they belong in times of need and seek organizational protection and support. Not surprisingly, findings also indicate that people feel and work best when they feel well-treated, valued, respected, and cared for by their organization. Interestingly, the same positive parental qualities that promote children's socioemotional and cognitive development also seem to support and enhance adults' emotional stability, social adjustment, and instrumental functioning within organizations: supportiveness, acceptance, appreciation, fairness, and respect. However, we still need research on the extent to which a responsive and supportive organization can enhance members' sense of attachment security and provide corrective, security-enhancing experiences for attachment-insecure members.

An Attachment-Informed Approach to Organizational Interventions

Although existing research supports the claim that responsive leaders and organizations can contribute to members' broaden-and-build processes, we know of no attachment-informed leadership or organizational development program designed to cultivate leaders' responsiveness or to promote a security-enhancing organizational culture. However, some attachment-theory principles can be found in organizational interventions based on the *theory of transformational leadership* (Bass, 1985; Bass & Riggio, 2006) or the *positive leadership approach* (Cameron, 2012). Although these programs do not explicitly address the attachment-like functions of a leader, they train leaders to attend to and validate subordinates' needs, recognize their accomplishments, and encourage their autonomous growth. Attachment-theoretical principles can also be found in organizational interventions aimed at creating a climate of care and support within organizations (e.g., Shanock et al., 2019).

It seems that organizational scientists and professionals are becoming more aware of the benefits of responsive leaders and emotionally safe organizations for both individual members and organizations as wholes. In a way, the ethos of attachment theory and research has been partially duplicated in the field of organizational behavior, but generally without linking up with the additional ideas, evidence, and applications developed in the attachment field.

In this section, we offer suggestions and guidelines based on attachment theory and research for applying attachment-theory principles to organizational practices and interventions. The aim is not to propose specific attachment-based interventions for leadership or organizational development, which stretches beyond our areas of expertise, but only to present the core themes derived from attachment theory that such interventions might include in an effort to create more security-enhancing leaders and organizations. We hope this will benefit organizational scholars and consultants who wish to promote organization members' well-being, engagement, and performance while also benefiting their organizations.

An Attachment-Informed Approach to Leadership Development

Leadership training programs are interventions aimed at enhancing "the collective capacity of organizational members to engage effectively in leadership roles and processes" (Day, 2000, p. 582). According to Day, the "roles" include both formal and informal authority positions, and the "processes" are those that facilitate successful individual or group performance and the attainment of organizational goals. These organizational interventions include managerial training and executive coaching programs designed to aid managers and supervisors in acquiring "various skills and knowledge that increase their effectiveness in a number of ways, which include leading and leadership, guiding, organizing, and influencing others, to name a few" (Klein & Ziegert, 2004, p. 360).

In recent decades, business, military, and governmental organizations have expended a great deal of time and money training managers, supervisors, and officers to become effective leaders, and they have viewed leadership development as an essential priority for enhancing organizational performance (Ho, 2016). Despite these considerable investments, however, organizations still frequently conclude that their members do not possess optimal leadership skills and express doubts about whether or not they are "equipping the leaders they are building with the critical capabilities and skills they need to succeed" (Schwartz et al., 2014, p. 26). To us, this indicates that organizational researchers should devote greater effort to figuring out what works and what doesn't work in the design and implementation of these programs. In the following pages, we consider the core attachment-theory principles that might be applied in leadership training programs to increase their effectiveness.

We should say at the outset that we don't mean to imply that existing leadership training programs are ineffective. In fact, the several meta-analyses published between 1986 and 2017 (Avolio et al., 2009; Burke & Day, 1986; Collins & Holton, 2004; Lacerenza et al., 2017; Powell & Yalcin, 2010; Taylor et al., 2009) have consistently shown that leadership training programs positively affect leaders' qualities, subordinates' well-being and instrumental performance, and organizational effectiveness. We are suggesting only that attachment theory and research might help to increase the effectiveness of existing leadership training programs and deliver a superior return on investment.

As in psychotherapy (see Chapter 6), insights from attachment theory and research should not necessarily be used to create a novel, attachment-based leadership development program. Rather, they can be used to improve outcomes of existing training programs that were originally derived from other compatible theoretical orientations (e.g., transformational leadership, positive leadership).

Understanding the Attachment-Related Nature of Leadership

From an attachment perspective, one of the initial tasks of an effective leadership training program is to cultivate potential leaders' (trainees') understanding of leadership as an attachment relationship. Consultants can assist trainees to recognize that "leadership has to do with relationships, the importance of which cannot be overstated" (Komives et al., 2013, p. 67). And in such workplace relationships, leaders possess more power than their subordinates and are expected to use this power benevolently to guide, direct, and empower subordinates so they can perform optimally, or at least beyond their expectations. In addition, consultants can assist trainees to understand that subordinates are not machines or objects but human beings with basic needs for safety and security, and that they feel and perform best when these needs are met by a leader.

Using concepts, graphs, and techniques from the COS program (see Chapter 4), trainees can learn that by being attentive and responsive to subordinates' needs for a safe haven and secure base, they can improve subordinates' engagement, performance, and creativity, and reach better organizational outcomes. Moreover, with the help of COS-related techniques, trainees can set aside any worries that serving as a caring, responsive leader might create needy and dependent, hence instrumentally ineffective, subordinates. The aim is to provide both a safe haven when needed and a secure base for optimal performance and further personal development.

Trainees learn that effective leadership is guided not only by instrumental motives but also by prosocial, other-oriented motives, and that caring for subordinates' welfare and personal growth is a prerequisite for attaining organizational goals. This perspective is similar to what Avolio and Hannah (2020), working within a transformational-leadership perspective, call shifting from "I" to "Them." In their own words, "a shift in focus from thinking about oneself or one's own needs to thinking about what one's actions mean for others . . . what it means to influence others to achieve an objective that may or may not be in the leaders' 'best' short-term interest" (p. 2). (This is the shift that Crocker & Canevello, 2015, call a move from "ego-system motivation" to "eco-system motivation.")

We believe that introducing trainees to the premise that an effective leader needs to be a responsive caregiver not only shifts the focus from "I" to "Them" but is also a foundational step in adopting a more psychologically beneficial stance toward leadership (Mayseless, 2016). Trainees might become more willing to adopt a caring, other-oriented attitude and to attend and sensitively respond to subordinates needs and feelings. Moreover, watching and reflecting on video clips of security-enhancing leader–subordinate interactions could be useful in helping trainees recognize the crucial role that sensitive provision of a safe haven and secure base plays in effective leadership.

Increasing Responsiveness to Subordinates' Needs

Cultivation of leaders' responsiveness to subordinates' needs, both instrumental and social-psychological, is another core component of an attachment-informed approach to leadership development. Using video clips of leader–subordinate interactions (including trainees' own interactions), or simulations of these kinds of interactions within the training group, consultants can provide constructive feedback and comments aimed at increasing trainees' awareness, attentiveness, and responsiveness to subordinates' needs (see similar techniques in attachment-based parenting interventions in Chapters 4 and 5). Moreover, consultants' own responsive stance toward trainees can improve trainees' responsiveness to subordinates' needs. By adopting an accepting, understanding, validating, and caring stance toward trainees, an attachment-informed consultant invites trainees to respond in a similar responsive manner to subordinates.

Cultivation of leaders' responsiveness resembles practices aimed at developing trainees' *individualized consideration* in transformational-leadership workshops—treatment of subordinates as individuals with unique needs, strengths, and weaknesses (Bass & Avolio, 1990). A transformational leader attempts to know subordinates' strengths and weaknesses, and to attend and respond to their needs individually. In attachment terms, perceiving subordinates as individuals is a fundamental but only preliminary step in being an effective leader. Adopting an attachment-informed approach, consultants would also encourage trainees to be consistently trustworthy, dependable, emotionally available, responsive, and engaged while interacting with subordinates and to create a safe and secure climate where subordinates can disclose their needs and concerns as freely as they are able. This managerial stance places an emphasis on accurate mentalizing, which we have discussed in relation to other kinds of caregiving roles.

Providing a Safe Haven

From an attachment perspective, functioning as an effective leader also includes assisting distressed subordinates to cope effectively and restore emotional equanimity (provision of safe-haven support). This may come in the form of emotional reassurance, nonjudgmental listening, emotion coaching (e.g., coaching subordinates in the use of effective ways of distress management), and tangible aids (e.g., time-out for calming oneself down). In this way, subordinates gradually become convinced that a kind, reliable, and engaged leader is on their side, and that they can move beyond their comfort zone and open themselves to novel perspectives and ideas with the confidence that a safe haven will be available when needed.

An attachment-informed approach to leadership development would place special emphasis on cultivating trainees' capacity to provide safe-haven forms of support. This requires fostering several attitudes, skills, and beliefs: (1) willingness to approach distressed subordinates in a compassionate manner, (2) genuine interest in comforting subordinates and alleviating their suffering, (3) the capacity to remain emotionally unperturbed by subordinates' distress, and (4) trainees' confidence in their capacity to soothe and reassure others ("I can effectively help others to manage distress"). Although the desired attitudes, skills, and beliefs can be negatively biased by trainees' attachment insecurities, attachment-informed interventions with parents, couples, therapists, and teachers have been effective in cultivating trainees' capacity to provide safe-haven forms of support. We are therefore confident that this capacity can also be strengthened when working with leaders.

In applying an attachment-informed approach to leadership development, organizational scholars and consultants should devote attention to what Feeney and Collins (2015) called *fortification* as a core component of safe-haven support. Safe-haven support involves not only providing emotional reassurance and comfort but also assisting a distressed person to recognize and expand his or her own strengths and capacities for coping with stress. Therefore, an effective leadership training program might include a module cultivating trainees' ability to fortify subordinates who are experiencing difficulties (whether directly related or not related to their job) by instilling confidence, coaching problem-solving strategies, helping to develop relevant skills, and providing opportunities for practicing the skills. In this way, trainees could not only learn how to provide emotional reassurance but also how to encourage subordinates to solve problems on their own, perform better in future tasks, and reach new heights in their career.

Following Feeney and Collins's (2015) conceptualization of safe-haven forms of support, trainees might learn how to assist distressed subordinates to "stay in the game" and not to dwell on self-related doubts and worries. They can learn about the importance of assisting subordinates to refrain from viewing a setback in job performance as a personal catastrophe, to put the setback in perspective, and to redefine it as an impetus for improving performance. (This would be a move away from attachment anxiety and other anxieties toward security and strength.) Trainees should understand that their role as leader involves not only helping subordinates return to baseline levels of functioning, but also assisting them to "grow, flourish, or prosper (to thrive) through the adversity" (Feeney & Collins, 2015, p. 118).

Providing a Secure Base

As demonstrated in previous chapters, providing effective safe-haven support in times of need is not enough for enhancing others' felt security and sustaining broaden-and-build processes. Attachment figures also need to be sensitive and responsive to others' needs for competence and autonomy, and to provide a solid scaffold for personal growth (secure-base provision). Therefore, an attachment-informed approach to leadership development should place special emphasis on the cultivation of a leader's capacity to provide a secure base for exploration and thriving.

Trainees can learn how to assist subordinates in taking on growth-promoting challenges and stretching themselves beyond their comfort zones. They can also practice other-empowering management practices, such as validating subordinates' aspirations, expressing enthusiasm for their engagement, celebrating their achievements, and responding sensitively and nonjudgmentally to failures. Trainees also need to learn to respect subordinates' choices and decisions, and to refrain from providing patronizing, intrusive, or coercive forms of support that interfere with subordinates' autonomy. They should understand that to be an effective leader, they need to provide an ethos and atmosphere that stresses management's approval of employees suggesting innovations and working toward higher job positions.

Cultivation of a leader's capacity to provide secure-base forms of support seems to be an integral part of the development of what Bass and others have called *transformational leadership*. Using concepts derived from transformational leadership theory (Bass, 1985; Bass & Riggio, 2006), what attachment theory calls secure-base provision can be equated with a leader's provision of intellectual stimulation, inspirational motivation, and idealized influence. *Intellectual stimulation* involves the leader stimulating subordinates to think creatively, explore new ideas and perspectives, and revise faulty assumptions. *Inspirational motivation* involves presenting subordinates with an optimistic and attainable view of the future and facilitating goal pursuit and attainment. *Idealized influence* includes celebrating subordinates' achievements, gaining their respect and trust, and serving as a role model for personal growth. In our view, these three characteristics are facets of secure-base provision, which allow subordinates to take on new opportunities and challenges, enjoy learning, and master new knowledge and skills.

Despite the strong emphasis that Bass and Avolio (1990) placed on the cultivation of these three transformational-leadership characteristics, we want to emphasize that cultivating the provision of a safe-haven is no less important for sustaining subordinates' engagement and growth. In fact, the secure-base function becomes evident only after a safe haven has been provided by a responsive attachment figure. Without responding supportively and constructively to distressed subordinates who seek emotional reassurance and comfort, any support for or encouragement of creativity and autonomy will be fruitless. In this case, subordinates will not consistently be able to comfortably explore and learn on their own.

In line with this reasoning, an attachment-informed approach to leadership development would emphasize cultivating the leader's sensitivity to what subordinates need at a given moment—safe haven, secure base, or time to be alone, reflect, or perform on their own. In this context, insights and practices from mentalization-based clinical and parenting interventions (see Chapters 4 and 7) could improve a leader's sensitivity to subordinates' needs; that is, leaders might be trained to make sense of subordinates' behaviors and subjective experiences and to adopt a *mentalization stance* toward subordinates. For example, trainees might learn about the importance of (1) asking a subordinate for descriptions and clarifications of what he or she is thinking and feeling at particular times, and (2) being attuned to how well they are conveying what they themselves are aiming at and thinking.

Being Aware of One's Own Attachment Insecurities

Beyond cultivating sensitivity and responsiveness to subordinates' needs, which is a goal shared with transformational-leadership training programs, an attachment-informed approach to leadership development would be unique in stressing the importance of working through leaders' own attachment insecurities. This is a crucial task in leadership development, because leaders' insecure working models can interfere with effective provision of a safe haven and secure base (see previous section for a review of relevant research). Therefore, trainees might be encouraged to be aware of, explore, and reflect on their own attachment fears and concerns, and which kind of subordinate or kind of interpersonal or group interaction activates or aggravates these insecurities.

Relying on Bowlby's (1988) five therapeutic tasks (see Chapter 7), Drake (2009) proposed an attachment-informed approach for coaching leaders to become aware of their attachment insecurities and manage them during interactions with subordinates. First, the coach (consultant) should create safe and secure coaching sessions in which leaders can relax and feel comfortable openly exploring and reflecting on their fears and defenses. Moreover, the coach should support and encourage leaders to reflect on and understand how they relate to subordinates, what they think and feel about themselves and subordinates when interacting with them, and how their attachment-related fears and defenses may negatively bias their thoughts, feelings, and behaviors.

According to Drake (2009), the coach should also assist leaders in reflecting on and understanding how their attachment-related fears and defenses are projected onto the coach and may be creating tension and relational ruptures during coaching sessions. In addition, the coach should help leaders reflect on how their thoughts, feelings, and responses to subordinates are rooted in past experiences with frustrating attachment figures. Finally, the coach would provide leaders with a secure base for exploring and experimenting with more secure relational patterns and would explain how they could reduce the intrusion of attachment-related fears and defenses during interactions with subordinates.

Managing Subordinates' Attachment Insecurities

Another unique feature of an attachment-informed approach to leadership development concerns the cultivation of the leader's capacity to manage or soften subordinates' attachment insecurities. This is an important task of a security-enhancing leader, because subordinates' insecure working models can interfere with organizational commitment and disrupt the quality of the leader–subordinate relationship (see previous section for a review of relevant research). Therefore, trainees can learn about the specific needs, fears, and defenses that characterize each kind of attachment insecurity (anxious, dismissingly avoidant, or fearfully avoidant/disorganized), and about specific leadership practices that can be helpful for managing them and softening their destructive consequences for organizational behavior.

For this purpose, a psychoeducational module on attachment working models might be integrated into leadership training programs, and leaders might be trained to use these concepts when thinking about specific subordinates. Moreover, leaders could be trained to respond more effectively to each kind of insecure subordinate based on Arriaga et al.'s (2018) model of attachment security enhancement (see Chapter 6). Although this model was originally developed in the realm of romantic and marital relationships, we believe that it can be tailored and applied for coaching leaders to manage subordinates' attachment insecurities.

Developing a Security-Enhancing Organization

Are there attachment-informed organizational changes that might provide members with greater feelings of safety and a secure base for personal growth? And would these changes result in heightened engagement, greater creativity, deeper engagement, and improved performance? From an attachment-theoretical viewpoint, every policy decision and communitywide gesture made by an organization and its leaders that reinforces perceptions of the organization as responsive and supportive might cause members to feel safer and more secure, which should have positive outcomes for both members and the organization. For example, organizations (government agencies, nongovernmental organizations [NGOs]) can provide a material safety net in times of economic or environmental crises, provide appropriate guidance for dealing with threats and dangers (e.g., media campaigns), or provide instrumental support for the pursuit of personal goals and interests (e.g., reducing unnecessary bureaucracy and restrictions on freedom of action). Moreover, organizations can frame their decisions and actions in terms of social solidarity and empowerment of individual members' or citizens' autonomy and talents. In addition, organizations can support members' autonomy by encouraging them to participate in decision-making processes and voice their personal views during the planning of organizational goals, strategies, and plans.

Shanock et al. (2019) discussed five principles for establishing and reinforcing perceptions of organizational support. The first principle deals with construing organizational support as voluntary. Organizations and their leaders need to honestly convey to members that their supportive, encouraging actions and policies are rooted in the organization's own values and are not merely due to external forces or regulations (discretionary support provision; Eisenberger et al., 2016). These messages could strengthen members' sense that the organization genuinely values and respects them. In a relevant study, Eisenberger et al. (1997) found that the association between favorable work experiences and perceived organizational support was six times stronger if employees believed that job conditions were under the voluntary control of the organization.

Eisenberger et al. (2016) provided two prototypical examples of discretionary support provision within a workplace. The first example concerns highly successful companies, including Google and Facebook when Eisenberger et al. were writing, which provide an array of human resource benefits (e.g., educational opportunities, facilities that allow employees to restore and maintain well-being in the workplace, time to work on personal projects) and devote a great deal of money and other resources to keep talented workers engaged and discourage them from moving to other organizations. The second example concerns organizations that provide employee assistance program (EAP) services, such as professional counseling and behavioral intervention programs, aimed at helping employees deal with personal problems. In both example cases, employees perceive that the benefits and services are voluntarily provided by the organization, and might then have more confidence in the availability of organizational support when needed.

The second principle deals with the stream of support and security flowing from the organization and its authorities to midlevel managers or supervisors, and from them to their subordinates. The main idea is that organizations should explicitly support midlevel managers' attempts to understand, validate, and care for their subordinates and ensure that safe-haven and secure-base forms of support are provided across all levels of the organization. In other words, organizations should treat managers well, genuinely care about their well-being, and provide a secure base for their personal growth (Shanock & Eisenberg, 2006).

In Chapters 10 and 11, we noted that being a responsive and supportive attachment figure in educational and medical settings (e.g., teachers, physicians, nurses) is a demanding job that can contribute to emotional burnout and alienation, particularly when an employee is caring for troubled, attachment-insecure students or patients. Similar emotional erosion can occur among organizational leaders who are expected to understand, validate, and care for their subordinates. In all of these contexts, teachers, health care workers, and leaders need to feel safe, secure, supported, respected, and valued by their organization in order to prevent these negative emotional outcomes. In short, an organizational culture of appreciation and validation of leaders' supportive efforts and caring about leaders' welfare can increase the security that leaders themselves require in order to serve as a secure base for subordinates.

The third principle deals with the authenticity of supportive organizational gestures. According to Shanock et al. (2019), organizational gestures of validation, appreciation, and support need to be authentic and reflect a genuine interest in members' well-being and personal growth. In fact, organizational expressions of understanding and positive regard can reinforce members' perceived organizational support only if they are sincere. Any sign of insincerity in organizational gestures can diminish members' trust in the organization's benevolence and kindness (Eisenberger & Stinglhamber, 2011).

The fourth principle deals with what Avolio and Bass (1988) called *individualized consideration* in their theory of transformational leadership. According to Shanock et al. (2019), organizations need to treat each individual member as a unique person and tailor supportive treatment to his or her personal needs. Like children who feel well treated by sensitive parents, organization members need to feel that the support they receive is given in a thoughtful, timely, and respectful manner.

The fifth principle deals with the perception that an organization is strong and competent enough to provide support and care. According to Shanock et al. (2019), organizations need to "convey organizational competence to give creditability to support provided: Supportive treatment by an organization that is perceived by employees as effective at reaching its goals or in day-to-day operations has a greater influence on perceived organizational support" (p. 172). This principle resonates with the two core features of any security-enhancing figure—benevolence and competence. From an attachment perspective, organizational members feel safe and secure mainly if they believe that their organization is strong enough to reach its goals, including the delivery of organizational support to its members.

Eisenberger et al. (2016) also noted the importance of three other organizational practices that can help to create a culture of organizational support and care. The first practice concerns fairness in the making, monitoring, and enforcement of organizational procedures and rules. Organizations that treat members fairly and equitably are likely to be perceived as supportive and genuinely concerned with members' well-being. Indeed, several studies have found that fair treatment is associated with positive perceptions of organizational support (e.g., Colquitt et al., 2001; Rhoades & Eisenberger, 2002). An organization can convey fairness in the distribution of organizational resources (e.g., job assignments, equipment and materials, promotions) among its members, in treating all of its members with respect and dignity, and in providing all of the necessary organization-related information and resources to all members.

The second practice concerns the promotion of strong and supportive social networks within organizations. A web of interpersonal relationships among organization members who provide support and comfort to each other in times of need can be an additional source of felt security and can further sustain members' well-being and organizational engagement (Berkman et al., 2000). Along these lines, Eisenberger et al. (2016) recommended the implementation of practices that facilitate the formation of social networks within the organization, for example, by arranging or promoting team projects, fostering informational social gatherings, and creating an intraorganization social media system. An organizational culture of respect, fairness, and support should guide the implementation of these practices in order to create security-enhancing social networks.

The third practice deals with anticipated organizational support prior to becoming a member of the organization, "the extent to which prospective employees expect they would be valued and cared for by the organization if they became employees" (Eisenberger et al., 2016, p. 17). The way an organization treats job applicants during the preemployment period influences their expectations about organizational responsiveness, and employees who were well-treated prior to being employed are likely to continue to perceive the organization as supportive of its employees. Anticipated organizational support can be fostered by informing candidates about human resource benefits offered by the organization (Casper & Buffardi, 2004) and by treating them with respect and dignity during the interview process (Smither et al., 1993).

From an attachment perspective, felt security in relation to an organization can also be increased by creating a mentalization-fostering organizational culture. By increasing organizational members' accurate reflection on their own and others' needs and feelings, an organization can promote more accepting, understanding, and validating interpersonal relationships and, thus, a more harmonious and secure organizational climate. In the service of improved mentalization, organizations can provide tangible resources (e.g., facilities, time), as well as learning methods and materials that encourage organization members' reflection on their own and each other's experiences and mental states. In addition, organization leaders can be trained to accurately reflect on subordinates' needs and feelings, and to help subordinates improve their own mentalizing capacities. For example, managers can introduce reflection periods during work time at the end of each day devoted to talking, reflecting on, and understanding what happened that day at work.

It may be especially beneficial to direct security-enhancing interventions and an organizational culture of respect, appreciation, and support to members who are insecure with respect to attachment. Because attachment-insecure people tend to be relatively poorly socially adjusted, have problems in social interactions, and be at increased risk for emotional and behavioral problems (Mikulincer & Shaver, 2016), fellow organization members might reflexively tend to ignore, devalue, or disrespect them. And these reactions might then aggravate and compound the insecure employees' insecurities and interpersonal difficulties, which would have damaging effects on everyone's work performances.

Therefore, organizations and their leaders should treat attachment-insecure people in an inclusive and responsive way so as to reduce their potentially damaging effects on organizational climate. It may help for leaders to learn about the positive contributions that attachment-insecure people can make to organizations (Ein-Dor, 2015), including rapid recognition of problems and setbacks that can endanger organizational performance (in the case of attachment-anxious members) and rapid problem-solving efforts (in the case of avoidant members). Recognizing the special proclivities and abilities of insecure members might allow fellow organization members to accept some of their quirks, which might allow the insecure members to gradually increase their sense security.

Concluding Remarks

Although we have offered a number of intervention suggestions based on attachment theory and research concerning other kinds of social relationships, we do not have good research evidence regarding the ability of an attachment-informed approach to leadership and organizational development to measurably contribute to members' felt security, health, well-being, and job performance. More thought and research are needed to integrate findings and insights from organizational-level interventions with the assessment of pre- to postintervention changes in members' felt security and working models in the organizational setting. Such a research program would not only provide data concerning security-enhancement processes in organizations but it would also help guide the development of more effective organizational interventions aimed at promoting members' well-being and job performance.

CHAPTER 13

Summing Up, Moving Forward

We had no idea what we were getting into when we first began thinking and talking informally about writing a book about applications of attachment theory and research. We were familiar with several of the applications and had even contributed to a few of them, and we knew that some had been evaluated in ambitious RCTs, which is an important part of creating a useful intervention. But the number and diversity of published and evaluated interventions based on attachment theory is truly remarkable. Reviewing and boiling down the enormous literature on this topic turned out to be a major undertaking, one that we hope readers find worthwhile.

There are, however, reasons to be cautious about it. Psychology, especially social psychology (our field), has been criticized for inventing or emphasizing catchy concepts (e.g., self-esteem, implicit racial bias, social priming, grit, nudges, power posing, embodied cognition), measuring them, making dramatic claims for their applicability, and marketing them to corporations, government agencies, and the general public, too often with expensive but disappointing results. Both journalists (e.g., Singal, 2021) and professional research psychologists (e.g., IJzerman et al., 2020) have questioned whether psychological research is really ready for, and deserving of, application. Singal's provocative book is titled *The Quick Fix: Why Fad Psychology Can't Cure Our Social Ills*, and the IJzerman et al. article (with 10 coauthors) in the prestigious journal *Nature Human Behaviour* is titled "Use Caution When Applying Behavioural Science to Policy."

This kind of writing is inspired, in part, by what is sometimes called the "replication crisis" in psychology (e.g., Open Science Collaboration, 2015). Many tantalizing one-off research findings, often described in articles and books by highly qualified, credible psychologists, get picked up by journalists, popularized in TED Talks, and viewed with great interest by people or corporations interested in applying the findings to cure personal or social ills. This can happen before the phenomena and claims about them can be replicated, dissected (including by rival researchers), and pilot-tested in trial applications. These misguided efforts often begin with a single simple variable or experimental effect. Claims that manipulation of a single variable (e.g., grit) will cure a social problem (e.g., educational disparities related to ethnicity or SES) are inherently questionable, because most persistent personal or social problems are far from simple (Singal, 2021).

Because "attachment" has become a popular concept in magazines and self-help books, and has often been presented in overly simplified forms, we hasten to point out that it is based on over 50 years of careful study, critical evaluation, and empirical testing. Its central claims are part of a rich and complex theoretical network that has been repeatedly challenged and reconfirmed, using a variety of carefully designed measures and research designs. As is evident in this book, the tests have included laboratory and field experiments, multivariate correlational studies, and longitudinal studies (some lasting over 30 years). In many cases, the replicability and strength of key findings have been assessed in large-scale meta-analyses, some of which we have referred to.

Thus, in this particular case, we believe that attempts to apply attachment theory and research are quite reasonable, although the value of the applications is always a matter to be assessed empirically. Throughout the book, we have provided whatever empirical evidence (or lack of evidence) is associated with a particular application or intervention. When the evidence is missing or incomplete, we have said so and specified what remains to be done. Often missing are measures of theoretically mediating processes. It will be important to examine this issue in future studies, because sometimes an intervention "works" for reasons other than the ones suggested by a particular theory.

There is also the problem, mentioned in Chapter 1, that most of attachment research, like most research in developmental and social psychology more generally, has been conducted with what are now, somewhat humorously but also derogatorily, called WEIRD samples (Western, educated, industrialized, rich, and democratic; Henrich et al., 2010). An additional *W* might be added for White. In the case of attachment theory and research, this restricted sampling raises questions about the applicability of concepts such as sensitivity and mentalization to parenting in other cultures and subcultures, where parenting may be more of a group responsibility than it is in WEIRD (and in particular WWEIRD) societies or subcultures (e.g., Keller, 2018), or where racism makes it wise for parents to be especially protective of their children and to prepare them for harsh experiences of race-based injustice (e.g., Stern et al., 2022).

This limitation, at least in the case of adult attachment studies like most of our own, may not be so severe. The two-factor (anxiety and avoidance) structure of adult attachment measures has been replicated in several non-Western countries and in different languages, as have many of the key research findings (e.g., Schmitt, 2010; Schmitt & Allik, 2005; Shaver et al., 2010). But this is obviously an important matter that should be pursued more thoroughly in future intervention research. Throughout this book, we have emphasized the importance of multiple, diverse tests of interventions and of the measures used to assess them. We have based our conclusions on whatever research is available, and most of it is based on WWEIRD samples. We do not speculate about how future findings in different cultures and subcultures might be different, and conclusions might need to be altered. We are personally inclined to expect cross-cultural similarities in findings from future attachment research. And when findings do differ, we would look first at issues of measurement—for example, of concepts such as sensitivity and responsiveness—before attempting to alter the core theory. But we will be interested in any required changes in the theory.

Attachment Theory in Brief

It may be worthwhile to review the core theory in light of all the applications we've considered. The main idea is that most human beings are born with a propensity to seek safety, security, solace, support, and encouragement in relationships with other human beings. They also have other propensities—for example, natural curiosity (an inclination to explore and understand their environment) and a natural capacity for empathy and compassion, which motivates them to care for others. Bowlby (1969/1982) attributed these propensities to innate behavioral systems: attachment, exploration, and caregiving. He was initially interested in the fact that troubled, especially delinquent, teenagers seemed always to have a history of unstable or absent parenting, which he called "maternal deprivation" (Bowlby, 1944). This led him to focus on the early mother–child relationship.

In that relationship, children are at first totally helpless and completely reliant on one or more "stronger and wiser" parents or caregivers, and usually become emotionally "attached" to the primary "figure," seeking him or her out for protection and support when frightened (e.g., by noises, pains, novel stimuli, or strangers) or uncertain about their own safety. If the caregiver is reliably present and consistently comforting and supportive, the child feels safe and secure, and naturally engages in exploration and play. This attachment relationship provides a scaffold for further healthy development, including increasing competence and autonomy.

Research by Ainsworth and her students showed early on that certain characteristics of a caregiver, which she called "sensitivity" and "responsiveness," are crucial for encouraging a secure attachment. The child's long path through interactions with original and subsequent attachment figures results in a complex personality structure—an attachment pattern, orientation, or style—that has continuing psychological and interpersonal effects.

In their 1978 book about "patterns of attachment," Ainsworth et al. showed that the patterns could be arrayed in a two-dimensional, anxiety-by-avoidance, conceptual space. Those two dimensions have since been measured in people of all ages, and the results of studies using such measures appear throughout this book. A great deal is now known about psychological and interpersonal correlates and consequences of a person's location in the two-dimensional space.

There are many ways to characterize what is "inside" the mind of a person that comprises his or her attachment pattern or style, and these mental contents have been named and measured in several ways: internal working models, the secure-base script, expectations (including biased expectations regarding relationship partners), characteristic self-protective defenses, and particular kinds of fantasies, dreams, and daydreams. There are also several well-identified characteristics of attachment figures that affect their influence on the people who are attached to them: their own attachment and caregiving patterns, their ability to empathize with and understand the people who depend on them, their ability to "mentalize" their own and their associates' thoughts and feelings, and their sensitive and responsive behavior (or lack thereof). An attachment relationship is a two-way street, so the security or insecurity of both partners matters for the quality of the relationship.

These are the kinds of issues on which applications of attachment theory and research focus. On the side of the attachment figure—whether parent, teacher, organizational manager or leader, or religious personage—the issues are similar in all cases. The desired outcome of an attachment-related intervention is, first, to improve the ability of the person (or group or organization) in the attachment-figure role to perform more optimally for the benefit of the attached person or persons (and perhaps also for the benefit of their organization). And second, the goal is to help attached individuals grow more secure under the responsive care of the attachment figure (*earned security*) and, as a result, cause them to be psychologically (and in some ways, physically) healthier, more creative, and more productive in whatever line of endeavor they choose to pursue. When applying attachment concepts in the ways we've considered in this book, it is always likely that the characteristics of insecure people, whether occupying the attachment figure or the attached individual role, will interfere in predictable ways with the planned intervention. Seeing how these ideas have been applied in the different domains we've explored in this book, we are left with a few lingering thoughts, hopes, and concerns.

Remaining Thoughts, Hopes, and Concerns

The Concept of Attachment

In this book, we have used the term *attachment* in a less specific way than the original attachment theorists and researchers intended. Although Bowlby (1979, 1969/1982) used the term *attachment* in a very inclusive manner (see Chapters 6, 7, and 9 in this book), Ainsworth and most of her disciples exclusively focused on the infant–mother relationship and were inclined to think of the "attachment behavioral system" as a specific evolved mechanism based on its adaptive advantage for infant survival. In the 1980s, the term *attachment*, and the key features of attachment theory as developed up to that point, were extended to apply to romantic love, pair bonding, or "romantic attachment." This was controversial at the time, but it followed Bowlby's (1979) "cradle to the grave" perspective on attachment relationships, and it fairly quickly became accepted by social-personality psychologists, resulting in an enormous number of extensions and empirical validations (reviewed in Mikulincer & Shaver, 2016). In the last 30 years, as shown throughout this book, the term *attachment* and the key concepts of attachment theory (safe haven, secure base, working models, attachment orientations or styles) have been extended to apply to other kinds of dyadic relationships (e.g., teacher–student, therapist–client, leader–follower) and to relationships between individuals, on one hand, and groups and larger social organizations, on the other (e.g., Pianta, 1992; Mallinckrodt, 2010; Mayseless & Popper, 2007).

This extension of the theory is based on the notion that there are common threat–security dynamics in the different kinds of relationships (Mikulincer & Shaver, 2023), even though these dynamics may not be rooted in a behavioral system evolved exclusively for infant–mother or adolescent and adult pair-bond attachment. The common element, or basic principle, is that the human brain evolved to respond to threats with a search for safety and security in the form of one or more other people. In the first years of life, these other people are likely to be parents or other nuclear or extended family members.

As a child grows and develops, the range of potential security providers expands. The underlying neural and hormonal processes are probably similar in some ways but different in other ways in the different kinds of relationships. If so, the notions of "attachment" and "attachment behavioral system" are used in somewhat abstract and function-oriented ways rather than concrete ways specifically rooted in a particular neural circuitry. This complex issue needs further thought and empirical study.

Safe Haven and Secure Base

Another important issue, which we have mentioned several times throughout the book, is that it is important when thinking about "attachment" to keep in mind both the safe-haven and secure-base functions of the process. Other theories, as well as some accounts of attachment theory, tend to emphasize only the safe-haven function, that is, people's tendency to seek safety in relationships and to become dependent on them. When this happens, the result may be a form of clinging or overdependency that we view as a form of insecure, rather than secure, attachment. At the dyadic level, this pattern is indicated by preoccupation, jealousy, intrusiveness, conflict, and acceptance of abuse. At the group level, it is indicated by overdependence on a group or group leader, sometimes resulting in a loss of independent identity and a vulnerability to abuse by the group or its leader.

Attachment theory and our extensions of it (Mikulincer & Shaver, 2023) include an emphasis on the secure base function of secure attachment, which supports an individual's movement toward individuality and autonomy. This positive outcome depends on the ability and unselfish inclination of an attachment figure to support the attached individual's moves toward competence and independence. If a parent, teacher, or leader takes advantage of an attached person to frighten, dominate, or abuse him or her, which unfortunately is not uncommon, neither safety nor a secure base is attained, and the person is likely to suffer long-term attachment injuries.

At the extreme, this is how some domestic abusers, gang leaders, cult leaders, and political leaders maintain control over their partners or followers. They are obviously not sensitive and responsive attachment figures, and they show at the extreme what the opposite of sensitivity and responsiveness is like. In the religious domain, this kind of reprehensible attachment figure is likely to proffer a view of God as angry, capricious, vindictive, and siding with the selfish attachment figure, thus ruling out God as a healthy alternative. Therefore, when choosing one's attachment figures (when choice is an option), it's important to be sensitive to the person's benevolence and competence. When designing and executing attachment-related interventions, it is important to make sure that the people occupying the role of attachment figure have, or can develop, the desired characteristics.

A secure and optimally functioning relationship involves trust on the parts of both the attached person and the attachment figure. The emerging sense of felt security encourages an attached person to trust the attachment figure's good intentions. But a good and worthy attachment figure also possesses a kind of trust in the person who is becoming attached: The worthy attachment figure has a generous faith in the attached person's value, goodness, and potential for growth. This kind of trust on the part of an attachment figure is evident in all of the different kinds of relationships we have discussed.

The sensitive and responsive teacher has faith in students' inherent value and potential, and this faith gets verbally and nonverbally communicated to the students. The sensitive and responsive group leader or manager has faith in his or her group members or employees, and this faith or trust contributes both to the employees' personal development and to the quality of the group's performance. The sensitive and responsive societal leader has faith in citizens' inherent value, deservingness, and potential for growth and contributions to a well-functioning society. Trust at each of these social levels contributes to trust and security at the other levels. It's more difficult to function as a caring, stabilizing attachment figure at the middle levels of an organization (e.g., a school or church or business) if the figures higher in the system are unreliable or unsupportive.

There are several differences in these respects between applications of attachment theory and applications of one-shot, single-variable social-psychological concepts. One of the reasons for Singal's (2021) dissatisfaction with single-variable "quick fixes" of social problems is that they misleadingly make it seem that the problems reside solely in the minds of individuals, when actually they are determined or heavily influenced by social and economic relationships between individuals and between individuals and groups, which are not under the individual's control. It's a long-standing feature of American culture to think that the secret to success and happiness lies somewhere in the isolated individual's mind. (The self-esteem movement was an example, as are all of the other "just believe in yourself" fads.) But the healthy individual mind has anchors in the healthy minds and actions of other people, just as the unhealthy mind has anchors in the unhealthy minds and actions of other people. Attachment-related interventions are aimed at making attachment figures and the people attached to them healthier and more secure. Often this requires altering the wider social networks and socioeconomic environments of both sides of the relationship.

Because attachment theory focuses on relationships between and among people, its applications are generally addressed to both individuals and the behavior of people who occupy the role of attachment figure. Although there is certainly nothing wrong with thinking about one's own attachment style and internal working models in hopes of altering them for the better, this is difficult to do on one's own, which is why we haven't written a self-help book. Changing people's attachment patterns for the better generally has to be done with the assistance, support, and encouragement of a sensitive and responsive attachment figure, whether this figure is a close relationship partner (e.g., parent, friend, romantic spouse), a "stronger and wiser" professional (e.g., teacher, mentor, therapist, nurse, physician), or a social group or organization. It isn't likely to be a quick or easy process.

Policy Implications

Beyond the specific applications and interventions considered in this book, are there other policy implications of attachment research? From the beginning, Bowlby and others were concerned that hospitals often denied parents and children an opportunity to meet with each other when one of them was hospitalized. This was an important example of the psychological pain and damage caused by separations, particularly in a time of illness. Robertson and Bowlby (1952) helped change this policy in Britain, and eventually it was changed in other countries as well. Today it is common for parents and children, or marital couples, to stay together overnight when one of them is hospitalized. That was an intervention that didn't require addressing or changing anyone's attachment pattern; it simply required changing a policy that got in the way of attachment processes that otherwise happen naturally. The old policy was an example of what happens when senior administrators in an organization fail to consider the attachment needs of people who use their services.

A more contemporary and complex American example is the separation of incarcerated parents from their children. As Cassidy, Poehlmann, and Shaver (2010) explained, when a parent, especially a mother, is incarcerated, the person's children have to be taken care of by someone else, either less invested or equally troubled relatives, or the foster care system. Looked at sadly but cynically, this is a policy inadvertently designed to increase the number of troubled and possibly criminal individuals in the next generation. Instead of reducing crime, it may be contributing to it, while causing unnecessary trauma to hundreds of thousands of individuals and families.

There are many ways in which this problem can be ameliorated if not solved: by avoiding unnecessary incarcerations, by creating better facilities for family visitations at prisons, and by making it possible for family members to communicate via video links with their imprisoned loved ones. Again, this doesn't require expensive efforts to change anyone's attachment pattern (although that would also be a worthy goal); it simply reduces barriers to natural attachment processes that have occurred or could occur over time if allowed to do so.

Another way in which attachment theory and research might have important beneficial effects is through education. As mentioned by Cassidy et al. (2013, p. 1428), "Far too many parents enter parenthood with insufficient knowledge about child development and the importance of the early parent–child relationship and without knowledge and skills needed to parent in a sensitive, responsive way. . . . In American schools, there seems to be a greater focus on education about sex than about successful parenting." To date, there is no attachment-informed, large-scale community intervention aimed at preparing youth for parenting tasks and helping them understand the nature of parent–child relationships. However, with a degree of creativity and flexibility, and enough funding for content development, implementation, and dissemination, the eight-session COS-P protocol (see Chapter 4) could be tailored to increase adolescents' and young adults' empathy and responsiveness, and prepare them to effectively provide a safe haven and secure base for their future children.

The same can be said about the absence of education concerning ways to create a successful, mutually satisfying marriage. Even the sex education in most public schools focuses more on anatomy and the dangers of pregnancy and sexually transmitted diseases than it does on the nature of a healthy relationship that includes sex. In this context, Johnson's (2008) Hold Me Tight (HmT) couple relationship education program (see Chapter 6), although originally created for young couples, can be used as a model for developing this kind of attachment-informed, school-level program. It wouldn't be terribly difficult to turn the HmT conversations into short didactic pieces for use as age-appropriate exercises for adolescents and young adults. Of course, this is the kind of intervention that might encounter resistance from parents who don't agree with the attachment-based conception of healthy relationships.

As explained in Chapter 3, there is good evidence that "security primes" of various sorts can temporarily increase a person's sense of felt security and his or her sensitivity and responsiveness to others (empathy and compassion), and if continued over time this might have more lasting effects on a person's prosocial orientation and altruistic behavior. Hence, any behavioral change program aimed at encouraging people's selfless engagement in volunteer actions on behalf of their community, humanity in general, or the earth as a whole (e.g., actions aimed at preventing neighborhood violence, the spread of deadly viruses, or destructive climate change) could benefit from the inclusion of security-priming components.

A first exemplary step in this direction was taken by Nisa et al. (2021), who used a security-enhancing banner (a picture of a pregnant woman with an Earth-shaped belly and the phrase "love your mother earth") at the entrance to a university cafeteria for several weeks and found reductions in students' daily food waste during the study period. Future behavioral change programs and social welfare campaigns could follow Nisa et al.'s lead and repeatedly and implicitly expose citizens to security reminders, which could increase their natural tendencies toward empathy, generosity, gratitude, and other social virtues. This is obviously what all major religions encourage believers to do but unfortunately, in some cases, their efforts do so by appealing to threats, fear, guilt, and rigidly hierarchical (usually male) leadership. The results might be more favorable if an emphasis were placed on attachment security (a safe haven and secure base).

Another example of the potential social impact of attachment-informed behavioral change programs concerns the fostering of intergroup positive and harmonious relationships. Since there is evidence (summarized by Mikulincer & Shaver, 2022) that attachment insecurity is associated with intergroup hostility, prejudice, discrimination, and racism, any program designed to reduce these destructive forces could include subtle or direct methods of enhancing felt security. This can be accomplished by not only using security reminders in media campaigns against intergroup violence, prejudice, or racism, but also by developing attachment-informed intergroup-contact interventions.

In a recent theoretical article, Tropp (2021) proposed viewing "intergroup contact itself as a question of attachment" and entertained the possibility that felt security can be enhanced not only by close relationship partners or in-groups but also by comforting interactions with out-group members during an appropriately designed intergroup-contact intervention. Specifically, Tropp suggested that if an out-group member with whom people come into contact is responsive to their needs for safety and security, people may feel more secure with regard to the out-group member and more likely to adopt a kind, other-oriented attitude toward him or her. In other words, out-group member responsiveness can contribute to "mutual growth cycles" (similar to our idea of security-supported broaden-and-build cycles at individual and dyadic levels) during intergroup contact and thus to the formation of mutually satisfying intergroup relationships. In this way, attachment-informed intergroup interventions aimed at creating comforting and empowering interactions with responsive out-group members could reduce intergroup hostility and increase positive responses to intergroup contact.

At the level of organizational leadership, as we have mentioned, leaders who are themselves secure with respect to attachment and who genuinely wish to contribute positively to their followers' security—with potential benefits to health, well-being, and organizational success—could apply attachment theory and research with large effects. But here again, it seems that (1) many people who attain positions of leadership do not have a history of attachment security, and (2) they often lead by instilling fear in their followers, deliberately saying, in effect, "You are weak, needy, and incompetent, and I am the only one who can save you." Because these appeals often arise in times of threat, or in times that the candidate for leadership can make seem threatening, the message can be persuasive to many people (perhaps including a disproportionate number of whom are insecure with respect to attachment). We have, unfortunately, seen distressing examples of this in both of our home countries.

In Chapters 10–12, we discussed the importance of designing attachment-based systemic interventions aimed at transforming entire schools, universities, hospitals, care centers, businesses, and governmental institutions into responsive, caring, and empowering social organizations. However, we don't as yet have much evidence concerning the feasibility and effectiveness of such programs. Moreover, these programs require a dramatic change in values and priorities at the societal level—a move from what Schwartz (1992) calls "self-enhancement values" (e.g., power, achievement) to self-transcendent values (benevolence, universalism).

In Gilbert's (2021) terms, the needed systemic programs are based on *caring and sharing* strategies, requiring societies to deemphasize, reject, and condemn organizations that rely excessively on *controlling and holding* strategies, strategies shaped by self-protection motives, egoistic self-focus, and attempts to obtain and accumulate resources without caring about others' welfare. Of course, this dramatic change in social values and priorities is hard to bring about, but we remain optimistic that human beings' natural capacities for empathy, compassion, and cooperation will eventually prevail and make possible the creation of security-enhancing organizations, institutions, and societies. As Pinker showed in an influential 2011 book, *The Better Angels of Our Nature*, when viewed from a long-term perspective on human history rather than the daily news, there has been a huge reduction in cruelty and violence over the millennia. This is compatible with Martin Luther King, Jr.'s famous optimistic claim that "the arc of the moral universe is long but it bends toward justice."

It seems possible to us that this gradual change for the better is related to gradual changes in childrearing and educational practices, combined with average improvements in people's standard of living (with many, many exceptions, of course). But this thesis would require another book to explore. (Pinker, 2019, has provided a good one, but it is more oriented toward education than attachment.)

Countervailing Factors

Given our optimistic account of many promising attachment-related interventions, we are left wondering: After 200,000 years as a species, if sensitivity, responsiveness, and felt security are so beneficial, why haven't human beings figured out how to make security the norm, thereby eliminating jealousy, cruelty, deception, corruption, and warfare? One part of the answer is that there are other forces—in individuals' minds and in group and intergroup processes—that militate against universal security.

First, there are often shortages of resources. At present there is a correlation, although far from a perfect one, between SES and the ability to provide safety and security for one's family and community members. And even those who are fairly secure at one point in societal development can become insecure later because of changes in the physical environment (as we see around the world today as the climate changes), the arrival of pandemics (e.g., COVID-19), or large-scale wars or economic collapses (as is happening, as we write, in Ukraine and parts of Africa and Latin America). In this sense, felt security is often outside the control of individuals, families, and local groups.

Second, when people are organized into groups, as they always are, competition and conflict between groups for status and resources are almost inevitable, and these conditions often foster insecurity, a search for a strong and powerful (hence possibly corruption-prone) leader, and willingness to inflict injury and sometimes death on members of other groups. There likely are evolved mechanisms other than attachment that serve the purposes of group survival and dominance, even if this interferes with kindness and security. (See Storr [2021] for a recent discussion of status seeking; see Shaver et al. [2011] for a discussion of a behavioral systems approach to power and aggression.) We can see examples of this all around the world, in all periods of history, including our own. In short, although we definitely believe it is possible and worthwhile to improve children's lives, adults' marriages, and the enjoyability and successful performance of larger social organizations, we are not oblivious to the unfortunate circumstances that often interfere with worthwhile improvement efforts.

The Nature of Threats

When Bowlby was conceptualizing the nature of infant–mother attachment, he was imagining a time in evolutionary history when infants could be victims of predation or severe accidents, so the "threat" was a threat to life or bodily integrity. He also saw and wrote insightfully about the threat of one's attachment figure's inattentiveness or absence (e.g., self-preoccupation, separation, abandonment, or death). When we consider attachment in the case of older children, adolescents, and adults, we recognize that there are also threats to the psychological self, not just the physical self. This is important to consider, because the threat of rejection or ostracism by one's close relationship partners or groups feels similar to death, and at many points in human history, rejection and abandonment would have actually led to physical death. More research is needed to clarify the diverse kinds of threats that trigger attachment needs and attachment behavior in people of different ages. To respond effectively to a particular threat, an attachment figure must often understand how he or she is perceived by and affects the attached person's seeking of safety and security. This is an important aspect of "mentalization."

It's worth thinking about the differences between safety, security, and self-esteem, the latter being the psychological variable that Singal (2021) criticized as the focus of massive and expensive interventions in schools for several years, especially in California. Those interventions included self-help statements such as "I AM LOVABLE. I AM LOVABLE" and group sessions in which students had to say what they liked about a particular classmate. Early in a person's life, "safety" and "security"—the foci of attachment theory—probably don't have much to do with self-esteem, because there isn't yet a psychological self to be esteemed. But even in that early period of life, a parent's touch, holding, warm approval, smiles, soft voice, and genuine appreciation and affection probably conveys something more than simple safety from threats. They convey that someone cares, and this implies, however vaguely at first, that "I am important and worthwhile."

Over the months and years, as a psychological self develops, what counts as safety and security has a great deal to do with the self being esteemed by others, because many of the threats concern the social safety and acceptability of one's person. But it's important to keep the idea of safety in mind, because it is probably still an important part of allowing one's self-defenses to relax. Attachment insecurity, increasingly beyond infancy, is tightly associated with self-protective defenses, and being safe in the arms (or mere presence) of a caring attachment figure has its beneficial effects partly by rendering defenses less necessary. This is partly a matter of felt safety and security, in addition to feelings of being esteemed and worthy of esteem.

The Importance of Theory

Two of the impressive features of attachment theory are its depth and coherence. The theory arose at a time when there were several competing psychoanalytic theories in play, and of these, only attachment theory inspired an explosion of research and detailed theoretical development that continues today. The others were fascinating and, in some cases, beautiful verbal constructions, but they didn't inspire sound measures or systematic empirical studies.

Because of the depth of attachment theory, attachment research is, for the most part, quite different from the single-variable, phenomenon-oriented research that is prominent in social psychology. Bowlby scoured the ethological literature for other phenomena like attachment, such as imprinting in precocial birds and the clinging of primate infants to their mother's fur. He was interested in the evolutionary history of the phenomena he studied (and late in his life actually wrote a psychobiography of Charles Darwin; Bowlby, 1990). He was a child psychiatrist who continued to do clinical work with children and families all of his life, which is not fertile ground for single-variable cure-alls. He was a wide reader whose theorizing was influenced by the emerging cognitive emphasis in psychology and by contemporary cybernetic devices and the control-systems theory that lay behind them.

As other people became familiar with his theory, beginning with Ainsworth, who was trained as a clinical and developmental researcher, Bowlby welcomed their measures, systematically gathered empirical findings, conceptual clarifications, and extensions. He kept track of the literatures on child development and community psychiatry, and was as interested in research on loss and grieving as he was in the process of attachment. He considered the full range of ideas and research findings related to attachment, separation, and loss, and he sought, quite successfully, to pull these ideas together into a coherent theoretical framework. Over 50 years later, his efforts and accomplishments are still remarkable, even awe-inspiring. And as shown in this book, his theory is still generating novel and important research and applications.- We are far from seeing the end of its development and influence.

References

Aarts, F., Hinnen, C., Gerdes, V. E. A., Brandjes, D. P. M., & Geenen, R. (2013). Mental healthcare utilization in patients seeking bariatric surgery: The role of attachment behavior. *Bariatric Surgical Practice and Patient Care, 8*, 134–138.

Aarts, H., & Dijksterhuis, A. (2003). The silence of the library: Environment, situational norm, and social behavior. *Journal of Personality and Social Psychology, 84*, 18–28.

Abrams, D., & Hogg, M. A. (1988). Comments on the motivational status of self-esteem in social identity and intergroup discrimination. *European Journal of Social Psychology, 18*, 317–334.

Abror, A., & Patrisia, D. (2020). Psychological safety and organizational performance: A systematic literature review. *International Journal of Advanced Science and Technology, 29*, 3634–3644.

Adams, G. C., & McWilliams, L. A. (2015). Relationships between adult attachment style ratings and sleep disturbances in a nationally representative sample. *Journal of Psychosomatic Research, 79*, 37–42.

Admoni, S. (2006). *Attachment security and eating disorders.* Unpublished doctoral dissertation, Bar-Ilan University, Ramat Gan, Israel.

Agostini, A., Rizzello, F., Ravegnani, G., Gionchetti, R., Tambasco, R., & Straforini, G. (2010). Adult attachment and early parental experiences in patients with Crohn's disease. *Psychosomatics, 51*, 208–215.

Agyapong, V. I. O., Hrabok, M., Juhas, M., Omeje, J., Denga, E., Nwaka, B., . . . Li, X.-M. (2018). Prevalence rates and predictors of generalized anxiety disorder symptoms in residents of Fort McMurray six months after a wildfire. *Frontiers in Psychiatry, 9*, Article 345.

Ahnert, L., Harwardt-Heinecke, E., Kappler, G., Eckstein-Madry, T., & Milatz, A. (2012). Student–teacher relationships and classroom climate in first grade: How do they relate to students' stress regulation? *Attachment and Human Development, 14*, 249–263.

Ahnert, L., Pinquart, M., & Lamb, M. E. (2006). Security of children's relationships with nonparental care providers: A meta-analysis. *Child Development, 74*, 664–679.

Ahrens, K. R., Ciechanowski, P., & Katon, W. (2012). Associations between adult attachment style and health risk behaviors in an adult female primary care population. *Journal of Psychosomatic Research, 72*, 364–370.

Ai, T., Gillath, O., & Karantzas, G. (2020). The dual function model of attachment security priming: Theoretical framework and empirical evidence. *International Journal of Environmental Research and Public Health, 17*, Article 8093.

Aikins, J. W., Howes, C., & Hamilton, C. (2009). Attachment stability and the emergence of unresolved representations during adolescence. *Attachment and Human Development, 11*, 491–512.

Ainsworth, M. D. S. (1940). *An evaluation of adjustment based on the concept of security.* Unpublished doctoral dissertation, University of Toronto, Ontario, Canada.

Ainsworth, M. D. S. (1967). *Infancy in Uganda: Infant care and the growth of love.* Johns Hopkins University Press.

Ainsworth, M. D. S. (1989). Attachments beyond infancy. *American Psychologist, 44*, 709–716.

Ainsworth, M. D. S. (1991). Attachment and other affectional bonds across the life cycle. In C. M. Parkes, J. Stevenson-Hinde, & P. Marris (Eds.), *Attachment across the life cycle* (pp. 33–51). Routledge.

Ainsworth, M. D. S., Bell, S. M., & Stayton, D. J.

(1971). Individual differences in strange-situation behavior of one-year-olds. In H. R. Schaffer (Ed.), *The origins of human social relations* (pp. 12–41). Academic Press.

Ainsworth, M. D. S., Bell, S. M., & Stayton, D. J. (1974). Infant–mother attachment and social development: Socialization as a product of reciprocal responsiveness to signals. In M. P. M. Richards (Ed.), *The integration of a child into a social world* (pp. 99–135). Cambridge University Press.

Ainsworth, M. D. S., Blehar, M. C., Waters, E., & Wall, S. (1978). *Patterns of attachment: Assessed in the Strange Situation and at home*. Erlbaum.

Al-Yagon, M., & Mikulincer, M. (2004). Socioemotional and academic adjustment among children with learning disorders: The mediational role of attachment-based factors. *Journal of Special Education, 38*, 111–123.

Alamos, P., Williford, A. P., & LoCasale-Crouch, J. (2018). Understanding Banking Time implementation in a sample of preschool children who display early disruptive behaviors. *School Mental Health, 10*, 437–449.

Alder, M. C., Dyer, W. J, Sandberg, J. G., Davis, S. Y., & Holt-Lunstad, J. (2018). Emotionally-focused therapy and treatment as usual comparison groups in decreasing depression: A clinical pilot study. *American Journal of Family Therapy, 46*, 541–555.

Algoe, S. B., Gable, S. L., & Maisel, N. C. (2010). It's the little things: Everyday gratitude as a booster shot for romantic relationships. *Personal Relationships, 17*, 217–233.

Allen, J. G. (2012). Reviving plain old therapy. Retrieved from *https://psychnews.psychiatryonline.org/doi/full/10.1176/pn.47.10.psychnews_47_10_3-a*.

Allen, J. G., Fonagy, P., & Bateman, A. W. (2008). *Mentalizing in clinical practice*. American Psychiatric Association.

Allen, J. P. (2021). Beyond stability: Toward understanding the development of attachment beyond childhood. In R. A. Thompson, J. A. Simpson, & L. J. Berlin (Eds.), *Attachment: The fundamental questions* (pp. 161–168). Guilford Press.

Allen, J. P., Costello, M., Kansky, J., & Loeb, E. L. (2022). When friendships surpass parental relationships as predictors of long-term outcomes: Adolescent relationship qualities and adult psychosocial functioning. *Child Development, 93*, 760–777.

Allen, J. P., Grande, L., Tan, J., & Loeb, E. (2018). Parent and peer predictors of change in attachment security from adolescence to adulthood. *Child Development, 89*, 1120–1132.

Allen, J. P., & Hauser, S. T. (1996). Autonomy and relatedness in adolescent–family interactions as predictors of young adults' states of mind regarding attachment. *Development and Psychopathology, 8*, 793–809.

Allen, J. P., McElhaney, K. B., Kuperminc, G. P., & Jodl, K. M. (2004). Stability and change in attachment security across adolescence. *Child Development, 75*, 1792–1805.

Allen, J. P., McElhaney, K. B., Land, D. J., Kuperminc, G. P., Moore, C. W., O'Beirne-Kelly, H., & Kilmer, S. L. (2003). A secure base in adolescence: Markers of attachment security in the mother–adolescent relationship. *Child Development, 74*, 292–307.

Allen, J. P., Narr, R. K., Nagel, A. G., Costello, M. A., & Guskin, K. (2021). The Connection Project: Changing the peer environment to improve outcomes for marginalized adolescents. *Development and Psychopathology, 33*, 647–657.

Allen, J. P., Pianta, R. C., Gregory, A., Mikami, A. Y., Lun, J. (2011). An interaction-based approach to enhancing secondary school instruction and student achievement. *Science, 333*, 1034–1037.

Allen, J. P., & Tan, J. (2016). The multiple facets of attachment in adolescence. In J. Cassidy & P. R. Shaver (Eds.), *Handbook of attachment: Theory, research, and clinical applications* (3rd ed., pp. 399–415). Guilford Press.

Allen, T. D., Shockley, K. M., & Poteat, L. (2010). Protégé anxiety attachment and feedback in mentoring relationships. *Journal of Vocational Behavior, 77*, 73–80.

Alsancak-Akbulut, C., Sahin-Acar, B., & Sumer, N. (2021). Effect of video-feedback intervention on Turkish mothers' sensitivity and physical intrusiveness: A randomized control trial. *Attachment and Human Development, 6*, 795–813.

Althobaiti, S., Kazantzis, N., Ofori-Asenso, R., Romero, L., Fisher, J., Mills, K. E., & Liew, D. (2020). Efficacy of interpersonal psychotherapy for post-traumatic stress disorder: A systematic review and meta-analysis. *Journal of Affective Disorders, 264*, 286–294.

Ames, M. E., Pratt, M. W., Pancer, S., Mark, W., Maxine, G., Polivy, J., . . . Adams, G. (2011). The moderating effects of attachment style on students' experience of a transition to university group facilitation program. *Canadian Journal of Behavioral Science, 43*, 1–12.

Ammaniti, M., van IJzendoorn, M. H., Speranza, A. M., & Tambelli, R. (2000). Internal working models of attachment during late childhood and early adolescence: An exploration of stability and change. *Attachment and Human Development, 2*, 328–346.

Amundsen, S., & Martinsen, Ø. L. (2014). Empowering leadership: Construct clarification, conceptualization, and validation of a new scale. *Leadership Quarterly, 25*, 487–511.

Andersen, S. M., & Chen, S. (2002). The relational self: An interpersonal social-cognitive theory. *Psychological Review, 109*, 619–645.

Andersen, T. E., Elklit, A., & Brink, O. (2013). PTSD

symptoms mediate the effect of attachment on pain and somatization after whiplash injury. *Clinical Practice and Epidemiology in Mental Health, 9*, 75–83.

Andersen, T. E., Ravn, S. L., Manniche, C., & O'Neill, S. (2018). The impact of attachment insecurity on pain and pain behaviors in experimental pain. *Journal of Psychosomatic Research, 111*, 127–132.

Andersen, T. E., Sterling, M., Maujean, A., & Meredith, P. (2019). Attachment insecurity as a vulnerability factor in the development of chronic whiplash associated disorder: A prospective cohort study. *Journal of Psychosomatic Research, 118*, 56–62.

Anderson, A. R., Christenson, S. L., Sinclair, M. F., & Lehr, C. A. (2004). Check & Connect: The importance of relationships for promoting engagement with school. *Journal of School Psychology, 42*, 95–113.

Anderson, B. J., Brackett, J., Ho, J., & Laffel, L. M. (1999). An office-based intervention to maintain parent–adolescent teamwork in diabetes management: Impact on parent involvement, family conflict, and subsequent glycemic control. *Diabetes Care, 22*, 713–721.

Anderson, N., Heywood-Everett, S., Siddiqi, N., Wright, J., Meredith, J., & McMillan, D. (2015). Faith-adapted psychological therapies for depression and anxiety: Systematic review and meta-analysis. *Journal of Affective Disorders, 176*, 183–196.

Andrews, N. E., Meredith, P. J., Strong, J., & Donohue, G. F. (2014). Adult attachment and approaches to activity engagement in chronic pain. *Pain Research and Management, 19*, 317–327.

Ano, G. G., & Pargament, K. I. (2013). Predictors of spiritual struggles: An exploratory study. *Mental Health, Religion and Culture, 16*, 419–434.

Ano, G. G., & Vasconcelles, E. B. (2005). Religious coping and psychological adjustment to stress: A meta-analysis. *Journal of Clinical Psychology, 61*, 461–480.

Ansari, A., & Pianta, R. C. (2018). Variation in the long-term benefits of child care: The role of classroom quality in elementary school. *Developmental Psychology, 54*, 1854–1867.

Arbuckle, R., Berry, K., Taylor, J., & Kennedy, S. (2012). Service user attachments to psychiatric key workers and teams. *Social Psychiatry and Psychiatric Epidemiology, 47*, 817–825.

Arndt, J., Schimel, J., Greenberg, J., & Pyszczynski, T. (2002). The intrinsic self and defensiveness: Evidence that activating the intrinsic self reduces self-handicapping and conformity. *Personality and Social Psychology Bulletin, 28*, 671–683.

Arnott, B., & Meins, E. (2007). Links between antenatal attachment representations, postnatal mind-mindedness, and infant attachment security: A preliminary study of mothers and fathers. *Bulletin of the Menninger Clinic, 71*, 132–149.

Arriaga, X. B., Eller, J., Kumashiro, M., Rholes, W. S., & Simpson, J. A. (2020). Self-efficacy and declines over time in attachment anxiety during the transition to parenthood. *Social Psychological and Personality Sciences, 12*, 658–666.

Arriaga, X. B., Kumashiro, M., Finkel, E. J., VanderDrift, L. E., & Luchies, L. B. (2014). Filling the void: Bolstering attachment security in committed relationships. *Social Psychological and Personality Science, 5*, 398–406.

Arriaga, X. B., Kumashiro, M., Simpson, J. A., & Overall, N. C. (2018). Revising working models across time: Relationship situations that enhance attachment security. *Personality and Social Psychology Review, 22*, 71–96.

Årseth, A. K., Kroger, J., Martinussen, M., & Marcia, J. E. (2009). Meta-analytic studies of identity status and the relational issues of attachment and intimacy. *Identity, 9*, 1–32.

Atkinson, L., Niccols, A., Paglia, A., Coolbear, J., Parker, K. C. H., Poulton, L., . . . Sitarenios, G. (2000). A meta-analysis of time between maternal sensitivity and attachment assessments: Implications for internal working models in infancy/toddlerhood. *Journal of Social and Personal Relationships, 17*, 791–810.

Atzil-Slonim, D., Bar-Kalifa, E., Fisher, H., Peri, T., Lutz, W., Rubel, J., & Rafaeli, E. (2018). Emotional congruence between clients and therapists and its effect on treatment outcome. *Journal of Counseling Psychology, 65*, 51–64.

Ávila, M., Brandão, T., Coimbra, J. L., Lopez, F., & Matos, P. M. (2016). Experiencing an intimate partner's breast cancer: Attachment, caregiving, and burden in men. *Psychiatry: Interpersonal and Biological Processes, 79*, 236–248.

Ávila, M., Cabral, J., & Matos, P. M. (2012). Identity in university students: The role of parental and romantic attachment. *Journal of Adolescence, 35*, 133–142.

Avolio, B. J., & Bass, B. M. (1988). Transformational leadership, charisma, and beyond. In J. G. Hunt, B. R. Baliga, H. P. Dachler, & C. A. Schriesheim (Eds.), *Emerging leadership vistas* (pp. 29–49). Lexington Books.

Avolio, B. J., & Hannah, S. T. (2020). An enduring leadership myth: Born a leader or made a leader? *Organizational Dynamics, 49*, Article 100730.

Avolio, B. J., Reichard, R. J., Hannah, S. T., Walumbwa, F. O., & Chan, A. (2009). A meta-analytic review of leadership impact research: Experimental and quasi-experimental studies. *Leadership Quarterly, 20*, 764–784.

Baccus, J. R., Baldwin, M. W., & Packer, D. J. (2004). Increasing implicit self-esteem through classical conditioning. *Psychological Science, 15*, 498–502.

Bachelor, A., Meunier, G., Laverdiere, O., & Gamache, D. (2010). Client attachment to therapist: Relation to client personality and symptomatology, and

their contributions to the therapeutic alliance. *Psychotherapy, 47,* 454–468.
Baer, R. A., Smith, G. T., Hopkins, J., Krietemeyer, J., & Toney, L. (2006). Using self-report assessment methods to explore facets of mindfulness. *Assessment, 13,* 27–45.
Bai, X., Chen, X., Zhou, M., Liu, C., & Hu, Y. (2019). The effects of negative context and attachment security priming on working memory updating among anxiously attached individuals. *Biological Psychology, 143,* 41–52.
Bailey, H. N., Bernier, A., Bouvette-Turcot, A.-A., Tarabulsy, G. M., Pederson, D. R., & Becker-Stoll, F. (2017). Deconstructing maternal sensitivity: Predictive relations to mother–child attachment in home and laboratory settings. *Social Development, 26,* 679–693.
Baker, W. D., & Oneal, J. R. (2001). Patriotism or opinion leadership?: The nature and origins of the "rally 'round the flag" effect. *Journal of Conflict Resolution, 45,* 661–687.
Bakermans-Kranenburg, M. J., Breddels-van Baardewijk, P., Juffer, F., Klein Velderman, M., & van IJzendoorn, M. H. (2008). Insecure mothers with temperamentally reactive infants: A chance for intervention. In F. Juffer, M. J. Bakermans-Kranenburg, & M. H. van IJzendoorn (Eds.), *Promoting positive parenting: An attachment-based intervention* (pp. 75–90). Taylor & Francis.
Bakermans-Kranenburg, M. J., & van IJzendoorn, M. H. (2009). The first 10,000 Adult Attachment Interviews: Distributions of adult attachment representations in clinical and non-clinical groups. *Attachment and Human Development, 11,* 223–263.
Bakermans-Kranenburg, M. J., van IJzendoorn, M. H., & Juffer, F. (2003). Less is more: Meta-analyses of sensitivity and attachment interventions in early childhood. *Psychological Bulletin, 129,* 195–215.
Bakermans-Kranenburg, M. J., van IJzendoorn, M. H., & Juffer, F. (2005). Disorganized infant attachment and preventive interventions: A review and meta-analysis. *Infant Mental Health Journal, 26,* 191–216.
Bakermans-Kranenburg, M. J., van IJzendoorn, M. H., & Kroonenberg, P. M. (2004). Differences in attachment security between African-American and white children: Ethnicity or socio-economic status? *Infant Behavior and Development, 27,* 417–433.
Bakermans-Kranenburg, M. J., van IJzendoorn, M. H., Mesman, J., Alink, L. R. A., & Juffer, F. (2008). Effects of an attachment-based intervention on daily cortisol moderated by dopamine receptor D4: A randomized control trial on 1- to 3-year-olds screened for externalizing behavior. *Development and Psychopathology, 20,* 805–820.
Baldwin, M. W., Fehr, B., Keedian, E., Seidel, M., & Thompson, D. W. (1993). An exploration of the relational schemata underlying attachment styles: Self-report and lexical decision approaches. *Personality and Social Psychology Bulletin, 19,* 746–754.
Baldwin, M. W., Keelan, J. P. R., Fehr, B., Enns, V., & Koh Rangarajoo, E. (1996). Social-cognitive conceptualization of attachment working models: Availability and accessibility effects. *Journal of Personality and Social Psychology, 71,* 94–109.
Bales, D. L., Timman, R., Andrea, H., Busschbach, J. J. V., Verheul, R., & Kamphuis, J. H. (2015). Effectiveness of day hospital mentalization-based treatment for patients with severe borderline personality disorder: A matched control study. *Clinical Psychology and Psychotherapy, 22,* 409–417.
Bales, D. L., van Beek, N., Smits, M., Willemsen, S., Busschbach, J. J. V., Verheul, R., & Andrea, H. (2012). Treatment outcome of 18-month, day hospital mentalization-based treatment (MBT) in patients with severe borderline personality disorder in the Netherlands. *Journal of Personality Disorders, 26,* 568–582.
Balestrieri, M., Zuanon, S., Pellizzari, J., Zappoli-Thyrion, E., & Ciano, R. (2015). Mentalization in eating disorders: A preliminary trial comparing mentalization-based treatment (MBT) with a psychodynamic-oriented treatment. *Eating and Weight Disorders, 20,* 525–528.
Balluerka, N., Muela, A., Amiano, N., & Caldentey, M. A. (2014). Influence of animal-assisted therapy (AAT) on the attachment representations of youth in residential care. *Children and Youth Services Review, 42,* 103–109.
Balluerka, N., Muela, A., Amiano, N., & Caldentey, M. A. (2015). Promoting psychosocial adaptation of youths in residential care through animal-assisted psychotherapy. *Child Abuse and Neglect, 50,* 193–205.
Bandura, A. (1986). *Social foundations of thought and action: A social cognitive theory.* Prentice-Hall.
Bangerter, A., Krings, F., Mouton, A., Gilles, I., Green, E. G. T., & Clémence, A. (2012). Longitudinal investigation of public trust in institutions relative to the 2009 H1N1 pandemic in Switzerland. *PLOS ONE, 7,* Article e49806.
Baran, B. E., Shanock, L. R., & Miller, L. R. (2012). Advancing organizational support theory into the twenty-first century world of work. *Journal of Business and Psychology, 27,* 123–147.
Barbarin, O. A. (2021). Racial disparities in the U.S. child protection system: Etiology and solutions. *International Journal on Child Maltreatment, 3,* 449–466.
Barber, B. K., & Olsen, J. A. (2004). Assessing the transitions to middle and high school. *Journal of Adolescent Research, 19,* 3–30.
Bargh, J. A., & Chartrand, T. L. (2014). The mind in the middle: A practical guide to priming and automaticity research. In H. T. Reis & C. M. Judd (Eds.), *Handbook of research methods in social and personality psychology* (pp. 311–344). Cambridge University Press.

Bargh, J. A., Chen, M., & Burrows, L. (1996). Automaticity of social behavior: Direct effects of trait construct and stereotype activation on action. *Journal of Personality and Social Psychology, 71,* 230–244.
Barnicot, K., Wampold, B., & Priebe, S. (2014). The effect of core clinician interpersonal behaviors on depression. *Journal of Affective Disorders, 167,* 112–117.
Barone, L., Barone, V., Dellagiulia, A., & Lionetti, F. (2018). Testing an attachment-based parenting intervention-VIPP-FC/A in adoptive families with post-institutionalized children: Do maternal sensitivity and genetic markers count? *Frontiers in Psychology, 9,* Article 156.
Barone, L., Carone, N., Costantino, A., Genschow, J., Merelli, S., Milloni, A., . . . Moretti, M. M. (2021). Effect of a parenting intervention on decreasing adolescents' behavioral problems via reduction in attachment insecurity: A longitudinal, multicenter, randomized controlled trial. *Journal of Adolescence, 91,* 82–96.
Barone, L., Carone, N., Salazar-Jimenez, J.-G., & Ortíz Muñoz, J. A. (2021). Enhancing food habits via sensitivity in rural low-SES mothers of children aged 1–3 living in Colombia: A randomized controlled trial using video-feedback intervention. *Attachment and Human Development, 23,* 831–852.
Barone, L., Ozturk, Y., & Lionetti, F. (2019). The key role of positive parenting and children's temperament in post-institutionalized children's socioemotional adjustment after adoption placement: A RCT study. *Social Development, 28,* 136–151.
Barry, M. J., & Edgman-Levitan, S. (2012). Shared decision making: The pinnacle patient-centered care. *New England Journal of Medicine, 366,* 780–781.
Barry, R. A., & Lawrence, E. (2013). "Don't stand so close to me": An attachment perspective of disengagement and avoidance in marriage. *Journal of Family Psychology, 27,* 484–494.
Barth, M., Masson, T., Fritsche, I., & Ziemer, C.-T. (2018). Closing ranks: Ingroup norm conformity as a subtle response to threatening climate change. *Group Processes and Intergroup Relations, 21,* 497–512.
Bartholomew, K. (1990). Avoidance of intimacy: An attachment perspective. *Journal of Social and Personal Relationships, 7,* 147–178.
Bartholomew, K., & Horowitz, L. M. (1991). Attachment styles among young adults: A test of a four-category model. *Journal of Personality and Social Psychology, 61,* 226–244.
Bartley, M., Head, J., & Stansfeld, S. (2007). Is attachment style a source of resilience against health inequalities at work? *Social Science and Medicine, 64,* 765–775.
Bartz, J. A., & Lydon, J. E. (2004). Close relationships and the working self-concept: Implicit and explicit effects of priming attachment on agency and communion. *Personality and Social Psychology Bulletin, 30,* 1389–1401.
Bass, B. M. (1985). *Leadership and performance beyond expectations.* Free Press.
Bass, B. M., & Avolio, B. J. (1990). Developing transformational leadership: 1992 and beyond. *Journal of European Industrial Training, 14,* 21–27.
Bass, B. M., Riggio, R. E. (2006). *Transformational leadership* (2nd ed.). Erlbaum.
Bastian, B., Jetten, J., Thai, H. A., & Steffens, N. K. (2018). Shared adversity increases team creativity through fostering supportive interaction. *Frontiers in Psychology, 9,* Article 2309.
Bateman, A., & Fonagy, P. (1999). Effectiveness of partial hospitalization in the treatment of borderline personality disorder: A randomized controlled trial. *American Journal of Psychiatry, 156,* 1563–1569.
Bateman, A., & Fonagy, P. (2001). Treatment of borderline personality disorder with psychoanalytically oriented partial hospitalization: An 18-month follow-up. *American Journal of Psychiatry, 158,* 36–42.
Bateman, A., & Fonagy, P. (2004). *Psychotherapy for borderline personality disorder: Mentalization-based treatment.* Oxford University Press.
Bateman, A., & Fonagy, P. (2008). 8-year follow-up of patients treated for borderline personality disorder: Mentalization-based treatment versus treatment as usual. *American Journal of Psychiatry, 165,* 631–638.
Bateman, A., & Fonagy, P. (2009). Randomized controlled trial of outpatient mentalization-based treatment versus structured clinical management for borderline personality disorder. *American Journal of Psychiatry, 166,* 1355–1364.
Bateman, A., & Fonagy, P. (2010). Mentalization based treatment for borderline personality disorder. *World Psychiatry, 9,* 11–15.
Bateman, A., & Fonagy, P. (Eds.). (2012). *Handbook of mentalizing in mental health practice.* American Psychiatric Publishing.
Bateman, A., & Fonagy, P. (2016). *Mentalization-based treatment for personality disorders: A practical guide.* Oxford University Press.
Batson, C. D. (1991). *The altruism question: Toward a social-psychological answer.* Erlbaum.
Batson, C. D., Schoenrade, P. A., & Ventis, W. L. (1993). *Religion and the individual: A social-psychological perspective.* Oxford University Press.
Baucom, D. H., Porter, L. S., Kirby, J. S., & Hudepohl, J. (2012). Couple-based interventions for medical problems. *Behavior Therapy, 43,* 61–76.
Bazzazian, S., & Besharat, M. A. (2012). An explanatory model of adjustment to type I diabetes based on attachment, coping, and self-regulation theories. *Psychology, Health and Medicine, 17,* 47–58.
Beal, D. J., Cohen, R. R., Burke, M. J., & McLendon, C. L. (2003). Cohesion and performance in groups: A meta-analytic clarification of construct relations. *Journal of Applied Psychology, 88,* 989–1004.

Beasley, C. C., & Ager, R. (2019). Emotionally focused couples therapy: A systematic review of its effectiveness over the past 19 years. *Journal of Evidence-Based Social Work, 16*, 144–159.

Beck, E., Bo, S., Jørgensen, M. S., Gondan, M., Poulsen, S., Storebø, O. J., . . . Simonsen, E. (2020). Mentalization-based treatment in groups for adolescents with borderline personality disorder: A randomized controlled trial. *Journal of Child Psychology and Psychiatry, 61*, 594–604.

Beck, L. A., Pietromonaco, P. R., DeBuse, C. J., Powers, S. I., & Sayer, A. G. (2013). Spouses' attachment pairings predict neuroendocrine, behavioral, and psychological responses to marital conflict. *Journal of Personality and Social Psychology, 105*, 388–424.

Beck, L. A., Pietromonaco, P. R., DeVito, C. C., Powers, S. I., & Boyle, A. M. (2014). Congruence between spouses' perceptions and observers' ratings of responsiveness: The role of attachment avoidance. *Personality and Social Psychology Bulletin, 40*, 164–174.

Beck, R. (2006). God as a secure base: Attachment to God and theological exploration. *Journal of Psychology and Theology, 34*, 125–132.

Beck, R., & McDonald, A. (2004). Attachment to God: The Attachment to God Inventory, tests of working model correspondence, and an exploration of faith group differences. *Journal of Psychology and Theology, 32*, 92–103.

Becker-Stoll, F., Fremmer-Bombik, E., Wartner, U., Zimmermann, P., & Grossmann, K. E. (2008). Is attachment at ages 1, 6 and 16 related to autonomy and relatedness behavior of adolescents in interaction towards their mothers? *International Journal of Behavioral Development, 32*, 372–380.

Bedics, J. D., Atkins, D. C., Comtois, K. A., & Linehan, M. M. (2012). Treatment differences in the therapeutic relationship and introject during a 2-year randomized controlled trial of dialectical behavior therapy versus non-behavioral psychotherapy experts for borderline personality disorder. *Journal of Consulting and Clinical Psychology, 80*, 66–77.

Bednar, R. L., Melnick, J., & Kaul, T. J. (1974). Risk, responsibility, and structure: A conceptual framework for initiating group counseling and psychotherapy. *Journal of Counseling Psychology, 21*, 31–37.

Beijersbergen, M. D., Juffer, F., Bakermans-Kranenburg, M. J., & van IJzendoorn, M. H. (2012). Remaining or becoming secure: Parental sensitive support predicts attachment continuity from infancy to adolescence in a longitudinal adoption study. *Developmental Psychology, 48*, 1277–1282.

Bélanger, J. J., Faber, T., & Gelfand, M. J. (2013). Supersize my identity: When thoughts of contracting swine flu boost one's patriotic identity. *Journal of Applied Social Psychology, 43*, E153–E155.

Belavich, T. G., & Pargament, K. I. (2002). The role of attachment in predicting spiritual coping with a loved one in surgery. *Journal of Adult Development, 9*, 13–29.

Belsky, J. (2005). Attachment theory and research in ecological perspective: Insights from the Pennsylvania Infant and Family Development Project and the NICHD Study of Early Child Care. In K. E. Grossmann, K. Grossmann, & E. Waters (Eds.), *Attachment from infancy to adulthood: The major longitudinal studies* (pp. 71–97). Guilford Press.

Ben David-Sela, T., Dolev-Amit, T., Eubanks, C. F., & Zilcha-Mano, S. (2021). Achieving successful resolution of alliance ruptures: For whom and when? *Psychotherapy Research, 31*, 870–881.

Ben-Gal Dahan, A., & Mikulincer, M. (2021). Attachment and task persistence: Attachment orientations, perception of teacher's responsiveness and adolescents' persistence in academic tasks. *Attachment and Human Development, 23*, 665–686.

Ben-Naim, S., Hirschberger, G., Ein-Dor, T., & Mikulincer, M. (2013). An experimental study of emotion regulation during relationship conflict interactions: The moderating role of attachment orientations. *Emotion, 13*, 506–519.

Benistri, A. (2019). *A secure base for flexibly responding to a changing world: The contribution of attachment security to task switching.* Unpublished MA thesis, Interdisciplinary Center (IDC) Herzliya, Herzliya, Israel.

Bennett, J. K., Fuertes, J. N., Keitel, M., & Phillips, R. (2011). The role of patient attachment and working alliance on patient adherence, satisfaction, and health-related quality of life in lupus treatment. *Patient Education Counseling, 85*, 53–59.

Berant, E., Mikulincer, M., & Florian, V. (2001). Attachment style and mental health: A 1-year follow-up study of mothers of infants with congenital heart disease. *Personality and Social Psychology Bulletin, 27*, 956–968.

Berg, C. A., Helgeson, V. S., Tracy, E. L., Butner, J. E., Kelly, C. S., Van Vleet, M., & Litchman, M. L. (2020). Daily illness appraisal and collaboration in couples with type 1 diabetes. *Health Psychology, 39*, 689–699.

Berk, M. S., & Andersen, S. M. (2000). The impact of past relationships on interpersonal behavior: Behavioral confirmation in the social-cognitive process of transference. *Journal of Personality and Social Psychology, 79*, 546–562.

Berkman, L. F., Glass, T., Brissette, I., Seeman, T. E. (2000). From social integration to health: Durkheim in the new millennium. *Social Science and Medicine, 51*, 843–857.

Berlin, L. J., Martoccio, T. L., Bryce, C. I., & Jones Harden, B. (2019). Improving infants' stress-induced cortisol regulation through attachment-based intervention: A randomized controlled trial. *Psychoneuroendocrinology, 103*, 225–232.

Berlin, L. J., Martoccio, T. L., & Jones Harden, B.

(2018). Improving early head start's impacts on parenting through attachment-based intervention: A randomized controlled trial. *Developmental Psychology, 54,* 2316–2327.

Berlin, L. J., Shanahan, M., & Carmody, K. A. (2014). Promoting supportive parenting in new mothers with substance-use problems: A pilot randomized trial of residential treatment plus an attachment-based parenting program. *Infant Mental Health Journal, 35,* 81–85.

Berlin, L. J., Zeanah, C. H., & Lieberman, A. (2016). Prevention and intervention programs to support early attachment security: A move to the level of community. In J. Cassidy & P. R. Shaver (Eds.), *Handbook of attachment: Theory, research, and clinical applications* (3rd ed., pp. 739–758). Guilford Press.

Bernard, K., Dozier, M., Bick, J., & Gordon, M. K. (2015). Intervening to enhance cortisol regulation among children at risk for neglect: Results of a randomized clinical trial. *Development and Psychopathology, 27,* 829–841.

Bernard, K., Dozier, M., Bick, J., Lewis-Morrarty, E., Lindhiem, O., & Carlson, E. (2012). Enhancing attachment organization among maltreated children: Results of a randomized clinical trial. *Child Development, 83,* 623–636.

Bernard, K., Hostinar, C. E., & Dozier, M. (2015). Intervention effects on diurnal cortisol rhythms of CPS-referred infants persist into early childhood: Preschool follow-up results of a randomized clinical trial. *JAMA Pediatrics, 169,* 112–119.

Bernard, K., Hostinar, C. E., & Dozier, M. (2019). Longitudinal associations between attachment quality in infancy, C-reactive protein in early childhood, and BMI in middle childhood: Preliminary evidence from a CPS-referred sample. *Attachment and Human Development, 21,* 5–22.

Bernard, K., Kuzava, S., Simons, R., & Dozier, M. (2018). CPS-referred mothers' psychophysiological responses to own versus other child predict sensitivity to child distress. *Developmental Psychology, 54,* 1255–1264.

Bernard, K., Lee, A. H., & Dozier, M. (2017). Effects of the ABC intervention on foster children's receptive vocabulary: Follow-up results from a randomized clinical trial. *Child Maltreatment, 22,* 174–179.

Bernard, K., Simons, R., & Dozier, M. (2015). Effects of an attachment-based intervention on child protective services-referred mothers' event-related potentials to children's emotions. *Child Development, 86,* 1673–1684.

Bernecker, S. L., Levy, K. N., & Ellison, W. D. (2014). A meta-analysis of the relation between patient adult attachment style and the working alliance. *Psychotherapy Research, 24,* 12–24.

Bernier, A., Beauchamp, M. H., Carlson, S. M., & Lalonde, G. (2015). A secure base from which to regulate: Attachment security in toddlerhood as a predictor of executive functioning at school entry. *Developmental Psychology, 51,* 1177–1189.

Bernier, A., Beauchamp, M. H., & Cimon-Paquet, C. (2020). From early relationships to preacademic knowledge: A sociocognitive developmental cascade to school readiness. *Child Development, 91,* e134–e145.

Bernier, A., Carlson, S. M., Deschênes, M., & Matte-Gagné, C. (2012). Social factors in the development of early executive functioning: A closer look at the caregiving environment. *Developmental Science, 15,* 12–24.

Bernier, A., & Dozier, M. (2003). Bridging the attachment transmission gap: The role of maternal mind-mindedness. *International Journal of Behavioral Development, 27,* 355–365.

Bernier, A., Larose, S., & Whipple, N. (2005). Leaving home for college: A potentially stressful event for adolescents with preoccupied attachment patterns. *Attachment and Human Development, 7,* 171–185.

Bernier, A., & Matte-Gagné, C. (2011). More bridges: Investigating the relevance of self-report and interview measures of adult attachment for marital and caregiving relationships. *International Journal of Behavioral Development, 35,* 307–316.

Bernier, A., McMahon, C. A., & Perrier, R. (2017). Maternal mind-mindedness and children's school readiness: A longitudinal study of developmental processes. *Developmental Psychology, 53,* 210–221.

Bernstein, R. E., Timmons, A. C., & Lieberman, A. F. (2019). Interpersonal violence, maternal perception of infant emotion, and child–parent psychotherapy. *Journal of Family Violence, 34,* 309–320.

Berry, J. K. M., & Drummond, P. D. (2014). Does attachment anxiety increase vulnerability to headache? *Journal of Psychosomatic Research, 76,* 113–120.

Berry, K., Shah, R., Cook, A., Geater, E., Barrowclough, C., & Wearden, A. (2008). Staff attachment styles: A pilot study investigating the influence of adult attachment styles on staff psychological mindedness and therapeutic relationships. *Journal of Clinical Psychology, 64,* 355–363.

Bick, J., & Dozier, M. (2013). The effectiveness of an attachment-based intervention in promoting foster mothers' sensitivity toward foster infants. *Infant Mental Health Journal, 34,* 95–103.

Bick, J., Palmwood, E. N., Zajac, L., Simons, R., & Dozier, M. (2019). Early parenting intervention and adverse family environments affect neural function in middle childhood. *Biological Psychiatry, 85,* 326–335.

Bindman, S. W., Pomerantz, E. M., & Roisman, G. I. (2015). Do children's executive functions account for associations between early autonomy-supportive parenting and achievement through high school? *Journal of Educational Psychology, 107,* 756–770.

Birgegard, A., & Granqvist, P. (2004). The correspondence between attachment to parents and God: Three experiments using subliminal separation cues. *Personality and Social Psychology Bulletin, 30*, 1122–1135.

Biringen, Z., Brown, D., Donaldson, L., Green, S., Krcmarik, S., & Lovas, G. (2000). Adult Attachment Interview: Linkages with dimensions of emotional availability for mothers and their prekindergarteners. *Attachment and Human Development, 2*, 188–202.

Birnbaum, G. E., Reis, H. T., Mikulincer, M., Gillath, O., & Orpaz, A. (2006). When sex is more than just sex: Attachment orientations, sexual experience, and relationship quality. *Journal of Personality and Social Psychology, 91*, 929–943.

Black, S., Hardy, G., Turpin, G., & Parry, G. (2005). Self-reported attachment styles and therapeutic orientation of therapists and their relationship with reported general alliance quality and problems in therapy. *Psychology and Psychotherapy, 78*, 363–377.

Blake Helms, C., Turan, J. M., Atkins, G., Kempf, M.-C., Clay, O. J., Raper, J. L., . . . Turan, B. (2017). Interpersonal mechanisms contributing to the association between HIV-related internalized stigma and medication adherence. *AIDS and Behavior, 21*, 238–247.

Blatt, S. J., Stayner, D. A., Auerbach, J. S., & Behrends, R. S. (1996). Change in object and self-representations in long-term, intensive, inpatient treatment of seriously disturbed adolescents and young adults. *Psychiatry, 59*, 82–107.

Bo, S., Sharp, C., Beck, E., Pedersen, J., Gondan, M., & Simonsen, E. (2017). First empirical evaluation of outcomes for mentalization-based group therapy for adolescents with BPD. *Personality Disorders: Theory, Research, and Treatment, 8*, 396–401.

Boag, E. M., & Carnelley, K. B. (2012). Self-reported discrimination and discriminatory behavior: The role of attachment security. *British Journal of Social Psychology, 51*, 393–403.

Boag, E. M., & Carnelley, K. B. (2016). Attachment and prejudice: The mediating role of empathy. *British Journal of Social Psychology, 55*, 337–356.

Bodenmann, G. (1997). Dyadic coping: A systemic-transactional view of stress and coping among couples: Theory and empirical findings. *European Review of Applied Psychology, 47*, 137–141.

Boelen, P. A., de Keijser, J., van den Hout, M. A., & van den Bout, J. (2007). Treatment of complicated grief: A comparison between cognitive-behavioral therapy and supportive counseling. *Journal of Consulting and Clinical Psychology, 75*, 277–284.

Bogaert, A. F., & Sadava, S. (2002). Adult attachment and sexual behavior. *Personal Relationships, 9*, 191–204.

Bohlin, G., Hagekull, B., & Rydell, A. M. (2000). Attachment and social functioning: A longitudinal study from infancy to middle childhood. *Social Development, 9*, 24–39.

Booth-LaForce, C., Groh, A. M., Burchinal, M. R., Roisman, G. I., Owen, M. T., & Cox, M. J. (2014). Caregiving and contextual sources of continuity and change in attachment security from infancy to late adolescence. *Monographs of the Society for Research in Child Development, 79*, 67–84.

Booth-LaForce, C., Kelly, J. F., Spieker, S. J., & Zuckerman, T. G. (2003). Toddlers' attachment security to child-care providers: The Safe and Secure Scale. *Early Education and Development, 14*, 83–100.

Booth-LaForce, C., & Roisman, G. I. (2021). Stability and change in attachment security. In R. A. Thompson, J. A. Simpson, & L. J. Berlin (Eds.), *Attachment: The fundamental questions* (pp. 154–160). Guilford Press.

Bordin, E. S. (1979). The generalizability of the psychoanalytic concept of the working alliance. *Psychotherapy, 16*, 252–260.

Borelli, J. L., Gaskin, G., Smiley, P., Chung, D., Shahar, B., & Bosmans, G. (2021, April 15). Multisystem physiological reactivity during help-seeking for attachment needs in school-aged children: Differences as a function of attachment. *Attachment and Human Development.* [Epub ahead of print].

Borelli, J. L., Lai, J., Smiley, P. A., Kerr, M. L., Buttitta, K., Hecht, H. K., & Rasmussen, H. F. (2021). Higher maternal reflective functioning is associated with toddlers' adaptive emotion regulation. *Infant Mental Health Journal, 42*, 473–487.

Borelli, J. L., Sbarra, D. A., & Mehl, M. (2019). Convergence of naïve coders and participant report ratings of attachment to a former partner: When we should be me. *Journal of Social and Personal Relationships, 36*, 977–999.

Borelli, J. L., Sbarra, D. A., Snavely, J. E., McMakin, D. L., Coffey, J. K., Ruiz, S. K., . . . Chung, S. Y. (2014). With or without you: Preliminary evidence that attachment avoidance predicts non-deployed spouses' reactions to relationship challenges during deployment. *Professional Psychology: Research and Practice, 45*, 478–487.

Bosman, R. J., Zee, M., de Jong, P. F., & Koomen, H. M. Y. (2021). Using relationship-focused reflection to improve teacher–child relationships and teachers' student-specific self-efficacy. *Journal of School Psychology, 87*, 28–47.

Bosmans, G., Bowles, D. P., Dewitte, M., De Winter, S., & Braet, C. (2014). An experimental evaluation of the State Adult Attachment Measure: The influence of attachment primes on the content of state attachment representations. *Journal of Experimental Psychopathology, 5*, 134–150.

Bosquet, M., & Egeland, B. (2001). Associations among maternal depressive symptomatology, state of mind, and parent and child behaviors: Implications for attachment-based interventions. *Attachment and Human Development, 3*, 173–199.

Bourassa, K. J., Ruiz, J. M., & Sbarra, D. A. (2019). The impact of physical proximity and attachment working models on cardiovascular reactivity: Comparing mental activation and romantic partner presence. *Psychophysiology, 56*, 1–12.

Bowlby, J. (1944). Forty-four juvenile thieves: Their characters and home life. *International Journal of Psychoanalysis, 25*, 19–52, 107–127.

Bowlby, J. (1958). The nature of the child's tie to his mother. *International Journal of Psychoanalysis, 39*, 350–373.

Bowlby, J. (1973). *Attachment and loss: Vol. 2. Separation: Anxiety and anger.* Basic Books.

Bowlby, J. (1979). *The making and breaking of affectional bonds.* Tavistock.

Bowlby, J. (1980). *Attachment and loss: Vol. 3. Sadness and depression.* Basic Books.

Bowlby, J. (1982). *Attachment and loss: Vol. 1. Attachment* (2nd ed.). Basic Books. (Original work published 1969)

Bowlby, J. (1988). *A secure base: Clinical applications of attachment theory.* Routledge.

Bowlby, J. (1990). *Charles Darwin: A new life.* Norton.

Bowles, D. P., & Meyer, B. (2008). Attachment priming and avoidant personality features as predictors of social-evaluation biases. *Journal of Personality Disorders, 22*, 72–88.

Bradshaw, M., & Kent, B. V. (2018). Prayer, attachment to God, and changes in psychological well-being in later life. *Journal of Aging and Health, 30*, 667–691.

Braun, M., Hales, S., Gilad, L., Mikulincer, M., Rydall, A., & Rodin, G. (2012). Caregiving styles and attachment orientations in couples facing advanced cancer. *Psycho-Oncology, 21*, 935–943.

Brennan, K. A., Clark, C. L., & Shaver, P. R. (1998). Self-report measurement of adult romantic attachment: An integrative overview. In J. A. Simpson & W. S. Rholes (Eds.), *Attachment theory and close relationships* (pp. 46–76). Guilford Press.

Brenning, K. M., Soenens, B., Braet, C., & Bal, S. (2012a). The role of parenting and mother–adolescent attachment in the intergenerational similarity of internalizing symptoms. *Journal of Youth and Adolescence, 41*, 802–816.

Brenning, K. M., Soenens, B., Braet, C., & Bosmans, G. (2012b). Attachment and depressive symptoms in middle childhood and early adolescence: Testing the validity of the emotion regulation model of attachment. *Personal Relationships, 19*, 445–464.

Bretherton, I. (1995). A communication perspective on attachment relationships and internal working models. *Monographs of the Society for Research in Child Development, 60*, 310–329.

Brewer, M. B. (2001). The many faces of social identity: Implications for political psychology. *Political Psychology, 22*, 115–125.

Brewer, M. B. (2007). The importance of being we: Human nature and intergroup relations. *American Psychologist, 62*, 728–738.

Brock, R. L., & Lawrence, E. (2014). Intrapersonal interpersonal and contextual risk factors for overprovision of partner support in marriage. *Journal of Family Psychology, 28*, 54–64.

Brooks, K. P., Robles, T. F., & Dunkel Schetter, C. (2011). Adult attachment and cortisol responses to discussions with a romantic partner. *Personal Relationships, 18*, 302–320.

Brubacher, L. L. (2018). *Stepping into emotionally focused couple therapy: Key ingredients of change.* Routledge.

Brubacher, L. L., & Wiebe, S. A. (2019). Process-research to practice in emotionally focused couple therapy: A map for reflective practice. *Journal of Family Psychotherapy, 30*, 292–313.

Brumbaugh, C. C., & Fraley, R. C. (2007). Transference of attachment patterns: How important relationships influence feelings toward novel people. *Personal Relationships, 14*, 513–530.

Bryant, R. A., & Bali, A. (2018). Activating attachment representations impact how we retrieve autobiographical memories. *Memory, 26*, 462–467.

Bryant, R. A., & Chan, L. (2015). Thinking of attachments reduces noradrenergic stress response. *Psychoneuroendocrinology, 60*, 39–45.

Bryant, R. A., & Chan, L. (2017). Activating attachment representations during memory retrieval modulates intrusive traumatic memories. *Consciousness and Cognition, 55*, 197–204.

Bryant, R. A., & Datta, S. (2019). Reconsolidating intrusive distressing memories by thinking of attachment figures. *Clinical Psychological Science, 7*, 1249–1256.

Bryant, R. A., & Foord, R. (2016). Activating attachments reduces memories of traumatic images. *PLOS ONE, 11*, Article e0162550.

Bryant, R. A., & Hutanamon, T. (2018). Activating attachments enhances heart rate variability. *PLOS ONE, 13*, Article e0151747.

Burchinal, M. R., Peisner-Feinberg, E., Pianta, R., & Howes, C. (2002). Development of academic skills from preschool through second grade: Family and classroom predictors of developmental trajectories. *Journal of School Psychology, 40*, 415–436.

Burge, D., Hammen, C., Davila, J., Daley, S. E., Paley, B., Herzberg, D., & Lindberg, N. (1997). Attachment cognitions and college and work functioning two years later in late adolescent women. *Journal of Youth and Adolescence, 26*, 285–301.

Burgess Moser, M., Johnson, S. M., Dalgleish, T. L., Lafontaine, M.-F., Wiebe, S. A., & Tasca, G. A. (2016). Changes in relationship-specific attachment in emotionally focused couple therapy. *Journal of Marital and Family Therapy, 42*, 231–245.

Burgess Moser, M., Johnson, S. M., Dalgleish, T. L., Wiebe, S. A., & Tasca, G. A. (2018). The impact of blamer-softening on romantic attachment in emotionally focused couples therapy. *Journal of Marital and Family Therapy, 44*, 640–654.

Burke, M. J., & Day, R. R. (1986). A cumulative study

of the effectiveness of managerial training. *Journal of Applied Psychology, 71*, 232–245.

Burkhart, M. L., Borelli, J. L., Rasmussen, H. F., Brody, R., & Sbarra, D. A. (2017). Parental mentalizing as an indirect link between attachment anxiety and parenting satisfaction. *Journal of Family Psychology, 31*, 203–213.

Burlingame, G. M., Fuhriman, A., & Johnson, J. E. (2001). Cohesion in group psychotherapy. *Psychotherapy, 38*, 373–379.

Burlingame, G. M., McClendon, D. T., & Yang, C. (2018). Cohesion in group therapy: A meta-analysis. *Psychotherapy, 55*, 384–398.

Butler, T. L., McKimmie, B. M., & Haslam, S. A. (2019). The approach-avoidance dilemma at the heart of group-based support: Evidence that group identification increases willingness to seek support at the same time that identity-based support threat reduces it. *European Journal of Social Psychology, 49*, 31–46.

Buyse, E., Verschueren, K., & Doumen, S. (2011). Preschoolers' attachment to mother and risk for adjustment problems in kindergarten: Can teachers make a difference? *Social Development, 20*, 33–50.

Byrd, K. R., & Boe, A. (2001). The correspondence between attachment dimensions and prayer in college students. *International Journal for the Psychology of Religion, 11*, 9–24.

Byrd, K. R., Patterson, C. L., & Turchik, J. A. (2010). Working alliance as a mediator of client attachment dimensions and psychotherapy outcome. *Psychotherapy, 47*, 631–636.

Byrne, Z., Albert, L., Manning, S., & Desir, R. (2017). Relational models and engagement: An attachment theory perspective. *Journal of Managerial Psychology, 32*, 30–44.

Caldwell, J. G., & Shaver, P. R. (2012). Exploring the cognitive-emotional pathways between adult attachment and ego-resiliency. *Individual Differences Research, 10*, 141–152.

Caldwell, J. G., Shaver, P. R., Li, C., & Minzenberg, M. J. (2011). Childhood maltreatment, adult attachment, and depression as predictors of parental self-efficacy in at-risk mothers. *Journal of Aggression, Maltreatment and Trauma, 20*, 595–616.

California Evidence-Based Clearinghouse Rating of ABC. (2014, September). Retrieved from *www.cebc4cw.org/program/attachment-and-biobehavioral-catch-up*.

California Evidence-Based Clearinghouse Rating of CPP. (2019, July). Retrieved from *www.cebc4cw.org/program/child-parent-psychotherapy*.

Callaci, M., Vaillancourt-Morel, M.-P., Labonté, T., Brassard, A., Tremblay, N., & Péloquin, K. (2021). Attachment insecurities predicting romantic disengagement over the course of couple therapy in a naturalistic setting. *Couple and Family Psychology: Research and Practice, 10*, 54–69.

Cameron, K. (2012). *Positive leadership*. Berrett-Koehler.

Campa, M. I., Hazan, C., & Wolfe, J. E. (2009). The form and function of attachment behavior in the daily lives of young adults. *Social Development, 18*, 288–304.

Campbell, L., Simpson, J. A., Boldry, J., & Kashy, D. A. (2005). Perceptions of conflict and support in romantic relationships: The role of attachment anxiety. *Journal of Personality and Social Psychology, 88*, 510–531.

Canterberry, M., & Gillath, O. (2013). Neural evidence for a multifaceted model of attachment security. *International Journal of Psychophysiology, 88*, 232–240.

Captari, L. E., Hook, J. N., Hoyt, W., Davis, D. E., McElroy-Heltzel, S. E., & Worthington, E. L., Jr. (2018). Integrating clients' religion and spirituality within psychotherapy: A comprehensive meta-analysis. *Journal of Clinical Psychology, 74*, 1938–1951.

Carcione, A., Riccardi, I., Bilotta, E., Leone, L., Pedone, R., Conti, L., . . . Semerari, A. (2019). Metacognition as a predictor of improvements in personality disorders. *Frontiers in Psychology, 10*, Article 170.

Carlson, E. A., Sroufe, L. A., & Egeland, B. (2004). The construction of experience: A longitudinal study of representation and behavior. *Child Development, 75*, 66–83.

Carmichael, C. L., Goldberg, M. H., & Coyle, M. A. (2021). Security-based differences in touch behavior and its relational benefits. *Social Psychological and Personality Sciences, 12*, 550–560.

Carnelley, K. B., Bejinaru, M.-M., Otway, L., Baldwin, D. S., & Rowe, A. C. (2018). Effects of repeated attachment security priming in outpatients with primary depressive disorders. *Journal of Affective Disorders, 234*, 201–206.

Carnelley, K. B., Israel, S., & Brennan, K. (2007). The role of attachment in influencing reactions to manipulated feedback from romantic partners. *European Journal of Social Psychology, 37*, 968–986.

Carnelley, K. B., Otway, L. J., & Rowe, A. C. (2016). The effects of attachment priming on depressed and anxious mood. *Clinical Psychological Science, 4*, 433–450.

Carnelley, K. B., & Rowe, A. C. (2007). Repeated priming of attachment security influences immediate and later views of self and relationships. *Personal Relationships, 14*, 307–320.

Carnelley, K. B., & Rowe, A. C. (2010). Priming a sense of security: What goes through people's minds. *Journal of Social and Personal Relationships, 27*, 253–261.

Caron, E. B., Bernard, K., & Dozier, M. (2018). *In vivo* feedback predicts parent behavior change in the attachment and biobehavioral catch-up intervention. *Journal of Clinical Child and Adolescent Psychology, 47*, S35–S46.

Caron, E. B., & Dozier, M. (2019). Effects of fidelity-focused consultation on clinicians' implementation: An exploratory multiple baseline design. *Administration and Policy in Mental Health and Mental Health Services Research, 46*, 445–457.

Caron, E. B., Weston-Lee, P., Haggerty, D., & Dozier, M. (2016). Community implementation outcomes of Attachment and Biobehavioral Catch-Up. *Child Abuse and Neglect, 53*, 128–137.

Carron, A. V., Brawley, L. R., & Widmeyer, W. N. (1998). The measurement of cohesiveness in sport groups. In J. L. Duda (Ed.), *Advances in sport and exercise psychology measurement* (pp. 213–226). Fitness Information Technology.

Carvallo, M., & Gabriel, S. (2006). No man is an island: The need to belong and dismissing avoidant attachment style. *Personality and Social Psychology Bulletin, 32*, 697–709.

Carver, C. S., & Scheier, M. F. (2012). A model of behavioral self-regulation. In P. A. M. Van Lange, A. W. Kruglanski, & E. T. Higgins (Eds.), *Handbook of theories of social psychology* (Vol. 1, pp. 505–525). SAGE.

Cash, A. H., Ansari, A., Grimm, K. J., & Pianta, R. C. (2019). Power of two: The impact of 2 years of high quality teacher child interactions. *Early Education and Development, 30*, 60–81.

Casper, W. J., & Buffardi, L. C. (2004). Work-life benefits and job pursuit intentions: The role of anticipated organizational support. *Journal of Vocational Behavior, 65*, 391–410.

Cassibba, R., Castoro, G., Costantino, E., Sette, G., & van IJzendoorn, M. H. (2015). Enhancing maternal sensitivity and infant attachment security with video feedback: An exploratory study in Italy. *Infant Mental Health Journal, 36*, 53–61.

Cassibba, R., Papagna, S., Calabrese, M. T., Costantino, E., Paterno, A., & Granqvist, P. (2014). The role of attachment to God in secular and religious/spiritual ways of coping with a serious disease. *Mental Health, Religion and Culture, 17*, 252–261.

Cassibba, R., Van IJzendoorn, M. H., & D'Odorico, L. (2000). Attachment and play in child care centers: Reliability and validity of the Attachment Q-sort for mothers and professional caregivers in Italy. *International Journal of Behavioral Development, 24*, 241–255.

Cassidy, J. (1994). Emotion regulation: Influences of attachment relationships. *Monographs of the Society for Research in Child Development, 59*, 228–283.

Cassidy, J. (2016). The nature of the child's ties. In J. Cassidy & P. R. Shaver (Eds.), *Handbook of attachment: Theory, research, and clinical applications* (3rd ed., pp. 3–24). Guilford Press.

Cassidy, J., Brett, B. E., Gross, J. T., Stern, J. A., Martin, D. R., Mohr, J. J., & Woodhouse, S. S. (2017). Circle of Security–Parenting: A randomized controlled trial in Head Start. *Development and Psychopathology, 29*, 651–673.

Cassidy, J., Jones, J. D., & Shaver, P. R. (2013). Contributions of attachment theory and research: A framework for future research, translation, and policy. *Development and Psychopathology, 25*, 1415–1434.

Cassidy, J., & Kobak, R. R. (1988). Avoidance and its relationship with other defensive processes. In J. Belsky & T. Nezworski (Eds.), *Clinical implications of attachment* (pp. 300–323). Erlbaum.

Cassidy, J., Poehlmann, J., & Shaver, P. R. (2010). An attachment perspective on incarcerated parents and their children. *Attachment and Human Development, 12*, 285–288.

Cassidy, J., & Shaver, P. R. (Eds.). (2016). *Handbook of attachment: Theory, research, and clinical applications* (3rd ed.). Guilford Press.

Cassidy, J., Shaver, P. R., Mikulincer, M., & Lavy, S. (2009). Experimentally induced security influences responses to psychological pain. *Journal of Social and Clinical Psychology, 28*, 463–478.

Cassidy, J., Stern, J. A., Mikulincer, M., Martin, D. R., & Shaver, P. R. (2018). Influences on care for others: Attachment security, personal suffering, and similarity between helper and care recipient. *Personality and Social Psychology Bulletin, 44*, 574–588.

Cassidy, J., Woodhouse, S. S., Cooper, G., Hoffman, K., Powell, B., & Rodenberg, M. (2005). Examination of the precursors of infant attachment security: Implications for early intervention and intervention research. In L. J. Berlin, Y. Ziv, L. Amaya-Jackson, & M. T. Greenberg (Eds.), *Enhancing early attachments: Theory, research, intervention, and policy* (pp. 34–60). Guilford Press.

Cassidy, J., Woodhouse, S. S., Sherman, L. J., Stupica, B., & Lejuez, C. W. (2011). Enhancing infant attachment security: An examination of treatment efficacy and differential susceptibility. *Development and Psychopathology, 23*, 131–148.

Cassidy, J., Ziv, Y., Stupica, B., Sherman, L. J., Butler, H., Karfgin, A., . . . Powell, B. (2010). Enhancing attachment security in the infants of women in a jail-diversion program. *Attachment and Human Development, 12*, 333–353.

Castano, E., & Dechesne, M. (2005). On defeating death: Group reification and social identification as immortality strategies. *European Review of Social Psychology, 16*, 221–255.

Castano, E., Yzerbyt, V., Paladino, M.-P., & Sacchi, S. (2002). I belong, therefore, I exist: Ingroup identification, ingroup entitativity, and ingroup bias. *Personality and Social Psychology Bulletin, 28*, 135–143.

Chandler, C. K. (2012). *Animal assisted therapy in counseling* (2nd ed.). Routledge.

Chang, S. J., Lee, J., An, H., Hong, W.-H., & Lee, J. Y. (2021). Animal-assisted therapy as an intervention for older adults: A systematic review and meta-analysis to guide evidence-based practice. *Worldviews on Evidence-Based Nursing, 18*, 60–67.

Charles-Sire, V., Guéguen, N., Pascual, A., & Meineri, S. (2012). Words as environmental cues: The effect of the word "loving" on compliance to a blood donation request. *Journal of Psychology: Interdisciplinary and Applied, 146*, 455–470.

Charles-Sire, V., Stefan, J., & Guéguen, N. (2016). Single exposure to the word "Loving" and implicit helping behavior. *Social Influence, 11*, 1–6.

Chen, E. C., & Mallinckrodt, B. (2002). Attachment, group attraction, and self–other agreement in interpersonal circumplex problems and perceptions of group members. *Group Dynamics, 6*, 311–324.

Cheng, H.-L., McDermott, R. C., & Lopez, F. G. (2015). Mental health, self-stigma, and help-seeking intentions among emerging adults: An attachment perspective. *Counseling Psychologist, 43*, 463–487.

Cheng, S. T., & Kwan, K. W. (2008). Attachment dimensions and contingencies of self-worth: The moderating role of culture. *Personality and Individual Differences, 45*, 509–514.

Cherry, M. G., Fletcher, I., Berridge, D., & O'Sullivan, H. (2018). Do doctors' attachment styles and emotional intelligence influence patients' emotional expressions in primary care consultations?: An exploratory study using multilevel analysis. *Patient Education and Counseling, 101*, 659–664.

Chida, Y., & Steptoe, A. (2010). Greater cardiovascular responses to laboratory mental stress are associated with poor subsequent cardiovascular risk status: A meta-analysis of prospective evidence. *Hypertension, 55*, 1026–1032.

Chiesa, M., Luyten, P., & Fonagy, P. (2021). Two-year follow-up and changes in reflective functioning in specialist and nonspecialist treatment models for personality disorder. *Personality Disorders: Theory, Research, and Treatment, 12*, 249–260.

Chong, S., Huang, Y., & Chang, C.-H. D. (2020). Supporting interdependent telework employees: A moderated-mediation model linking daily COVID-19 task setbacks to next-day work withdrawal. *Journal of Applied Psychology, 105*, 1408–1422.

Chopik, W. J. (2015). Relational attachment and ethical workplace decisions: The mediating role of emotional burnout. *Personality and Individual Differences, 75*, 160–164.

Chopik, W. J., Moors, A. C., & Edelstein, R. S. (2014). Maternal nurturance predicts decreases in attachment avoidance in emerging adulthood. *Journal of Research in Personality, 53*, 47–53.

Cicchetti, D., Rogosch, F. A., & Toth, S. L. (2000). The efficacy of toddler–parent psychotherapy for fostering cognitive development in offspring. *Journal of Abnormal Child Psychology, 28*, 135–148.

Cicchetti, D., Rogosch, F. A., & Toth, S. L. (2006). Fostering secure attachment in infants in maltreating families through preventive interventions. *Development and Psychopathology, 18*, 623–649.

Cicchetti, D., Rogosch, F. A., & Toth, S. L. (2011). The effects of child maltreatment and polymorphisms of the serotonin transporter and dopamine D4 receptor genes on infant attachment and intervention efficacy. *Development and Psychopathology, 23*, 357–372.

Cicchetti, D., Rogosch, F. A., Toth, S. L., & Sturge-Apple, M. L. (2011). Normalizing the development of cortisol regulation in maltreated infants through preventive interventions. *Development and Psychopathology, 23*, 789–800.

Ciechanowski, P. S., Katon, W. J., Russo, J. E., & Walker, E. A. (2001). The patient–provider relationship: Attachment theory and adherence to treatment in diabetes. *American Journal of Psychiatry, 158*, 29–35.

Ciechanowski, P. S., Russo, J., Katon, W., Von Korff, M., Ludman, E., Lin, E., . . . Bush, T. (2004). Influence of patient attachment style on self-care and outcomes in diabetes. *Psychosomatic Medicine, 66*, 720–728.

Clark, M. S., Greenberg, A., Hill, E., Lemay, E. P., Clark-Polner, E., & Roosth, D. (2011). Heightened interpersonal security diminishes the monetary value of possessions. *Journal of Experimental Social Psychology, 47*, 359–364.

Coan, J. A., Kasle, S., Jackson, A., Schaefer, H. S., & Davidson, R. J. (2013). Mutuality and the social regulation of neural threat responding. *Attachment and Human Development, 15*, 303–315.

Coan, J. A., Schaefer, H. S., & Davidson, R. J. (2006). Lending a hand: Social regulation of the neural response to threat. *Psychological Science, 17*, 1032–1039.

Cobb, R. J., & Davila, J. (2009). Internal working models and change. In J. Obegi & E. Berant (Eds.), *Clinical applications of adult attachment* (pp. 209–234). Guilford Press.

Coffey, J. K., Xia, M., & Fosco, G. M. (2022). When do adolescents feel loved?: A daily within-person study of parent–adolescent relations. *Emotion, 22*, 861–873.

Cohen, E., Zerach, G., & Solomon, Z. (2011). The implication of combat-induced stress reaction, PTSD, and attachment in parenting among war veterans. *Journal of Family Psychology, 25*, 688–698.

Cohen, N. J., Muir, E., Lojkasek, M., Muir, R., Parker, C. J., Barwick, M., & Brown, M. (1999). Watch, wait, and wonder: Testing the effectiveness of a new approach to mother–infant psychotherapy. *Infant Mental Health Journal, 20*, 429–451.

Cohen, S., Janicki-Deverts, D., Turner, R. B., & Doyle, W. J. (2015). Does hugging provide stress-buffering social support?: A study of susceptibility to upper respiratory infection and illness. *Psychological Science, 26*, 135–147.

Collins, A. M., & Loftus, E. F. (1975). A spreading-activation theory of semantic processing. *Psychological Review, 82*, 407–428.

Collins, D. B., & Holton, E. F., III. (2004). The effectiveness of managerial leadership development programs: A meta-analysis of studies from 1982 to 2001. *Human Resource Development Quarterly, 15*, 217–248.

Collins, N. L. (1996). Working models of attachment: Implications for explanation, emotion, and behavior. *Journal of Personality and Social Psychology, 71*, 810–832.

Collins, N. L., Cooper, M., Albino, A., & Allard, L. (2002). Psychosocial vulnerability from adolescence to adulthood: A prospective study of attachment style differences in relationship functioning and partner choice. *Journal of Personality, 70*, 965–1008.

Collins, N. L., & Feeney, B. C. (2000). A safe haven: An attachment theory perspective on support seeking and caregiving in intimate relationships. *Journal of Personality and Social Psychology, 78*, 1053–1073.

Collins, N. L., & Feeney, B. C. (2004). Working models of attachment shape perceptions of social support: Evidence from experimental and observational studies. *Journal of Personality and Social Psychology, 87*, 363–383.

Collins, N. L., Ford, M. B., Guichard, A. C., & Allard, L. M. (2006). Working models of attachment and attribution processes in intimate relationships. *Personality and Social Psychology Bulletin, 32*, 201–219.

Collins, N. L., Ford, M. B., Guichard, A. C., Kane, H. S., & Feeney, B. C. (2010). Responding to need in intimate relationships: Social support and caregiving processes in couples. In M. Mikulincer & P. R. Shaver (Eds.), *Prosocial motives, emotions, and behavior: The better angels of our nature* (pp. 367–389). American Psychological Association.

Collins, N. L., & Read, S. J. (1990). Adult attachment, working models, and relationship quality in dating couples. *Journal of Personality and Social Psychology, 58*, 644–663.

Collins, N. L., & Read, S. J. (1994). Cognitive representations of attachment: The structure and function of working models. In K. Bartholomew & D. Perlman (Eds.), *Advances in personal relationships: Attachment processes in adulthood* (Vol. 5, pp. 53–92). Jessica Kingsley.

Collins, T. J., & Gillath, O. (2012). Attachment, breakup strategies, and associated outcomes: The effects of security enhancement on the selection of breakup strategies. *Journal of Research in Personality, 46*, 210–222.

Colonnesi, C., Zeegers, M. A. J., Majdandžić, M., van Steensel, F. J. A., & Bögels, S. M. (2019). Fathers' and mothers' early mind-mindedness predicts social competence and behavior problems in childhood. *Journal of Abnormal Child Psychology, 47*, 1421–1435.

Colquitt, J. A., Conlon, D. E., Wesson, M. J., Porter, C. O., & Ng, K. Y. (2001). Justice at the millennium: A meta-analytic review of 25 years of organizational justice research. *Journal of Applied Psychology, 86*, 425–445.

Commodari, E. (2013). Preschool teacher attachment, school readiness and risk of learning difficulties. *Early Childhood Research Quarterly, 28*, 123–133.

Compare, A., Maxwell, H., Brugnera, A., Zarbo, C., Dalle Grave, R., & Tasca, G. A. (2018). Change in attachment dimensions and reflective functioning following emotionally focused group therapy for binge eating disorder. *International Journal of Group Psychotherapy, 68*, 385–406.

Conduct Problems Prevention Research Group. (2011). The effects of the Fast Track preventive intervention on the development of conduct disorder across childhood. *Child Development, 82*, 331–345.

Conger, J. A., & Kanungo, R. N. (1988). The empowerment process: Integrating theory and practice. *Academy of Management Review, 13*, 471–482.

Conradi, H. J., Dingemanse, P., Noordhof, A., Finkenauer, C., & Kamphuis, J. H. (2018). Effectiveness of the "Hold me Tight" relationship enhancement program in a self-referred and a clinician-referred sample: An emotionally focused couples therapy-based approach. *Family Process, 57*, 613–628.

Consedine, N. S., Tuck, N. L., & Fiori, K. L. (2013). Attachment and health care utilization among middle-aged and older African-descent men: Dismissiveness predicts less frequent digital rectal examination and prostate-specific antigen screening. *American Journal of Men's Health, 7*, 382–393.

Cook, C. R., Little, S. G., & Akin-Little, A. (2007). Interventions based on attachment theory: A critical analysis. *Journal of Early Childhood and Infant Psychology, 3*, 61–73.

Cook, S. W., Aten, J. D., Moore, M., Hook, J. N., & Davis, D. E. (2013). Resource loss, religiousness, health, and posttraumatic growth following Hurricane Katrina. *Mental Health, Religion and Culture, 16*, 352–366.

Cooper, G., Hoffman, K., & Powell, B. (2000). *The COS–Home Visiting-4 Intervention (COSHV4)*. Unpublished manuscript, COS International, Spokane, WA.

Cooper, G., Hoffman, K., & Powell, B. (2003). *The COS Perinatal Protocol (COS-PP)*. Unpublished manuscript, COS International, Spokane, WA.

Cooper, G., Hoffman, K., & Powell, B. (2009). *COS Parenting: A relationship-based parenting program (DVD)*. (More information at *http://circleofsecurity.com*)

Cooper, G., Hoffman, K., & Powell, B. (2017). Circle of Security in child care: Putting attachment theory into practice in preschool classrooms. *Zero to Three, 37*, 27–34.

Cooper, L. B., Bruce, A. J., Harman, M. J., & Boccaccini, M. T. (2009). Differentiated styles of attachment to God and varying religious coping efforts. *Journal of Psychology and Theology, 37*, 134–141.

Cooper, M. L., Shaver, P. R., & Collins, N. L. (1998). Attachment styles, emotion regulation, and adjustment in adolescence. *Journal of Personality and Social Psychology, 74*, 1380–1397.

Costello, A. H., Roben, C. K. P., Schein, S. S., Blake, F., & Dozier, M. (2019). Monitoring provider fidelity of a parenting intervention using observational methods. *Professional Psychology: Research and Practice, 50*, 264–271.

Costello, M. A., Nagel, A. G., Hunt, G. L., Rivens, A. J., Hazelwood, O. A., Pettit, C., & Allen, J. P. (2022). Facilitating connection to enhance college student well-being: Evaluation of an experiential group program. *American Journal of Community Psychology, 70*, 314–326.

Costello, P. C. (2013). *Attachment-based psychotherapy: Helping patients develop adaptive capacities.* American Psychological Association.

Couture-Lalande, M. -E., Greenman, P. S., Naaman, S., & Johnson, S. M. (2007). Emotionally focused therapy (EFT) for couples with a female partner who suffers from breast cancer: An exploratory study. *Psycho-Oncologie, 1*, 257–264.

Cowan, P. A., & Cowan, C. P. (2002). Interventions as tests of family systems theories: Marital and family relationships in children's development and psychopathology. *Development and Psychopathology, 14*, 731–759.

Coyne, A. E., Constantino, M. J., Ravitz, P., & McBride, C. (2018). The interactive effect of patient attachment and social support on early alliance quality in interpersonal psychotherapy. *Journal of Psychotherapy Integration, 28*, 46–59.

Craik, K. (1943). *The nature of explanation.* Cambridge University Press.

Crangle, C. J., Torbit, L. A., Ferguson, S. E., & Hart, T. L. (2020). Dyadic coping mediates the effects of attachment on quality of life among couples facing ovarian cancer. *Journal of Behavioral Medicine, 43*, 564–575.

Crasta, D., Rogge, R. D., Maniaci, M. R., & Reis, H. T. (2021). Toward an optimized measure of perceived partner responsiveness: Development and validation of the perceived responsiveness and insensitivity scale. *Psychological Assessment, 33*, 338–355.

Creasey, G. (2014). Conflict-management behavior in dual trauma couples. *Psychological Trauma: Theory, Research, Practice, and Policy, 6*, 232–239.

Crocker, J., & Canevello, A. (2015). Relationships and the self: Egosystem and ecosystem. In M. Mikulincer, P. R. Shaver, J. Simpson, & J. F. Dovidio (Eds.), *Handbook of personality and social psychology: Vol. 3. Interpersonal relationships and group processes* (pp. 93–116). American Psychological Association.

Cross, E. J., Overall, N. C., Low, R. S. T., & Henderson, A. M. E. (2021). Relationship problems, agreement and bias in perceptions of partners' parental responsiveness, and family functioning. *Journal of Family Psychology, 35*, 510–522.

Crowell, J. A., & Feldman, S. (1989). Assessment of mothers' working models of relationships: Some clinical implications. *Infant Mental Health Journal, 10*, 173–184.

Crowell, J. A., & Feldman, S. (1991). Mothers' working models of attachment relationships and mother and child behavior during separation and reunion. *Developmental Psychology, 27*, 597–605.

Crowell, J. A., Fraley, R. C., & Roisman, G. I. (2016). Measurement of individual differences in adult attachment. In J. Cassidy & P. R. Shaver (Eds.), *Handbook of attachment: Theory, research, and clinical applications* (3rd ed., pp. 598–638). Guilford Press.

Crowell, J. A., Treboux, D., Gao, Y., Fyffe, C., Pan, H., & Waters, E. (2002). Assessing secure base behavior in adulthood: Development of a measure, links to adult attachment representations, and relations to couples' communication and reports of relationships. *Developmental Psychology, 38*, 679–693.

Crowell, J. A., Warner, D. E., Davis, C. R., Marraccini, M., & Dearing, E. (2010). The influence of childhood adversity on mothers' behavior with preschoolers: Role of maternal attachment coherence, dissociative symptoms, and marital behaviors. *Research in Human Development, 7*, 274–291.

Cuevas, A. G., O'Brien, K., & Saha, S. (2019). Can patient-centered communication reduce the effects of medical mistrust on patients' decision making? *Health Psychology, 38*, 325–333.

Cuijpers, P., Donker, T., Weissman, M. M., Ravitz, P., & Cristea, I. A. (2016). Interpersonal psychotherapy for mental health problems: A comprehensive meta-analysis. *American Journal of Psychiatry, 173*, 680–687.

Cuijpers, P., Geraedts, A. S., van Oppen, P., Andersson, G., Markowitz, J. C., & van Straten, A. (2011). Interpersonal psychotherapy for depression: A meta-analysis. *American Journal of Psychiatry, 168*, 581–592.

Cuijpers, P., van Straten, A., Andersson, G., & van Oppen, P. (2008). Psychotherapy for depression in adults: A meta-analysis of comparative outcome studies. *Journal of Consulting and Clinical Psychology, 76*, 909–922.

Cummings, E. M., & Davies, P. T. (2002). Effects of marital conflict on children: Recent advances and emerging themes in process-oriented research. *Journal of Child Psychology and Psychiatry, 43*, 31–63.

Cusack, O. (1988). *Pets and mental health.* Haworth Press.

Cutrona, C. E., Bodenmann, G., Randall, A. K., Clavél, F. D., & Johnson, M. (2018). Stress, dyadic coping, and social support: Moving toward integration. In A. L. Vangelisti & D. Perlman (Eds.), *The Cambridge handbook of personal relationships* (pp. 341–352). Cambridge University Press.

Cutrona, C. E., & Russell, D. (1990). Type of social support and specific stress: Toward a theory of optimal matching. In I. G. Sarason, B. R. Sarason, & G. R. Pierce (Eds.), *Social support: An interactional view* (pp. 319–366). Wiley.

Cutrona, C. E., Russell, D. W., Hessling, R. M., Brown, P. A., & Murry, V. (2000). Direct and moderating effects of community context on the psychological well-being of African American women. *Journal of Personality and Social Psychology, 79*, 1088–1101.

Cuyvers, B., Verhees, M. W. F. T., van IJzendoorn, M., Bakermans-Kranenburg, M., Rowe, A., Cuelemans, E., . . . Bosmans, G. (2023). The effect of attachment priming on state attachment security in middle childhood: The moderating roles of trait attachment and state attachment volatility. *Journal of Early Adolescence, 43*, 164–193.

Cyr, C., Dubois-Comtois, K., Paquette, D., Lopez, L., & Bigras, M. (2022). An attachment-based parental capacity assessment to orient decision-making in child protection cases: A randomized control trial. *Child Maltreatment, 27*, 66–77.

Dagan, O., Asok, A., Steele, H., Steele, M., & Bernard, K. (2018). Attachment security moderates the link between adverse childhood experiences and cellular aging. *Development and Psychopathology, 30*, 1211–1223.

Dahl, R. E., & El-Sheikh, M. (2007). Considering sleep in a family context: Introduction to the special issue. *Journal of Family Psychology, 21*, 1–3.

Dalgleish, T. L., Johnson, S. M., Burgess Moser, M., Lafontaine, M.-F., Wiebe, S. A., & Tasca, G. A. (2015). Predicting change in marital satisfaction throughout emotionally focused couple therapy. *Journal of Marital and Family Therapy, 41*, 276–291.

Dalgleish, T. L., Johnson, S. M., Burgess Moser, M., Wiebe, S. A., & Tasca, G. A. (2015). Predicting key change events in emotionally focused couple therapy. *Journal of Marital and Family Therapy, 41*, 260–275.

Dalton, E. J., Greenman, P. S., Classen, C. C., & Johnson, S. M. (2013). Nurturing connections in the aftermath of childhood trauma: A randomized controlled trial of emotionally focused couple therapy for female survivors of childhood abuse. *Couple and Family Psychology: Research and Practice, 2*, 209–221.

Daly, K. D., & Mallinckrodt, B. (2009). Experienced therapists' approach to psychotherapy for adults with attachment avoidance or attachment anxiety. *Journal of Counseling Psychology, 56*, 549–563.

Dandeneau, M. L., & Johnson, S. M. (1994). Facilitating intimacy: Interventions and effects. *Journal of Marital and Family Therapy, 20*, 17–33.

Dandeneau, S. D., Baldwin, M. W., Baccus, J. R., Sakellaropoulo, M., & Pruessner, J. C. (2007). Cutting stress off at the pass: Reducing vigilance and responsiveness to social threat by manipulating attention. *Journal of Personality and Social Psychology, 93*, 651–666.

Danesh, J., Collins, R., Appleby, P., & Peto, R. (1998). Association of fibrinogen, C-reactive protein, albumin, or leukocyte count with coronary heart disease: Meta-analyses of prospective studies. *Journal of the American Medical Association, 279*, 1477–1482.

Daniel, S. I. F., Folke, S., Lunn, S., Gondan, M., & Poulsen, S. (2018). Mind the gap: In-session silences are associated with client attachment insecurity, therapeutic alliance, and treatment outcome. *Psychotherapy Research, 28*, 203–216.

Davidovitz, R., Mikulincer, M., Shaver, P. R., Ijzak, R., & Popper, M. (2007). Leaders as attachment figures: Their attachment orientations predict leadership-related mental representations and followers' performance and mental health. *Journal of Personality and Social Psychology, 93*, 632–650.

Davila, J., & Cobb, R. J. (2003). Predicting change in self-reported and interviewer-assessed adult attachment: Tests of the individual difference and life stress models of attachment change. *Personality and Social Psychology Bulletin, 29*, 859–870.

Davila, J., Karney, B. R., & Bradbury, T. N. (1999). Attachment change processes in the early years of marriage. *Journal of Personality and Social Psychology, 76*, 783–802.

Davila, J., & Kashy, D. (2009). Secure base processes in couples: Daily associations between support experiences and attachment security. *Journal of Family Psychology, 23*, 76–88.

Davis, C. R., Usher, N., Dearing, E., Barkai, A. R., Crowell-Doom, C., Neupert, S. D., . . . Crowell, J. A. (2014). Attachment and the metabolic syndrome in midlife: The role of interview-based discourse patterns. *Psychosomatic Medicine, 76*, 611–621.

Davis, E. B., Granqvist, P., & Sharp, C. (2021). Theistic relational spirituality: Development, dynamics, health, and transformation. *Psychology of Religion and Spirituality, 13*, 401–415.

Davis, E. B., Kimball, C. N., Aten, J. D., Hamilton, C., Andrews, B., Lemke, A., . . . Chung, J. (2019). Faith in the wake of disaster: A longitudinal qualitative study of religious attachment following a catastrophic flood. *Psychological Trauma: Theory, Research, Practice, and Policy, 11*, 578–587.

Davis, H. A. (2001). The quality and impact of relationships between elementary school students and teachers. *Contemporary Educational Psychology, 26*, 431–453.

Dawson, E., Hartwig, M., & Brimbal, L. (2015). Interviewing to elicit information: Using priming to promote disclosure. *Law and Human Behavior, 39*, 443–450.

Dawson, N. (2018). From Uganda to Baltimore to Alexandra Township: How far can Ainsworth's theory stretch? *South African Journal of Psychiatry, 24*, Article 1137.

Day, D. V. (2000). Leadership development: A review in context. *Leadership Quarterly, 11*, 581–613.

de Lange, T. (2002). Protection of mammalian telomeres. *Oncogene, 21*, 532–540.

De Meulemeester, C., Vansteelandt, K., Luyten, P., & Lowyck, B. (2018). Mentalizing as a mechanism of change in the treatment of patients with borderline personality disorder: A parallel process growth modeling approach. *Personality Disorders: Theory, Research, and Treatment, 9,* 22–29.

de Wolff, M., & van IJzendoorn, M. H. (1997). Sensitivity and attachment: A meta-analysis on parental antecedents of infant attachment. *Child Development, 68,* 571–591.

Deci, E. L., Connell, J. P., & Ryan, R. M. (1989). Self-determination in a work organization. *Journal of Applied Psychology, 74,* 580–590.

DeMarco, T. C., & Newheiser, A.-K. (2019). Attachment to groups: Relationships with group esteem, self-esteem, and investment in ingroups. *European Journal of Social Psychology, 49,* 63–75.

Deng, Y., Yan, M., Chen, H., Sun, X., Zhang, P., Zeng, X., . . . Lye, Y. (2016). Attachment security balances perspectives: Effects of security priming on highly optimistic and pessimistic explanatory styles. *Frontiers in Psychology, 7,* Article 1269.

Denton, W. H., Burleson, B. R., Clark, T. E., Rodriguez, C. P., & Hobbs, B. V. (2000). A randomized trial of emotion-focused therapy for couples in a training clinic. *Journal of Marital and Family Therapy, 26,* 65–78.

Denton, W. H., Wittenborn, A. K., & Golden, R. N. (2012). Augmenting antidepressant medication treatment of depressed women with emotionally focused therapy for couples: A randomized pilot study. *Journal of Marital and Family Therapy, 38,* 23–38.

Dessaulles, A., Johnson, S. M., & Denton, W. H. (2003). Emotion-focused therapy for couples in the treatment of depression: A pilot study. *American Journal of Family Therapy, 31,* 345–353.

Dewitte, M., & De Houwer, J. (2011). Attachment-style differences in the appraisal of the attachment figure. *European Journal of Personality, 25,* 173–183.

Dewitte, M., De Houwer, J., & Buysse, A. (2008). On the role of the implicit self-concept in adult attachment. *European Journal of Psychological Assessment, 24,* 282–289.

Dewitte, M., De Houwer, J., Goubert, L., & Buysse, A. (2010). A multi-modal approach to the study of attachment-related distress. *Biological Psychology, 85,* 149–162.

Diamond, D., Stovall-McClough, C., Clarkin, J. F., & Levy, K. N. (2003). Patient–therapist attachment in the treatment of borderline personality disorder. *Bulletin of the Menninger Clinic, 67,* 227–259.

Diamond, G. M., Boruchovitz-Zamir, R., Gat, I., & Nir-Gottlieb, O. (2019). Relationship focused therapy for sexual minority individuals and their parents. In J. Panchankis & S. Safren (Eds.), *Handbook of evidence-based mental health practice with sexual and gender minorities* (pp. 314–327). Oxford University Press.

Diamond, G. M., Boruchovitz-Zamir, R., Nir-Gotlieb, O., Gat, I., Bar-Kalifa, E., Fitoussi, P.-Y., & Katz, S. (2022). Attachment-based family therapy for sexual and gender minority young adults and their non-accepting parents. *Family Process, 61,* 530–548.

Diamond, G. M., Diamond, G. S., Levy, S., Closs, C., Ladipo, T., & Siqueland, L. (2012). Attachment-based family therapy for suicidal lesbian, gay, and bisexual adolescents: A treatment development study and open trial with preliminary findings. *Psychotherapy, 49,* 62–71.

Diamond, G. M., Shahar, B., Sabo, D., & Tsvieli, N. (2016). Attachment-based family therapy and emotion-focused therapy for unresolved anger: The role of productive emotional processing. *Psychotherapy, 53,* 34–44.

Diamond, G. S., Creed, T., Gillham, J., Gallop, R., Hamilton, J. L. (2012). Sexual trauma history does not moderate treatment outcome in attachment-based family therapy (ABFT) for adolescents with suicide ideation. *Journal of Family Psychology, 26,* 595–605.

Diamond, G. S., Diamond, G. M., & Levy, S. (2021). Attachment-based family therapy: Theory, clinical model, outcomes, and process research. *Journal of Affective Disorders, 294,* 286–295.

Diamond, G. S., Diamond, G. M., & Levy, S. A. (2014). *Attachment-based family therapy for depressed adolescents.* American Psychological Association.

Diamond, G. S., Kobak, R. R., Krauthamer Ewing, E. S., Levy, S. A., Herres, J. L., Russon, J. M., & Gallop, R. J. (2019). A randomized controlled trial: Attachment-based family and nondirective supportive treatments for youth who are suicidal. *Journal of the American Academy of Child and Adolescent Psychiatry, 58,* 721–731.

Diamond, G. S., Reis, B. F., Diamond, G. M., Siqueland, L., & Isaacs, L. (2002). Attachment-based family therapy for depressed adolescents: A treatment development study. *Journal of the American Academy of Child and Adolescent Psychiatry, 41,* 1190–1196.

Diamond, G. S., Siqueland, L., & Diamond, G. M. (2003). Attachment-based family therapy for depressed adolescents: Programmatic treatment development. *Clinical Child and Family Psychology Review, 6,* 107–127.

Diamond, G. S., Wintersteen, M. B., Brown, G. K., Diamond, G. M., Gallop, R., Shelef, K., & Levy, S. (2010). Attachment-based family therapy for adolescents with suicidal ideation: A randomized controlled trial. *Journal of the American Academy of Child and Adolescent Psychiatry, 41,* 122–131.

Diamond, L. M., & Hicks, A. M. (2005). Attachment style, current relationship security, and negative emotions: The mediating role of physiological regulation. *Journal of Social and Personal Relationships, 22,* 499–518.

Diamond, L. M., Hicks, A. M., & Otter-Henderson, K. D. (2006). Physiological evidence for repressive coping among avoidantly attached adults. *Journal of Social and Personal Relationships, 23,* 205–229.

Diamond, L. M., Hicks, A. M., & Otter-Henderson,

K. D. (2008). Every time you go away: Changes in affect, behavior, and physiology associated with travel-related separations from romantic partners. *Journal of Personality and Social Psychology, 95*, 385–403.

Diebels, K. J., & Leary, M. R. (2019). The psychological implications of believing that everything is one. *Journal of Positive Psychology, 14*, 463–473.

Diener, M. J., Geenen, R., Koelen, J. A., Aarts, F., Gerdes, V. E. A., Brandjes, D. P. M., & Hinnen, C. (2016). The significance of attachment quality for obesity: A meta-analytic review. *Canadian Journal of Behavioral Science, 48*, 255–265.

Diener, M. J., Hilsenroth, M. J., & Weinberger, J. (2009). A primer on meta-analysis of correlation coefficients: The relationship between patient-reported therapeutic alliance and adult attachment style as an illustration. *Psychotherapy Research, 19*, 519–526.

Diener, M. J., & Monroe, J. M. (2011). The relationship between adult attachment style and therapeutic alliance in individual psychotherapy: A meta-analytic review. *Psychotherapy, 48*, 237–248.

Dijksterhuis, A., & van Knippenberg, A. (1998). Inhibition, Aberdeen, and other cloudy subjects. In R. S. Wyer, Jr. (Ed.), *Advances in social cognition: Vol. 11. Stereotype activation and inhibition* (pp. 83–96). Erlbaum.

Dimri, S. (2018). *Lost and found: The contribution of the sense of attachment security to spatial navigation.* Unpublished MA thesis, Interdisciplinary Center (IDC) Herzliya, Herzliya, Israel.

Dinero, R. E., Conger, R. D., Shaver, P. R., Widaman, K. F., & Larsen-Rife, D. (2008). Influence of family of origin and adult romantic partners on romantic attachment security. *Journal of Family Psychology, 22*, 622–632.

Dinger, U., Strack, M., Sachsse, T., & Schauenburg, H. (2009). Therapists' attachment, patients' interpersonal problems, and alliance development over time in inpatient psychotherapy. *Psychotherapy, 46*, 277–290.

Ditzen, B., Schmidt, S., Strauss, B., Nater, U. M., Ehlert, U., & Heinrichs, M. (2008). Adult attachment and social support interact to reduce psychological but not cortisol responses to stress. *Journal of Psychosomatic Research, 64*, 479–486.

Doherty, N. A., & Feeney, J. A. (2004). The composition of attachment networks throughout the adult years. *Personal Relationships, 11*, 469–488.

Dollberg, D. G. (2022). Mothers' parental mentalization, attachment dimensions and mother–infant relational patterns. *Attachment and Human Development, 24*, 189–207.

Doosje, B., Ellemers, N., & Spears, R. (1995). Perceived intragroup variability as a function of group status and identification. *Journal of Experimental Social Psychology, 31*, 410–436.

Doron, G., Sar-El, D., Mikulincer, M., & Talmor, D. (2012). Experimentally-enhanced attachment security influences obsessive compulsive related washing tendencies in a non-clinical sample. *E-Journal of Applied Psychology, 8*, 1–8.

Douglas, V. J., Kwan, M. Y., & Gordon, K. H. (2021, August 31). Pet attachment and the interpersonal theory of suicide. *Crisis.* [Epub ahead of print].

Downer, J. T., Pianta, R. C., Burchinal, M., Field, S., Hamre, B. K., LoCasale-Crouch, J., & Scott-Little, C. (2014). *Coaching and coursework focused on teacher–child interactions during language/literacy instruction: Effects on teacher beliefs, knowledge, skills, and practice.* Unpublished manuscript. University of Virginia, Charlottesville, VA.

Downer, J. T., Pianta, R. C., Fan, X., Hamre, B. K., Mashburn, A., & Justice, L. (2011). Effects of web-mediated teacher professional development on the language and literacy skills of children enrolled in prekindergarten programs. *NHSA Dialog, 14*, 189–212.

Doyle, A. B., & Markiewicz, D. (2005). Parenting, marital conflict, and adjustment from early- to mid-adolescence: Mediated by adolescent attachment style? *Journal of Youth and Adolescence, 34*, 97–110.

Dozier, M., & Bernard, K. (2019). *Coaching parents of vulnerable infants: The attachment and biobehavioral catch-up approach.* Guilford Press.

Dozier, M., Cue, K. L., & Barnett, L. (1994). Clinicians as caregivers: Role of attachment organization in treatment. *Journal of Consulting and Clinical Psychology, 62*, 793–800.

Dozier, M., Lindhiem, O., & Ackerman, J. (2005). Attachment and Biobehavioral Catch-Up. In L. Berlin, Y. Ziv, L. Amaya-Jackson, & M. T. Greenberg (Eds.), *Enhancing early attachments: Theory, research, intervention, and policy* (pp. 178–194). Guilford Press.

Dozier, M., Meade, E. B., & Bernard, K. (2014). Attachment and Biobehavioral Catch-Up: An intervention for parents at risk of maltreating their infants and toddlers. In S. Timmer & A. Urquiza (Eds.), *Evidence-based approaches for the treatment of child maltreatment* (pp. 43–60). Springer.

Dozier, M., Peloso, E., Lewis, E., Laurenceau, J.-P., & Levine, S. (2008). Effects of an attachment-based intervention of the cortisol production of infants and toddlers in foster care. *Development and Psychopathology, 20*, 845–859.

Dozier, M., Peloso, E., Lindhiem, O., Gordon, M. K., Manni, M., Sepulveda, S., . . . Levine, S. (2006). Developing evidence-based interventions for foster children: An example of a randomized clinical trial with infants and toddlers. *Journal of Social Issues, 62*, 767–785.

Dozier, M., & Tyrrell, C. (1998). The role of attachment in therapeutic relationships. In J. A. Simpson & W. S. Rholes (Eds.), *Attachment theory and close relationships* (pp. 221–248). Guilford Press.

Drake, D. B. (2009). Using attachment theory in coaching leaders: The search for a coherent narrative. *International Coaching Psychology Review, 4,* 49–58.

Drake, K., Belsky, J., & Fearon, R. M. P. (2014). From early attachment to engagement with learning in school: The role of self-regulation and persistence. *Developmental Psychology, 50,* 1350–1361.

Driscoll, K. C., & Pianta, R. C. (2010). Banking time in head start: Early efficacy of an intervention designed to promote supportive teacher–child relationships. *Early Education and Development, 21,* 38–64.

Driscoll, K. C., Wang, L., Mashburn, A. J., & Pianta, R. C. (2011). Fostering supportive teacher–child relationships Intervention implementation in a state-funded preschool program. *Early Education and Development, 22,* 593–619.

Duan, C., & Kivlighan, D. M., Jr. (2002). Relationships among therapist pre-session mood, therapist empathy, and session evaluation. *Psychotherapy Research, 12,* 23–37.

Dujardin, A., Santens, T., Braet, C., De Raedt, R., Vos, P., Maes, B., & Bosmans, G. (2016). Middle childhood support-seeking behavior during stress: Links with self-reported attachment and future depressive symptoms. *Child Development, 87,* 326–340.

Dunkley, D. M., Berg, J. L., & Zuroff, D. C. (2012). The role of perfectionism in daily self-esteem, attachment, and negative affect. *Journal of Personality, 80,* 633–663.

Dutton, D. G., Lane, R. A., Koren, T., & Bartholomew, K. (2016). Secure base priming diminishes conflict-based anger and anxiety. *PLOS ONE, 11,* Article e0162374.

Dykas, M. J., & Cassidy, J. (2011). Attachment and the processing of social information across the life span: Theory and evidence. *Psychological Bulletin, 137,* 19–46.

Dykas, M. J., Woodhouse, S. S., Cassidy, J., & Waters, H. S. (2006). Narrative assessment of attachment representations: Links between secure base scripts and adolescent attachment. *Attachment and Human Development, 8,* 221–240.

Dykas, M. J., Woodhouse, S. S., Jones, J. D., & Cassidy, J. (2014). Attachment-related biases in adolescents' memory. *Child Development, 85,* 2185–2201.

Dziobek, I., Fleck, S., Kalbe, E., Rogers, K., Hassenstab, J., Brand, M., . . . Convit, A. (2006). Introducing MASC: A movie for the assessment of social cognition. *Journal of Autism and Developmental Disorders, 36,* 623–636.

Eagle, M. N. (2017). Attachment theory and research and clinical work. *Psychoanalytic Inquiry, 37,* 284–297.

Eames, V., & Roth, A. (2000). Patient attachment orientation and the early working alliance: A study of patient and therapist reports of alliance quality and ruptures. *Psychotherapy Research, 10,* 421–434.

Early, D. M., Maxwell, K. L., Ponder, B. D., & Pan, Y. (2017). Improving teacher–child interactions: A randomized controlled trial of Making the Most of Classroom Interactions and my teaching partner professional development models. *Early Childhood Research Quarterly, 38,* 57–70.

Edelstein, R. S., Alexander, K. W., Shaver, P. R., Schaaf, J. M., Quas, J. A., Lovas, G. S., & Goodman, G. S. (2004). Adult attachment style and parental responsiveness during a stressful event. *Attachment and Human Development, 6,* 31–52.

Edelstein, R. S., Ghetti, S., Quas, J. A., Goodman, G. S., Alexander, K. W., Redlich, A. D., & Cordon, I. M. (2005). Individual differences in emotional memory: Adult attachment and long-term memory for child sexual abuse. *Personality and Social Psychology Bulletin, 31,* 1537–1548.

Edmondson, A. (1999). Psychological safety and learning behavior in work teams. *Administrative Science Quarterly, 44,* 350–383.

Egozi, S., Tishby, O., & Wiseman, H. (2021). Changes in clients and therapists experiences of therapeutic distance during psychodynamic therapy. *Journal of Clinical Psychology, 77,* 910–926.

Ehrhardt, K., & Ragins, B. R. (2019). Relational attachment at work: A complementary fit perspective on the role of relationships in organizational life. *Academy of Management Journal, 62,* 248–282.

Ehrlich, K. B., Miller, G. E., Jones, J. D., & Cassidy, J. (2016). Attachment and psychoneuroimmunology. In J. Cassidy & P. R. Shaver (Eds.), *Handbook of attachment: Theory, research, and clinical applications* (3rd ed., pp. 180–201). Guilford Press.

Ehrlich, K. B., Miller, G. E., Rogosch, F. A., & Cicchetti, D. (2021). Maltreatment exposure across childhood and low-grade inflammation: Considerations of exposure type, timing, and sex differences. *Developmental Psychobiology, 63,* 529–537.

Ehrlich, K. B., Stern, J. A., Eccles, J., Dinh, J. V., Hopper, E. A., Kemeny, M. E., . . . Cassidy, J. (2019). A preliminary investigation of attachment style and inflammation in African-American young adults. *Attachment and Human Development, 21,* 57–69.

Ein-Dor, T. (2015). Attachment dispositions and human defensive behavior. *Personality and Individual Differences, 81,* 112–116.

Ein-Dor, T., Hirschberger, G., Tsur, N., Mikulincer, M., Bazak, S. B., & Solomon, Z. (2020). The link between attachment orientations and cellular aging among former prisoners of war. *Attachment and Human Development, 22,* 352–366.

Ein-Dor, T., Mikulincer, M., & Shaver, P. R. (2011a). Attachment insecurities and the processing of threat-related information: Studying schemas involved in insecure people's coping strategies. *Journal of Personality and Social Psychology, 101,* 78–93.

Ein-Dor, T., Mikulincer, M., & Shaver, P. R. (2011b). Effective reaction to danger: Attachment insecurities predict behavioral reactions to an experimentally induced threat above and beyond general personality traits. *Social Psychological and Personality Science, 2,* 467–473.

Ein-Dor, T., & Orgad, T. (2012). Scared saviours: Evidence that people high in attachment anxiety are more effective in alerting others to threat. *European Journal of Social Psychology, 42,* 667–671.

Eisenberger, N. I., Lieberman, M. D., & Williams, K. D. (2003). Does rejection hurt?: An fMRI study of social exclusion. *Science, 302,* 290–292.

Eisenberger, N. I., Master, S. L., Inagaki, T. K., Taylor, S. E., Shirinyan, D., Lieberman, M. D., & Naliboff, B. D. (2011). Attachment figures activate a safety signal-related neural region and reduce pain experience. *Proceedings of the National Academy of Sciences USA, 108,* 11721–11726.

Eisenberger, R., Cummings, J., Armeli, S., & Lynch, P. (1997). Perceived organizational support, discretionary treatment, and job satisfaction. *Journal of Applied Psychology, 82,* 812–820.

Eisenberger, R., Huntington, R., Hutchison, S., & Sowa, D. (1986). Perceived organizational support. *Journal of Applied Psychology, 71,* 500–507.

Eisenberger, R., Malone, G. P., & Presson, W. D. (2016). Optimizing perceived organizational support to enhance employee engagement (SHRM-SIOP Science of HR series, 1–22). Retrieved from *www.shrm.org/hr-today/trends-and-forecasting/special-reports-and-expert-views/documents/shrm-siop%20perceived%20organizational%20support.pdf.*

Eisenberger, R., & Stinglhamber, F. (2011). *Perceived organizational support: Fostering enthusiastic and productive employees.* American Psychological Association.

Elkin, I., Shea, M. T., Watkins, J. T., Imber, S. D., Sotsky, S. M., Collins, J. F., . . . Parloff, M. B. (1989). National Institute of Mental Health Treatment of Depression Collaborative Research Program: General effectiveness of treatments. *Archives of General Psychiatry, 46,* 971–982.

Elliott, R., Bohart, A. C., Watson, J. C., & Murphy, D. (2018). Therapist empathy and client outcome: An updated meta-analysis. *Psychotherapy, 55,* 399–410.

Ellison, C. G., Bradshaw, M., Flannelly, M. J., & Galek, K. C. (2014). Prayer, attachment to God, and symptoms of anxiety-related disorders. *Sociology of Religion, 75,* 208–233.

Ellison, C. G., Deangelis, R. T., Hill, T. D., & Froese, P. (2019). Sleep quality and the stress-buffering role of religious involvement: A mediated moderation analysis. *Journal for the Scientific Study of Religion, 58,* 251–268.

Elsey, T., Keller, P. S., & El-Sheikh, M. (2019). The role of couple sleep concordance in sleep quality: Attachment as a moderator of associations. *Journal of Sleep Research, 28,* Article e12825.

Englund, M. M., Kuo, S., Puig, J., & Collins, W. (2011). Early roots of adult competence: The significance of close relationships from infancy to early adulthood. *International Journal of Behavioral Development, 35,* 490–496.

Epitropaki, O., & Martin, R. (2005). From ideal to real: A longitudinal study of the role of implicit leadership theories on leader–member exchanges and employee outcomes. *Journal of Applied Psychology, 90,* 659–676.

Epstein, R. M., & Street, R. L., Jr. (2007). *Patient-centered communication in cancer care: Promoting healing and reducing suffering.* National Cancer Institute.

Erdman, P., Ng, K. M., & Metzger, S. (Eds.). (2010). *Attachment: Expanding the cultural connections.* Routledge.

Eubanks, C. F., Sergi, J., & Muran, J. C. (2021). Responsiveness to ruptures and repairs in psychotherapy. In J. C. Watson & H. Wiseman (Eds.), *The responsive psychotherapist: Attuning to clients in the moment* (pp. 83–103). American Psychological Association.

Euser, S., Vrijhof, C. I., Van den Bulk, B. G., Vermeulen, R., Bakermans-Kranenburg, M. J., & van IJzendoorn, M. H. (2021). Video-feedback promotes sensitive limit-setting in parents of twin preschoolers: A randomized controlled trial. *BMC Psychology, 9,* Article 468.

Evans, C. R., & Dion, K. L. (1991). Group cohesion and performance: A meta-analysis. *Small Group Research, 22,* 175–186.

Faber, A., Dubé, L., & Knäuper, B. (2018). Attachment and eating: A meta-analytic review of the relevance of attachment for unhealthy and healthy eating behaviors in the general population. *Appetite, 123,* 410–438.

Fagundes, C. P., Diamond, L. M., & Allen, K. P. (2012). Adolescent attachment insecurity and parasympathetic functioning predict future loss adjustment. *Personality and Social Psychology Bulletin, 38,* 821–832.

Fagundes, C. P., Jaremka, L. M., Glaser, R., Alfano, C. M., Povoski, S. P., Lipari, A. M., . . . Kiecolt-Glaser, J. K. (2014). Attachment anxiety is related to Epstein–Barr virus latency. *Brain, Behavior, and Immunity, 41,* 232–238.

Fagundes, C. P., & Wu, E. L. (2020). Matters of the heart: Grief, morbidity, and mortality. *Current Directions in Psychological Science, 29,* 235–241.

Fairbairn, C. E., Briley, D. A., Kang, D., Fraley, R. C., Hankin, B. L., & Ariss, T. (2018). A meta-analysis of longitudinal associations between substance use and interpersonal attachment security. *Psychological Bulletin, 144,* 532–555.

Farber, B. A., Suzuki, J. Y., & Lynch, D. A. (2018). Positive regard and psychotherapy outcome: A meta-analytic review. *Psychotherapy, 55,* 411–423.

Farrell, A. K., Simpson, J. A., Overall, N. C., & Shallcross, S. L. (2016). Buffering the responses of avoidantly attached romantic partners in strain test situations. *Journal of Family Psychology, 30,* 580–591.

Farrell, A. K., Waters, T. E. A., Young, E. S., Englund, M. M., Carlson, E. E., Roisman, G. I., & Simpson, J. A. (2019). Early maternal sensitivity, attachment security in young adulthood, and cardiometabolic risk at midlife. *Attachment and Human Development, 21*, 70–86.

Fearon, R. M. P., & Belsky, J. (2016). Precursors of attachment security. In J. Cassidy & P. R. Shaver (Eds.), *Handbook of attachment: Theory, research, and clinical applications* (3rd ed., pp. 291–313). Guilford Press.

Feder, M. M., & Diamond, G. M. (2016). Parent-therapist alliance and parent attachment-promoting behavior in attachment-based family therapy for suicidal and depressed adolescents. *Journal of Family Therapy, 38*, 82–101.

Feeney, B. C. (2004). A secure base: Responsive support of goal strivings and exploration in adult intimate relationships. *Journal of Personality and Social Psychology, 87*, 631–648.

Feeney, B. C. (2007). The dependency paradox in close relationships: Accepting dependence promotes independence. *Journal of Personality and Social Psychology, 92*, 268–285.

Feeney, B. C., Cassidy, J., & Ramos-Marcuse, F. (2008). The generalization of attachment representations to new social situations: Predicting behavior during initial interactions with strangers. *Journal of Personality and Social Psychology, 95*, 1481–1498.

Feeney, B. C., & Collins, N. L. (2001). Predictors of caregiving in adult intimate relationships: An attachment theoretical perspective. *Journal of Personality and Social Psychology, 80*, 972–994.

Feeney, B. C., & Collins, N. L. (2003). Motivations for caregiving in adult intimate relationships: Influences on caregiving behavior and relationship functioning. *Personality and Social Psychology Bulletin, 29*, 950–968.

Feeney, B. C., & Collins, N. L. (2015). A new look at social support. *Personality and Social Psychology Review, 19*, 113–147.

Feeney, B. C., & Collins, N. L. (2019). The importance of relational support for attachment and exploration needs. *Current Opinion in Psychology, 25*, 182–186.

Feeney, B. C., Collins, N. L., van Vleet, M., & Tomlinson, J. M. (2013). Motivations for providing a secure base: Links with attachment orientation and secure base support behavior. *Attachment and Human Development, 15*, 261–280.

Feeney, B. C., & Kirkpatrick, L. A. (1996). Effects of adult attachment and presence of romantic partners on physiological responses to stress. *Journal of Personality and Social Psychology, 70*, 255–270.

Feeney, B. C., & Monin, J. K. (2016). Divorce through the lens of attachment theory. In J. Cassidy & P. R. Shaver (Eds.), *Handbook of attachment: Theory, research, and clinical applications* (3rd ed., pp. 941–965). Guilford Press.

Feeney, B. C., & Thrush, R. L. (2010). Relationship influences on exploration in adulthood: The characteristics and function of a secure base. *Journal of Personality and Social Psychology, 98*, 57–76.

Feeney, B. C., Van Vleet, M., Jakubiak, B. K., & Tomlinson, J. M. (2017). Predicting the pursuit and support of challenging life opportunities. *Personality and Social Psychology Bulletin, 43*, 1171–1187.

Feeney, J. A. (1995). Adult attachment, coping style, and health locus of control as predictors of health behavior. *Australian Journal of Psychology, 47*, 171–177.

Feeney, J. A. (2002). Early parenting and parental attachment: Links with offspring's attachment and perceptions of social support. *Journal of Family Studies, 8*, 5–23.

Feeney, J. A. (2006). Parental attachment and conflict behavior: Implications for offspring's attachment, loneliness, and relationship satisfaction. *Personal Relationships, 13*, 19–36.

Feeney, J. A., Hohaus, L., Noller, P., & Alexander, R. (2001). *Becoming parents: Exploring the bonds between mothers, fathers, and their infants.* Cambridge University Press.

Feeney, J. A., Kelly, L., Gallois, C., Peterson, C., & Terry, D. J. (1999). Attachment style, assertive communication, and safer-sex behavior. *Journal of Applied Social Psychology, 29*, 1964–1983.

Feeney, J. A., Peterson, C., Gallois, C., & Terry, D. J. (2000). Attachment style as a predictor of sexual attitudes and behavior in late adolescence. *Psychology and Health, 14*, 1105–1122.

Feeney, J. A., & Ryan, S. M. (1994). Attachment style and affect regulation: Relationships with health behavior and family experiences of illness in a student sample. *Health Psychology, 13*, 334–345.

Feeney, J. R., Gellatly, I. R., Goffin, R. D., & Inness, M. (2020). Organizational attachment: Conceptualization, measurement, and incremental prediction of work attitudes and outcomes. *Journal of Personnel Psychology, 19*, 113–124.

Fein, E. C., Benea, D., Idzadikhah, Z., & Tziner, A. (2020). The security to lead: A systematic review of leader and follower attachment styles and leader-member exchange. *European Journal of Work and Organizational Psychology, 29*, 106–125.

Field, N. P., & Filanosky, C. (2010). Continuing bonds, risk factors for complicated grief, and adjustment to bereavement. *Death Studies, 34*, 1–29.

Field, N. P., Orsini, L., Gavish, R., & Packman, W. (2009). Role of attachment in response to pet loss. *Death Studies, 33*, 334–355.

Field, N. P., Packman, J. D., Ronen, R., Pries, A., Davies, B., & Kramer, R. (2013). Type of continuing bonds expression and its comforting versus distressing nature: Implications for adjustment among bereaved mothers. *Death Studies, 37*, 889–912.

Field, N. P., & Sundin, E. C. (2001). Attachment style

in adjustment to conjugal bereavement. *Journal of Social and Personal Relationships, 18*, 347–361.

Field, N. P., Tzadikario, E., Pel, D., & Ret, T. (2014). Attachment and mother–child communication in adjustment to the death of a father among Cambodian adolescents. *Journal of Loss and Trauma, 19*, 314–330.

Figley, C. R. (2002). Compassion fatigue and the psychotherapist's chronic lack of self-care. *Journal of Clinical Psychology, 58*, 1433–1441.

Fine, A. H. (2000). Animals and therapists: Incorporating animals in outpatient psychotherapy. In A. H. Fine (Ed.), *Handbook on animal-assisted therapy: Theoretical foundations and guidelines for practice* (pp. 179–211). Academic Press.

Fischer-Kern, M., Doering, S., Taubner, S., Hörz, S., Zimmermann, J., Rentrop, M., . . . Buchheim, A. (2015). Transference-focused psychotherapy for borderline personality disorder: Change in reflective function. *British Journal of Psychiatry, 207*, 173–174.

Fisher, H., Rafaeli, E., Bar-Kalifa, E., Barber, J. P., Solomonov, N., Peri, T., & Atzil-Slonim, D. (2020). Therapists' interventions as a predictor of clients' emotional experience, self-understanding, and treatment outcomes. *Journal of Counseling Psychology, 67*, 66–78.

Fletcher, I., McCallum, R., & Peters, S. (2016). Attachment styles and clinical communication performance in trainee doctors. *Patient Education and Counseling, 99*, 1852–1857.

Florian, V., & Mikulincer, M. (1998). Terror management in childhood: Does death conceptualization moderate the effects of mortality salience on acceptance of similar and different others? *Personality and Social Psychology Bulletin, 24*, 1104–1112.

Folke, S., Daniel, S. I. F., Poulsen, S., & Lunn, S. (2016). Client attachment security predicts alliance in a randomized controlled trial of two psychotherapies for bulimia nervosa. *Psychotherapy Research, 26*, 459–471.

Fonagy, P., Gergely, G., Jurist, E. L., & Target, M. (2002). *Affect regulation, mentalization, and the development of the self.* Other Press.

Fonagy, P., Leigh, T., Steele, M., Steele, H., Kennedy, R., Mattoon, G., . . . Gerber, A. (1996). The relation of attachment status, psychiatric classification, and response to psychotherapy. *Journal of Consulting and Clinical Psychology, 64*, 22–31.

Fonagy, P., Luyten, P., Moulton-Perkins, A., Lee, Y.-W., Warren, F., Howard, S., . . . Lowyck, B. (2016). Development and validation of a self-report measure of mentalizing: The Reflective Functioning Questionnaire. *PLOS ONE, 11*, Article e0158678.

Fonagy, P., Steele, M., Steele, H., Moran, G. S., & Higgitt, P. (1991). The capacity for understanding mental states: The reflective self in parent and child and its significance for security of attachment. *Infant Mental Health Journal, 12*, 201–218.

Fonagy, P., & Target, M. (1997). Attachment and reflective function: Their role in self-organization. *Development and Psychopathology, 9*, 679–700.

Fonagy, P., Target, M., Steele, M., & Gerber, A. (1995). Psychoanalytic perspectives on developmental psychopathology. In D. Cicchetti & D. J. Cohen (Eds.), *Developmental psychopathology: Vol. 1. Theory and methods* (pp. 504–554). Wiley.

Fonagy, P., Twemlow, S. W., Vernberg, E. M., Nelson, J. M., Dill, E. J., Little, T. D., & Sargent, J. A. (2009). A cluster randomized controlled trial of child-focused psychiatric consultation and a school systems-focused intervention to reduce aggression. *Journal of Child Psychology and Psychiatry, 50*, 607–616.

Forsythe, L. P., Romano, J. M., Jensen, M. P., & Thorn, B. E. (2012). Attachment style is associated with perceived spouse responses and pain-related outcomes. *Rehabilitation Psychology, 57*, 290–300.

Fosha, D. (2000). *The transforming power of affect: A model for accelerated change.* Basic Books.

Fosha, D. (2002). The activation of affective change processes in accelerated experiential-dynamic psychotherapy (AEDP). In F. W. Kaslow & J. J. Magnavita (Eds.), *Comprehensive handbook of psychotherapy: Psychodynamic/object relations* (pp. 309–343). Wiley.

Fosha, D. (2004). "Nothing that feels bad is ever the last step": The role of positive emotions in experiential work with difficult emotional experiences. *Clinical Psychology and Psychotherapy, 11*, 30–43.

Fosha, D. (2005). Emotion, true self, true other, core state: Toward a clinical theory of affective change process. *Psychoanalytic Review, 92*, 513–552.

Fosha, D. (2021). How AEDP works. In D. Fosha (Ed.), *Undoing aloneness and the transformation of suffering into flourishing: AEDP 2.0* (pp. 27–52). American Psychological Association.

Fosha, D., Thoma, N., & Yeung, D. (2019). Transforming emotional suffering into flourishing: Meta-therapeutic processing of positive affect as a trans-theoretical vehicle for change. *Counselling Psychology Quarterly, 32*, 563–593.

Fossati, A., Feeney, J., Maffei, C., & Borroni, S. (2014). Thinking about feelings: Affective state mentalization, attachment styles, and borderline personality disorder features among Italian nonclinical adolescents. *Psychoanalytic Psychology, 31*, 41–67.

Foulkes-Bert, D., Volk, F., Garzon, F., & Pride, M. (2019). The relationship between transformational leadership behavior, adult attachment, and God attachment. *Journal of Psychology and Theology, 47*, 20–33.

Fraiberg, S. (1980). *Clinical studies in infant mental health.* Tavistock.

Fraley, R. C. (2002). Attachment stability from infancy to adulthood: Meta-analysis and dynamic modeling of developmental mechanisms. *Personality and Social Psychology Review, 6*, 123–151.

Fraley, R. C. (2019). Attachment in adulthood: Recent developments, emerging debates, and future directions. *Annual Review of Psychology, 70,* 401–422.

Fraley, R. C., & Bonanno, G. A. (2004). Attachment and loss: A test of three competing models on the association between attachment-related avoidance and adaptation to bereavement. *Personality and Social Psychology Bulletin, 30,* 878–890.

Fraley, R. C., & Brumbaugh, C. C. (2004). A dynamical systems approach to conceptualizing and studying stability and change in attachment security. In W. S. Rholes & J. A. Simpson (Eds.), *Adult attachment: Theory, research, and clinical implications* (pp. 86–132). Guilford Press.

Fraley, R. C., & Davis, K. E. (1997). Attachment formation and transfer in young adults' close friendships and romantic relationships. *Personal Relationships, 4,* 131–144.

Fraley, R. C., Heffernan, M. E., Vicary, A. M., & Brumbaugh, C. C. (2011). The experiences in close relationships-relationship structures questionnaire: A method for assessing attachment orientations across relationships. *Psychological Assessment, 23,* 615–625.

Fraley, R. C., Hudson, N. W., Heffernan, M. E., & Segal, N. (2015). Are adult attachment styles categorical or dimensional?: A taxometric analysis of general and relationship-specific attachment orientations. *Journal of Personality and Social Psychology, 109,* 354–368.

Fraley, R. C., & Roisman, G. I. (2019). The development of adult attachment styles: Four lessons. *Current Opinion in Psychology, 25,* 26–30.

Fraley, R. C., Roisman, G. I., Booth-LaForce, C., Owen, M. T., & Holland, A. S. (2013). Interpersonal and genetic origins of adult attachment styles: A longitudinal study from infancy to early adulthood. *Journal of Personality and Social Psychology, 104,* 817–838.

Fraley, R. C., & Shaver, P. R. (1998). Airport separations: A naturalistic study of adult attachment dynamics in separating couples. *Journal of Personality and Social Psychology, 75,* 1198–1212.

Fraley, R. C., & Shaver, P. R. (2000). Adult romantic attachment: Theoretical developments, emerging controversies, and unanswered questions. *Review of General Psychology, 4,* 132–154.

Fraley, R. C., & Shaver, P. R. (2016). Attachment, loss, and grief: Bowlby's views, new developments, and current controversies. In J. Cassidy & P. R. Shaver (Eds.), *Handbook of attachment: Theory, research, and clinical applications* (3rd ed., pp. 40–62). Guilford Press.

Fraley, R. C., Vicary, A. M., Brumbaugh, C. C., & Roisman, G. I. (2011). Patterns of stability in adult attachment: An empirical test of two models of continuity and change. *Journal of Personality and Social Psychology, 101,* 974–992.

Frederiksen, H. B., Kragstrup, J., & Dehlholm-Lambertsen, B. (2010). Attachment in the doctor-patient relationship in general practice: A qualitative study. *Scandinavian Journal of Primary Health Care, 28,* 185–190.

Fredrickson, B. L. (2001). The role of positive emotions in positive psychology: The broaden-and-build theory of positive emotions. *American Psychologist, 56,* 218–226.

Fredrickson, M., Howie, A. R. (2000). Methods, standards, guidelines, and considerations in selecting animal in animal-assisted therapy. In A. H. Fine (Ed.), *Handbook on animal-assisted therapy: Theoretical foundations and guidelines for practice* (pp. 99–114). Academic Press.

Frei, J. R., & Shaver, P. R. (2002). Respect in close relationships: Prototype definition, self-report assessment, and initial correlates. *Personal Relationships, 9,* 121–139.

Freud, S. (1961). Address delivered [in 1930] at the Goethe House at Frankfurt. In J. Strachey (Ed. & Trans.), *The standard edition of the complete psychological works of Sigmund Freud* (Vol. 22, pp. 208–212). Hogarth Press. (Original work published 1930)

Frías, M. T., & Shaver, P. R. (2014). The moderating role of attachment insecurities in the association between social and physical pain. *Journal of Research in Personality, 53,* 193–200.

Fritsche, I., Jonas, E., Ablasser, C., Beyer, M., Kuban, J., Manger, A. M., & Schultz, M. (2013). The power of we: Evidence for group-based control. *Journal of Experimental Social Psychology, 49,* 19–32.

Fritsche, I., Jonas, E., & Fankhänel, T. (2008). The role of control motivation in mortality salience effects on ingroup support and defense. *Journal of Personality and Social Psychology, 95,* 524–541.

Fuchs, N. F., & Taubner, S. (2019). Exploring the interplay of attachment style and attachment-related mood on short-term change in mentalization: A pilot study. *Personality and Individual Differences, 144,* 94–99.

Fuertes, J. N., Mislowack, A., Brown, S., Gur-Arie, S., Wilkinson, S., & Gelso, C. J. (2007). Correlates of the real relationship in psychotherapy: A study of dyads. *Psychotherapy Research, 17,* 423–430.

Fuertes, J. N., Moore, M., & Ganley, J. (2019). Therapists' and clients' ratings of real relationship, attachment, therapist self-disclosure, and treatment progress. *Psychotherapy Research, 29,* 594–606.

Fukkink, R., Helmerhorst, K., Deynoot-Schaub, M. G., & Sluiter, R. (2019). Training interaction skills of pre-service ECEC teachers: Moving from in-service to pre-service professional development. *Early Childhood Education Journal, 47,* 497–507.

Furman, W., & Buhrmester, D. (1992). Age and sex differences in perceptions of networks of personal relationships. *Child Development, 63,* 103–115.

Gabriel, S., Kawakami, K., Bartak, C., Kang, S.-J., & Mann, N. (2010). Negative self-synchronization: Will I change to be like you when it is bad for me? *Journal of Personality and Social Psychology, 98,* 857–871.

Gall, T. L., & Bilodeau, C. (2018). The role of relationship with God in couples' adjustment to the threat of breast cancer. *Psychology of Religion and Spirituality, 10,* 375–385.

Gall, T. L., Kristjansson, E., Charbonneau, C., & Florack, P. (2009). A longitudinal study on the role of spirituality in response to the diagnosis and treatment of breast cancer. *Journal of Behavioral Medicine, 32,* 174–186.

Gallagher, M. E., Tasca, G. A., Ritchie, K., Balfour, L., & Bissada, H. (2014). Attachment anxiety moderates the relationship between growth in group cohesion and treatment outcomes in group psychodynamic interpersonal psychotherapy for women with binge eating disorder. *Group Dynamics, 18,* 38–52.

Gallarin, M., & Alonso-Arbiol, I. (2012). Parenting practices, parental attachment and aggressiveness in adolescence: A predictive model. *Journal of Adolescence, 35,* 1601–1610.

Gallo, L. C., & Matthews, K. A. (2006). Adolescents' attachment orientation influences ambulatory blood pressure responses to everyday social interactions. *Psychosomatic Medicine, 68,* 253–261.

Gama, G., Barbosa, F., & Vieira, M. (2014). Personal determinants of nurses' burnout in end of life care. *European Journal of Oncology Nursing, 18,* 527–533.

Gan, Y., Ma, J., Wu, J., Chen, Y., Zhu, H., & Hall, B. J. (2022). Immediate and delayed psychological effects of province-wide lockdown and personal quarantine during the COVID-19 outbreak in China. *Psychological Medicine, 52,* 1321–1332.

García-Ruiz, M., Rodrigo, M. J., Hernández-Cabrera, J. A., & Máiquez, M. L. (2013). Contribution of parents' adult attachment and separation attitudes to parent–adolescent conflict resolution. *Scandinavian Journal of Psychology, 54,* 459–467.

Garnett, M., Bernard, K., Hoye, J., Zajac, L., & Dozier, M. (2020). Parental sensitivity mediates the sustained effect of Attachment and Biobehavioral Catch-Up on cortisol in middle childhood: A randomized clinical trial. *Psychoneuroendocrinology, 121,* Article 104809.

Garrison, A. M., Kahn, J. H., Sauer, E. M., & Florczak, M. A. (2012). Disentangling the effects of depression symptoms and adult attachment on emotional disclosure. *Journal of Counseling Psychology, 59,* 230–239.

Geller, J. D., & Farber, B. A. (2015). Attachment style, representations of psychotherapy, and clinical interventions with insecurely attached clients. *Journal of Clinical Psychology, 71,* 457–468.

George, C., Kaplan, N., & Main, M. (1985). *The Adult Attachment Interview.* Unpublished protocol, Department of Psychology, University of California, Berkeley.

George-Levi, S., Peleg, S., Vilchinsky, N., Rafaeli, E., Khaskiaa, A., Mosseri, M., & Hod, H. (2020). Attachment insecurity hinders cardiac patients' ability to receive partners' care: A longitudinal dyadic study. *Journal of Social and Personal Relationships, 37,* 1494–1512.

Georgiou, S. N., Demetriou, A. P., & Stavrinides, P. (2008). Attachment style and mentoring relationships in adolescence. *Educational Psychology, 28,* 603–614.

Georgopoulou, S., Prothero. L., & D'Cruz, D. P. (2018). Physician–patient communication in rheumatology: A systematic review. *Rheumatology International, 38,* 763–775.

Ghochani, M., Saffarian Toosi, M., & Khoynezhad, G. (2020). A comparison between the effectiveness of the combined couple therapy and emotionally focused therapy for couples on the improvement of intimacy and PTSD. *Learning and Motivation, 71,* Article 101637.

Ghosh Ippen, C., Harris, W. W., Van Horn, P., & Lieberman, A. F. (2011). Traumatic and stressful events in early childhood: Can treatment help those at highest risk? *Child Abuse and Neglect, 35,* 504–513.

Giannotta, F., Ortega, E., & Stattin, H. (2013). An attachment parenting intervention to prevent adolescents' problem behaviors: A pilot study in Italy. *Child and Youth Care Forum, 42,* 71–85.

Gick, M. L., & Sirois, F. M. (2010). Insecure attachment moderates women's adjustment to inflammatory bowel disease severity. *Rehabilitation Psychology, 55,* 170–179.

Gilbert, P. (2021). Creating a compassionate world: Addressing the conflicts between *sharing and caring* versus *controlling and holding* evolved strategies. *Frontiers in Psychology, 11,* Article 582090.

Gillath, O., Atchley, R., Imran, A., Haj-Mohamadi, P., & El-Hodiri, M. (2020). Attachment and resource sharing. *Personal Relationships, 27,* 228–250.

Gillath, O., Bunge, S. A., Shaver, P. R., Wendelken, C., Mikulincer, M. (2005). Attachment-style differences in the ability to suppress negative thoughts: Exploring the neural correlates. *NeuroImage, 28,* 835–847.

Gillath, O., Hart, J., Noftle, E. E., & Stockdale, G. D. (2009). Development and validation of a state adult attachment measure (SAAM). *Journal of Research in Personality, 43,* 362–373.

Gillath, O., & Karantzas, G. C. (2015). Attachment security and prosociality: Dynamics, underlying mechanisms, and implications. In P. Caroll, R. Arkin, & A. Wichman (Eds.), *Handbook of personal security* (pp. 159–172). Psychology Press.

Gillath, O., & Karantzas, G. C. (2019). Attachment security priming: A systematic review. *Current Opinion in Psychology, 25,* 86–95.

Gillath, O., Karantzas, G. C., Romano, D., & Karantzas, K. M. (2022). Attachment security priming:

A meta-analysis. *Personality and Social Psychology Review, 26,* 183–241.

Gillath, O., Karantzas, G. C., & Selcuk, E. (2017). A net of friends: Investigating friendship by integrating attachment theory and social network analysis. *Personality and Social Psychology Bulletin, 43,* 1546–1565.

Gillath, O., Mikulincer, M., Fitzsimons, G. M., Shaver, P. R., Schachner, D. A., & Bargh, J. A. (2006). Automatic activation of attachment-related goals. *Personality and Social Psychology Bulletin, 32,* 1375–1388.

Gillath, O., Sesko, A. K., Shaver, P. R., & Chun, D. S. (2010). Attachment, authenticity, and honesty: Dispositional and experimentally induced security can reduce self- and other-deception. *Journal of Personality and Social Psychology, 98,* 841–855.

Gillath, O., & Shaver, P. R. (2007). Effects of attachment style and relationship context on selection among relational strategies. *Journal of Research in Personality, 41,* 968–976.

Gillath, O., Shaver, P. R., Mikulincer, M., Nitzberg, R. A., Erez, A., & van IJzendoorn, M. H. (2005). Attachment, caregiving, and volunteering: Placing volunteerism in an attachment-theoretical framework. *Personal Relationships, 12,* 425–446.

Giraldo-O'Meara, M., & Doron, G. (2021). Can self-esteem be improved using short daily training on mobile applications?: Examining real world data of GG Self-esteem users. *Clinical Psychologist, 25,* 131–139.

Girme, Y. U., Overall, N. C., Simpson, J. A., & Fletcher, G. J. O. (2015). "All or nothing": Attachment avoidance and the curvilinear effects of partner support. *Journal of Personality and Social Psychology, 108,* 450–475.

Gjerde, P. F., Onishi, M., & Carlson, K. S. (2004). Personality characteristics associated with romantic attachment: A comparison of interview and self-report methodologies. *Personality and Social Psychology Bulletin, 30,* 1402–1415.

Goagoses, N., Bolz, T., Eilts, J., Schipper, N., Schütz, J., Rademache, A., . . . Koglin, U. (2022). Parenting dimensions/styles and emotion dysregulation in childhood and adolescence: A systematic review and meta-analysis. *Current Psychology.* [Epub ahead of print].

Goffin, K. C., Kochanska, G., & Yoon, J. E. (2020). Children's theory of mind as a mechanism linking parents' mind-mindedness in infancy with children's conscience. *Journal of Experimental Child Psychology, 193,* Article 104784.

Goldberg, A., & Scharf, M. (2020). How do highly sensitive persons parent their adolescent children?: The role of sensory processing sensitivity in parenting practices. *Journal of Social and Personal Relationships, 37,* 1825–1842.

Goldsmith, H. H., & Alansky, J. A. (1987). Maternal and infant temperamental predictors of attachment: A meta-analytic review. *Journal of Consulting and Clinical Psychology, 55,* 805–816.

Gonçalves, J. P. B., Lucchetti, G., Menezes, P. R., & Vallada, H. (2015). Religious and spiritual interventions in mental health care: A systematic review and meta-analysis of randomized controlled clinical trials. *Psychological Medicine, 45,* 2937–2949.

Gosnell, C. L., & Gable, S. L. (2013). Attachment and capitalizing on positive events. *Attachment & Human Development, 15,* 281–302.

Gouin, J. P., Glaser, R., Loving, T. J., Malarkey, W. B., Stowell, J., Houts, C., & Kiecolt-Glaser, J. K. (2009). Attachment avoidance predicts inflammatory responses to marital conflict. *Brain, Behavior, and Immunity, 23,* 898–904.

Gouin, J. P., & MacNeil, S. (2019). Attachment style and changes in systemic inflammation following migration to a new country among international students. *Attachment and Human Development, 21,* 38–56.

Grady, J., Grady, V., McCreesh, P., & Noakes, I. (2020). *Workplace attachments: Managing beneath the surface.* Routledge.

Granqvist, P. (2002). Attachment and religiosity in adolescence: Cross-sectional and longitudinal evaluations. *Personality and Social Psychology Bulletin, 28,* 260–270.

Granqvist, P. (2020). *Attachment in religion and spirituality.* Guilford Press.

Granqvist, P., Lantto, S., Ortiz, L., & Andersson, G. (2001). Adult attachment, perceived family support, and problems experienced by tinnitus patients. *Psychology and Health, 16,* 357–366.

Granqvist, P., Mikulincer, M., Gurwitz, V., & Shaver, P. R. (2012). Experimental findings on God as an attachment figure: Normative processes and moderating effects of internal working models. *Journal of Personality and Social Psychology, 103,* 804–818.

Green, J. D., & Campbell, W. (2000). Attachment and exploration in adults: Chronic and contextual accessibility. *Personality and Social Psychology Bulletin, 26,* 452–461.

Green, J., Charman, T., Pickles, A., Wan, M. W., Elsabbagh, M., Slonims, V., . . . BASIS Team. (2015). Parent-mediated intervention versus no intervention for infants at high risk of autism: A parallel, single-blind randomized trial. *Lancet Psychiatry, 2,* 133–140.

Green, J., Pickles, A., Pasco, G., Bedford, R., Wan, M. W., Elsabbagh, M., . . . BASIS Team. (2017). Randomized trial of a parent-mediated intervention for infants at high risk for autism: Longitudinal outcomes to age 3 years. *Journal of Child Psychology and Psychiatry, and Allied Disciplines, 58,* 1330–1340.

Green-Hennessy, S., & Reis, H. T. (1998). Openness in processing social information among attachment types. *Personal Relationships, 5,* 449–466.

Greenaway, K. H., & Aknin, L. B. (2018). Do people turn to visible reminders of group identity under stress? *Journal of Applied Social Psychology, 48,* 205–216.

Greenberg, J., Pyszczynski, T., Solomon, S., Rosenblatt, A., Veeder, M., Kirkland, S., & Lyon, D. (1990). Evidence for terror management theory II: The effects of mortality salience on reactions to those who threaten or bolster the cultural worldview. *Journal of Personality and Social Psychology, 58,* 308–318.

Greenberg, L. S., Ford, C. L., Alden, L. S., & Johnson, S. M. (1993). In-session change in emotionally focused therapy. *Journal of Consulting and Clinical Psychology, 61,* 78–84.

Greenberg, L. S., & Johnson, S. M. (1988). *Emotionally focused therapy for couples.* Guilford Press.

Greenfield, E. A., & Marks, N. F. (2010). Sense of community as a protective factor against long-term psychological effects of childhood violence. *Social Service Review, 84,* 129–147.

Greenleaf, R. K. (1977). *Servant leadership: A journey into the nature of legitimate power and greatness.* Paulist Press.

Greenman, P. S., & Johnson, S. M. (2013). Process research on emotionally focused therapy (EFT) for couples: Linking theory to practice. *Family Process, 52,* 46–61.

Greenman, P. S., Johnson, S. M., & Wiebe, S. (2019). Emotionally focused therapy for couples: At the heart of science and practice. In B. H. Fiese, M. Celano, K. Deater-Deckard, E. N. Jouriles, & M. A. Whisman (Eds.), *APA handbook of contemporary family psychology: Family therapy and training* (pp. 291–305). American Psychological Association.

Greenson, R. R. (1967). *The technique and practice of psychoanalysis* (Vol. 1). International Universities Press.

Gregersen, S. C., & Gillath, O. (2020). How food brings us together: The ties between attachment and food behaviors. *Appetite, 151,* Article 104654.

Gregory, A., Allen, J. P., Mikami, A. Y., Hafen, C. A., & Pianta, R. C. (2014). Effects of a professional development program on behavioral engagement of students in middle and high school. *Psychology in the Schools, 51,* 143–163.

Groeneveld, M. G., Vermeer, H. J., van IJzendoorn, M. H., & Linting, M. (2011). Enhancing home-based child care quality through video-feedback intervention: A randomized controlled trial. *Journal of Family Psychology, 25,* 86–96.

Groh, A. M., & Haydon, K. C. (2018). Mothers' neural and behavioral responses to their infants' distress cues: The role of secure base script knowledge. *Psychological Science, 29,* 242–253.

Gruneau Brulin, J. (2021). *Security in the welfare state: Attachment, religion, and secularity.* PhD dissertation. Stockholm University, Stockholm, Sweden.

Gruneau Brulin, J., Hill, P. C., Laurin, K., Mikulincer, M., & Granqvist, P. (2018). Religion vs. the welfare state: The importance of cultural context for religious schematicity and priming. *Psychology of Religion and Spirituality, 10,* 276–287.

Gruneau Brulin, J., Shaver, P. R., Mikulincer, M., & Granqvist, P. (2022). Attachment in the time of COVID-19: Insecure attachment orientations are associated with defiance of authorities' guidelines during the pandemic. *Journal of Social and Personal Relationships, 39,* 2528–2548.

Guéguen, N., Jacob, C., & Charles-Sire, V. (2011). The effect of the word "loving" on compliance to a fundraising request: Evidence from a French field study. *International Journal of Nonprofit and Voluntary Sector Marketing, 16,* 371–380.

Guerra, P., Sánchez-Adam, A., Anllo-Vento, L., Ramírez, I., & Vila, J. (2012). Viewing loved faces inhibits defense reactions: A health-promotion mechanism? *PLOS ONE, 7,* Article e41631.

Guerrero, L. K. (1996). Attachment-style differences in intimacy and involvement: A test of the four-category model. *Communication Monographs, 63,* 269–292.

Guild, D. J., Alto, M. E., Handley, E. D., Rogosch, F., Cicchetti, D., & Toth, S. L. (2021). Attachment and affect between mothers with depression and their children: Longitudinal outcomes of child parent psychotherapy. *Research on Child and Adolescent Psychopathology, 49,* 563–577.

Guild, D. J., Toth, S. L., Handley, E. D., Rogosch, F. A., & Cicchetti, D. (2017). Attachment security mediates the longitudinal association between child–parent psychotherapy and peer relations for toddlers of depressed mothers. *Development and Psychopathology, 29,* 587–600.

Gully, S. M., Devine, D. J., & Whitney, D. J. (1995). A meta-analysis of cohesion and performance: Effects of levels of analysis and task interdependence. *Small Group Research, 26,* 497–520.

Gunlicks-Stoessel, M., Westervelt, A., Reigstad, K., Mufson, L., & Lee, S. (2019). The role of attachment style in interpersonal psychotherapy for depressed adolescents. *Psychotherapy Research, 29,* 78–85.

Gupta, S., Hill, C. E., & Kivlighan, D. M., Jr. (2018). Client laughter in psychodynamic psychotherapy: Not a laughing matter. *Journal of Counseling Psychology, 65,* 463–473.

Gur-Yaish, N., Cohen, D., & Shochat, T. (2020). Attachment orientations and sleep patterns: The moderating role of exchanges with spouse. *Journal of Social and Personal Relationships, 37,* 1282–1295.

Gurland, S. T., & Grolnick, W. S. (2003). Children's expectancies and perceptions of adults: Effects on rapport. *Child Development, 74,* 1212–1224.

Haas, J. W, Rief, W., Weiß, F., Doering, B. K, Kleinstäuber, M., Ruwoldt, S., . . . Rheker, J. (2022). The effect of patient-centered communication on medication intake: An experimental study. *Psychology, Health and Medicine, 27,* 2138–2151.

Hackney, C. H., & Sanders, G. S. (2003). Religiosity and mental health: A meta-analysis of recent studies. *Journal for the Scientific Study of Religion, 42*, 43–55.

Haft, W. L., & Slade, A. (1989). Affect attunement and maternal attachment: A pilot study. *Infant Mental Health Journal, 10*, 157–172.

Hagan, M. J., Browne, D. T., Sulik, M., Ippen, C. G., Bush, N., & Lieberman, A. F. (2017). Parent and child trauma symptoms during child–parent psychotherapy: A prospective cohort study of dyadic change. *Journal of Traumatic Stress, 30*, 690–697.

Halchuk, R. A., Makinen, J. A., & Johnson, S. M. (2010). Resolving attachment injuries in couples using emotionally focused therapy: A three-year follow-up. *Journal of Couple and Relationship Therapy, 9*, 31–47.

Halford, W. K., & Sweeper, S. (2013). Trajectories of adjustment to couple relationship separation. *Family Process, 52*, 228–243.

Haltigan, J. D., Leerkes, E. M., Supple, A. J., & Calkins, S. D. (2014). Infant negative affect and maternal interactive behavior during the still-face procedure: The moderating role of adult attachment states of mind. *Attachment and Human Development, 16*, 149–173.

Hamilton, W. (1971). Geometry for the selfish herd. *Journal of Theoretical Biology, 31*, 295–311.

Hamre, B. K., Justice, L. M., Pianta, R. C., Kilday, C., Sweeney, B., Downer, J. T., & Leach, A. (2010). Implementation fidelity of MyTeachingPartner literacy and language activities: Association with preschoolers' language and literacy growth. *Early Childhood Research Quarterly, 25*, 329–347.

Hamre, B. K., & Pianta, R. C. (2001). Early teacher–child relationships and the trajectory of children's school outcomes through eighth grade. *Child Development, 72*, 625–638.

Hamre, B. K., Pianta, R. C., Burchinal, M., Field, S., LoCasale-Crouch, J., Downer, J. T., . . . Scott-Little, C. (2012). A course on effective teacher–child interactions: Effects on teacher beliefs, knowledge, and observed practice. *American Educational Research Journal, 49*, 88–123.

Harden, B. J., Martoccio, T. L., & Berlin, L. J. (2021, August 26). Maternal psychological risk moderates the impacts of attachment-based intervention on mother–toddler mutuality and toddler behavior problems: A randomized controlled trial. *Prevention Science*. [Epub ahead of print].

Harding, R., Beesley, H., Holcombe, C., Fisher, J., & Salmon, P. (2015). Are patient–nurse relationships in breast cancer linked to adult attachment style? *Journal of Advanced Nursing, 71*, 2305–2314.

Hardy, G. E., Aldridge, J., Davidson, C., Rowe, C., & Reilly, S. (2004). Assessing and formulating attachment issues and styles in psychotherapy. *British Journal of Psychotherapy, 20*, 493–512.

Hare, A. L., Szwedo, D. E., Schad, M. M., & Allen, J. P. (2015). Undermining adolescent autonomy with parents and peers: The enduring implications of psychologically controlling parenting. *Journal of Research on Adolescence, 25*, 739–752.

Harel, Y., Shechtman, Z., & Cutrona, C. (2011). Individual and group process variables that affect social support in counseling groups. *Group Dynamics, 15*, 297–310.

Harlow, H. F. (1959). Love in infant monkeys. *Scientific American, 200*, 68–86.

Harmon-Jones, E., Greenberg, J., Solomon, S., & Simon, L. (1996). The effects of mortality salience on intergroup bias between minimal groups. *European Journal of Social Psychology, 26*, 677–681.

Harms, P. D., Bai, Y., & Han, G. H. (2016). How leader and follower attachment styles are mediated by trust. *Human Relations, 69*, 1853–1876.

Harpaz-Rotem, I., & Blatt, S. J. (2005). Changes in representations of a self-designated significant other in long-term intensive inpatient treatment of seriously disturbed adolescents and young adults. *Psychiatry, 68*, 266–282.

Hart, J. J., Shaver, P. R., & Goldenberg, J. L. (2005). Attachment, self-esteem, worldviews, and terror management: Evidence for a tripartite security system. *Journal of Personality and Social Psychology, 88*, 999–1013.

Haslam, C., Haslam, S. A., Knight, C., Gleibs, I., Ysseldyk, R., & McCloskey, L.-G. (2014). We can work it out: Group decision-making builds social identity and enhances the cognitive performance of care residents. *British Journal of Psychology, 105*, 17–34.

Haslam, C., Haslam, S. A., Ysseldyk, R., McCloskey, L.-G., Pfisterer, K., & Brown, S. G. (2014). Social identification moderates cognitive health and well-being following story-and song-based reminiscence. *Aging and Mental Health, 18*, 425–434.

Haslam, S. A., Jetten, J., O'Brien, A., & Jacobs, E. (2004). Social identity, social influence and reactions to potentially stressful tasks: Support for the self-categorization model of stress. *Stress and Health, 20*, 3–9.

Haslam, S. A., Jetten, J., Postmes, T., & Haslam, C. (2009). Social identity, health and well-being: An emerging agenda for applied psychology. *Applied Psychology, 58*, 1–23.

Haslam, S. A., & Reicher, S. (2006). Stressing the group: Social identity and the unfolding dynamics of responses to stress. *Journal of Applied Psychology, 91*, 1037–1052.

Haslam, S. A., Reicher, S. D., & Platow, M. J. (2015). Leadership: Theory and practice. In M. Mikulincer, P. R. Shaver, J. F. Dovidio, & J. A. Simpson (Eds.), *APA handbook of personality and social psychology: Vol. 2. Group processes* (pp. 67–94). American Psychological Association.

Hatfield, B. E., & Williford, A. P. (2017). Cortisol patterns for young children displaying disruptive behavior: Links to a teacher–child, relationship-focused intervention. *Prevention Science, 18*, 40–49.

Hauber, K., Boon, A. E., & Vermeiren, R. (2017). Examining changes in personality disorder and symptomology in an adolescent sample receiving intensive mentalization based treatment: A pilot study. *Child and Adolescent Psychiatry and Mental Health, 11,* Article 58.

Håvås, E., Svartberg, M., & Ulvenes, P. (2015). Attuning to the unspoken: The relationship between therapist nonverbal attunement and attachment security in adult psychotherapy. *Psychoanalytic Psychology, 32,* 235–254.

Haviland, J., Sodergren, S., Calman, L., Corner, J., Din, A., Fenlon, D., . . . Study Advisory Committee. (2017). Social support following diagnosis and treatment for colorectal cancer and associations with health-related quality of life: Results from the UK Colorectal Wellbeing (CREW) cohort study. *Psycho-Oncology, 26,* 2276–2284.

Hawkins, A. J., Blanchard, V. L., Baldwin, S. A., & Fawcett, E. B. (2008). Does marriage and relationship education work?: A meta-analytic study. *Journal of Consulting and Clinical Psychology, 76,* 723–734.

Haydon, K. C., Collins, W. A., Salvatore, J. E., Simpson, J. A., & Roisman, G. I. (2012). Shared and distinctive origins and correlates of adult attachment representations: The developmental organization of romantic functioning. *Child Development, 83,* 1689–1702.

Hazan, C., & Shaver, P. R. (1987). Romantic love conceptualized as an attachment process. *Journal of Personality and Social Psychology, 52,* 511–524.

Hazan, C., & Shaver, P. R. (1990). Love and work: An attachment-theoretical perspective. *Journal of Personality and Social Psychology, 59,* 270–280.

Hazan, C., & Zeifman, D. (1994). Sex and the psychological tether. In K. Bartholomew & D. Perlman (Eds.), *Advances in personal relationships: Attachment processes in adulthood* (Vol. 5, pp. 151–177). Jessica Kingsley.

Hediger, K., Wagner, J., Künzi, P., Haefeli, A., Theis, F., Grob, C., . . . Gerger, H. (2021). Effectiveness of animal-assisted interventions for children and adults with post-traumatic stress disorder symptoms: A systematic review and meta-analysis. *European Journal of Psychotraumatology, 12,* Article 1879713.

Helgeson, V. S., Jakubiak, B., Van Vleet, M., & Zajdel, M. (2018). Communal coping and adjustment to chronic illness: Theory update and evidence. *Personality and Social Psychology Review, 22,* 170–195.

Helgeson, V. S., Zajdel, M., Tracy, E. L., Allen, N. A., Kent de Grey, R. G., Litchman, M. L., & Berg, C. A. (2022). Observed dyadic collaboration among couples coping with type 1 diabetes. *Journal of Family Psychology, 36,* 147–152.

Hendrick, C., & Hendrick, S. S. (1986). A theory and method of love. *Journal of Personality and Social Psychology, 50,* 392–402.

Henrich, J., Heine, S. J., & Norenzayan, A. (2010). The weirdest people in the world? *Behavioral and Brain Sciences, 33,* 61–83.

Hepper, E. G., & Carnelley, K. B. (2012). The self-esteem roller coaster: Adult attachment moderates the impact of daily feedback. *Personal Relationships, 19,* 504–520.

Hepworth, A. D., Berlin, L. J., Martoccio, T. L., Cannon, E. N., Berger, R. H., & Harden, B. J. (2020). Supporting infant emotion regulation through attachment-based intervention: A randomized controlled trial. *Prevention Science, 21,* 702–713.

Hepworth, A. D., Berlin, L. J., Salas, K., Pardue-Kim, M., Martoccio, T. L., & Jones Harden, B. (2021). Increasing maternal sensitivity to infant distress through attachment-based intervention: A randomized controlled trial. *Attachment and Human Development, 23,* 953–968.

Herrler, A., Kukla, H., Vennedey, V., & Stock, S. (2021). What matters to people aged 80 and over regarding ambulatory care?: A systematic review and meta-synthesis of qualitative studies. *European Journal of Ageing, 19,* 325–339.

Hertz, R. M., Laurent, H. K., & Laurent, S. M. (2015). Attachment mediates effects of trait mindfulness on stress responses to conflict. *Mindfulness, 6,* 483–489.

Hertzmann, L., Target, M., Hewison, D., Casey, P., Fearon, P., & Lassri, D. (2016). Mentalization-based therapy for parents in entrenched conflict: A random allocation feasibility study. *Psychotherapy, 53,* 388–401.

Hesse, E. (2016). The Adult Attachment Interview: Protocol, method of analysis, and selected empirical studies: 1985–2015. In J. Cassidy & P. R. Shaver (Eds.), *Handbook of attachment: Theory, research, and clinical applications* (3rd ed., pp. 553–557). Guilford Press.

Hicks, A. M., & Diamond, L. M. (2011). Don't go to bed angry: Attachment, conflict, and affective and physiological reactivity. *Personal Relationships, 18,* 266–284.

Hill, E. M., & Gick, M. L. (2013). Attachment and barriers to cervical screening. *Journal of Health Psychology, 18,* 648–657.

Hillen, M. A., de Haes, H. C. J. M., Stalpers, L. J. A., Klinkenbijl, J. H. G., Eddes, E. H., Verdam, M. G. E., & Smets, E. M. A. (2014). How attachment style and locus of control influence patients' trust in their oncologist. *Journal of Psychosomatic Research, 76,* 221–226.

Hinde, R. (1966). *Animal behavior: A synthesis of ethology and comparative psychology.* McGraw-Hill.

Hirschberger, G., Srivastava, S., Marsh, P., Cowan, C., & Cowan, P. (2009). Attachment, marital satisfaction, and divorce during the first 15 years of parenthood. *Personal Relationships, 16,* 401–420.

Ho, M. (2016). Investment in learning increases for fourth straight year. Retrieved from *www.td.org/publications/magazines/td/td-archive/2016/11/investment-in-learning-increases-for-fourth-straight-year.*

Hodes, M. W., Meppelder, M., de Moor, M., Kef, S., & Schuengel, C. (2017). Alleviating parenting stress in parents with intellectual disabilities: A randomized controlled trial of a video-feedback intervention to promote positive parenting. *Journal of Applied Research in Intellectual Disabilities, 30*, 423–432.

Hodes, M. W., Meppelder, M., de Moor, M., Kef, S., & Schuengel, C. (2018). Effects of video-feedback intervention on harmonious parent–child interaction and sensitive discipline of parents with intellectual disabilities: A randomized controlled trial. *Child: Care, Health and Development, 44*, 304–311.

Hofer, M. K., & Chen, F. S. (2020). The scent of a good night's sleep: Olfactory cues of a romantic partner improve sleep efficiency. *Psychological Science, 31*, 449–459.

Hofer, M. K., Collins, H. K., Whillans, A. V., & Chen, F. S. (2018). Olfactory cues from romantic partners and strangers influence women's responses to stress. *Journal of Personality and Social Psychology, 114*, 1–9.

Hoffman, K., Marvin, R., Cooper, G., & Powell, B. (2006). Changing toddlers' and preschoolers' attachment classifications: The COS Intervention. *Journal of Consulting and Clinical Psychology, 74*, 1017–1026.

Hoffmann, R., Lagerkvist, C. J., Hagberg Gustavsson, M., & Holst, B. S. (2018). An empirical examination of the conceptualization of companion animals. *BMC Psychology, 6*, Article 15.

Hofstra, J., van Oudenhoven, J. P., & Buunk, B. P. (2005). Attachment styles and majority members' attitudes towards adaptation strategies of immigrants. *International Journal of Intercultural Relations, 29*, 601–619.

Hogg, M. A. (2007). Uncertainty-identity theory. In M. P. Zanna (Ed.), *Advances in experimental social psychology* (Vol. 39, pp. 69–126). Academic Press.

Högström, J., Olofsson, V., Özdemir, M., Enebrink, P., & Stattin, H. (2017). Two-year findings from a national effectiveness trial: Effectiveness of behavioral and non-behavioral parenting programs. *Journal of Abnormal Child Psychology, 45*, 527–542.

Hojat, M., Gonnella, J. S., Nasca, T. J., Mangione, S., Vergare, M., & Magee, M. (2002). Physician empathy: Definition, components, measurement, and relationship to gender and specialty. *American Journal of Psychiatry, 159*, 1563–1569.

Hojat, M., Louis, D. Z., Markham, F. W., Wender, R., Rabinowitz, C., & Gonnella, J. S. (2011). Physicians' empathy and clinical outcomes for diabetic patients. *Academic Medicine, 86*, 359–364.

Holmes, J. (2001). *The search for the secure base: Attachment theory and psychotherapy*. Brunner-Routledge.

Holwerda, N., Sanderman, R., Pool, G., Hinnen, C., Langendijk, J. A., Bemelman, W. A., . . . Sprangers, M. A. (2013). Do patients trust their physician?: The role of attachment style in the patient–physician relationship within one year after a cancer diagnosis. *Acta Oncologica, 52*, 110–117.

Hood, R. W., Jr., Spilka, B., Hunsberger, B., & Gorsuch, R. (1996). *The psychology of religion: An empirical approach* (2nd ed.). Guilford Press.

Hoogendijk, C., Holland, J. G., Tick, N. T., Hofman, A. W. H., Severiens, S. E., Vuijk, P., . . . van Veen, D. (2020). Effect of Key2Teach on Dutch teachers' relationships with students with externalizing problem behavior: A randomized controlled trial. *European Journal of Psychology of Education, 35*, 111–135.

Hoogendijk, C., Tick, N. T., Hofman, W. H. A., Holland, J. G., Severiens, S. E., Vuijk, P., & van Veen, A. F. D. (2018). Direct and indirect effects of Key2Teach on teachers' sense of self-efficacy and emotional exhaustion, a randomized controlled trial. *Teaching and Teacher Education, 76*, 1–13.

Hoogendijk, C., Tick, N. T., Holland, J. G., Hofman, W. H. A., Severiens, S. E., Vuijk, P., & van Veen, A. F. D. (2020). Effects of Key2Teach on students' externalizing and social–emotional problem behaviors, mediated by the teacher–student relationship. *Emotional and Behavioural Difficulties, 25*, 304–320.

Hornstein, E. A., & Eisenberger, N. I. (2017). Unpacking the buffering effect of social support figures: Social support attenuates fear acquisition. *PLOS ONE, 12*, Article e0175891.

Hornstein, E. A., Fanselow, M. S., & Eisenberger, N. I. (2016). A safe haven: Investigating social-support figures as prepared safety stimuli. *Psychological Science, 27*, 1051–1060.

Hornstein, E. A., Haltom, K. E. B., Shirole, K., & Eisenberger, N. I. (2018). A unique safety signal: Social-support figures enhance rather than protect from fear extinction. *Clinical Psychological Science, 6*, 407–415.

Horton, E., & Murray, C. (2015). A quantitative exploratory evaluation of the COS-parenting program with mothers in residential substance-abuse treatment. *Infant Mental Health Journal, 36*, 320–336.

Hospel, V., & Galand, B. (2016). Are both classroom autonomy support and structure equally important for students' engagement?: A multilevel analysis. *Learning and Instruction, 41*, 1–10.

Howell, J. M. (1988). Two faces of charisma: Socialized and personalized leadership in organizations. In J. A. Conger & R. N. Kanungo (Eds.), *Charismatic leadership: The elusive factor in organizational effectiveness* (pp. 213–236). Jossey-Bass.

Howes, C., & Hamilton, C. E. (1992). Children's relationships with child care teachers: Stability and concordance with parental attachments. *Child Development, 63*, 867–878.

Howes, C., & Ritchie, S. (1998). Changes in child–teacher relationships in a therapeutic preschool program. *Early Education and Development, 9*, 411–422.

Howes, C., & Ritchie, S. (1999). Attachment organizations in children with difficult life circumstances. *Development and Psychopathology, 11*, 251–268.

Howes, C., & Smith, E. W. (1995a). Relations among child care quality, teacher behavior, children's play activities, emotional security, and cognitive activity in child care. *Early Childhood Research Quarterly, 10*, 381–404.

Howes, C., & Smith, E. W. (1995b). Children and their child care caregivers: Profiles of relationships. *Social Development, 7*, 77–51.

Huang, Y., Tan, N. T., & Liu, J. (2016). Support, sense of community, and psychological status in the survivors of the Yaan earthquake. *Journal of Community Psychology, 44*, 919–936.

Huber, A., McMahon, C. A., & Sweller, N. (2015a). Efficacy of the 20-week COS intervention: Changes in caregiver reflective functioning, representations, and child attachment in an Australian clinical sample. *Infant Mental Health Journal, 36*, 556–574.

Huber, A., McMahon, C. A., & Sweller, N. (2015b). Improved child behavioral and emotional functioning after COS 20-week intervention. *Attachment and Human Development, 17*, 547–569.

Huber, A., McMahon, C., & Sweller, N. (2016). Improved parental emotional functioning after Circle of Security 20-week parent–child relationship intervention. *Journal of Child and Family Studies, 25*, 2526–2540.

Hudson, N. W., & Fraley, R. C. (2018). Moving toward greater security: The effects of repeatedly priming attachment security and anxiety. *Journal of Research in Personality, 74*, 147–157.

Humfress, H., O'Connor, T. G., Slaughter, J., Target, M., & Fonagy, P. (2002). General and relationship-specific models of social cognition: Explaining the overlap and discrepancies. *Journal of Child Psychology and Psychiatry, 43*, 873–883.

Hunter, J. J., & Maunder, R. G. (2001). Using attachment theory to understand illness behavior. *General Hospital Psychiatry, 23*, 177–182.

Huth-Bocks, A. C., Muzik, M., Beeghly, M., Earls, L., & Stacks, A. M. (2014). Secure base scripts are associated with maternal parenting behavior across contexts and reflective functioning among trauma-exposed mothers. *Attachment and Human Development, 16*, 535–556.

Hutton, J., Ellett, L., & Berry, K. (2017). Adult attachment and paranoia: An experimental investigation. *Cognitive Behavior Therapist, 10*, Article e4.

IJzerman, H., Lewis, N. A., Jr., Przybylski, A. K., Weinstein, N., DeBruine, L., Ritchie, S. J., . . . Anvari, F. (2020). Use caution when applying behavioral science to policy. *Nature Human Behaviour, 4*, 1092–1094.

Illing, V., Tasca, G. A., Balfour, L., & Bissada, H. (2011). Attachment dimensions and group climate growth in a sample of women seeking treatment for eating disorders. *Psychiatry: Interpersonal and Biological Processes, 74*, 255–269.

Impett, E. A., & Gordon, A. M. (2010). Why do people sacrifice to approach rewards versus to avoid costs?: Insights from attachment theory. *Personal Relationships, 17*, 299–315.

Israel, P., & Diamond, G. S. (2013). Feasibility of attachment based family therapy for depressed clinic-referred Norwegian adolescents. *Clinical Child Psychology and Psychiatry, 18*, 334–350.

Iwakabe, S., Edlin, J., Fosha, D., Gretton, H., Joseph, A. J., Nunnink, S. E., . . . Thoma, N. C. (2020). The effectiveness of accelerated experiential dynamic psychotherapy (AEDP) in private practice settings: A transdiagnostic study conducted within the context of a practice-research network. *Psychotherapy, 57*, 548–561.

Iwakabe, S., Edlin, J., Fosha, D., Thoma, N. C., Gretton, H., Joseph, A. J., & Nakamura, K. (2022). The long-term outcome of accelerated experiential dynamic psychotherapy: 6- and 12-month follow-up results. *Psychotherapy, 59*, 431–446.

Jacobs, W. J., & Lolardo, V. M. (1977). The sensory basis of avoidance responding in the rat: Relative dominance of auditory or visual warning signals and safety signals. *Learning and Motivation, 8*, 448–466.

Jacobsen, M. N., Ha, C., & Sharp, C. (2015). A mentalization-based treatment approach to caring for youth in foster care. *Journal of Infant, Child, and Adolescent Psychotherapy, 14*, 440–454.

Jakubiak, B. K., Debrot, A., Kim, J., & Impett, E. A. (2021). Approach and avoidance motives for touch are predicted by attachment and predict daily relationship well-being. *Journal of Personal and Social Relationships, 38*, 256–278.

Jakubiak, B. K., & Feeney, B. C. (2016). Daily goal progress is facilitated by spousal support and promotes psychological, physical, and relational well-being throughout adulthood. *Journal of Personality and Social Psychology, 111*, 317–340.

Jakubiak, B. K., & Feeney, B. C. (2019). Interpersonal touch as a resource to facilitate positive personal and relational outcomes during stress discussions. *Journal of Social and Personal Relationships, 36*, 2918–2936.

James, P. S. (1991). Effects of a communication training component added to an emotionally focused couples therapy. *Journal of Marital and Family Therapy, 17*, 263–275.

Jankowski, P. J., & Sandage, S. J. (2011). Meditative prayer, hope, adult attachment, and forgiveness: A proposed model. *Psychology of Religion and Spirituality, 3*, 115–131.

Jaremka, L. M., Glaser, R., Loving, T. J., Malarkey, W. B., Stowell, J. R., & Kiecolt-Glaser, J. K. (2013). Attachment anxiety is linked to alterations in cortisol production and cellular immunity. *Psychological Science, 24*, 272–279.

Jarvinen, M. J., & Paulus, T. B. (2017). Attachment and cognitive openness: Emotional underpinnings of intellectual humility. *Journal of Positive Psychology, 12*, 74–86.

Jennissen, S., Huber, J., Ehrenthal, J. C., Schauenburg, H., & Dinger, U. (2018). Association between insight and outcome of psychotherapy: Systematic review and meta-analysis. *American Journal of Psychiatry, 175*, 961–969.

Jerga, C., Shaver, P. R., & Wilkinson, R. B. (2011). Attachment insecurities and identification of at-risk individuals following the death of a loved one. *Journal of Social and Personal Relationships, 28*, 891–914.

Jetten, J., Branscombe, N. R., Haslam, S. A., Haslam, C., Cruwys, T., Jones, J. M., . . . Zhang, A. (2015). Having a lot of a good thing: Multiple important group memberships as a source of self-esteem. *PLOS ONE, 10*, e0131035.

Jetten, J., Haslam, C., & Haslam, S. A. (Eds.). (2012). *The social cure: Identity, health and well-being.* Psychology Press.

Jetten, J., Haslam, S. A., Cruwys, T., Greenaway, K. H., Haslam, C., & Steffens, N. K. (2017). Advancing the social identity approach to health and well-being: Progressing the social cure research agenda. *European Journal of Social Psychology, 47*, 789–802.

Jimenez, X. F. (2017). Attachment in medical care: A review of the interpersonal model in chronic disease management. *Chronic Illness, 13*, 14–27.

Johnson, S. M. (2004). *The practice of emotionally focused couple therapy: Creating connection* (2nd ed.). Routledge.

Johnson, S. M. (2008). *Hold me tight: Seven conversations for a lifetime of love.* Little, Brown Spark.

Johnson, S. M. (2010). *The hold me tight program: Conversations for connection: Facilitator's guide for small groups.* International Centre for Excellence in Emotionally Focused Therapy.

Johnson, S. M. (2019a). *Attachment theory in practice: Emotionally focused therapy (EFT) with individuals, couples, and families.* Guilford Press.

Johnson, S. M. (2019b). Attachment in action: Changing the face of 21st century couple therapy. *Current Opinion in Psychology, 25*, 101–104.

Johnson, S. M., Burgess Moser, M., Beckes, L., Smith, A., Dalgleish, T., Halchuk, R., . . . Coan, J. A. (2013). Soothing the threatened brain: Leveraging contact comfort with emotionally focused therapy. *PLOS ONE, 8*, e79314.

Johnson, S. M., & Campbell, T. L. (2022). *A primer of emotionally focused individual therapy (EFIT): Cultivating fitness and growth in every client.* Routledge.

Johnson, S. M., & Greenberg, L. S. (1985a). Differential effects of experiential and problem-solving interventions in resolving marital conflict. *Journal of Consulting and Clinical Psychology, 53*, 175–184.

Johnson, S. M., & Greenberg, L. S. (1985b). Emotionally focused couples therapy: An outcome study. *Journal of Marital and Family Therapy, 11*, 313–317.

Johnson, S. M., & Greenberg, L. S. (1988). Relating process to outcome in marital therapy. *Journal of Marital and Family Therapy, 14*, 175–183.

Johnson, S. M., & Greenman, P. S. (2006). The path to a secure bond: Emotionally focused couple therapy. *Journal of Clinical Psychology, 62*, 597–609.

Johnson, S. M., Hunsley, J., Greenberg, L., & Schindler, D. (1999). Emotionally focused couples therapy: Status and challenges. *Clinical Psychology: Science and Practice, 6*, 67–79.

Johnson, S. M., & Talitman, E. (1997). Predictors of success in emotionally focused marital therapy. *Journal of Marital and Family Therapy, 23*, 135–152.

Johnston, M. A. (2000). Delegation and organizational structure in small businesses: Influences of manager's attachment patterns. *Group and Organization Management, 25*, 4–21.

Jonas, E., Kauffeld, S., Sullivan, D., & Fritsche, I. (2011). Dedicate your life to the company!: A terror management perspective on organizations. *Journal of Applied Social Psychology, 41*, 2858–2882.

Jones, J. D., Brett, B. E., Ehrlich, K. B., Lejuez, C. W., & Cassidy, J. (2014). Maternal attachment style and responses to adolescents' negative emotions: The mediating role of maternal emotion regulation. *Parenting: Science and Practice, 14*, 235–257.

Jones, J. D., & Cassidy, J. (2014). Parental attachment style: Examination of links with parent secure base provision and adolescent secure base use. *Attachment and Human Development, 16*, 437–461.

Jones, J. D., Cassidy, J., & Shaver, P. R. (2015a). Parents' self-reported attachment styles: A review of links with parenting behaviors, emotions, and cognitions. *Personality and Social Psychology Review, 19*, 44–76.

Jones, J. D., Cassidy, J., & Shaver, P. R. (2015b). Adult attachment style and parenting. In J. A. Simpson & W. S. Rholes (Eds.), *Attachment theory and research: New directions and emerging themes* (pp. 234–260). Guilford Press.

Jones, J. D., Ehrlich, K. B., Brett, B. E., Gross, J. T., Mohr, J. J., Hopper, E. A., . . . Cassidy, J. (2017). Perceptions of parental secure base support in African American adolescents and young adults: A preliminary study of predictive links to adult C-reactive protein. *Journal of Social and Personal Relationships, 34*, 1168–1185.

Jones, J. D., Ehrlich, K. B., Lejuez, C. W., & Cassidy, J. (2015). Parental knowledge of adolescent activities: Links with parental attachment style and adolescent substance use. *Journal of Family Psychology, 29*, 191–200.

Jones, J. D., Fraley, R. C., Ehrlich, K. B., Stern, J. A., Lejuez, C. W., Shaver, P. R., & Cassidy, J. (2018). Stability of attachment style in adolescence: An empirical test of alternative developmental processes. *Child Development, 89*, 871–880.

Jones, J. D., Stern, J. A., Fitter, M., Mikulincer, M., Shaver, P. R., & Cassidy, J. (2022). Attachment and attitudes toward children: Effects of security priming in parents and non-parents. *Attachment and Human Development, 24*, 147–168.

Jørgensen, M. S., Storebø, O. J., Bo, S., Poulsen, S., Gondan, M., Beck, E., . . . Simonsen, E. (2021). Mentalization-based treatment in groups for adolescents with borderline personality disorder: 3- and 12-month follow-up of a randomized controlled trial. *European Child and Adolescent Psychiatry, 30*, 699–710.

Joseph, M. A., O'Connor, T. G., Briskman, J. A., Maughan, B., & Scott, S. (2014). The formation of secure new attachments by children who were maltreated: An observational study of adolescents in foster care. *Development and Psychopathology, 26*, 67–80.

Juffer, F., Bakermans-Kranenburg, M. J., & van IJzendoorn, M. H. (2005). The importance of parenting in the development of disorganized attachment: Evidence from a preventive intervention study in adoptive families. *Journal of Child Psychology and Psychiatry, 46*, 263–274.

Juffer, F., Bakermans-Kranenburg, M. J., & van IJzendoorn, M. H. (2015). *Manual Video-Feedback Intervention to promote Positive Parenting and Sensitive Discipline (VIPP-SD) (version 3.0)*. Leiden University, Centre for Child and Family Studies.

Juffer, F., BakermansKranenburg, M. J., & van IJzendoorn, M. H. (2018). Videofeedback intervention to promote positive parenting and sensitive discipline: Development and meta-analytic evidence for its effectiveness. In H. Steele & M. Steele (Eds.), *Handbook of attachment-based interventions* (pp. 1–26). Guilford Press.

Juffer, F., & Steele, M. (2014). What words cannot say: The telling story of video in attachment-based interventions. *Attachment and Human Development, 16*, 307–314.

Juffer, F., van IJzendoorn, M. H., & Bakermans-Kranenburg, M. J. (2008). Supporting adoptive families with video-feedback intervention. In F. Juffer, M. J. Bakermans-Kranenburg, & M. H. van IJzendoorn (Eds.), *Promoting positive parenting: An attachment-based intervention* (pp. 139–153). Taylor & Francis.

Julal, F. S., & Carnelley, K. B. (2012). Attachment, perceptions of care and caregiving to romantic partners and friends. *European Journal of Social Psychology, 42*, 832–843.

Jungert, T., & Koestner, R. (2015). Science adjustment, parental and teacher autonomy support and the cognitive orientation of science students. *Educational Psychology, 35*, 361–376.

Kabat-Zinn, J. (1994). *Wherever you go, there you are: Mindfulness meditation in everyday life*. Hyperion.

Kachadourian, L. K., Fincham, F., & Davila, J. (2004). The tendency to forgive in dating and married couples: The role of attachment and relationship satisfaction. *Personal Relationships, 11*, 373–393.

Kafetsios, K., Athanasiadou, M., & Dimou, N. (2014). Leaders' and subordinates' attachment orientations, emotion regulation capabilities and affect at work: A multilevel analysis. *Leadership Quarterly, 25*, 512–527.

Kafetsios, K., Hantzara, K., Anagnostopoulos, F., & Niakas, D. (2016). Doctors' attachment orientations, emotion regulation strategies, and patient satisfaction: A multilevel analysis. *Health Communication, 31*, 772–777.

Kafetsios, K., & Nezlek, J. B. (2002). Attachment styles in everyday social interaction. *European Journal of Social Psychology, 32*, 719–735.

Kalinauskiene, L., Cekuoliene, D., van IJzendoorn, M. H., Bakermans-Kranenburg, M. J., Juffer, F., & Kusakovskaja, I. (2009). Supporting insensitive mothers: The Vilnius randomized control trial of video feedback intervention to promote maternal sensitivity and infant attachment. *Child: Care, Health and Development, 35*, 613–623.

Kammrath, L. K., Armstrong, B. F., III, Lane, S. P., Francis, M. K., Clifton, M., McNab, K. M., . . . Baumgarten, O. M. (2020). What predicts who we approach for social support?: Tests of the attachment figure and strong ties hypotheses. *Journal of Personality and Social Psychology, 118*, 481–500.

Kane, H. S., McCall, C., Collins, N., & Blascovich, J. B. (2012). Mere presence is not enough: Responsive support in a virtual world. *Journal of Experimental Social Psychology, 48*, 37–44.

Kaniasty, K. (2020). Social support, interpersonal, and community dynamics following disasters caused by natural hazards. *Current Opinion in Psychology, 32*, 105–109.

Karl, A, Carnelley, K. B., Arikan, G., Baldwin, D. S., Heinrichs, M., & Stopa, L. (2021). The effect of attachment security priming and oxytocin on physiological responses to trauma films and subsequent intrusions. *Behaviour Research and Therapy, 141*, Article e103845.

Karreman, A., Vingerhoets, A. J. J. M., & Bekker, M. H. J. (2019). Attachment styles and secure base priming in relation to emotional reactivity after frustration induction. *Cognition and Emotion, 33*, 428–441.

Karremans, J. C., & Aarts, H. (2007). The role of automaticity in determining the inclination to forgive close others. *Journal of Experimental Social Psychology, 43*, 902–917.

Karremans, J. C., Heslenfeld, D. J., van Dillen, L. F., & Van Lange, P. A. M. (2011). Secure attachment partners attenuate neural responses to social exclusion: An fMRI investigation. *International Journal of Psychophysiology, 81*, 44–50.

Karterud, S. (2015). *Mentalization-based group therapy (MBT-G): A theoretical, clinical, and research manual*. Oxford University Press.

Katon, W. J., Lin, E. H. B., Von Korff, M., Ciechanowski, P., Ludman, E., Young, B., . . . McCulloch, D. (2010). Collaborative care for patients with depression and chronic illnesses. *New England Journal of Medicine, 363*, 2611–2620.

Katznelson, H. (2014). Reflective functioning: A review. *Clinical Psychology Review, 34*, 107–117.

Katznelson, H., Falkenström, F., Daniel, S. I. F., Lunn, S., Folke, S., Pedersen, S. H., & Poulsen, S. (2020). Reflective functioning, psychotherapeutic alliance, and outcome in two psychotherapies for bulimia nervosa. *Psychotherapy, 57*, 129–140.

Kay, A. C., Gaucher, D., Napier, J. L., Callan, M. J., & Laurin, K. (2008). God and the government: Testing a compensatory control mechanism for the support of external systems. *Journal of Personality and Social Psychology, 95*, 18–35.

Kay, A. C., Wheeler, S. C., Bargh, J. A., & Ross, L. (2004). Material priming: The influence of mundane physical objects on situational construal and competitive behavioral choice. *Organizational Behavior and Human Decision Processes, 95*, 83–96.

Kealy, D., Rice, S. M., Chartier, G. B., & Cox, D. W. (2021). Investigating attachment insecurity and somatosensory amplification, and the mediating role of interpersonal problems. *European Journal of Health Psychology, 28*, 120–130.

Keating, L., Tasca, G., Gick, M., Ritchie, T., Balfour, L., & Bissada, H. (2014). Change in attachment to the therapy group generalizes to change in individual attachment among women with binge-eating disorder. *Psychotherapy, 51*, 78–87.

Kedia, S. K., Collins, A., Dillon, P. J., Akkus, C., Ward, K. D., & Jackson, B. M. (2020). Psychosocial interventions for informal caregivers of lung cancer patients: A systematic review. *Psycho-Oncology, 29*, 251–262.

Keefe, F. J., Affleck, G., Lefebvre, J., Underwood, L., Caldwell, D. S., Drew, J., . . . Pargament, K. (2001). Living with rheumatoid arthritis: The role of daily spirituality and daily religious and spiritual coping. *Journal of Pain, 2*, 101–110.

Keller, C. J., & Brown, C. (2014). Conflictual independence, adult attachment orientation, and career indecision among Asian American students. *Journal of Career Development, 41*, 426–444.

Keller, H. (2018). Universality claim of attachment theory: Children's socioemotional development across cultures. *Proceedings of the National Academy of Sciences of the USA, 115*, 11414–11419.

Keller, T. (2003). Parental images as a guide to leadership sense-making: An attachment perspective on implicit leadership theories. *Leadership Quarterly, 14*, 141–160.

Kelley, H. H., Berscheid, E., Christensen, A., Harvey, J. A., Huston, T. L., Levinger, G., . . . Peterson, D. R. (1983). *Close relationships*. New York: Freeman.

Kelm, Z., Womer, J., Walter, J. K., & Feudtner, C. (2014). Interventions to cultivate physician empathy: A systematic review. *BMC Medical Education, 14*, Article 219.

Kennedy, N., Johnson, S. M., Wiebe, S. A., Willett, J. B., & Tasca, G. A. (2019). Conversations for connection: An outcome assessment of the Hold-Me-Tight relationship-education program, and recommendations for improving future research methodology in relationship education. *Journal of Marital and Family Therapy, 45*, 431–446.

Kent de Grey, R. G., Uchino, B. N., Pietromonaco, P. R., Hogan, J. N., Smith, T. W., Cronan, S., & Trettevik, R. (2019). Strained bedfellows: An actor-partner analysis of spousal attachment insecurity and sleep quality. *Annals of Behavioral Medicine, 53*, 115–125.

Kerns, K. A., Aspelmeier, J. E., Gentzler, A. L., & Grabill, C. M. (2001). Parent–child attachment and monitoring in middle childhood. *Journal of Family Psychology, 15*, 69–81.

Kerns, K. A., Tomich, P. L., & Kim, P. (2006). Normative trends in children's perceptions of availability and utilization of attachment figures in middle childhood. *Social Development, 15*, 1–22.

Kestenbaum, R., Farber, E. A., & Sroufe, L. A. (1989). Individual differences in empathy among preschoolers: Relation to attachment history. In N. Eisenberg (Ed.), *Empathy and related emotional competence. New Directions for child development* (pp. 51–64). Jossey-Bass.

Kidd, T., Hamer, M., & Steptoe, A. (2011). Examining the association between adult attachment style and cortisol responses to acute stress. *Psychoneuroendocrinology, 36*, 771–779.

Kidd, T., Hamer, M., & Steptoe, A. (2013). Adult attachment style and cortisol responses across the day in older adults. *Psychophysiology, 50*, 841–847.

Kidd, T., Poole, L., Leigh, E., Ronaldson, A., Jahangiri, M., & Steptoe, A. (2014). Attachment anxiety predicts IL-6 and length of hospital stay in coronary artery bypass graft surgery (CABG) patients. *Journal of Psychosomatic Research, 77*, 155–157.

Kilmann, P. R., Laughlin, J. E., Carranza, L. V., Downer, J. T., Major, S., & Parnell, M. M. (1999). Effects of an attachment-focused group preventive intervention on insecure women. *Group Dynamics, 3*, 138–147.

Kilmann, P. R., Vendemia, J. M. C., Parnell, M. M., & Urbaniak, G. C. (2009). Parent characteristics linked with daughters' attachment styles. *Adolescence, 44*, 557–568.

Kim, K. J., Feeney, B. C., & Jakubiak, B. K. (2018). Touch reduces romantic jealousy in the anxiously attached. *Journal of Social and Personal Relationships, 35*, 1019–1041.

Kim, S., Fonagy, P., Allen, J., Martinez, S., Iyengar, U., & Strathearn, L. (2014). Mothers who are securely attached in pregnancy show more attuned infant mirroring 7 months postpartum. *Infant Behavior and Development, 37*, 491–504.

Kim, Y. (2006). Gender, attachment, and relationship duration on cardiovascular reactivity to stress in a laboratory study of dating couples. *Personal Relationships, 13*, 103–114.

Kim, Y., & Carver, C. S. (2007). Frequency and difficulty in caregiving among spouses of individuals with cancer: Effects of adult attachment and gender. *Psycho-Oncology, 16*, 714–728.

Kim, Y., Carver, C. S., Deci, E. L., & Kasser, T. (2008). Adult attachment and psychological well-being in cancer caregivers: The meditational role of spouses' motives for caregiving. *Health Psychology, 27*, S144–S154.

Kinley, J. L., & Reyno, S. M. (2013). Attachment style changes following intensive short-term group psychotherapy. *International Journal of Group Psychotherapy, 63*, 53–75.

Kirchmann, H., Steyer, R., Mayer, A., Joraschky, P., Schreiber-Willnow, K., & Strauss, B. (2012). Effects of adult inpatient group psychotherapy on attachment characteristics: An observational study comparing routine care to an untreated comparison group. *Psychotherapy Research, 22*, 95–114.

Kirkpatrick, L. A. (1994). The role of attachment in religious belief and behavior. In D. Perlman & K. Bartholomew (Eds.), *Advances in personal relationships* (Vol. 5, pp. 239–265). Jessica Kingsley.

Kirkpatrick, L. A. (2005). *Attachment, evolution, and the psychology of religion*. Guilford Press.

Kirkpatrick, L. A., & Shaver, P. R. (1992). An attachment-theoretical approach to romantic love and religious belief. *Personality and Social Psychology Bulletin, 18*, 266–275.

Kiss, O., Kis, A., Scheiling, K., & Topál, J. (2020). Behavioral and neurophysiological correlates of dogs' individual sensitivities to being observed by their owners while performing a repetitive fetching task. *Frontiers in Psychology, 11*, Article 1461.

Kitagawa, M., Iwamoto, S., Umemura, T., Kudo, S., Kazui, M., Matsuura, H., & Mesman, J. (2022). Attachment-based intervention improves Japanese parent–child relationship quality: A pilot study. *Current Psychology, 41*, 8568–8578.

Kivlighan, D. M., Jr., Lo Coco, G. L., & Gullo, S. (2012). Attachment anxiety and avoidance and perceptions of group climate: An actor–partner interdependence analysis. *Journal of Counseling Psychology, 59*, 518–527.

Kivlighan, D. M., Jr., Lo Coco, G., Gullo, S., Pazzagli, C., & Mazzeschi, C. (2017). Attachment anxiety and attachment avoidance: Members' attachment fit with their group and group relationships. *International Journal of Group Psychotherapy, 67*, 223–239.

Kivlighan, D. M., Jr., Multon, K. D., & Patton, M. J. (2000). Insight and symptom reduction in time-limited psychoanalytic counseling. *Journal of Counseling Psychology, 47*, 50–58.

Klein, K. J., & Ziegert, J. C. (2004). Leader development and change over time: A conceptual integration and exploration of research challenges. In D. V. Day, S. J. Zaccaro, & S. M. Halpin (Eds.), *Leader development for transforming organizations: Growing leaders for tomorrow* (pp. 359–382). Erlbaum.

Klein Velderman, M. K., Bakermans-Kranenburg, M. J., Juffer, F., van IJzendoorn, M. H., Mangelsdorf, S. C., & Zevalkink, J. (2006). Preventing preschool externalizing behavior problems through video-feedback intervention in infancy. *Infant Mental Health Journal, 27*, 466–493.

Klerman, G. L., Weissman, M. M. (1994). *Interpersonal psychotherapy of depression: A brief, focused, specific strategy*. Rowman & Littlefield.

Klerman, G. L., Weissman, M. M., Rounsaville, B. J., Chevron, E. S. (1984). *Interpersonal psychotherapy for depression*. Basic Books.

Klohnen, E. C., & Bera, S. (1998). Behavioral and experiential patterns of avoidantly and securely attached women across adulthood: A 31-year longitudinal perspective. *Journal of Personality and Social Psychology, 74*, 211–223.

Knabb, J. J., & Pelletier, J. (2014). The relationship between problematic Internet use, God attachment, and psychological functioning among adults at a Christian university. *Mental Health, Religion and Culture, 17*, 239–251.

Knabb, J. J., Vazquez, V. E., Wang, K. T., & Pate, R. A. (2021). The Christian Gratitude Scale: An emic approach to measuring thankfulness in every season of life. *Spirituality in Clinical Practice*. [Epub ahead of print].

Kobak, R. R., Abbott, C., Zisk, A., & Bounoua, N. (2017). Adapting to the changing needs of adolescents: Parenting practices and challenges to sensitive attunement. *Current Opinion in Psychology, 15*, 137–142.

Kobak, R. R., Cole, H. E., Ferenz-Gillies, R., Fleming, W. S., & Gamble, S. (1993). Attachment and emotion regulation during mother–teen problem solving: A control theory analysis. *Child Development, 64*, 231–245.

Kobak, R. R., Ferenz-Gillies, R., Everhart, E., & Seabrook, L. (1994). Maternal attachment strategies and emotion regulation with adolescent offspring. *Journal of Research on Adolescence, 4*, 553–566.

Kobak, R., Herres, J., Gaskins, C., & Laurenceau, J.-P. (2012). Teacher–student interactions and attachment states of mind as predictors of early romantic involvement and risky sexual behaviors. *Attachment and Human Development, 14*, 289–303.

Kobak, R. R., & Kerig, P. K. (2015). Introduction to the special issue: Attachment-based treatments for adolescents. *Attachment and Human Development, 17*, 111–118.

Kochanska, G., Boldt, L. J., & Goffin, K. C. (2019). Early relational experience: A foundation for the unfolding dynamics of parent–child socialization. *Child Development Perspectives, 13*, 41–47.

Koehn, A. J., & Kerns, K. A. (2018). Parent–child attachment: Meta-analysis of associations with parenting behaviors in middle childhood and adolescence. *Attachment and Human Development, 20*, 378–405.

Koenig, H. G., King, D. E., & Carson, V. B. (2012).

Handbook of religion and health (2nd ed.). Oxford University Press.

Kogut, T., & Kogut, E. (2013). Exploring the relationship between adult attachment style and the identifiable victim effect in helping behavior. *Journal of Experimental Social Psychology, 49*, 651–660.

Kolijn, L., den Bulk, B. G., van IJzendoorn, M. H., Bakermans-Kranenburg, M. J., & Huffmeijer, R. (2021). Does maternal inhibitory control mediate effects of a parenting intervention on maternal sensitive discipline?: Evidence from a randomized-controlled trial. *Infant Mental Health Journal, 42*, 749–766.

Komives, S. R., Lucas, N., & McMahon, T. R. (2013). *Exploring leadership*. Jossey-Bass.

Koomen, H. M. Y., & Hoeksma, J. B. (2003). Regulation of emotional security by children after entry to special and regular kindergarten classes. *Psychological Reports, 93*, 1319–1334.

Kor, A., Mikulincer, M., & Pirutinsky, S. (2012). Family functioning among returnees to Orthodox Judaism in Israel. *Journal of Family Psychology, 26*, 149–158.

Kordahji, H., Bar-Kalifa, E., & Rafaeli, E. (2015). Attachment insecurity as a moderator of cardiovascular arousal effects following dyadic support. *Journal of Research in Personality, 57*, 89–99.

Koren-Karie, N., Oppenheim, D. (2001). *Insightfulness procedure administration and coding manual*. Unpublished manual, University of Haifa, Haifa, Israel.

Koren-Karie, N., Oppenheim, D., Dolev, S., Sher, E., & Etzion-Carasso, A. (2002). Mothers' insightfulness regarding their infants' internal experience: Relations with maternal sensitivity and infant attachment. *Developmental Psychology, 38*, 534–542.

Korom, M., Goldstein, A., Tabachnick, A. R., Palmwood, E. N., Simons, R. F., & Dozier, M. (2021). Early parenting intervention accelerates inhibitory control development among CPS-involved children in middle childhood: A randomized clinical trial. *Developmental Science, 24*, Article e13054.

Kosminsky, P. S., & Jordan, J. R. (2016). *Attachment-informed grief therapy: The clinician's guide to foundations and applications*. Routledge.

Krahé, C., Paloyelis, Y., Condon, H., Jenkinson, P. M., Williams, S. C. R., & Fotopoulou, A. (2015). Attachment style moderates partner presence effects on pain: A laser-evoked potentials study. *Social Cognitive and Affective Neuroscience, 10*, 1030–1037.

Kratz, A. L., Davis, M. C., & Zautra, A. J. (2012). Attachment predicts daily catastrophizing and social coping in women with pain. *Health Psychology, 31*, 278–285.

Kraus, M. W., & Chen, S. (2009). Striving to be known by significant others: Automatic activation of self-verification goals in relationship contexts. *Journal of Personality and Social Psychology, 97*, 58–73.

Krishnamoorthy, G., Hessing, P., Middeldorp, C., & Branjerdporn, M. (2020). Effects of the "Circle of Security" group parenting program (COS-P) with foster carers: An observational study. *Children and Youth Services Review, 115*, Article 105082.

Krpalek, D., Meredith, P., & Ziviani, J. (2014). Investigating mediated pathways between adult attachment patterns and reported rates of absenteeism and presenteeism. *Journal of Workplace Behavioral Health, 29*, 259–280.

Kruger, K. A., & Serpell, J. A. (2006). Animal-assisted interventions in mental health: Definitions and theoretical foundations. In A. H. Fine (Ed.), *Handbook on animal-assisted therapy: Theoretical foundations and guidelines for practice* (2nd ed., pp. 21–38). Academic Press.

Kuhn, R., Milek, A., Meuwly, N., Bradbury, T. N., & Bodenmann, G. (2017). Zooming in: A microanalysis of couples' dyadic coping conversations after experimentally induced stress. *Journal of Family Psychology, 31*, 1063–1073.

Kumashiro, M., & Sedikides, C. (2005). Taking on board liability-focused information: Close positive relationships as a self-bolstering resource. *Psychological Science, 16*, 732–739.

Kunce, L. J., & Shaver, P. R. (1994). An attachment-theoretical approach to caregiving in romantic relationships. In K. Bartholomew & D. Perlman (Eds.), *Advances in personal relationships: Attachment processes in adulthood* (Vol. 5, pp. 205–237). Jessica Kingsley.

Kupor, D. M., Laurin, K., & Levav, J. (2015). Anticipating divine protection?: Reminders of god can increase non-moral risk taking. *Psychological Science, 26*, 374–384.

Kurdek, L. A. (2008). Pet dogs as attachment figures. *Journal of Social and Personal Relationships, 25*, 247–266.

Kurtessis, J. N., Eisenberger, R., Ford, M. T., Buffardi, L. C., Stewart, K. A., & Adis, C. S. (2017). Perceived organizational support: A meta-analytic evaluation of organizational support theory. *Journal of Management, 43*, 1854–1884.

Kwon, K. I., & Jo, S. Y. (2012). The relationship among counselor experience level, empathic accuracy, and counseling outcome in the early phase of counseling. *Asia Pacific Education Review, 13*, 771–777.

Kwong, M., & Bartholomew, K. (2011). "Not just a dog": An attachment perspective on relationships with assistance dogs. *Attachment and Human Development, 13*, 421–436.

La Guardia, J. G., Ryan, R. M., Couchman, C. E., & Deci, E. L. (2000). Within-person variation in security of attachment: A self-determination theory perspective on attachment, need fulfillment, and well-being. *Journal of Personality and Social Psychology, 79*, 367–384.

La Valley, A. G., & Guerrero, L. K. (2012). Perceptions

of conflict behavior and relational satisfaction in adult parent–child relationships: A dyadic analysis from an attachment perspective. *Communication Research, 39,* 48–78.
Labella, M. H., Lind, T., Sellers, T., Roben, C. K. P., & Dozier, M. (2020). Emotion regulation among children in foster care versus birth parent care: Differential effects of an early home-visiting intervention. *Journal of Abnormal Child Psychology, 48,* 995–1006.
Lacerenza, C. N., Reyes, D. L., Marlow, S. L., Joseph, D. L., & Salas, E. (2017). Leadership training design, delivery, and implementation: A meta-analysis. *Journal of Applied Psychology, 102,* 1686–1718.
Lafontaine, M. F., Brassard, A., Lussier, Y., Valois, P., Shaver, P. R., & Johnson, S. M. (2015). Selecting the best items for a short-form of the Experiences in Close Relationships questionnaire. *European Journal of Psychological Assessment, 32,* 140–154.
Lamb, M. E. (2005). Attachments, social networks, and developmental contexts. *Human Development, 48,* 108–112.
Lambert, A. J., Schott, J. P., & Scherer, L. (2011). Threat, politics, and attitudes: Toward a greater understanding of rally-'round-the-flag effects. *Current Directions in Psychological Science, 20,* 343–348.
Larose, S., Bernier, A., & Tarabulsy, G. M. (2005). Attachment state of mind, learning dispositions, and academic performance during the college transition. *Developmental Psychology, 41,* 281–289.
Larose, S., Tarabulsy, G. M., Boisclair-Châteauvert, G., & Karcher, M. (2019). When insecure attachment dispositions affect mentoring relationship quality: An exploration of interactive mentoring contexts. *Journal of Relationships Research, 10,* Article e6.
Lasher, M. (1998). A relational approach to the human–animal bond. *Anthrozoös, 11,* 130–133.
Lattifian, M., & Delavarpour, M. A. (2012). An investigation into the relationship between attachment style and mental health by the mediating role of emotional creativity. *Advances in Cognitive Science, 14,* 45–62.
Lau, K. K. H., Randall, A. K., Duran, N. D., & Tao, C. (2019). Examining the effects of couples' real-time stress and coping processes on interaction quality: Language use as a mediator. *Frontiers in Psychology, 9,* Article 2598.
Laurenssen, E. M. P., Hutsebaut, J., Feenstra, D. J., Bales, D. L., Noom, M. J., Busschbach, J. J. V., . . . Luyten, P. (2014). Feasibility of mentalization-based treatment for adolescents with borderline symptoms: A pilot study. *Psychotherapy, 51,* 159–166.
Laurenssen, E. M. P., Luyten, P., Kikkert, M. J., Westra, D., Peen, J., Soons, M. B. J., . . . Dekker, J. J. M. (2018). Day hospital mentalization-based treatment v. specialist treatment as usual in patients with borderline personality disorder: Randomized controlled trial. *Psychological Medicine, 48,* 2522–2529.
Laurent, H., & Powers, S. (2007). Emotion regulation in emerging adult couples: Temperament, attachment, and HPA response to conflict. *Biological Psychology, 76,* 61–71.
Lavi, I., Gard, A. M., Hagan, M., Van Horn, P., & Lieberman, A. F. (2015). Child–parent psychotherapy examined in a perinatal sample: Depression, posttraumatic stress symptoms and child-rearing attitudes. *Journal of Social and Clinical Psychology, 34,* 64–82.
Lavi, N. (2007). *Bolstering attachment security in romantic relationships: The long-term contribution of partner's sensitivity, expressiveness, and supportiveness.* Unpublished doctoral dissertation, Bar-Ilan University, Ramat Gan, Israel.
Lavy, S. (2014). Supervisor security provision: Correlates and related mechanisms. *Psychological Reports, 114,* 758–783.
Lavy, S., Bareli, Y., & Ein-Dor, T. (2015). The effects of attachment heterogeneity and team cohesion on team functioning. *Small Group Research, 46,* 27–49.
Lavy, S., Mikulincer, M., & Shaver, P. R. (2013). Intrusiveness from an attachment theory perspective: A dyadic diary study. *Personality and Individual Differences, 55,* 972–977.
Lawson, D., Barnes, A. D., Madkins, J. P., & Francois-Lamonte, B. M. (2006). Changes in male partner abuser attachment styles in group treatment. *Psychotherapy, 43,* 232–237.
Le, T. L., Conklin, C. A., George, T. P., Levitan, R. D., Mann, R. E., & Maunder, R. G. (2020). Exposure to attachment figure cue reduces cigarette craving. *Experimental and Clinical Psychopharmacology, 28,* 81–86.
Lee, A., Lyubovnikova, J., Tian, A. W., & Knight, C. (2020). Servant leadership: A meta-analytic examination of incremental contribution, moderation, and mediation. *Journal of Occupational and Organizational Psychology, 93,* 1–44.
Lee, A. A., Piette, J. D., Heisler, M., Janevic, M. R., & Rosland, A.-M. (2019). Diabetes self-management and glycemic control: The role of autonomy support from informal health supporters. *Health Psychology, 38,* 122–132.
Lee, A., Willis, S., & Tian, A. W. (2018). Empowering leadership: A meta-analytic examination of incremental contribution, mediation, and moderation. *Journal of Organizational Behavior, 39,* 306–325.
Leerkes, E. M., & Zhou, N. (2018). Maternal sensitivity to distress and attachment outcomes: Interactions with sensitivity to nondistress and infant temperament. *Journal of Family Psychology, 32,* 753–761.
Legood, A., van der Werff, L., Lee, A., & Den Hartog,

D. (2021). A meta-analysis of the role of trust in the leadership-performance relationship. *European Journal of Work and Organizational Psychology, 30*, 1–22.

Leitemo, K., Vestbø, H. S. B., Bakali, J. V., & Nissen-Lie, H. A. (2020). The role of attachment anxiety and avoidance for reduced interpersonal problems in training group analytic therapy. *Group Dynamics, 24*, 26–41.

Lemche, E., Giampietro, V. P., Surguladze, S. A., Amaro, E. J., Andrew, C. M., Williams, S. C., . . . Phillips, M. L. (2006). Human attachment security is mediated by the amygdala: Evidence from combined fMRI and psychophysiological measures. *Human Brain Mapping, 27*, 623–635.

LeRoy, A. S., Gabert, T., Garcini, L., Murdock, K. W., Heijnen, C., & Fagundes, C. P. (2020). Attachment orientations and loss adjustment among bereaved spouses. *Psychoneuroendocrinology, 112*, Article 104401.

Levinson, B. M. (1972). *Pets and human development.* Charles C Thomas.

Levy, K. N., Ellison, W. D., Scott, L. N., & Bernecker, S. L. (2011). Attachment style. In J. C. Norcross (Ed.), *Psychotherapy relationships that work: Evidence-based responsiveness* (pp. 377–401). Oxford University Press.

Levy, K. N., & Johnson, B. N. (2019). Attachment and psychotherapy: Implications from empirical research. *Canadian Psychology, 60*, 178–193.

Levy, K. N., Kivity, Y., Johnson, B. N., & Gooch, C. V. (2018). Adult attachment as a predictor and moderator of psychotherapy outcome: A meta-analysis. *Journal of Clinical Psychology, 74*, 1996–2013.

Levy, K. N., Meehan, K. B., Kelly, K. M., Reynoso, J. S., Weber, M., Clarkin, J. F., & Kernberg, O. F. (2006). Change in attachment patterns and reflective function in a randomized control trial of transference-focused psychotherapy for borderline personality disorder. *Journal of Consulting and Clinical Psychology, 74*, 1027–1040.

Lewis-Morrarty, E., Dozier, M., Bernard, K., Terracciano, S. M., & Moore, S. V. (2012). Cognitive flexibility and theory of mind outcomes among foster children: Preschool follow-up results of a randomized clinical trial. *Journal of Adolescent Health, 51*, S17–S22.

Li, C., Liu, J., Zhang, S., Huo, Y., You, J., & Wang, K. (2016). Effects of dispositional and temporarily primed attachment security on response inhibition following ego-depletion among Chinese college students. *Personality and Individual Differences, 99*, 368–375.

Li, J.-B., Willems, Y. E, Stok, F. M., Deković, M., Bartels, M., & Finkenauer, C. (2019). Parenting and self-control across early to late adolescence: A three-level meta-analysis. *Perspectives on Psychological Science, 14*, 967–1005.

Li, Q., & Brewer, M. B. (2004). What does it mean to be an American?: Patriotism, nationalism, and merican identity after 9/11. *Political Psychology, 25*, 727–739.

Li, R., Bunke, S., & Psouni, E. (2016). Attachment relationships and physical activity in adolescents: The mediation role of physical self-concept. *Psychology of Sport and Exercise, 22*, 160–169.

Liao, R., Wang, S., Zhang, P., Zhou, Y., & Liu, X. (2017). Effect of priming with attachment security on positive affect among individuals with depression. *Social Behavior and Personality, 45*, 331–338.

Liddell, B. J., & Courtney, B. S. (2018). Attachment buffers the physiological impact of social exclusion. *PLOS ONE, 13*, Article e0203287.

Liden, R. C., Wayne, S. J., Zhao, H., & Henderson, D. (2008). Servant leadership: Development of a multidimensional measure and multi-level assessment. *Leadership Quarterly, 19*, 161–177.

Lieberman, A. F., Ippen, C. G., & Van Horn, P. (2006). Child-parent psychotherapy: 6-month follow-up of a randomized controlled trial. *Journal of the American Academy of Child and Adolescent Psychiatry, 45*, 913–918.

Lieberman, A. F., Ippen, C. G., & Van Horn, P. (2015). *"Don't hit my mommy!": A manual for child–parent psychotherapy with young children exposed to violence and other trauma.* ZERO TO THREE Press.

Lieberman, A. F., & Van Horn, P. (2005). *"Don't hit my mommy!": A manual for child–parent psychotherapy with young witnesses of family violence.* ZERO TO THREE Press.

Lieberman, A. F., & Van Horn, P. (2008). *Psychotherapy with infants and young children: Repairing the effects of stress and trauma on early attachment.* Guilford Press.

Lieberman, A. F., Van Horn, P., & Ippen, C. G. (2005). Toward evidence-based treatment: Child-parent psychotherapy with preschoolers exposed to marital violence. *Journal of the American Academy of Child and Adolescent Psychiatry, 44*, 1241–1248.

Lieberman, A. F., Weston, D. R., & Pawl, J. H. (1991). Preventive intervention and outcome with anxiously attached dyads. *Child Development, 62*, 199–209.

Lieberman, M. D. (2013). *Social: Why our brains are wired to connect.* Random House.

Lifshin, U., Binyamin Kleinerman, I., Shaver, P. R., & Mikulincer, M. (2020). Teachers' attachment orientations and children's school adjustment: Evidence from a longitudinal study of first graders. *Journal of Social and Personal Relationships, 37*, 559–580.

Lifshitz, C., Tsvieli, N., Bar-Kalifa, E., Abbott, C., Diamond, G. S., Kobak, R. R., & Diamond, G. M. (2021). Emotional processing in attachment-based family therapy for suicidal adolescents. *Psychotherapy Research, 31*, 267–279.

Lind, T., Bernard, K., Ross, E., & Dozier, M. (2014). Intervention effects on negative affect of CPS-referred children: Results of a randomized clinical trial. *Child Abuse and Neglect, 38*, 1459–1467.

Lind, T., Bernard, K., Yarger, H. A., & Dozier, M. (2020). Promoting compliance in children referred to child protective services: A randomized clinical trial. *Child Development, 91*, 563–576.

Lind, T., Raby, K. L., Caron, E. B., Roben, C. K. P., & Dozier, M. (2017). Enhancing executive functioning among toddlers in foster care with an attachment-based intervention. *Development and Psychopathology, 29*, 575–586.

Lind, T., Raby, K. L., Goldstein, A., Bernard, K., Caron, E., Yarger, H. A., . . . Dozier, M. (2021). Improving social-emotional competence in internationally adopted children with the Attachment and Biobehavioral Catch-up intervention. *Development and Psychopathology, 33*, 957–969.

Lipsitz, J. D., & Markowitz, J. C. (2013). Mechanisms of change in interpersonal therapy (IPT). *Clinical Psychology Review, 33*, 1134–1147.

Little, K. C., McNulty, J. K., & Russell, V. M. (2010). Sex buffers intimates against the negative implications of attachment insecurity. *Personality and Social Psychology Bulletin, 36*, 484–498.

Littman-Ovadia, H., Oren, L., & Lavy, S. (2013). Attachment and autonomy in the workplace: New insights. *Journal of Career Assessment, 21*, 502–518.

Liu, D., Zhang, S., Wang, L., & Lee, T. W. (2011). The effects of autonomy and empowerment on employee turnover: Test of a multilevel model in teams. *Journal of Applied Psychology, 96*, 1305–1316.

Lo Coco, G., Gullo, S., Oieni, V., Giannone, F., Di Blasi, M., & Kivlighan, D. M., Jr. (2016). The relationship between attachment dimensions and perceptions of group relationships over time: An actor-partner interdependence analysis. *Group Dynamics, 20*, 276–293.

LoCasale-Crouch, J., Kraft-Sayre, M., Pianta, R. C., Hamre, B. K., Downer, J. T., Leach, A., . . . Scott-Little, C. (2011). Implementing an early childhood professional development course across 10 sites and 15 sections: Lessons learned. *NHSA Dialog, 14*, 275–292.

Loeb, E. L., Kansky, J., Tan, J. S., Costello, M. A., & Allen, J. P. (2021). Perceived psychological control in early adolescence predicts lower levels of adaptation into mid-adulthood. *Child Development, 92*, e158–e172.

Londono Tobon, A., Condon, E., Sadler, L., Holland, M., Mayes, L., & Slade, A. (2022). School age effects of Minding the Baby—an attachment-based home-visiting intervention—on parenting and child behaviors. *Development and Psychopathology, 34*, 55–67.

Lopez, F. G. (2001). Adult attachment orientations, self-other boundary regulation, and splitting tendencies in a college sample. *Journal of Counseling Psychology, 48*, 440–446.

Lorenz, K. Z. (1952). *King Solomon's ring.* Crowell.

Lowell, D. I., Carter, A. S., Godoy, L., Paulicin, B., & Briggs-Gowan, M. J. (2011). A randomized controlled trial of Child FIRST: A comprehensive home-based intervention translating research into early childhood practice. *Child Development, 82*, 193–208.

Lowery, B. S., Eisenberger, N. I., Hardin, C. D., & Sinclair, S. (2007). Long-term effects of subliminal priming on academic performance. *Basic and Applied Social Psychology, 29*, 151–157.

Lucassen, N., Tharner, A., van IJzendoorn, M. H., Bakermans-Kranenburg, M. J., Volling, B. L., Verhulst, F. C., . . . Tiemeier, H. (2011). The association between paternal sensitivity and infant–father attachment security: A meta-analysis of three decades of research. *Journal of Family Psychology, 25*, 986–992.

Luke, M. A., Maio, G. R., & Carnelley, K. B. (2004). Attachment models of the self and others: Relations with self-esteem, humanity-esteem, and parental treatment. *Personal Relationships, 11*, 281–303.

Luke, M. A., Sedikides, C., & Carnelley, K. (2012). Your love lifts me higher!: The energizing quality of secure relationships. *Personality and Social Psychology Bulletin, 38*, 721–733.

Lun, J., Kesebir, S., & Oishi, S. (2008). On feeling understood and feeling well: The role of interdependence. *Journal of Research in Personality, 42*, 1623–1628.

Luyten, P., Blatt, S. J., & Mayes, L. C. (2012). Process and outcome in psychoanalytic psychotherapy research: The need for a (relatively) new paradigm. In R. A. Levy, J. S. Ablon, & H. Kächele (Eds.), *Psychodynamic psychotherapy research: Evidence-based practice and practice-based evidence* (pp. 345–359). Springer.

Luyten, P., & Fonagy, P. (2014). Mentalising in attachment contexts. In P. Holmes & S. Farnfield (Eds.), *The Routledge handbook of attachment: Theory* (pp. 109–126). Routledge.

Lynch, M., & Cicchetti, D. (1997). Children's relationships with adults and peers: An examination of elementary and junior high school students. *Journal of School Psychology, 35*, 81–99.

Lyon, A. R., Gershenson, R. A., Farahmand, F. K., Thaxter, P. J., Behling, S., & Budd, K. S. (2009). Effectiveness of teacher–child interaction training (TCIT) in a preschool setting. *Behavior Modification, 33*, 855–884.

Lyons, R. F., Mickelson, K. D., Sullivan, M. J., & Coyne, J. C. (1998). Coping as a communal process. *Journal of Social and Personal Relationships, 15*, 579–605.

Lyons-Ruth, K., Bronfman, E., & Parsons, E. (1999). Maternal frightened, frightening, or atypical behavior and disorganized infant attachment patterns. *Monographs of the Society for Research in Child Development, 64*, 67–96.

Lyons-Ruth, K., & Jacobvitz, D. (2016). Attachment disorganization from infancy to adulthood: Neurobiological correlates, parenting contexts, and pathways to disorder. In J. Cassidy & P. R. Shaver (Eds.), *Handbook of attachment: Theory, research, and clinical applications* (3rd ed., pp. 667–695). Guilford Press.

Ma, Y., Long, W., Liu, G., & Ma, H. (2021). Boosting attachment security promotes giving behavior in higher attachment anxiety. *Australian Journal of Psychology, 73,* 452–461.

Maciejewski, P. K., Maercker, A., Boelen, P. A., Prigerson, H. G. (2016). "Prolonged grief disorder" and "persistent complex bereavement disorder," but not "complicated grief," are one and the same diagnostic entity: An analysis of data from the Yale Bereavement Study. *World Psychiatry, 15,* 266–275.

MacIntosh, H. B. (2013). Mentalising: An exploration of its potential contribution to understanding the challenges faced by childhood sexual abuse survivors in couple therapy. *Journal of Couple and Family Psychoanalysis, 3,* 188–207.

MacIntosh, H. B., Fletcher, K., & Ainsworth, L. (2019). Measuring mentalizing in emotionally focused therapy for couples with childhood sexual abuse survivors and their partners. *Journal of Couple and Relationship Therapy, 18,* 303–329.

MacIntosh, H. B., & Johnson, S. (2008). Emotionally focused therapy for couples and childhood sexual abuse survivors. *Journal of Marital and Family Therapy, 34,* 298–315.

MacPhee, D. C., Johnson, S. M., & van der Veer, M. M. C. (1995). Low sexual desire in women: The effects of marital therapy. *Journal of Sex and Marital Therapy, 21,* 159–182.

Magro, S. W., Fraley, R. C., & Roisman, G. I. (2020). Early maternal sensitivity and teacher–student relationship quality across grade school: Enduring or transient associations? *Child Development, 91,* e883–e901.

Maillard, P., Dimaggio, G., Berthoud, L., de Roten, Y., Despland, J.-N., & Kramer, U. (2020). Metacognitive improvement and symptom change in a 3-month treatment for borderline personality disorder. *Psychology and Psychotherapy: Theory, Research and Practice, 93,* 309–325.

Main, M., Kaplan, N., & Cassidy, J. (1985). Security in infancy, childhood, and adulthood: A move to the level of representation. *Monographs of the Society for Research in Child Development, 50,* 66–104.

Main, M., & Solomon, J. (1990). Procedures for identifying infants as disorganized/disoriented during the Ainsworth Strange Situation. In M. T. Greenberg, D. Cicchetti, & M. Cummings (Eds.), *Attachment in the preschool years: Theory, research, and intervention* (pp. 121–160). University of Chicago Press.

Maki, K. G. (2020). Social support, strain, and glycemic control: A path analysis. *Personal Relationships, 27,* 592–612.

Makinen, J. A., & Johnson, S. M. (2006). Resolving attachment injuries in couples using emotionally focused therapy: Steps toward forgiveness and reconciliation. *Journal of Consulting and Clinical Psychology, 74,* 1055–1064.

Malda, M., & Mesman, J. (2017). Parental sensitivity and attachment in ethnic minority families. In N. J. Cabrera & B. Leyendecker (Eds.), *Handbook on positive development of minority children and youth* (pp. 71–88). Springer.

Malda-Castillo, J., Browne, C., & Perez-Algorta, G. (2019). Mentalization-based treatment and its evidence-base status: A systematic literature review. *Psychology and Psychotherapy: Theory, Research and Practice, 92,* 465–498.

Malin, A. J., & Pos, A. E. (2015). The impact of early empathy on alliance building, emotional processing, and outcome during experiential treatment of depression. *Psychotherapy Research, 25,* 445–459.

Mallinckrodt, B. (2000). Attachment, social competencies, social support, and interpersonal process in psychotherapy. *Psychotherapy Research, 10,* 239–266.

Mallinckrodt, B. (2010). The psychotherapy relationship as attachment: Evidence and implications. *Journal of Social and Personal Relationships, 27,* 262–270.

Mallinckrodt, B., Anderson, M. Z., Choi, G., Levy, K. N., Petrowski, K., Sauer, E. M., . . . Wiseman, H. (2017). Pseudo-secure vs. individuated-secure client attachment to therapist: Implications for therapy process and outcome. *Psychotherapy Research, 27,* 677–691.

Mallinckrodt, B., & Chen, E. C. (2004). Attachment and interpersonal impact perceptions of group members: A social relations model analysis of transference. *Psychotherapy Research, 14,* 210–230.

Mallinckrodt, B., Choi, G., & Daly, K. D. (2015). Pilot test of a measure to assess therapeutic distance and its association with client attachment and corrective experience in therapy. *Psychotherapy Research, 25,* 505–517.

Mallinckrodt, B., Daly, K., & Wang, C. D. C. (2009). An attachment approach to adult psychotherapy. In J. H. Obegi & E. Berant (Eds.), *Attachment theory and research in clinical work with adults* (pp. 234–268). Guilford Press.

Mallinckrodt, B., Gantt, D. L., & Coble, H. M. (1995). Attachment patterns in the psychotherapy relationship: Development of the Client Attachment to Therapist Scale. *Journal of Counseling Psychology, 42,* 307–317.

Mallinckrodt, B., & Jeong, J. (2015). Meta-analysis of client attachment to therapist: Associations with working alliance and client pretherapy attachment. *Psychotherapy, 52,* 134–139.

Mallinckrodt, B., McNett, A. M. S., Celebi, E., Birks, K. M., Tsai, C.-L., & Williams, B. E. (2013). Cognitive primes for attachment security can increase cultural empathy, but also interact negatively with attachment anxiety. *Journal of Social and Clinical Psychology, 32,* 1013–1039.

Mallinckrodt, B., Porter, M. J., & Kivlighan, D. M., Jr. (2005). Client attachment to therapist, depth of in-session exploration, and object relations in brief psychotherapy. *Psychotherapy, 42,* 85–100.

Mancini, A. D., Robinaugh, D., Shear, K., & Bonanno, G. A. (2009). Does attachment avoidance help people cope with loss?: The moderating effects of relationship quality. *Journal of Clinical Psychology, 65,* 1127–1136.

Markman, H. J., Floyd, F. J., Stanley, S. M., & Storaasli, R. D. (1988). Prevention of marital distress: A longitudinal investigation. *Journal of Consulting and Clinical Psychology, 56,* 210–217.

Markman, H. J., Williams, T., Einhorn, L., & Stanley, S. M. (2008). The new frontier in relationship education: Innovations and challenges in dissemination. *Behavior Therapist, 31,* 14–17.

Markowitz, J. C. (2010). The cutting edge: IPT and PTSD. *Depression and Anxiety, 27,* 879–884.

Markowitz, J. C., Lipsitz, J., & Milrod, B. L. (2014). Critical review of outcome research on interpersonal psychotherapy for anxiety disorders. *Depression and Anxiety, 31,* 316–325.

Markowitz, J. C., & Weissman, M. M. (2004). Interpersonal psychotherapy: Principles and applications. *World Psychiatry, 3,* 136–139.

Markowitz, J. C., & Weissman, M. M. (Eds.). (2012). *Casebook of interpersonal psychotherapy.* Oxford University Press.

Marmarosh, C. L., & Markin, R. D. (2007). Group and personal attachments: Two is better than one when predicting college adjustment. *Group Dynamics, 11,* 153–164.

Marmarosh, C. L., Markin, R., & Spiegel, E. (2013). *Attachment in group psychotherapy.* American Psychological Association.

Marmarosh, C. L., Schmidt, E., Pembleton, J., Rotbart, E., Muzyk, N., Liner, A., & Salmen, K. (2015). Novice therapist attachment and perceived ruptures and repairs: A pilot study. *Psychotherapy, 52,* 140–144.

Marmarosh, C. L., Whipple, R., Schettler, M., Pinhas, S., Wolf, J., & Sayit, S. (2009). Adult attachment styles and group psychotherapy attitudes. *Group Dynamics, 13,* 255–264.

Martin, A. M., III, Paetzold, R. L., & Rholes, W. S. (2010). Adult attachment and exploration: Linking attachment style to motivation and perceptions of support in adult exploration. *Basic and Applied Social Psychology, 32,* 196–205.

Martire, L. M., & Helgeson, V. S. (2017). Close relationships and the management of chronic illness: Associations and interventions. *American Psychologist, 72,* 601–612.

Martire, L. M., Stephens, M. A. P., Mogle, J., Schulz, R., Brach, J., & Keefe, F. J. (2013). Daily spousal influence on physical activity in knee osteoarthritis. *Annals of Behavioral Medicine, 45,* 213–223.

Mashburn, A. J., Downer, J. T., Hamre, B. K., Justice, L. M., & Pianta, R. C. (2010). Consultation for teachers and children's language and literacy development during pre-kindergarten. *Applied Developmental Science, 14,* 179–196.

Maslow, A. H. (1971). *The farther reaches of human nature.* Viking.

Massengale, M., Davis, D. E., DeBlaere, C., Zelaya, D. G., Shannonhouse, L., Van Tongeren, D. R., . . . Hill, P. C. (2017). Attachment avoidance to God exacerbates the negative effect of tangible resource loss on psychological resource loss. *Mental Health, Religion and Culture, 20,* 489–501.

Mathieu, M., Eschleman, K. J., & Cheng, D. (2019). Meta-analytic and multiwave comparison of emotional support and instrumental support in the workplace. *Journal of Occupational Health Psychology, 24,* 387–409.

Matte-Gagné, C., Bernier, A., Sirois, M.-S., Lalonde, G., & Hertz, S. (2018). Attachment security and developmental patterns of growth in executive functioning during early elementary school. *Child Development, 89,* e167–e182.

Maunder, R. G., & Hunter, J. J. (2001). Attachment and psychosomatic medicine: Developmental contributions to stress and disease. *Psychosomatic Medicine, 63,* 556–567.

Maunder, R. G., & Hunter, J. J. (2015). *Love, fear, and health: How our attachments to others shape health and health care.* University of Toronto Press.

Maunder, R. G., & Hunter, J. J. (2016). Can patients be "attached" to healthcare providers?: An observational study to measure attachment phenomena in patient–provider relationships. *BMJ Open, 6,* Article e011068.

Maunder, R. G., Hunter, J. J., Atkinson, L., Steiner, M., Wazana, A., Fleming, A. S., . . . Levitan, R. D. (2017). An attachment-based model of the relationship between childhood adversity and somatization in children and adults. *Psychosomatic Medicine, 79,* 506–513.

Maunder, R. G., Lancee, W. J., Greenberg, G., Hunter, J. J., & Fernandes, B. (2000). Insecure attachment in a subgroup of ulcerative colitis defined by ANCA status. *Digestive Diseases Science, 45,* 2127–2132.

Maunder, R. G., Lancee, W. J., Nolan, R. P., Hunter, J. J., & Tannenbaum, D. W. (2006). The relationship of attachment insecurity to subjective stress and autonomic function during standardized acute stress in healthy adults. *Journal of Psychosomatic Research, 60,* 283–290.

Maunder, R. G., Panzer, A., Viljoen, M., Owen, J., Human, S., & Hunter, J. J. (2006). Physicians' difficulty with emergency department patients is related to patients' attachment style. *Social Science and Medicine, 63*, 552–562.

Mawson, A. R. (2005). Understanding mass panic and other collective responses to threat and disaster. *Psychiatry: Interpersonal and Biological Processes, 68*, 95–113.

Maxwell, A.-M., McMahon, C., Huber, A., Reay, R. E., Hawkins, E., & Barnett, B. (2021). Examining the effectiveness of circle of security parenting (COS-P): A multi-site non-randomized study with wait-list control. *Journal of Child and Family Studies, 30*, 1123–1140.

Maxwell, H., Compare, A., Brugnera, A., Zarbo, C., Rabboni, M., Dalle Grave, R., & Tasca, G. A. (2018). Reflective functioning and growth in therapeutic alliance during emotionally focused group therapy for binge-eating disorder. *Group Dynamics, 22*, 32–44.

Maxwell, H., Tasca, G. A., Gick, M., Ritchie, K., Balfour, L., & Bissada, H. (2012). The impact of attachment anxiety on interpersonal complementarity in early group therapy interactions among women with binge eating disorder. *Group Dynamics: Theory, Research, and Practice, 16*, 255–271.

Maxwell, H., Tasca, G. A., Grenon, R., Faye, M., Ritchie, K., Bissada, H., & Balfour, L. (2018). Change in attachment dimensions in women with binge-eating disorder following group psychodynamic interpersonal psychotherapy. *Psychotherapy Research, 28*, 887–901.

Maxwell, H., Tasca, G. A., Grenon, R., Ritchie, K., Bissada, H., & Balfour, L. (2017). Change in attachment states of mind of women with binge-eating disorder. *Clinical Psychology and Psychotherapy, 24*, 1292–1303.

Maxwell, H., Tasca, G. A., Ritchie, K., Balfour, L., & Bissada, H. (2014). Change in attachment insecurity is related to improved outcomes 1-year post group therapy in women with binge eating disorder. *Psychotherapy, 51*, 57–65.

Mayseless, O. (2005). Ontogeny of attachment in middle childhood: Conceptualization of normative changes. In K. A. Kerns & R. A. Richardson (Eds.), *Attachment in middle childhood* (pp. 1–23). Guilford Press.

Mayseless, O. (2016). *The caring motivation: An integrated theory.* Oxford University Press.

Mayseless, O., & Popper, M. (2007). Reliance on leaders and social institutions: An attachment perspective. *Attachment and Human Development, 9*, 73–93.

Mayseless, O., & Popper, M. (2019). Attachment and leadership: Review and new insights. *Current Opinion in Psychology, 25*, 157–161.

McBride, C., Atkinson, L., Quilty, L. C., & Bagby, R. M. (2006). Attachment as moderator of treatment outcome in major depression: A randomized control trial of interpersonal psychotherapy versus cognitive behavior therapy. *Journal of Consulting and Clinical Psychology, 74*, 1041–1054.

McClintock, A. S., Anderson, T., Patterson, C. L, & Wing, E. H. (2018). Early psychotherapeutic empathy, alliance, and client outcome: Preliminary evidence of indirect effects. *Journal of Clinical Psychology, 74*, 839–848.

McClure, M. J., Bartz, J. A., & Lydon, J. E. (2013). Uncovering and overcoming ambivalence: The role of chronic and contextually activated attachment in two-person social dilemmas. *Journal of Personality, 81*, 103–117.

McCluskey, U. (2002). The dynamics of attachment and systems-centered group psychotherapy. *Group Dynamics, 6*, 131–142.

McCoyd, J. L. M., Koller, J. M., & Walter, C. A. (2021). *Grief and loss across the lifespan: A biopsychosocial perspective* (3rd ed.). Springer.

McGregor, H., Leiberman, J., Greenberg, J., Solomon, S., Arndt, J., Simon, L., & Pyszczynski, T. (1998). Terror management and aggression: Evidence that mortality salience promotes aggression against worldview-threatening individuals. *Journal of Personality and Social Psychology, 74*, 590–605.

McGuire, A., Gillath, O., Jackson, Y., & Ingram, R. (2018). Attachment security priming as a potential intervention for depressive symptoms. *Journal of Social and Clinical Psychology, 37*, 44–68.

McIntosh, D. E., Rizza, M. G., & Bliss, L. (2000). Implementing empirically supported interventions: Teacher–child interaction therapy. *Psychology in the Schools, 37*, 453–462.

McLean, H. R., Bailey, H. N., & Lumley, M. N. (2014). The secure base script: Associated with early maladaptive schemas related to attachment. *Psychology and Psychotherapy, 87*, 425–446.

McLean, L. M., Walton, T., Rodin, G., Esplen, M. J., & Jones, J. M. (2013). A couple-based intervention for patients and caregivers facing end-stage cancer: Outcomes of a randomized controlled trial. *Psycho-Oncology, 22*, 28–38.

McNeely, C. A., & Barber, B. K. (2010). How do parents make adolescents feel loved?: Perspectives on supportive parenting from adolescents in 12 cultures. *Journal of Adolescent Research, 25*, 601–631.

McWilliams, L. A. (2018). Relationships between adult attachment dimensions and patient–physician relationship quality. *Journal of Relationships Research, 9*, Article e15.

McWilliams, L. A., & Bailey, S. J. (2010). Associations between adult attachment ratings and health conditions: Evidence from the National Comorbidity Survey Replication. *Health Psychology, 29*, 446–453.

McWilliams, L. A., & Holmberg, D. (2010). Adult attachment and pain catastrophizing for self and significant other. *Pain, 149*, 278–283.

Meins, E. H. (1997). Security of attachment and maternal tutoring strategies: Interaction within the zone of proximal development. *British Journal of Developmental Psychology, 15*, 129–144.

Meins, E. H., Bureau, J.-F., & Fernyhough, C. (2018). Mother–child attachment from infancy to the preschool years: Predicting security and stability. *Child Development, 89*, 1022–1038.

Meins, E. H., & Fernyhough, C. (2015). *Mind-mindedness coding manual, Version 2.2*. Unpublished manuscript, University of York, York, UK.

Meins, E. H., Fernyhough, C., & Centifanti, L. C. M. (2019). Mothers' early mind-mindedness predicts educational attainment in socially and economically disadvantaged British children. *Child Development, 90*, e454–e467.

Meins, E. H., Fernyhough, C., de Rosnay, M., Arnott, B., Leekam, S. R., & Turner, M. (2012). Mind-mindedness as a multidimensional construct: Appropriate and non-attuned mind-related comments independently predict infant–mother attachment in a socially diverse sample. *Infancy, 17*, 393–415.

Meins, E. H., Fernyhough, C., Wainwright, R., Gupta, M. D., Fradley, E., & Tuckey, M. (2002). Maternal mind-mindedness and attachment security as predictors of theory of mind understanding. *Child Development, 73*, 1715–1726.

Melen, S., Pepping, C. A., & O'Donovan, A. (2017). Social foundations of mindfulness: Priming attachment anxiety reduces emotion regulation and mindful attention. *Mindfulness, 8*, 136–143.

Meneses, C. W., & Greenberg, L. S. (2011). The construction of a model of the process of couples' forgiveness in emotion-focused therapy for couples. *Journal of Marital and Family Therapy, 37*, 491–502.

Mercer, S. W., Higgins, M., Bikker, A. M., Fitzpatrick, B., McConnachie, A., Lloyd, S. M., . . . Watt, G. C. M. (2016). General practitioners' empathy and health outcomes: A prospective observational study of consultations in areas of high and low deprivation. *Annals of Family Medicine, 14*, 117–124.

Meredith, P. J., Andrews, N. E., Thackeray, J., Bowen, S., Poll, C., & Strong. J. (2021). Can sensory- and attachment-informed approaches modify the perception of pain?: An experimental study. *Pain Research and Management*, Article 5527261.

Meredith, P. J., Ownsworth, T., & Strong, J. (2008). A review of the evidence linking adult attachment theory and chronic pain: Presenting a conceptual model. *Clinical Psychology Review, 28*, 407–429.

Meredith, P. J., & Strong, J. (2019). Attachment and chronic illness. *Current Opinion in Psychology, 25*, 132–138.

Meredith, P. J., Strong, J., & Feeney, J. A. (2006). Adult attachment, anxiety, and pain self-efficacy as predictors of pain intensity and disability. *Pain, 123*, 146–154.

Mesman, J. (2021). Attachment theory's universality claims: Asking different questions. In R. A. Thompson, J. A. Simpson, & L. J. Berlin (Eds.), *Attachment: The fundamental questions* (pp. 245–251). Guilford Press.

Mesman, J., Minter, T., Angnged, A., Cissé, I. A. H., Salali, G. D., & Migliano, A. B. (2018). Universality without uniformity: A culturally inclusive approach to sensitive responsiveness in infant caregiving. *Child Development, 89*, 837–850.

Mesman, J., van IJzendoorn, M., & Sagi-Schwartz, A. (2016). Cross-cultural patterns of attachment: Universal and contextual dimensions. In J. Cassidy & P. R. Shaver (Eds.), *Handbook of Attachment: Theory, Research, and Clinical Applications* (3rd ed., pp. 790–815). Guilford Press.

Midgley, N., & Vrouva, I. (Eds.). (2012). *Minding the child: Mentalization-based interventions with children, young people and their families*. Routledge/Taylor & Francis.

Mikail, S. F., Henderson, P. R., & Tasca, G. A. (1994). An interpersonally based model of chronic pain: An application of attachment theory. *Clinical Psychology Review, 14*, 1–16.

Mikami, A. Y., Gregory, A., Allen, J. P., Pianta, R. C., & Lun, J. (2011). Effects of a teacher professional development intervention on peer relationships in secondary classrooms. *School Psychology Review, 40*, 367–385.

Mikulincer, M. (1995). Attachment style and the mental representation of the self. *Journal of Personality and Social Psychology, 69*, 1203–1215.

Mikulincer, M. (1997). Adult attachment style and information processing: Individual differences in curiosity and cognitive closure. *Journal of Personality and Social Psychology, 72*, 1217–1230.

Mikulincer, M. (1998a). Adult attachment style and affect regulation: Strategic variations in self-appraisals. *Journal of Personality and Social Psychology, 75*, 420–435.

Mikulincer, M. (1998b). Attachment working models and the sense of trust: An exploration of interaction goals and affect regulation. *Journal of Personality and Social Psychology, 74*, 1209–1224.

Mikulincer, M. (1998c). Adult attachment style and individual differences in functional versus dysfunctional experiences of anger. *Journal of Personality and Social Psychology, 74*, 513–524.

Mikulincer, M., Agam, T., & Shaver, P. R. (2020). A secure base for mindful dreaming: Dispositional and contextually variable attachment security and the experiential quality of dreams. *Attachment and Human Development, 22*, 606–626.

Mikulincer, M., & Arad, D. (1999). Attachment working models and cognitive openness in close relationships: A test of chronic and temporary accessibility effects. *Journal of Personality and Social Psychology, 77*, 710–725.

Mikulincer, M., Florian, V., & Tolmacz, R. (1990). Attachment styles and fear of personal death: A case study of affect regulation. *Journal of Personality and Social Psychology, 58*, 273–280.

Mikulincer, M., Gillath, O., Halevy, V., Avihou, N., Avidan, S., & Eshkoli, N. (2001). Attachment theory and reactions to others' needs: Evidence that activation of the sense of attachment security promotes empathic responses. *Journal of Personality and Social Psychology, 81*, 1205–1224.

Mikulincer, M., Gillath, O., Sapir-Lavid, Y., Yaakobi, E., Arias, K., Tal-Aloni, L., & Bor, G. (2003). Attachment theory and concern for others' welfare: Evidence that activation of the sense of secure base promotes endorsement of self-transcendence values. *Basic and Applied Social Psychology, 25*, 299–312.

Mikulincer, M., Gillath, O., & Shaver, P. R. (2002). Activation of the attachment system in adulthood: Threat-related primes increase the accessibility of mental representations of attachment figures. *Journal of Personality and Social Psychology, 83*, 881–895.

Mikulincer, M., Hirschberger, G., Nachmias, O., & Gillath, O. (2001). The affective component of the secure base schema: Affective priming with representations of attachment security. *Journal of Personality and Social Psychology, 81*, 305–321.

Mikulincer, M., Orbach, I., & Iavnieli, D. (1998). Adult attachment style and affect regulation: Strategic variations in subjective self-other similarity. *Journal of Personality and Social Psychology, 75*, 436–448.

Mikulincer, M., & Shaver, P. R. (2001). Attachment theory and intergroup bias: Evidence that priming the secure base schema attenuates negative reactions to out-groups. *Journal of Personality and Social Psychology, 81*, 97–115.

Mikulincer, M., & Shaver, P. R. (2003). The attachment behavioral system in adulthood: Activation, psychodynamics, and interpersonal processes. In M. P. Zanna (Ed.), *Advances in experimental social psychology* (Vol. 35, pp. 53–152). Academic Press.

Mikulincer, M., & Shaver, P. R. (2004). Security-based self-representations in adulthood: Contents and processes. In W. S. Rholes & J. A. Simpson (Eds.), *Adult attachment: Theory, research, and clinical implications* (pp. 159–195). Guilford Press.

Mikulincer, M., & Shaver, P. R. (2007). Boosting attachment security to promote mental health, prosocial values, and inter-group tolerance. *Psychological Inquiry, 18*, 139–156.

Mikulincer, M., & Shaver, P. R. (2013). Attachment insecurities and disordered patterns of grief. In M. Stroebe, H. Schut, P. Boelen, & J. van den Bout (Eds.), *Complicated grief: Scientific foundations for health care professionals* (pp. 190–203). Routledge.

Mikulincer, M., & Shaver, P. R. (2016). *Attachment in adulthood: Structure, dynamics, and change* (2nd ed.). Guilford Press.

Mikulincer, M., & Shaver, P. R. (2020). Enhancing the "broaden and build" cycle of attachment security in adulthood: From the laboratory to relational contexts and societal systems. *International Journal of Environmental Research and Public Health, 17*, Article 2054.

Mikulincer, M., & Shaver, P. R. (2022). Enhancing the "broaden-and-build" cycle of attachment security as a means of overcoming prejudice, discrimination, and racism. *Attachment and Human Development, 24*, 260–273.

Mikulincer, M., & Shaver, P. R. (2023). *Attachment theory expanded: Security dynamics in individuals, dyads, groups, and societies.* Guilford Press.

Mikulincer, M., Shaver, P. R., Bar-On, N., & Sahdra, B. K. (2014). Security enhancement, self-esteem threat, and mental depletion affect provision of a safe haven and secure base to a romantic partner. *Journal of Social and Personal Relationships, 31*, 630–650.

Mikulincer, M., Shaver, P. R., Gillath, O., & Nitzberg, R. A. (2005). Attachment, caregiving, and altruism: Boosting attachment security increases compassion and helping. *Journal of Personality and Social Psychology, 89*, 817–839.

Mikulincer, M., Shaver, P. R., & Rom, E. (2011). The effects of implicit and explicit security priming on creative problem solving. *Cognition and Emotion, 25*, 519–531.

Mikulincer, M., Shaver, P. R., Sahdra, B. K., & Bar-On, N. (2013). Can security-enhancing interventions overcome psychological barriers to responsiveness in couple relationships? *Attachment & Human Development, 15*, 246–260.

Mikulincer, M., Shaver, P. R., Sapir-Lavid, Y., & Avihou-Kanza, N. (2009). What's inside the minds of securely and insecurely attached people?: The secure-base script and its associations with attachment-style dimensions. *Journal of Personality and Social Psychology, 97*, 615–633.

Mikulincer, M., Shaver, P. R., & Slav, K. (2006). Attachment, mental representations of others, and gratitude and forgiveness in romantic relationships. In M. Mikulincer & G. S. Goodman (Eds.), *Dynamics of romantic love: Attachment, caregiving, and sex* (pp. 190–215). Guilford Press.

Mikulincer, M., Solomon, Z., Shaver, P. R., & Ein-Dor, T. (2014). Attachment-related consequences of war captivity and trajectories of posttraumatic stress disorder: A 17-year longitudinal study. *Journal of Social and Clinical Psychology, 33*, 207–228.

Miller, G. E., Chen, E., & Parker, K. J. (2011). Psychological stress in childhood and susceptibility to the chronic diseases of aging: Moving toward a model of behavioral and biological mechanisms. *Psychological Bulletin, 137*, 959–997.

Miller, J. D., Gentile, B., & Campbell, W. K. (2013). A test of the construct validity of the five-factor narcissism inventory. *Journal of Personality Assessment, 95*, 377–387.

Miller, J. E., Kim, S., Boldt, L. J., Goffin, K. C., & Kochanska, G. (2019). Long-term sequelae of mothers' and fathers' mind-mindedness in infancy: A developmental path to children's attachment at age 10. *Developmental Psychology, 55*, 675–686.

Miller-Bottome, M., Talia, A., Eubanks, C. F., Safran, J. D., & Muran, J. C. (2019). Secure in-session attachment predicts rupture resolution: Negotiating a secure base. *Psychoanalytic Psychology, 36*, 132–138.

Milligan, K., Khoury, J. E., Benoit, D., & Atkinson, L. (2015). Maternal attachment and mind-mindedness: The role of emotional specificity. *Attachment and Human Development, 17*, 302–318.

Millings, A., Carnelley, K. B., Cavanagh, K., Wilderspin, A., Wiseman, H., & Rowe, A. C. (2019). Priming attachment security improves attitudes towards a range of therapies. *British Journal of Psychology, 110*, 15–39.

Millings, A., Walsh, J., Hepper, E., & O'Brien, M. (2013). Good partner, good parent: Responsiveness mediates the link between romantic attachment and parenting style. *Personality and Social Psychology Bulletin, 39*, 170–180.

Milyavskaya, M., McClure, M. J., Ma, D., Koestner, R., & Lydon, J. (2012). Attachment moderates the effects of autonomy-supportive and controlling interpersonal primes on intrinsic motivation. *Canadian Journal of Behavioral Science, 44*, 278–287.

Miranda, R., & Andersen, S. M. (2010). The social psychology of transference. In J. E. Maddux & J. P. Tangney (Eds.), *Social psychological foundations of clinical psychology* (pp. 476–496). Guilford Press.

Mohr, J. J., Gelso, C. J., & Hill, C. E. (2005). Client and counselor trainee attachment as predictors of session evaluation and countertransference behavior in first counseling sessions. *Journal of Counseling Psychology, 52*, 298–309.

Molden, D. C. (Ed.). (2014). *Understanding priming effects in social psychology*. Guilford Press.

Molero, F., Mikulincer, M., Shaver, P. R., Laguía, A., & Moriano, J. A. (2019). The development and validation of the Leader as Security Provider Scale. *Journal of Work and Organizational Psychology, 35*, 183–193.

Molero, F., Moriano, J. A., & Shaver, P. R. (2013). The Influence of leadership style on subordinates' attachment to the leader. *Spanish Journal of Psychology, 16*, Article E62.

Monroe, N., & Jankowski, P. J. (2016). The effectiveness of a prayer intervention in promoting change in perceived attachment to God, positive affect, and psychological distress. *Spirituality in Clinical Practice, 3*, 237–249.

Montano, D., Reeske, A., Franke, F., & Hüffmeier, J. (2017). Leadership, followers' mental health and job performance in organizations: A comprehensive meta-analysis from an occupational health perspective. *Journal of Organizational Behavior, 38*, 327–350.

Monteleone, A. M., Ruzzi, V., Pellegrino, F., Patriciello, G., Cascino, G., Del Giorno, C., . . . Maj, M. (2019). The vulnerability to interpersonal stress in eating disorders: The role of insecure attachment in the emotional and cortisol responses to the Trier Social Stress Test. *Psychoneuroendocrinology, 101*, 278–285.

Moon, J. R., Glymour, M. M., Vable, A. M., Liu, S. Y., & Subramanian, S. V. (2014). Short- and long-term associations between widowhood and mortality in the United States: Longitudinal analyses. *Journal of Public Health, 36*, 382–389.

Moran, G., Diamond, G. M., & Diamond, G. S. (2005). The relational reframe and parents' problem constructions in attachment-based family therapy. *Psychotherapy Research, 15*, 226–235.

Moran, G., & Diamond, G. S. (2008). Generating nonnegative attitudes among parents of depressed adolescents: The power of empathy, concern, and positive regard. *Psychotherapy Research, 18*, 97–107.

Moreau, E., & Mageau, G. A. (2012). The importance of perceived autonomy support for the psychological health and work satisfaction of health professionals: Not only supervisors count, colleagues too! *Motivation and Emotion, 36*, 268–286.

Moretti, M. M., Holland, R., Moore, K., & McKay, S. (2004). An attachment-based parenting program for caregivers of severely conduct-disordered adolescents. *Journal of Child and Youth Care Work, 19*, 170–178.

Moretti, M. M., & Obsuth, I. (2009). Effectiveness of an attachment-focused manualized intervention for parents of teens at risk for aggressive behavior: The Connect Program. *Journal of Adolescence, 32*, 1347–1357.

Moretti, M. M., Obsuth, I., Craig, S. G., & Bartolo, T. (2015). An attachment-based intervention for parents of adolescents at risk: Mechanisms of change. *Attachment and Human Development, 17*, 119–135.

Moretti, M. M., Obsuth, I., Mayseless, O., & Scharf, M. (2012). Shifting internal parent–child representations among caregivers of teens with serious behavior problems: An attachment-based approach. *Journal of Child and Adolescent Trauma, 5*, 191–204.

Moretti, M. M., Pasalich, D. S., & O'Donnell, K. A. (2018). Connect: An attachmentbased program for parents of teens. In H. Steele & M. Steele (Eds.), *Handbook of attachment-based interventions* (pp. 375–400). Guilford Press.

Morgis, B. L., Ewing, E. S. K., Liu, T., Slaughter-Acey, J., Fisher, K., & Jampol, R. (2019). A Hold Me Tight workshop for couple attachment and sexual intimacy. *Contemporary Family Therapy, 41*, 368–383.

Moriano, J. A., Molero, F., Mikulincer, M., Laguía, A., & Shaver, P. R. (2021). Security providing leadership and employees' job burnout: The mediating role of psychological safety climate and organizational dehumanization. *International Journal of Environmental Research and Public Health, 18*, Article 12551.

Morris, B. A., Chambers, S. K., Campbell, M., Dwyer,

M., & Dunn, J. (2012). Motorcycles and breast cancer: The influence of peer support and challenge on distress and posttraumatic growth. *Supportive Care in Cancer, 20*, 1849–1858.

Morse, J. Q., Shaffer, D. R., Williamson, G. M., Dooley, W. K., & Schulz, R. (2012). Models of self and others and their relation to positive and negative caregiving responses. *Psychology and Aging, 27*, 211–218.

Moss, E., Dubois-Comtois, K., Cyr, C., Tarabulsy, G. M., St-Laurent, D., & Bernier, A. (2011). Efficacy of a home-visiting intervention aimed at improving maternal sensitivity, child attachment, and behavioral outcomes for maltreated children: A randomized control trial. *Development and Psychopathology, 23*, 195–210.

Moss, K. M., Healy, K. L., Ziviani, J., Newcombe, P., Cobham, V. E., McCutcheon, H., . . . Kenardy, J. (2019). Trauma-informed care in practice: Observed use of psychosocial care practices with children and families in a large pediatric hospital. *Psychological Services, 16*, 16–28.

Moss, S. (2009). Cultivating the regulatory focus of followers to amplify their sensitivity to transformational leadership. *Journal of Leadership and Organizational Studies, 15*, 241–259.

Muela, A., Balluerka, N., Amiano, N., Caldentey, M. A., & Aliri, J. (2017). Animal-assisted psychotherapy for young people with behavioral problems in residential care. *Clinical Psychology and Psychotherapy, 24*, O1485–O1494.

Mueller, J. E. (1970). Presidential popularity from Truman to Johnson. *American Political Science Review, 64*, 18–34.

Mufson, L., Moreau, D., Weissman, M. M., & Klerman, G. L. (1993). *Interpersonal psychotherapy for depressed adolescents*. Guilford Press.

Muller, R. T., & Rosenkranz, S. E. (2009). Attachment and treatment response among adults in inpatient treatment for posttraumatic stress disorder. *Psychotherapy, 46*, 82–96.

Murase, H., Simons, R. M., & Simons, J. S. (2021). Distinct paths to alcohol problems: Impacts of childhood maltreatment, attachment insecurity, and interpersonal problems. *Addictive Behaviors, 115*, Article 106780.

Murdock, K. W., Seiler, A., Chirinos, D. A., Garcini, L. M., Acebo, S. L., Cohen, S., & Fagundes, C. P. (2018). Low childhood subjective social status and telomere length in adulthood: The role of attachment orientations. *Developmental Psychobiology, 60*, 340–346.

Murdock, K. W., Zilioli, S., Ziauddin, K., Heijnen, C. J., & Fagundes, C. P. (2018). Attachment and telomere length: More evidence for psychobiological connections between close relationships, health, and aging. *Journal of Behavioral Medicine, 41*, 333–343.

Murphy, D., & Cramer, D. (2014). Mutuality of Rogers's therapeutic conditions and treatment progress in the first three psychotherapy sessions. *Psychotherapy Research, 24*, 651–661.

Murray, C., & Greenberg, M. T. (2001). Relationships with teachers and bonds with school: Social emotional adjustment correlates for children with and without disabilities. *Psychology in the Schools, 38*, 25- 41.

Mychailyszyn, M. P., & Elson, D. M. (2018). Working through the blues: A meta-analysis on interpersonal psychotherapy for depressed adolescents (IPT-A). *Children and Youth Services Review, 87*, 123–129.

Nagar, S., Mikulincer, M., Nitsan, G., & Ben-David, B. (2022). Safe and sound: The effects of experimentally priming the sense of attachment security on pure tone audiometric thresholds among young and older adults. *Psychological Science, 33*, 424–432.

Neff, K. D., & McGehee, P. (2010). Self-compassion and psychological resilience among adolescents and young adults. *Self and Identity, 9*, 225–240.

Negrão, M., Pereira, M., Soares, I., & Mesman, J. (2014). Enhancing positive parent–child interactions and family functioning in a poverty sample: A randomized control trial. *Attachment and Human Development, 16*, 315–328.

Neimeyer, R. A. (2012). Presence, process, and procedure: A relational frame for technical proficiency in grief therapy. In R. A. Neimeyer (Ed.), *Techniques of grief therapy: Creative practices for counseling the bereaved* (pp. 3–11). Routledge/Taylor & Francis Group.

Neimeyer, R. A., & Jordan, J. R. (2013). Historical and contemporary perspectives on assessment and intervention. In D. K. Meagher & D. E. Balk (Eds.), *Handbook of thanatology: The essential body of knowledge for the study of death, dying, and bereavement* (pp. 219–237). Routledge.

Nelson, B. W., Bernstein, R., Allen, N. B., & Laurent, H. K. (2020). The quality of early infant–caregiver relational attachment and longitudinal changes in infant inflammation across 6 months. *Developmental Psychobiology, 62*, 674–683.

Nelson, J. M., Hardy, S. A., & Watkins, P. (2022). Transcendent indebtedness to God: A new construct in the psychology of religion and spirituality. *Psychology of Religion and Spirituality*. [Epub ahead of print].

Newman-Taylor, K., Sood, M., Rowe, A. C., & Carnelley, K. B. (2021). The impact of repeated attachment priming on paranoia, mood and help-seeking intentions in an analogue sample. *Brain Sciences, 11*, Article 1257.

Newsom, C., Schut, H., Stroebe, M. S., Wilson, S., Birrell, J., Moerbeek, M., & Eisma, M. C. (2017). Effectiveness of bereavement counselling through a community-based organization: A naturalistic, controlled trial. *Clinical Psychology and Psychotherapy, 24*, O1512–O1523.

Ng, T. W. H., & Sorensen, K. L. (2008). Toward a further understanding of the relationships between perceptions of support and work attitudes: A meta-analysis. *Group and Organization Management, 33*, 243–268.

Nguyen, T., Ansari, A., Pianta, R. C., Whittaker, J. V., Vitiello, V. E., & Ruzek, E. (2020). The classroom relational environment and children's early development in preschool. *Social Development, 29*, 1071–1091.

NICHD Early Child Care Research Network. (1999). Child care and mother–child interaction in the first three years of life. *Developmental Psychology, 35*, 1399–1413.

Nichols, A. L., & Cottrell, C. A. (2014). What do people desire in their leaders?: The role of leadership level on trait desirability. *Leadership Quarterly, 25*, 711–729.

Nisa, C. F., Bélanger, J. J., Schumpe, B. M., & Sasin, E. M. (2021). Secure human attachment can promote support for climate change mitigation. *Proceedings of the National Academy of Sciences of the USA, 118*, Article e2101046118.

Njus, D. M., & Scharmer, A. (2020). Evidence that god attachment makes a unique contribution to psychological well-being. *International Journal for the Psychology of Religion, 30*, 178–201.

Norman, L., Lawrence, N., Iles, A., Benattayallah, A., & Karl, A. (2015). Attachment-security priming attenuates amygdala activation to social and linguistic threat. *Social Cognitive and Affective Neuroscience, 10*, 832–839.

Obegi, J. H., & Berant, E. (2009). Introduction. In J. H. Obegi & E. Berant (Eds.), *Attachment theory and research in clinical work with adults* (pp. 1–14). Guilford Press.

O'Bertos, S. E., Holmberg, D., Shields, C. A., & Matheson, L. P. (2020). Partners' attachment styles and overprotective support as predictors of patient outcomes in cardiac rehabilitation. *Rehabilitation Psychology, 65*, 258–267.

O'Connor, E. E., Collins, B. A., & Supplee, L. (2012). Behavior problems in late childhood: The roles of early maternal attachment and teacher–child relationship trajectories. *Attachment and Human Development, 14*, 265–288.

O'Connor, E. E., & McCartney, K. (2006). Testing associations between young children's relationships with mothers and teachers. *Journal of Educational Psychology, 98*, 87–98.

O'Connor, E. E., & McCartney, K. (2007). Examining teacher–child relationships and achievement as part of an ecological model of development. *American Educational Research Journal, 44*, 340–369.

O'Connor, M.-F. (2022). *The grieving brain: The surprising science of how we learn from love and loss.* HarperOne.

O'Farrelly, C., Watt, H., Babalis, D., Bakermans-Kranenburg, M. J., & Ramchandani, P. G. (2021). A brief home-based parenting intervention to reduce behavior problems in young children: A pragmatic randomized clinical trial. *JAMA Pediatrics, 175*, 567–576.

Obsuth, I., Moretti, M. M., Holland, R., Braber, K., & Cross, S. (2006). Conduct disorder: New directions in promoting effective parenting and strengthening parent–adolescent relationships. *Journal of the Canadian Academy of Child and Adolescent Psychiatry, 15*, 6–15.

Odendaal, J. S. J., Meintjes, R. A. (2003). Neurophysiological correlates of affiliative behavior between humans and dogs. *Veterinary Journal, 165*, 296–301.

Oehler, M., & Psouni, E. (2019). "Partner in prime"?: Effects of repeated mobile security priming on attachment security and perceived stress in daily life. *Attachment and Human Development, 21*, 638–657.

Olds, D. L. (2002). Prenatal and infancy home visiting by nurses: From randomized trials to community replication. *Prevention Science, 3*, 153–172.

Oliveira, P., & Costa, E. (2009). Interrelationships of adult attachment orientations, health status and worrying among Fibromyalgia patients. *Journal of Health Psychology, 14*, 1184–1195.

Olsson, C. A., Moyzis, R. K., Williamson, E., Ellis, J. E., Parkinson-Bates, M., Patton, G. C., . . . Moore, E. E. (2013). Gene–environment interaction in problematic substance use: Interaction between DRD4 and insecure attachments. *Addiction Biology, 18*, 717–726.

Open Science Collaboration. (2015). Estimating the reproducibility of psychological science. *Science, 349*, Article 4716.

Oppenheim, D., & Koren-Karie, N. (2002). Mothers' insightfulness regarding their children's internal worlds: The capacity underlying secure child–mother relationships. *Infant Mental Health Journal, 23*, 593–605.

Oppenheim, D., Koren-Karie, N., Dolev, S., & Yirmiya, N. (2012). Maternal sensitivity mediates the link between maternal insightfulness/resolution and child–mother attachment: The case of children with autism spectrum disorder. *Attachment and Human Development, 14*, 567–584.

Ordway, M. R., Sadler, L. S., Dixon, J., Close, N., Mayes, L., Slade, A. (2014). Lasting effects of an interdisciplinary home visiting program on child behavior: Preliminary follow-up results of a randomized trial. *Journal of Pediatric Nursing, 29*, 3–13.

Ordway, M. R., Sadler, L. S., Holland, M. L., Slade, A., Close, N., & Mayes, L. C. (2018). A home visiting parenting program and child obesity: A randomized trial. *Pediatrics, 141*, 1–9.

Organ, D. W. (1997). Organizational citizenship behavior: It's construct clean-up time. *Human Performance, 10*, 85–97.

Oriña, M. M., Collins, W. A., Simpson, J. A., Salvatore, J. E., Haydon, K. C., & Kim, J. S. (2011). Developmental and dyadic perspectives on commitment in adult romantic relationships. *Psychological Science, 22,* 908–915.

Osman, F., Flacking, R., Schön, U. K., & Klingberg-Allvin, M. (2017). A support program for Somali-born parents on children's behavioral problems. *Pediatrics, 139,* Article e20162764.

Osman, F., Salari, R., Klingberg-Allvin, M., Schön, U. K., & Flacking, R. (2017). Effects of a culturally tailored parenting support program in Somali-born parents' mental health and sense of competence in parenting: A randomized controlled trial. *BMJ Open, 7,* Article e017600.

Osman, F., Vixner, L., Flacking, R., Klingberg-Allvin, M., Schön, U. K., & Salari, R. (2021). Impact of a culturally tailored parenting program on the mental health of Somali parents and children living in Sweden: A longitudinal cohort study. *BMJ Open, 11,* Article e045067.

Otway, L. J., Carnelley, K. B., & Rowe, A. C. (2014). Texting "boosts" felt security. *Attachment and Human Development, 16,* 93–101.

Overall, N. C., Fletcher, G. J. O., & Friesen, M. D. (2003). Mapping the intimate relationship mind: Comparisons between three models of attachment representations. *Personality and Social Psychology Bulletin, 29,* 1479–1493.

Overall, N. C., Fletcher, G. J. O., Simpson, J. A., & Fillo, J. (2015). Attachment insecurity, biased perceptions of romantic partners' negative emotions, and hostile relationship behavior. *Journal of Personality and Social Psychology, 108,* 730–749.

Overall, N., Simpson, J. A., & Struthers, H. (2013). Buffering attachment-related avoidance: Softening emotional and behavioral defenses during conflict discussions. *Journal of Personality and Social Psychology, 104,* 854–871.

Ozturk, Y., Moretti, M., & Barone, L. (2019). Addressing parental stress and adolescents' behavioral problems through an attachment-based program: An intervention study. *International Journal of Psychology and Psychological Therapy, 19,* 89–100.

Papa, A., Rummel, C., Garrison-Diehn, C., & Sewell, M. T. (2013). Behavioral activation for pathological grief. *Death Studies, 37,* 913–936.

Parenteau, S. C., Hurd, K., Wu, H., & Feck, C. (2019). Attachment to god and psychological adjustment: God's responses and our coping strategies. *Journal of Religion and Health, 58,* 1286–1306.

Pargament, K. I. (1997). *The psychology of religion and coping.* Guilford Press.

Pargament, K. I. (2011). *Spiritually integrated psychotherapy: Understanding and addressing the sacred.* Guilford Press.

Pargament, K. I., & Exline, J. J. (2022). *Working with spiritual struggles in psychotherapy: From research to practice.* Guilford Press.

Parish-Plass, N. (2008). Animal-assisted therapy with children suffering from insecure attachment due to abuse and neglect: A method to lower the risk of intergenerational transmission of abuse? *Clinical Child Psychology and Psychiatry, 13,* 7–30.

Park, L. E. (2007). Appearance-based rejection sensitivity: Implications for mental and physical health, affect, and motivation. *Personality and Social Psychology Bulletin, 33,* 490–504.

Park, Y., Impett, E. A., MacDonald, G., & Lemay, E. P., Jr. (2019). Saying "thank you": Partners' expressions of gratitude protect relationship satisfaction and commitment from the harmful effects of attachment insecurity. *Journal of Personality and Social Psychology, 117,* 773–806.

Park, Y., Johnson, M. D., MacDonald, G., & Impett, E. A. (2019). Perceiving gratitude from a romantic partner predicts decreases in attachment anxiety. *Developmental Psychology, 55,* 2692–2700.

Parkes, C. M., & Weiss, R. S. (1983). *Recovery from bereavement.* Basic Books.

Partee, A., Williford, A., & Whittaker, J. (2022). Implementing Banking Time with teachers and preschoolers displaying disruptive behaviors: Links between consultant–teacher relationship quality, implementation fidelity and dosage, and dyadic teacher–child interactions. *School Mental Health, 14,* 341–356.

Pasalich, D. S., Craig, S. G., Goulter, N., O'Donnell, K. A., Sierra Hernandez, C., & Moretti, M. M. (2022). Patterns and predictors of different youth responses to attachment-based parent intervention. *Journal of Clinical Child and Adolescent Psychology, 51,* 796–809.

Pasalich, D. S., Moretti, M. M., Hassall, A., & Curcio, A. (2021). Pilot randomized controlled trial of an attachment- and trauma-focused intervention for kinship caregivers. *Child Abuse and Neglect, 120,* Article 105178.

Patel, S., Pelletier-Bui, A., Smith, S., Roberts, M. B., Kilgannon, H., Trzciak, S., & Roberts, B. W. (2019). Curricula for empathy and compassion training in medical education: A systematic review. *PLOS ONE, 14,* Article e0221412.

Pearce, M. J., Koenig, H. G., Robins, C. J., Nelson, B., Shaw, S. F., Cohen, H. J., & King, M. B. (2015). Religiously integrated cognitive behavioral therapy: A new method of treatment for major depression in patients with chronic medical illness. *Psychotherapy, 52,* 56–66.

Péloquin, K., Brassard, A., Lafontaine, M.-F., & Shaver, P. R. (2014). Sexuality examined through the lens of attachment theory: Attachment, caregiving, and sexual satisfaction. *Journal of Sex Research, 51,* 561–576.

Peltz, J. S., Rogge, R. D., Rogosch, F. A., Cicchetti, D., & Toth, S. L. (2015). The benefits of child–parent psychotherapy to marital satisfaction. *Families, Systems, and Health, 33,* 372–382.

Pennebaker, J. W., Booth, R. J., & Francis, M. E.

(2007). *LIWC2007: Linguistic Inquiry and Word Count.* liwc.net.

Peplau, L. A., & Perlman, D. (Eds.). (1982). *Loneliness: A sourcebook of current theory, research, and therapy.* Wiley.

Pepping, C. A., Davis, P. J., & O'Donovan, A. (2015a). The association between state attachment security and state mindfulness. *PLOS ONE, 10,* Article e0116779.

Pepping, C. A., Davis, P. J., O'Donovan, A., & Pal, J. (2015b). Individual differences in self-compassion: The role of attachment and experiences of parenting in childhood. *Self and Identity, 14,* 104–117.

Perren, S., Schmid, R., Herrmann, S., & Wettstein, A. (2007). The impact of attachment on dementia-related problem behavior and spousal caregivers' well-being. *Attachment and Human Development, 9,* 163–178.

Perrone, L., Imrisek, S. D., Dash, A., Rodriguez, M., Monticciolo, E., & Bernard, K. (2021). Changing parental depression and sensitivity: Randomized clinical trial of ABC's effectiveness in the community. *Development and Psychopathology, 33,* 1026–1040.

Petrowski, K., Berth, H., Schurig, S., & Probst, T. (2019). Suppressor effects in associations between patient attachment to therapist and psychotherapy outcome. *Clinical Psychology and Psychotherapy, 26,* 105–109.

Philips, B., Wennberg, P., Konradsson, P., & Franck, J. (2018). Mentalization-based treatment for concurrent borderline personality disorder and substance use disorder: A randomized controlled feasibility study. *European Addiction Research, 24,* 1–8.

Pianta, R. C. (Ed.). (1992). *Beyond the parent: The role of other adults in children's lives.* Jossey-Bass.

Pianta, R. C. (1993). *The Student–Teacher Relationship Scale.* University of Virginia.

Pianta, R. C. (1999). Assessing child–teacher relationships. In R. C. Pianta (Ed.), *Enhancing relationships between children and teachers* (pp. 85–104). American Psychological Association.

Pianta, R. C., Belsky, J., Vandergrift, N., Houts, R., & Morrison, F. J. (2008). Classroom effects on children's achievement trajectories in elementary school. *American Educational Research Journal, 45,* 365–397.

Pianta, R. C., DeCoster, J., Cabell, S., Burchinal, M., Hamre, B. K., Downer, J., . . . Howes, C. (2014). Dose–response relations between preschool teachers' exposure to components of professional development and increases in quality of their interactions with children. *Early Childhood Research Quarterly, 29,* 499–508.

Pianta, R. C., & Hamre, B. (2001). *Students, teachers, and relationship support (STARS).* Psychological Assessment Resources.

Pianta, R. C., Hamre, B., Downer, J., Burchinal, M., Williford, A., LoCasale-Crouch, J., . . . Cabell, S. Q. (2017). Early childhood professional development: Coaching and coursework effects on indicators of children's school readiness. *Early Education and Development, 28,* 956–975.

Pianta, R. C., La Paro, K. M., & Hamre, B. K. (2007). *Classroom Assessment Scoring System [CLASS] manual: Pre-K.* Brookes.

Pianta, R. C., Lipscomb, D., & Ruzek, E. (2021). Coaching teachers to improve students' school readiness skills: Indirect effects of teacher–student interaction. *Child Development, 92,* 2509–2528.

Pianta, R. C., Mashburn, A. J., Downer, J. T., Hamre, B. K., Justice, L. (2008). Effects of web-mediated professional development resources on teacher–child interactions in pre-kindergarten classrooms. *Early Childhood Research Quarterly, 23,* 431–451.

Pianta, R. C., & Steinberg, M. (1992). Teacher–child relationships and the process of adjusting to school. In R. C. Pianta (Ed.), *Beyond the parent: The role of other adults in children's lives* (pp. 61–80). Jossey-Bass.

Pianta, R. C., & Stuhlman, M. W. (2004). Teacher–child relationships and chi'dren's success in the first years of school. *School Psychology Review, 33,* 444–458.

Pianta, R. C., Whittaker, J. E., Vitiello, V., Ruzek, E., Ansari, A., Hofkens, T., & DeCoster, J. (2020). Children's school readiness skills across the pre-K year: Associations with teacher–student interactions, teacher practices, and exposure to academic content. *Journal of Applied Developmental Psychology, 66,* Article 101084.

Picardi, A., Battisti, F., Tarsitani, L., Baldassari, M., Copertaro, A., Mocchegiani, E., & Biandi, M. (2007). Attachment security and immunity in healthy women. *Psychosomatic Medicine, 69,* 40–46.

Picardi, A., Miglio, R., Tarsitani, L., Battisti, F., Baldassari, M., Copertaro, A., . . . Biondi, M. (2013). Attachment style and immunity: A 1-year longitudinal study. *Biological Psychology, 92,* 353–358.

Pierce, T., & Lydon, J. (1998). Priming relational schemas: Effects of contextually activated and chronically accessible interpersonal expectations on responses to a stressful event. *Journal of Personality and Social Psychology, 75,* 1441–1448.

Pietromonaco, P. R., & Collins, N. L. (2017). Interpersonal mechanisms linking close relationships to health. *American Psychologist, 72,* 531–542.

Pietromonaco, P. R., DeVito, C. C., Ge, F., & Lembke, J. (2015). Health and attachment processes. In J. A. Simpson & W. S. Rholes (Eds.), *Attachment theory and research: New directions and emerging themes* (pp. 287–318). Guilford Press.

Pinker, S. (2011). *The better angels of our nature: Why violence has declined.* Viking.

Pinker, S. (2019). *Enlightenment now: The case for reason, science, humanism, and progress.* Penguin

Pinquart, M. (2016). Associations of parenting styles and dimensions with academic achievement in children and adolescents: A meta-analysis. *Educational Psychology Review, 28*, 475–493.

Pinquart, M. (2017a). Associations of parenting dimensions and styles with internalizing symptoms in children and adolescents: A meta-analysis. *Marriage and Family Review, 53*, 613–640.

Pinquart, M. (2017b). Associations of parenting dimensions and styles with externalizing problems of children and adolescents: An updated meta-analysis. *Developmental Psychology, 53*, 873–932.

Pinquart, M., Feußner, C., & Ahnert, L. (2013). Meta-analytic evidence for stability in attachments from infancy to early adulthood. *Attachment and Human Development, 15*, 189–218.

Pinsof, W. M., & Catherall, D. R. (1986). The integrative psychotherapy alliance: Family, couple and individual therapy scales. *Journal of Marital and Family Therapy, 12*, 137–151.

Pistole, M. C. (1997). Attachment theory: Contributions to group work. *Journal for Specialists in Group Work, 22*, 7–21.

Pitillas, C. (2020). Common therapeutic elements of interventions aimed at enhancing parent–child early relationships. *Psychoanalytic Psychology, 37*, 28–36.

Pizzano, P. A., Sherblom, J. C., & Umphrey, L. R. (2013). Being secure means being willing to say you're sorry: Attachment style and the communication of relational dissatisfaction and disengagement. *Journal of Relationships Research, 4*, Article E7.

Planalp, E. M., O'Neill, M., & Braungart-Rieker, J. M. (2019). Parent mind-mindedness, sensitivity, and infant affect: Implications for attachment with mothers and fathers. *Infant Behavior and Development, 57*, Article 101330.

Platje, E., Sterkenburg, P., Overbeek, M., Kef, S., & Schuengel, C. (2018). The efficacy of VIPP-V parenting training for parents of young children with a visual or visual-and-intellectual disability: A randomized controlled trial. *Attachment and Human Development, 20*, 455–472.

Platt, J. M., Lowe, S. R., Galea, S., Norris, F. H., & Koenen, K. C. (2016). A longitudinal study of the bidirectional relationship between social support and posttraumatic stress following a natural disaster. *Journal of Traumatic Stress, 29*, 205–213.

Poortvliet, P. M., Anseel, F., & Theuwis, F. (2015). Mastery-approach and mastery-avoidance goals and their relation with exhaustion and engagement at work: The roles of emotional and instrumental support. *Work and Stress, 29*, 150–170.

Popper, M., & Mayseless, O. (2003). Back to basics: Applying a parenting perspective to transformational leadership. *Leadership Quarterly, 14*, 41–65.

Popper, M., Mayseless, O., & Castelnovo, O. (2000). Transformational leadership and attachment. *Leadership Quarterly, 11*, 267–289.

Poslawsky, I. E., Naber, F. B. A., Bakermans-Kranenburg, M. J., De Jonge, M. V., van Engeland, H., & van IJzendoorn, M. H. (2014). Development of a Video-Feedback Intervention to promote Positive Parenting for Children with Autism (VIPP-AUTI). *Attachment and Human Development, 16*, 343–355.

Poslawsky, I. E., Naber, F. B. A., Bakermans-Kranenburg, M. J., van Daalen, E., van Engeland, H., & van IJzendoorn, M. H. (2015). Video-Feedback Intervention to promote Positive Parenting adapted to Autism (VIPP-AUTI): A randomized controlled trial. *Autism, 19*, 588–603.

Post, B. C., & Wade, N. G. (2009). Religion and spirituality in psychotherapy: A practice-friendly review of research. *Journal of Clinical Psychology, 65*, 131–146.

Postmes, T., Wichmann, L. J., van Valkengoed, A. M., & Hoef, H. (2019). Social identification and depression: A meta-analysis. *European Journal of Social Psychology, 49*, 110–126.

Poteat, L. F., Shockley, K. M., & Allen, T. D. (2015). Attachment anxiety in mentoring: The role of commitment. *Career Development International, 20*, 119–132.

Powell, B., Cooper, G., Hoffman, K., & Marvin, B. (2014). *The Circle of Security intervention: Enhancing attachment in early parent–child relationships*. Guilford Press.

Powell, K. S., & Yalcin, S. (2010). Managerial training effectiveness: A meta-analysis 1952–2002. *Personnel Review, 39*, 227–241.

Powers, S. I., Pietromonaco, P. R., Gunlicks, M., & Sayer, A. (2006). Dating couples' attachment styles and patterns of cortisol reactivity and recovery in response to a relationship conflict. *Journal of Personality and Social Psychology, 90*, 613–628.

Price, L. H., Kao, H.-T., Burgers, D. E., Carpenter, L. L., & Tyrka, A. R. (2013). Telomeres and early-life stress: An overview. *Biological Psychiatry, 73*, 15–23.

Prusova, I., & Gulevich, O. (2019). *The effect of mortality salience on attitudes toward national outgroups* (Higher School of Economics Research Paper No. WP BRP 105/PSY/2019). National Research University.

Pu, J., Zhou, X., Liu, L., Zhang, Y., Yang, L., Yuan, S., . . . Xie, P. (2017). Efficacy and acceptability of interpersonal psychotherapy for depression in adolescents: A meta-analysis of randomized controlled trials. *Psychiatry Research, 253*, 226–232.

Puig, J., Englund, M. M., Simpson, J. A., & Collins, W. A. (2013). Predicting adult physical illness from infant attachment: A prospective longitudinal study. *Health Psychology, 32*, 409–417.

Pyszczynski, T., Wicklund, R. A., Floresku, S., Koch, H., Gauch, G., Solomon, S., & Greenberg, J. (1996). Whistling in the dark: Exaggerated consensus estimates in response to incidental reminders of mortality. *Psychological Science, 7*, 332–336.

Quinn, K., Spiby, H., & Slade, P. (2015). A longitudinal study exploring the role of adult attachment in relation to perceptions of pain in labor, childbirth memory and acute traumatic stress responses. *Journal of Reproductive and Infant Psychology, 33*, 256–267.

Quinn, S. C., Parmer, J., Freimuth, V. S., Hilyard, K. M., Musa, D., & Kim, K. H. (2013). Exploring communication, trust in government, and vaccination intention later in the 2009 H1N1 pandemic: Results of a national survey. *Biosecurity and Bioterrorism, 11*, 96–106.

Raby, K. L., Freedman, E., Yarger, H. A., Lind, T., & Dozier, M. (2019). Enhancing the language development of toddlers in foster care by promoting foster parents' sensitivity: Results from a randomized controlled trial. *Developmental Science, 22*, Article e12753.

Raby, K. L., Lawler, J. M., Shlafer, R. J., Hesemeyer, P. S., Collins, W. A., & Sroufe, L. A. (2015). The interpersonal antecedents of supportive parenting: A prospective, longitudinal study from infancy to adulthood. *Developmental Psychology, 51*, 115–123.

Raby, K. L., Roisman, G. I., Fraley, R. C., & Simpson, J. A. (2015). The enduring predictive significance of early maternal sensitivity: Social and academic competence through age 32 years. *Child Development, 86*, 695–708.

Raby, K. L., Roisman, G. I., Simpson, J. A., Collins, W. A., & Steele, R. D. (2015). Greater maternal insensitivity in childhood predicts greater electrodermal reactivity during conflict discussions with romantic partners in adulthood. *Psychological Science, 26*, 348–353.

Raby, K. L., Waters, T. E. A., Tabachnick, A. R., Zajac, L., & Dozier, M. (2021). Increasing secure base script knowledge among parents with attachment and biobehavioral catch-up. *Development and Psychopathology, 33*, 554–564.

Raikes, H. A., & Thompson, R. A. (2006). Family emotional climate, attachment security and young children's emotion knowledge in a high risk sample. *British Journal of Developmental Psychology, 24*, 89–104.

Rakel, D. P., Hoeft, T. J., Barrett, B. P., Chewning, B. A., Craig, B. M., & Niu, M. (2009). Practitioner empathy and the duration of the common cold. *Family Medicine, 41*, 494–501.

Ramsauer, B., Lotzin, A., Quitmann, J. H., Becker-Stoll, F., Tharner, A., & Romer, G. (2014). Insightfulness and later infant attachment in clinically depressed and nonclinical mothers. *Infant Mental Health Journal, 35*, 210–219.

Ramsauer, B., Mühlhan, C., Lotzin, A., Achtergarde, S., Mueller, J., Krink, S., . . . Romer, G. (2020). Randomized controlled trial of the Circle of Security-intensive intervention for mothers with postpartum depression: Maternal unresolved attachment moderates changes in sensitivity. *Attachment and Human Development, 22*, 705–726.

Ramseyer, F., & Tschacher, W. (2011). Nonverbal synchrony in psychotherapy: Coordinated body movement reflects relationship quality and outcome. *Journal of Consulting and Clinical Psychology, 79*, 284–295.

Randall, A. K., & Butler, E. A. (2013). Attachment and emotion transmission within romantic relationships: Merging intrapersonal and interpersonal perspectives. *Journal of Relationships Research, 4*, Article ID e10.

Raposo, S., & Muise, A. (2021). Perceived partner sexual responsiveness buffers anxiously attached individuals' relationship and sexual quality in daily life. *Journal of Family Psychology, 35*, 500–509.

Ravitz, P., Maunder, R., & McBride, C. (2008). Attachment, contemporary interpersonal theory, and IPT: An integration of theoretical, clinical, and empirical perspectives. *Journal of Contemporary Psychotherapy, 38*, 11–21.

Reichert, E. (1998). Individual counseling for sexually abused children: A role for animal and storytelling. *Child and Adolescence Social Work Journal, 15*, 177–185.

Reid, J., & Scharfe, E. (2019). University blues: Role of attachment and distress on students' evaluations of instructors' teaching performance. *Journal of Relationships Research, 10*, Article e23.

Reid, M., Landesman, S., Treder, R., & Jaccard, J. (1989). "My family and friends": Six- to twelve-year-old children's perceptions of social support. *Child Development, 60*, 896–910.

Reiner, I., Bakermans-Kranenburg, M. J., van IJzendoorn, M. H., Fremmer-Bombik, E., & Beutel, M. (2016). Adult attachment representation moderates psychotherapy treatment efficacy in clinically depressed inpatients. *Journal of Affective Disorders, 195*, 163–171.

Reis, H. T. (2014). Responsiveness: Affective interdependence in close relationships. In M. Mikulincer & P. R. Shaver (Eds.), *Mechanisms of social connection: From brain to group* (pp. 255–271). American Psychological Association.

Reis, H. T., Clark, M. S., Gray, D. J. P., Tsai, F.-F., Brown, J. B., Stewart, M., & Underwood, L. G. (2008). Measuring responsiveness in the therapeutic relationship: A patient perspective. *Basic and Applied Social Psychology, 30*, 339–348.

Reis, H. T., Lee, K. Y., O'Keefe, S. D., & Clark, M. S. (2018). Perceived partner responsiveness promotes intellectual humility. *Journal of Experimental Social Psychology, 79*, 21–33.

Reis, H. T., & Shaver, P. R. (1988). Intimacy as an interpersonal process. In S. Duck (Ed.), *Handbook of research in personal relationships* (pp. 367–389). Wiley.

Reizer, A. (2019). Bringing self-kindness into the workplace: Exploring the mediating role of self-compassion in the associations between attachment and organizational outcomes. *Frontiers in Psychology, 10*, Article 1148.

Reizer, A., Oren, L., & Hornik, Y. (2022). Does group cohesion moderate associations between attachment, caregiving, and OCB? *Journal of Management and Organization, 28*, 715–732.

Remien, R. H., Stirratt, M. J., Dolezal, C., Dognin, J. S., Wagner, G. J., Carballo-Dieguez, A., . . . Jung, T. M. (2005). Couple-focused support to improve HIV medication adherence: A randomized controlled trial. *AIDS, 19*, 807–814.

Repacholi, B., & Trapolini, T. (2004). Attachment and preschool children's understanding of maternal versus non-maternal psychological states. *British Journal of Developmental Psychology, 22*, 395–415.

Rhoades, L., & Eisenberger, R. (2002). Perceived organizational support: A review of the literature. *Journal of Applied Psychology, 87*, 698–714.

Rholes, W. S., Eller, J., Simpson, J. A., & Arriaga, X. B. (2021). Support processes predict declines in attachment avoidance across the transition to parenthood. *Personality and Social Psychology Bulletin, 47*, 810–825.

Rholes, W. S., Kohn, J. L., & Simpson, J. A. (2014). A longitudinal study of conflict in new parents: The role of attachment. *Personal Relationships, 21*, 1–21.

Rholes, W. S., Simpson, J. A., Campbell, L., & Grich, J. (2001). Adult attachment and the transition to parenthood. *Journal of Personality and Social Psychology, 81*, 421–435.

Riem, M. M. E., Doedée, E. N. E. M., Broekhuizen-Dijksman, S. C., & Beijer, E. (2018). Attachment and medically unexplained somatic symptoms: The role of mentalization. *Psychiatry Research, 268*, 108–113.

Rifkin-Graboi, A. (2008). Attachment status and salivary cortisol in a normal day and during simulated interpersonal stress in young men. *Stress, 11*, 210–224.

Riggle, R. J., Edmondson, D. R., & Hansen, J. D. (2009). A meta-analysis of the relationship between perceived organizational support and job outcomes: 20 years of research. *Journal of Business Research, 62*, 1027–1030.

Rimm-Kaufman, S. E., Voorhees, M. D., Snell, M. E., & La Paro, K. M. (2003). Improving the sensitivity and responsivity of preservice teachers toward young children with disabilities. *Topics in Early Childhood Special Education, 23*, 151–163.

Risholm Mothander, P., Furmark, C., & Neander, K. (2018). Adding "Circle of Security-Parenting" to treatment as usual in three Swedish infant mental health clinics: Effects on parents' internal representations and quality of parent–infant interaction. *Scandinavian Journal of Psychology, 59*, 262–272.

Roben, C. K. P., Dozier, M., Caron, E. B., & Bernard, K. (2017). Moving an evidence-based parenting program into the community. *Child Development, 88*, 1447–1452.

Robertson, J., & Bowlby, J. (1952). Responses of young children to separation from their mothers. *Courier of the International Children's Center, Paris, 2*, 131–140.

Robinson, P., Hellier, J., Barrett, B., Barzdaitiene, D., Bateman, A., Bogaardt, A., . . . Fonagy, P. (2016). The NOURISHED randomized controlled trial comparing mentalisation-based treatment for eating disorders (MBT-ED) with specialist supportive clinical management (SSCM-ED) for patients with eating disorders and symptoms of borderline personality disorder. *Trials, 17*, 1–15.

Robles, T. F., Brooks, K. P., Kane, H. S., & Schetter, C. D. (2013). Attachment, skin deep?: Relationships between adult attachment and skin barrier recovery. *International Journal of Psychophysiology, 88*, 241–252.

Rockett, B., & Carr, S. (2014). Animals and attachment theory. *Society and Animals: Journal of Human–Animal Studies, 22*, 415–433.

Rockliff, H., Gilbert, P., McEwan, K., Lightman, S., & Glover, D. (2008). A pilot exploration of heart rate variability and salivary cortisol responses to compassion-focused imagery. *Journal of Clinical Neuropsychiatry, 5*, 132–139.

Rodin, G., Walsh, A., Zimmermann, C., Gagliese, L., Jones, J., Shepherd, F. A., . . . Mikulincer, M. (2007). The contribution of attachment security and social support to depressive symptoms in patients with metastatic cancer. *Psycho-Oncology, 16*, 1080–1091.

Rogers, C. R. (1961). *On becoming a person*. Houghton Mifflin.

Rognli, E. W., Waraan, L., Czajkowski, N. O., & Aalberg, M. (2020). Moderation of treatment effects by parent–adolescent conflict in a randomized controlled trial of attachment-based family therapy for adolescent depression. *Scandinavian Journal of Child and Adolescent Psychiatry and Psychology, 8*, 110–122.

Rohmann, E., Neumann, E., Herner, M. J., & Bierhoff, M. H. W. (2012). Grandiose and vulnerable narcissism: Self-construal, attachment, and love in romantic relationship. *European Psychologist, 17*, 279–290.

Roisman, G. I. (2007). The psychophysiology of adult attachment relationships: Autonomic reactivity in marital and premarital interactions. *Developmental Psychology, 43*, 39–53.

Roisman, G. I., Madsen, S. D., Hennighausen, K. H., Sroufe, L. A., & Collins, W. A. (2001). The coherence of dyadic behavior across parent–child and romantic relationships as mediated by the internalized representation of experience. *Attachment and Human Development, 3*, 156–172.

Rollnick, S., Miller, W. R., & Butler, C. C. (2008). *Motivational interviewing in health care: Helping patients change behavior.* Guilford Press.

Rom, E., & Benatov, J. (2018). Adult attachment and perceived parental style may shape leadership behaviors. *Leadership and Organization Development Journal, 39*, 261–275.

Rom, E., & Mikulincer, M. (2003). Attachment theory and group processes: The association between attachment style and group-related representations, goals, memories, and functioning. *Journal of Personality and Social Psychology, 84*, 1220–1235.

Romano, V., Fitzpatrick, M., & Janzen, J. (2008). The secure-base hypothesis: Global attachment, attachment to counselor, and session exploration in psychotherapy. *Journal of Counseling Psychology, 55*, 495–504.

Romano, V., Janzen, J. I., & Fitzpatrick, M. R. (2009). Volunteer client attachment moderates the relationship between trainee therapist attachment and therapist interventions. *Psychotherapy Research, 19*, 666–676.

Ronen, S., & Mikulincer, M. (2009). Attachment orientations and work outcomes: The mediating role of employees' appraisals of organizational fairness, team cohesion, and manager's leadership. *Journal of Social and Personal Relationships, 26*, 549–567.

Ronen, S., & Mikulincer, M. (2012). Predicting employees' satisfaction and burnout from managers' attachment and caregiving orientations. *European Journal of Work and Organizational Psychology, 21*, 828–849.

Ronen, S., & Zuroff, D. C. (2017). How does secure attachment affect job performance and job promotion?: The role of social-rank behaviors. *Journal of Vocational Behavior, 100*, 137–148.

Roorda, D. L., Jak, S., Zee, M., Oort, F. J., & Koomen, H. M. Y. (2017). Affective teacher–student relationships and students' engagement and achievement: A meta-analytic update and test of the mediating role of engagement. *School Psychology Review, 46*, 239–261.

Roorda, D. L., Koomen, H. M. Y., Spilt, J. L., & Oort, F. J. (2011). The influence of affective teacher–student relationships on students' school engagement and achievement: A meta-analytic approach. *Review of Educational Research, 81*, 493–529.

Rose, J., McGuire-Snieckus, R., Gilberta, L., & McInnes, K. (2019). Attachment Aware Schools: The impact of a targeted and collaborative intervention. *Pastoral Care in Education, 37*, 162–184.

Rosenberg, T., & Shields, C. (2009). The role of parent-adolescent attachment in the glycemic control of adolescents with type 1 diabetes: A pilot study. *Families, Systems and Health 27*, 237–248.

Rosenthal, H. E. S., Somers, N., Fleming, P., & Walsh, J. (2014). The contributions of interpersonal attachment and friendship group identification to depressive symptoms in a nonclinical sample. *Journal of Applied Social Psychology, 44*, 409–414.

Rosenthal, N. L., & Kobak, R. (2010). Assessing adolescents' attachment hierarchies: Differences across developmental periods and associations with individual adaptation. *Journal of Research on Adolescence, 20*, 678–706.

Rosland, A.-M., Heisler, M., & Piette, J. D. (2012). The impact of family behaviors and communication patterns on chronic illness outcomes: A systematic review. *Journal of Behavioral Medicine, 35*, 221–239.

Rosmarin, D. H. (2018). *Spirituality, religion, and cognitive-behavioral therapy: A guide for clinicians.* Guilford Press.

Rosso, A. M., & Airaldi, C. (2016). Intergenerational transmission of reflective functioning. *Frontiers in Psychology, 7*, Article 1903.

Rossouw, T. (2018). Mentalizationbased therapy for adolescents: Managing storms in youth presenting with self-harm and suicidal states. In H. Steele & M. Steele (Eds.), *Handbook of attachment-based interventions* (pp. 419–440). Guilford Press.

Rossouw, T. I., & Fonagy, P. (2012). Mentalization-based treatment for self-harm in adolescents: A randomized controlled trial. *Journal of the American Academy of Child and Adolescent Psychiatry, 51*, 1304–1313.

Rowatt, W. C., & Kirkpatrick, L. A. (2002). Two dimensions of attachment to God and their relation to affect, religiosity, and personality constructs. *Journal for the Scientific Study of Religion, 41*, 637–651.

Rowe, A. C., & Carnelley, K. B. (2003). Attachment style differences in the processing of attachment-relevant information: Primed-style effects on recall, interpersonal expectations, and affect. *Personal Relationships, 10*, 59–75.

Rowe, A. C., Carnelley, K. B., Harwood, J., Micklewright, D., Russouw, L., Rennie, C. L., & Liossi, C. (2012). The effect of attachment orientation priming on pain sensitivity in pain-free individuals. *Journal of Social and Personal Relationships, 29*, 488–507.

Rowe, A. C., Gold, E. R., & Carnelley, K. B. (2020). The effectiveness of attachment security priming in improving positive affect and reducing negative affect: A systematic review. *International Journal of Environmental Research and Public Health, 17*, Article 968.

Rowe, A. C., Shepstone, L., Carnelley, K. B., Cavanagh, K., & Millings, A. (2016). Attachment security and self-compassion priming increase the likelihood that first-time engagers in mindfulness meditation will continue with mindfulness training. *Mindfulness, 7*, 642–650.

Rubenstein, C., & Shaver, P. R. (1982). The experience of loneliness. In L. A. Peplau & D. Perlman (Eds.), *Loneliness: A sourcebook of current theory, research, and therapy* (pp. 206–223). Wiley.

Rubin, S. S., Malkinson, R., & Witztum, E. (2012). *Working with the bereaved: Multiple lenses on loss and mourning.* Routledge.

Rubino, G., Barker, C., Roth, T., & Fearon, P. (2000). Therapist empathy and depth of interpretation in response to potential alliance ruptures: The role of therapist and patient attachment styles. *Psychotherapy Research, 10*, 408–420.

Ruhl, H., Dolan, E. A., & Buhrmester, D. (2015). Adolescent attachment trajectories with mothers and fathers: The importance of parent-child relationship experiences and gender. *Journal of Research on Adolescence, 25*, 427–442.

Rujoiu, O., & Rujoiu, V. (2014). Pet loss and human emotion: Romanian students' reflections on pet loss. *Journal of Loss and Trauma, 19*, 474–483.

Runze, J., van Ijzendoorn, M. H., Vrijhof, C. I., & Bakermans-Kranenburg, M. J. (2022). Replicating a randomized trial with video-feedback to promote positive parenting in parents of school-aged twins. *Journal of Family Psychology, 36*, 490–501.

Russon, J., Morrissey, J., Dellinger, J., Jin, B., & Diamond, G. (2022). Implementing attachment-based family therapy for depressed and suicidal adolescents and young adults in LGBTQ+ services: Feasibility, acceptability, and preliminary effectiveness. *Crisis, 43*, 500–507.

Ryan, R. M., & Deci, E. L. (2017). *Self-determination theory: Basic psychological needs in motivation, development, and wellness.* Guilford Press.

Rydell, A.-M., Bohlin, G., & Thorell, L. B. (2005). Representations of attachment to parents and shyness as predictors of children's relationships with teachers and peer competence in preschool. *Attachment and Human Development, 7*, 187–204.

Sabol, T. J., & Pianta, R. C. (2012). Recent trends in research on teacher–child relationships. *Attachment and Human Development, 14*, 213–231.

Sadava, S. W., Busseri, M. A., Molnar, D. S., Perrier, C. P. K., & DeCourville, N. (2009). Investigating a four pathway model of adult attachment orientation and health. *Journal of Social and Personal Relationships, 26*, 604–633.

Sadler, L. S., Slade, A., Close, N., Webb, D. L., Simpson, T., Fennie, K., & Mayes, L. C. (2013). Minding the Baby: Enhancing reflectiveness to improve early health and relationship outcomes in an interdisciplinary home visiting program. *Infant Mental Health Journal, 34*, 391–405.

Sadler, L. S., Slade, A., & Mayes, L. C. (2006). Minding the Baby: A mentalization based parenting program. In J. G. Allen & P. Fonagy (Eds.), *Handbook of mentalization-based treatment* (pp. 271–288). Wiley.

Sakman, E., & Sümer, N. (2018). Attachment (in) security and threat priming influence signal detection performance. *Journal of Social and Personal Relationships, 35*, 889–916.

Saleem, M., Prot, S., Cikara, M., Lam, B. C. P., Anderson, C. A., & Jelic, M. (2015). Cutting Gordian knots: Reducing prejudice through attachment security. *Personality and Social Psychology Bulletin, 41*, 1560–1574.

Salmanian, M., Ghobari-Bonab, B., Hooshyari, Z., & Mohammadi, M.-R. (2020). Effectiveness of spiritual psychotherapy on attachment to God among adolescents with conduct disorder: A randomized controlled trial. *Psychology of Religion and Spirituality, 12*, 269–275.

Salvatore, J. E., Kuo, S. I., Steele, R. D., Simpson, J. A., & Collins, W. A. (2011). Recovering from conflict in romantic relationships: A developmental perspective. *Psychological Science, 22*, 376–383.

Sambo, C. F., Howard, M., Kopelman, M., Williams, S., & Fotopoulou, A. (2010). Knowing you care: Effects of perceived empathy and attachment style on pain perception. *Pain, 151*, 687–693.

Sandage, S. J., Jankowski, P., Crabtree, S. A., & Schweer, M. (2015). Attachment to God, adult attachment, and spiritual pathology: Mediator and moderator effects. *Mental Health, Religion and Culture, 18*, 795–808.

Santascoy, N., Burke, S. E., & Dovidio, J. F. (2018). Avoidant attachment style predicts less positive evaluations of warm (but not cold) social groups. *Group Processes and Intergroup Relations, 21*, 19–36.

Sauer, E. M., Anderson, M. Z., Gormley, B., Richmond, C. J., & Preacco, L. (2010). Client attachment orientations, working alliances, and responses to therapy: A psychology training clinic study. *Psychotherapy Research, 20*, 702–711.

Sauer, E. M., Lopez, F. G., & Gormley, B. (2003). Respective contributions of therapist and client adult attachment orientations to the development of the early working alliance: A preliminary growth modeling study. *Psychotherapy Research, 13*, 371–382.

Sauer, E. M., Rice, K. G., Roberts, K. E., & Richardson, C. M. E. (2020). Client attachment and change in mental health during psychotherapy. *Psychotherapy, 57*, 574–579.

Saypol, E., & Farber, B. A. (2010). Attachment style and patient disclosure in psychotherapy. *Psychotherapy Research, 20*, 462–471.

Sbarra, D. A. (2006). Predicting the onset of emotional recovery following nonmarital relationship dissolution: Survival analyses of sadness and anger. *Personality and Social Psychology Bulletin, 32*, 298–312.

Sbarra, D. A., & Borelli, J. L. (2019). Attachment reorganization following divorce: Normative processes and individual differences. *Current Opinion in Psychology, 25*, 71–75.

Sbarra, D. A., Bourassa, K. J., & Manvelian, A. (2019). Marital separation and divorce: Correlates and consequences. In B. H. Fiese, M. Celano, K. Deater-Deckard, E. N. Jouriles, & M. A. Whisman (Eds.), *APA handbook of contemporary family psychology: Foundations, methods, and contemporary issues across the lifespan* (pp. 687–705). American Psychological Association.

Schachner, D. A., Shaver, P. R., & Gillath, O. (2008). Attachment style and long-term singlehood. *Personal Relationships, 15*, 479–491.

Scharf, M., Mayseless, O., & Kivenson-Baron, I. (2004). Adolescents' attachment representations and developmental tasks in emerging adulthood. *Developmental Psychology, 40*, 430–444.

Schermer, V. L., & Pines, F. (1994). *Ring of fire: Primitive affects and object relations in group psychotherapy.* Routledge.

Schimel, J., Arndt, J., Pyszczynski, T., & Greenberg, J. (2001). Being accepted for who we are: Evidence that social validation of the intrinsic self reduces general defensiveness. *Journal of Personality and Social Psychology, 80*, 35–52.

Schmidt, G. B. (2016). How adult attachment styles relate to perceived psychological contract breach and affective organizational commitment. *Employee Responsibilities and Rights Journal, 28*, 147–170.

Schmitt, D. P. (2010). Romantic attachment from Argentina to Zimbabwe: Patterns of adaptive variation across contexts, cultures, and local ecologies. In P. Erdman & K.-M. Ng (Eds.), *Attachment: Expanding the cultural connections* (pp. 211–226). Routledge.

Schmitt, D. P., & Allik, J. (2005). Simultaneous administration of the Rosenberg Self-Esteem Scale in 53 nations: Exploring the universal and culture-specific features of global self-esteem. *Journal of Personality and Social Psychology, 89*, 623–642.

Schnall, S., Harber, K. D., Stefanucci, J. K., & Proffitt, D. R. (2008). Social support and the perception of geographical slant. *Journal of Experimental Social Psychology, 44*, 1246–1255.

Schoemaker, N. K., Juffer, F., Rippe, R. C. A., Vermeer, H. J., Stoltenborgh, M., Jagersma, G. J., . . . Alink, L. R. A. (2020). Positive parenting in foster care: Testing the effectiveness of a video-feedback intervention program on foster parents' behavior and attitudes. *Children and Youth Services Review, 110*, Article 104779.

Schoemann, A. M., Gillath, O., & Sesko, A. K. (2012). Regrets, I've had a few: Effects of dispositional and manipulated attachment on regret. *Journal of Social and Personal Relationships, 29*, 795–819.

Schoenherr, D., Strauss, B., Paulick, J., Deisenhofer, A.-K., Schwartz, B., Rubel, J., . . . Altmann, U. (2021). Movement synchrony and attachment related anxiety and avoidance in social anxiety disorder. *Journal of Psychotherapy Integration, 31*, 163–189.

Schrage, K. M., Le, B. M., Stellar, J. E., & Impett, E. A. (2022, September 20). Feeling appreciated predicts prosocial motivation in avoidantly attached individuals. *Personality and Social Psychology Bulletin.* [Epub ahead of print].

Schrage, K. M., Maxwell, J. A., Impett, E. A., Keltner, D., & MacDonald, G. (2020). Effects of verbal and nonverbal communication of affection on avoidantly attached partners' emotions and message receptiveness. *Personality and Social Psychology Bulletin, 46*, 1567–1580.

Schwartz, J., Bersin, J., & Pelster, B. (2014). Human Capital Trends 2014 Survey. Retrieved from *http://dupress.com/articles/human-capital-trends-2014-survey-top-10-findings.*

Schwartz, S. H. (1992). Universals in the content and structure of values: Theoretical advances and empirical tests in 20 countries. In M. P. Zanna (Ed.), *Advances in experimental social psychology* (Vol. 25, pp. 1–65). Academic Press.

Scott, S., Briskman, J., Woolgar, M., Humayun, S., & O'Connor, T. G. (2011). Attachment in adolescence: Overlap with parenting and unique prediction of behavioral adjustment. *Journal of Child Psychology and Psychiatry, 52*, 1052–1062.

Scrima, F., Di Stefano, G., Guarnaccia, C., & Lorito, L. (2015). The impact of adult attachment style on organizational commitment and adult attachment in the workplace. *Personality and Individual Differences, 86*, 432–437.

Seibert, A. C., & Kerns, K. A. (2009). Attachment figures in middle childhood. *International Journal of Behavioral Development, 33*, 347–355.

Selcuk, E., Zayas, V., Günaydin, G., Hazan, C., & Kross, E. (2012). Mental representations of attachment figures facilitate recovery following upsetting autobiographical memory recall. *Journal of Personality and Social Psychology, 103*, 362–378.

Seligman, M. E. P. (2002). *Authentic happiness: Using the new positive psychology to realize your potential for lasting fulfillment.* Free Press.

Selterman, D. F., Apetroaia, A., & Waters, E. (2012). Script-like attachment representations in dreams containing current romantic partners. *Attachment and Human Development, 14*, 501–515.

Selterman, D. F., & Maier, M. A. (2013). Secure attachment and material reward both attenuate romantic jealousy. *Motivation and Emotion, 37*, 765–775.

Shalit, A., Popper, M., & Zakay, D. (2010). Followers' attachment styles and their preference for social or personal charismatic leaders. *Leadership and Organizational Development Journal, 31*, 458–472.

Shang, F., Kaniasty, K., Cowlishaw, S., Wade, D., Ma, H., & Forbes, D. (2019). Social support following a natural disaster: A longitudinal study of survivors of the 2013 Lushan earthquake in China. *Psychiatry Research, 273*, 641–646.

Shanock, L. R., & Eisenberger, R. (2006). When supervisors feel supported: Relationships with subordinates' perceived supervisor support, perceived organizational support, and performance. *Journal of Applied Psychology, 91*, 689–695.

Shanock, L. R., Eisenberger, R., Heggestad, E. D.,

Malone, G., Clark, L., Dunn, A., . . . Woznyj, H. (2019). Treating employees well: The value of organizational support theory in human resource management. *Psychologist-Manager Journal, 22*, 168–191.

Shaver, P. R., Collins, N. L., & Clark, C. L. (1996). Attachment styles and internal working models of self and relationship partners. In G. J. O. Fletcher & J. Fitness (Eds.), *Knowledge structures in close relationships: A social psychological approach* (pp. 25–61). Erlbaum.

Shaver, P. R., & Hazan, C. (1984). Incompatibility, loneliness, and limerence. In W. Ickes (Ed.), *Compatible and incompatible relationships* (pp. 163–184). Springer.

Shaver, P. R., Hazan, C., & Bradshaw, D. (1988). Love as attachment: The integration of three behavioral systems. In R. J. Sternberg & M. Barnes (Eds.), *The psychology of love* (pp. 68–99). Yale University Press.

Shaver, P. R., Lavy, S., Saron, C. D., & Mikulincer, M. (2007). Social foundations of the capacity for mindfulness: An attachment perspective. *Psychological Inquiry, 18*, 264–271.

Shaver, P. R., & Mikulincer, M. (2002). Attachment-related psychodynamics. *Attachment and Human Development, 4*, 133–161.

Shaver, P. R., & Mikulincer, M. (2011). An attachment perspective on self-protection and self-enhancement. In C. Sedikides & M. Alicke (Eds.), *Handbook of self-enhancement and self-protection* (pp. 279–297). Guilford Press.

Shaver, P. R., Mikulincer, M., Alonso-Arbiol, I., & Lavy, S. (2010). Assessment of adult attachment across cultures: Conceptual and methodological considerations. In P. Erdman & K.-M. Ng (Eds.), *Attachment: Expanding the cultural connections* (pp. 89–108). Routledge.

Shaver, P. R., Mikulincer, M., Gross, J. T., Stern, J. A., & Cassidy, J. (2016). A life perspective on attachment and care for others: Empathy, altruism, and prosocial behavior. In J. Cassidy & P. R. Shaver (Eds.), Handbook of attachment: Theory, research and clinical applications (3rd ed., pp. 878–916). Guilford Press.

Shaver, P. R., Segev, M., & Mikulincer, M. (2011). A behavioral systems perspective on power and aggression. In P. R. Shaver & M. Mikulincer (Eds.), *Human aggression and violence: Causes, manifestations, and consequences* (pp. 71–87). American Psychological Association.

Shechtman, Z., & Dvir, V. (2006). Attachment style as a predictor of behavior in group counseling with preadolescents. *Group Dynamics, 10*, 29–42.

Shechtman, Z., & Rybko, J. (2004). Attachment style and observed initial self-disclosure as explanatory variables of group functioning. *Group Dynamics, 8*, 207–220.

Shlafer, R. J., Raby, K. L., Lawler, J. M., Hesemeyer, P. S., & Roisman, G. I. (2015). Longitudinal associations between adult attachment states of mind and parenting quality. *Attachment and Human Development, 17*, 83–95.

Shpigel, M. S., Diamond, G. M., & Diamond, G. S. (2012). Changes in parenting behaviors, attachment, depressive symptoms, and suicidal ideation in attachment-based family therapy for depressive and suicidal adolescents. *Journal of Marital and Family Therapy, 38*, 271–283.

Sibley, C. G., & Bulbulia, J. (2012). Faith after an earthquake: A longitudinal study of religion and perceived health before and after the 2011 Christchurch New Zealand Earthquake. *PLOS ONE, 7*, Article e49648.

Sibley, C. G., Fischer, R., & Liu, J. H. (2005). Reliability and validity of the revised Experiences in Close Relationships (ECR-R) self-report measure of adult romantic attachment. *Personality and Social Psychology Bulletin, 31*, 1524–1536.

Sibley, C. G., Greaves, L. M., Satherley, N., Wilson, M. S., Overall, N. C., Lee, C. H. J., . . . Barlow, F. K. (2020). Effects of the COVID-19 pandemic and nationwide lockdown on trust, attitudes toward government, and well-being. *American Psychologist, 75*, 618–630.

Sime, J. D. (1985). Movement toward the familiar: Person and place affiliation in a fire entrapment setting. *Environment and Behavior, 17*, 697–724.

Simpson, J. A., Collins, W. A., Salvatore, J. E., & Sung, S. (2014). The impact of early interpersonal experience on adult romantic relationship functioning. In M. Mikulincer & P. R. Shaver (Eds.), *Mechanisms of social connection: From brain to group* (pp. 221–234). American Psychological Association.

Simpson, J. A., Collins, W. A., Tran, S., & Haydon, K. C. (2007). Attachment and the experience and expression of emotions in adult romantic relationships: A developmental perspective. *Journal of Personality and Social Psychology, 92*, 355–367.

Simpson, J. A., Rholes, W. S., Campbell, L., & Wilson, C. L. (2003). Changes in attachment orientations across the transitions to parenthood. *Journal of Experimental Social Psychology, 39*, 317–331.

Simpson, J. A., Rholes, W. S., & Nelligan, J. S. (1992). Support seeking and support giving within couples in an anxiety-provoking situation: The role of attachment styles. *Journal of Personality and Social Psychology, 62*, 434–446.

Simpson, J. A., Winterheld, H. A., Rholes, W. S., & Oriña, M. M. (2007). Working models of attachment and reactions to different forms of caregiving from romantic partners. *Journal of Personality and Social Psychology, 93*, 466–477.

Singal, J. (2021). *The quick fix: Why fad psychology can't cure our social ills.* Farrar, Straus & Giroux.

Siqueland, L., Rynn, M., & Diamond, G. S. (2005). Cognitive behavioral and attachment based family therapy for anxious adolescents: Phase I and II studies. *Journal of Anxiety Disorders, 19*, 361–381.

Sirois, M.-S., & Bernier, A. (2018). Mother–child relationships and children's psychosocial functioning: The specific roles of attachment security and maternal behavior. *Parenting: Science and Practice, 18*, 172–189.

Slade, A. (2004). Two therapies: Attachment organization and the clinical process. In L. Atkinson & S. Goldberg (Eds.), *Attachment issues in psychopathology and intervention* (pp. 181–206). Erlbaum.

Slade, A., Aber, J. L., Berger, B., Bresgi, I., & Kaplan, M. (2003). *The Parent Development Interview—Revised*. City University of New York.

Slade, A., Grienenberger, J., Bernbach, E., Levy, D., & Locker, A. (2005). Maternal reflective functioning and attachment: Considering the transmission gap. *Attachment and Human Development, 7*, 283–292.

Slade, A., Holland, M. L., Ordway, M. R., Carlson, E. A., Jeon, S., Close, N., . . . Sadler, L. S. (2020). Minding the Baby®: Enhancing parental reflective functioning and infant attachment in an attachment-based, interdisciplinary home visiting program. *Development and Psychopathology, 32*, 123–137.

Slade, A., & Holmes, J. (2019). Attachment and psychotherapy. *Current Opinion in Psychology, 25*, 152–156.

Slade, A., Sadler, L. S., & Mayes, L. C. (2005). Minding the Baby: Enhancing parental reflective functioning in a nursing/mental health home visiting program. In L. J. Berlin, Y. Ziv, L. Amaya-Jackson, & M. T. Greenberg (Eds.), *Enhancing early attachments: Theory, research, intervention, and policy* (pp. 152–177). Guilford Press.

Slade, A., Simpson, T. E., Webb, D., Albertson, J. G., Sadler, L. S., & Close, N. (2018). Minding the Baby: Complex trauma and attachment-based home intervention. In H. Steele & M. Steele (Eds.), *Handbook of attachment-based interventions* (pp. 151–173). Guilford Press.

Slatcher, R. B., Selcuk, E., & Ong, A. D. (2015). Perceived partner responsiveness predicts diurnal cortisol profiles 10 years later. *Psychological Science, 26*, 972–982.

Slemp, G. R., Kern, M. L., Patrick, K. J., & Ryan, R. M. (2018). Leader autonomy support in the workplace: A meta-analytic review. *Motivation and Emotion, 42*, 706–724.

Sloan, E., Maunder, R. G., Hunter, J. J., & Moldofsky, H. (2007). Insecure attachment is associated with the alpha-EEG anomaly during sleep. *Biopsychology Medicine, 1*, Article 20.

Smeets, T. (2010). Autonomic and hypothalamic-pituitary-adrenal stress resilience: Impact of cardiac vagal tone. *Biological Psychology, 84*, 290–295.

Smith, E. R., Murphy, J., & Coats, S. (1999). Attachment to groups: Theory and management. *Journal of Personality and Social Psychology, 77*, 94–110.

Smith, P. N., Gamble, S. A., Cort, N. A., Ward, E. A., He, H., & Talbot, N. L. (2012). Attachment and alliance in the treatment of depressed, sexually abused women. *Depression and Anxiety, 29*, 123–130.

Smith, T. B., McCullough, M. E., & Poll, J. (2003). Religiousness and depression: Evidence for a main effect and the moderating influence of stressful life events. *Psychological Bulletin, 129*, 614–636.

Smither, J. W., Reilly, R. R., Millsap, R. E., Pearlman, K., & Stoffey, R. W. (1993). Applicant reactions to selection procedures. *Personnel Psychology, 46*, 49–76.

Smyth, N., Thorn, L., Oskis, A., Hucklebridge, F., Evans, P., & Clow, A. (2015). Anxious attachment style predicts an enhanced cortisol response to group psychosocial stress. *Stress, 18*, 143–148.

Sockol, L. E. (2018). A systematic review and meta-analysis of interpersonal psychotherapy for perinatal women. *Journal of Affective Disorders, 232*, 316–328.

Solomon, Z., Tsur, N., Levin, Y., Uziel, O., Lahav, M., & Ohry, A. (2017). The implications of war captivity and long-term psychopathology trajectories for telomere length. *Psychoneuroendocrinology, 81*, 122–128.

Somers, J. A., & Luecken, L. J. (2021). Socioemotional mechanisms of children's differential response to the effects of maternal sensitivity on child adjustment. *Parenting: Science and Practice, 21*, 241–275.

Sood, M., Carnelley, K. B., & Newman-Taylor, K. (2021). How does attachment imagery for paranoia work?: Cognitive fusion and beliefs about self and others mediate the impact on paranoia and anxiety. *Psychology and Psychotherapy: Theory, Research and Practice, 94*, 973–993.

Sood, M., Carnelley, K. B., & Newman-Taylor, K. (2022). Do emotion regulation strategies mediate the attachment–paranoia association?: An experimental study of repeated attachment imagery priming and stress buffering. *Psychology and Psychotherapy: Theory, Research and Practice, 95*, 781–806.

Sood, M., & Newman-Taylor, K. (2020). Cognitive fusion mediates the impact of attachment imagery on paranoia and anxiety. *Cognitive Therapy and Research, 44*, 1150–1161.

Sorkin, D. H., Mavandadi, S., Rook, K. S., Biegler, K. A., Kilgore, D., Dow, E., & Ngo-Metzger, Q. (2014). Dyadic collaboration in shared health behavior change: The effects of a randomized trial to test a lifestyle intervention for high-risk Latinas. *Health Psychology, 33*, 566–575.

Spielmann, S. S., Maxwell, J. A., MacDonald, G., & Baratta, P. L. (2013). Don't get your hopes up: Avoidantly attached individuals perceive lower social reward when there is potential for intimacy. *Personality and Social Psychology Bulletin, 39*, 219–236.

Spilt, J. L., Koomen, H. M. Y., & Mantzicopoulos, P. Y. (2010). Young children's perceptions of teacher–child relationships: An evaluation of two instruments and the role of child gender in kindergarten. *Journal of Applied Developmental Psychology, 31,* 428–438.

Spilt, J. L., Koomen, H. M. Y., Thijs, J. T., & van der Leij, A. (2012). Supporting teachers' relationships with disruptive children: The potential of relationship-focused reflection. *Attachment and Human Development, 14,* 305–318.

Spilt, J. L., Vervoort, E., & Verschueren, K. (2018). Teacher–child dependency and teacher sensitivity predict engagement of children with attachment problems. *School Psychology Quarterly, 33,* 419–427.

Sroufe, A. (2020). *A compelling idea: How we become the persons we are.* Safer Society Press.

Sroufe, L. A., Egeland, B., Carlson, E., & Collins, W. A. (2005). *The development of the person: The Minnesota study of risk and adaptation from birth to adulthood.* Guilford Press.

Sroufe, L. A., Fox, N. E., & Pancake, V. R. (1983). Attachment and dependency in developmental perspective. *Child Development, 54,* 1615–1627.

Sroufe, L. A., & Waters, E. (1977). Attachment as an organizational construct. *Child Development, 48,* 1184–1199.

Srull, T. K., & Wyer, R. S. (1979). The role of category accessibility in the interpretation of information about persons: Some determinants and implications. *Journal of Personality and Social Psychology, 37,* 1660–1672.

Stacks, A. M., Muzik, M., Wong, K., Beeghly, M., Huth-Bocks, A., Irwin, J. L., & Rosenblum, K. L. (2014). Maternal reflective functioning among mothers with childhood maltreatment histories: Links to sensitive parenting and infant attachment security. *Attachment and Human Development, 16,* 515–533.

Stams, G.-J. J. M., Juffer, F., van IJzendoorn, M. H., & Hocksbergen, R. C. (2001). Attachment-based intervention in adoptive families in infancy and children's development at age 7: Two follow-up studies. *British Journal of Developmental Psychology, 19,* 159–180.

Stanovich, K. E., & West, R. F. (1983). On priming by a sentence context. *Journal of Experimental Psychology: General, 112,* 1–36.

Stanton, S. C. E., & Campbell, L. (2014). Perceived social support moderates the link between attachment anxiety and health outcomes. *PLOS ONE, 9,* Article e95358.

Stanton, S. C. E., Campbell, L., & Pink, J. C. (2017). Benefits of positive relationship experiences for avoidantly attached individuals. *Journal of Personality and Social Psychology, 113,* 568–588.

Stattin, H., Enebrink, P., Özdemir, M., & Giannotta, F. (2015). A national evaluation of parenting programs in Sweden: The short-term effects using an RCT effectiveness design. *Journal of Consulting and Clinical Psychology, 83,* 1069–1084.

Stavrianopoulos, K. (2015). Enhancing relationship satisfaction among college student couples: An Emotionally Focused Therapy (EFT) approach. *Journal of Couple and Relationship Therapy, 14,* 1–16.

Steele, H., & Steele, M. (Eds.). (2018). *Handbook of attachment-based interventions.* Guilford Press.

Steele, R. D., Waters, T. E. A., Bost, K. K., Vaughn, B. E., Truit, W., Waters, H. S., . . . Roisman, G. I. (2014). Caregiving antecedents of secure base script knowledge: A comparative analysis of young adult attachment representations. *Developmental Psychology, 50,* 2526–2538.

Steffens, N. K., LaRue, C. J., Haslam, C., Walter, Z. C., Cruwys, T., Munt, K. A., . . . Tarrant, M. (2021). Social identification-building interventions to improve health: A systematic review and meta-analysis. *Health Psychology Review, 15,* 85–112.

Stein, A., Netsi, E., Lawrence, P. J., Granger, C., Kempton, C., Craske, M. G., . . . Murray, L. (2018). Mitigating the effect of persistent postnatal depression on child outcomes through an intervention to treat depression and improve parenting: A randomised controlled trial. *Lancet Psychiatry, 5,* 134–144.

Stein, A., Woolley, H., Senior, R., Hertzmann, L., Lovel, M., Lee, J., . . . Fairburn, C. G. (2006). Treating disturbances in the relationship between mothers with bulimic eating disorders and their infants: A randomized controlled trial of video feedback. *American Journal of Psychiatry, 163,* 899–906.

Steinberg, L. D. (2019). *Adolescence* (12th ed.). McGraw-Hill.

Stephens, M. A. P., Franks, M. M., Rook, K. S., Iida, M., Hemphill, R. C., & Salem, J. K. (2013). Spouses' attempts to regulate day-to-day dietary adherence among patients with type 2 diabetes. *Health Psychology, 32,* 1029–1037.

Steptoe, A., Hamer, M., Lin, J., Blackburn, E. H., & Erusalimsky, J. D. (2016). The longitudinal relationship between cortisol responses to mental stress and leukocyte telomere attrition. *Journal of Clinical Endocrinology and Metabolism, 102,* 962–969.

Stern, J. A., Barbarin, O., & Cassidy, J. (2022). Working toward anti-racist perspectives in attachment theory, research, and practice. *Attachment and Human Development, 24,* 392–422.

Stern, J. A., Fraley, R. C., Jones, J. D., Gross, J. T., Shaver, P. R., & Cassidy, J. (2018). Developmental processes across the first two years of parenthood: Stability and change in adult attachment style. *Developmental Psychology, 54,* 975–988.

Sternberg, R. J. (1986). A triangular theory of love. *Psychological Review, 93,* 119–135.

Stevenson, J. C., Emerson, L.-M., & Millings, A. (2017). The relationship between adult attachment orientation and mindfulness: A systematic review and meta-analysis. *Mindfulness, 8,* 1438–1455.

Stevenson, J. C., Millings, A., Emerson, L.-M., Sirois, F., & Rowe, A. C. (2021). Adult attachment and mindfulness: Examining directionality, causality, and theoretical implications. *Journal of Research in Personality, 90,* Article 104043.

Stewart, M., Brown, J. B., Weston, W. W., McWhinney, I. R., McWilliam, C. L., & Freeman, T. R. (1995). *Patient-centered medicine: Transforming the clinical method.* SAGE.

Stockdale, S. E., Wells, K. B., Tang, L., Belin, T. R., Zhang, L., & Sherbourne, C. D. (2007). The importance of social context: Neighborhood stressors, stress-buffering mechanisms, and alcohol, drug, and mental health disorders. *Social Science and Medicine, 65,* 1867–1881.

Stollberg, J., Fritsche, I., & Jonas, E. (2017). The groupy shift: Conformity to liberal in-group norms as a group-based response to threatened personal control. *Social Cognition, 35,* 374–394.

Storr, W. (2021). *The status game: On social position and how we use it.* HarperCollins.

Strachman, A., & Impett, E. A. (2009). Attachment orientations and daily condom use in dating relationships. *Journal of Sex Research, 46,* 1–11.

Strauss, B. M., Mestel, R., & Kirchmann, H. (2011). Changes of attachment status among women with personality disorders undergoing inpatient treatment. *Counseling and Psychotherapy Research, 11,* 275–283.

Stroebe, M., & Schut, H. (2010). The dual process model of coping with bereavement: A decade on. *Omega: Journal of Death and Dying, 61,* 273–289.

Stroebe, M., Schut, H., & Stroebe, W. (2005). Attachment in coping with bereavement: A theoretical integration. *Review of General Psychology, 9,* 48–66.

Stronach, E. P., Toth, S. L., Rogosch, F., & Cicchetti, D. (2013). Preventive interventions and sustained attachment security in maltreated children. *Development and Psychopathology, 25,* 919–930.

Stulp, H. P., Koelen, J., Schep-Akkerman, A., Glas, G. G., & Eurelings-Bontekoe, L. (2019). God representations and aspects of psychological functioning: A meta-analysis. *Cogent Psychology, 6,* Article 1647926.

Stupica, B., Brett, B. E., Woodhouse, S. S., & Cassidy, J. (2019). Attachment security priming decreases children's physiological response to threat. *Child Development, 90,* 1254–1271.

Suchman, N. E., DeCoste, C. L., Castiglioni, N., McMahon, T. J., Rounsaville, B., & Mayes, L. C. (2010). The Mothers and Toddlers Program, an attachment-based parenting intervention for substance using women: Post-treatment results from a randomized clinical pilot. *Attachment and Human Development, 12,* 483–504.

Suchman, N. E., DeCoste, C. L., McMahon, T. J., Dalton, R., Mayes, L. C., & Borelli, J. (2017). Mothering from the Inside Out: Results of a second randomized clinical trial testing a mentalization-based intervention for mothers in addiction treatment. *Development and Psychopathology, 29,* 617–636.

Sultan, S., Attali, C., Gilberg, S., Zenasni, F., & Hartemann, A. (2011). Physicians' understanding of patients' personal representations of their diabetes: Accuracy and association with self-care. *Psychology and Health, 26,* 101–117.

Sun, Y., Wang, L., Jiang, J., & Wang, R. (2020). Your love makes me feel more secure: Boosting attachment security decreases materialistic values. *International Journal of Psychology, 55,* 33–41.

Sutin, A. R., & Gillath, O. (2009). Autobiographical memory phenomenology and content mediate attachment style and psychological distress. *Journal of Counseling Psychology, 56,* 351–364.

Tabachnick, A. R., Raby, K. L., Goldstein, A., Zajac, L., & Dozier, M. (2019). Effects of an attachment-based intervention in infancy on children's autonomic regulation during middle childhood. *Biological Psychology, 143,* 22–31.

Tajfel, H., & Turner, J. C. (1979). An integrative theory of inter-group conflict. In W. G. Austin & S. Worchel (Eds.), *The social psychology of inter-group relations* (pp. 33–47). Brooks/Cole.

Talia, A., Daniel, S. I. F., Miller-Bottome, M., Brambilla, D., Miccoli, D., Safran, J. D, & Lingiardi, V. (2014). AAI predicts patients' in-session interpersonal behavior and discourse: A "move to the level of the relation" for attachment-informed psychotherapy research. *Attachment and Human Development, 16,* 192–209.

Tang, C. S.-K. (2007). Trajectory of traumatic stress symptoms in the aftermath of extreme natural disaster: A study of adult Thai survivors of the 2004 Southeast Asian earthquake and tsunami. *Journal of Nervous and Mental Disease, 195,* 54–59.

Tang, Q., Chen, X., Hu, J., & Liu, Y. (2017). Priming the secure attachment schema affects the emotional face processing bias in attachment anxiety: An fMRI research. *Frontiers in Psychology, 8,* Article 624.

Tangney, J. P., Baumeister, R. F., & Boone, A. L. (2004). High self-control predicts good adjustment, less pathology, better grades, and interpersonal success. *Journal of Personality, 72,* 271–322.

Tarabeh, G., Zreik, G., Oppenheim, D., Sagi-Schwartz, A., & Koren-Karie, N. (2019). Maternal mind-mindedness and its association with attachment: The case of Arab infants and mothers in Israel. *Attachment and Human Development, 21,* 571–581.

Tarabulsy, G. M., Bernier, A., Provost, M. A., Maranda, J., Larose, S., Moss, M., . . . Tessier, R. (2005). Another look inside the gap: Ecological contributions to the transmission of attachment in a sample of adolescent mother–infant dyads. *Developmental Psychology, 41,* 212–224.

Tasca, G. A., Balfour, L., Ritchie, K., & Bissada, H. (2006). Developmental changes in group climate in two types of group therapy for binge-eating disorder: A growth curve analysis. *Psychotherapy Research, 16,* 499–514.

Tasca, G. A., Balfour, L., Ritchie, K., & Bissada, H. (2007). Change in attachment anxiety is associated with improved depression among women with binge eating disorder. *Psychotherapy, 44*, 423–433.

Tasca, G. A., Koszycki, D., Brugnera, A., Chyurlia, L., Hammond, N., Francis, K., . . . Balfour, L. (2019). Testing a stepped care model for binge-eating disorder: A two-step randomized controlled trial. *Psychological Medicine, 49*, 598–606.

Tasca, G. A., & Maxwell, H. (2021). Attachment and group psychotherapy: Applications to work groups and teams. In C. D. Parks & G. A. Tasca (Eds.), *The psychology of groups: The intersection of social psychology and psychotherapy research* (pp. 149–167). American Psychological Association.

Tasca, G. A., Mikail, S. F., & Hewitt, P. L. (2005). Group psychodynamic interpersonal psychotherapy: Summary of a treatment model and outcomes for depressive symptoms. In M. E. Abehan (Ed.), *Focus on psychotherapy research* (pp. 159–188). Nova Science.

Tasca, G. A., Mikail, S. F., & Hewitt, P. L. (2021). *Group psychodynamic-interpersonal psychotherapy*. American Psychological Association.

Tasca, G. A., Ritchie, K., Conrad, G., Balfour, L., Gayton, J., Lybanon, V., & Bissada, H. (2006). Attachment scales predict outcome in a randomized controlled trial of two group therapies for binge eating disorder: An aptitude by treatment interaction. *Psychotherapy Research, 16*, 106–121.

Taubman-Ben-Ari, O., & Mikulincer, M. (2007). The effects of dispositional attachment orientations and contextual priming of attachment security on reckless driving. *Transportation Research Part F: Traffic Psychology and Behavior, 10*, 123–138.

Taylor, P., Rietzschel, J., Danquah, A., & Berry, K. (2015). Changes in attachment representations during psychological therapy. *Psychotherapy Research, 25*, 222–238.

Taylor, P. J., Russ-Eft, D. F., & Taylor, H. (2009). Transfer of management training from alternative perspectives. *Journal of Applied Psychology, 94*, 104–121.

Thibault, J. W., & Kelley, H. H. (1959). *The social psychology of groups*. Wiley.

Thompson, D., & Ciechanowski, P. S. (2003). Attaching a new understanding to the patient–physician relationship in family practice. *Journal of the American Board of Family Practice, 16*, 219–226.

Thompson, P.-M. M., Fosse, T. H., & Skouverøe, J. B. (2021). Leaders that don't care: Investigating leader caregiving from an attachment-theoretical perspective. *Psychologist-Manager Journal, 24*, 141–161.

Thompson, P.-M. M., Glasø, L., & Matthiesen, S. B. (2018). The way I see you: Implicit followership theories explored through the lens of attachment. *Psychologist-Manager Journal, 21*, 85–105.

Thompson, R., & Zuroff, D. C. (2004). The levels of self-criticism scale: Comparative self-criticism and internalized self-criticism. *Personality and Individual Differences, 36*, 419–430.

Thomsen, M. S., Ruocco, A. C., Uliaszek, A. A., Mathiesen, B. B., & Simonsen, E. (2017). Changes in neurocognitive functioning after 6 months of mentalization-based treatment for borderline personality disorder. *Journal of Personality Disorders, 31*, 306–324.

Tmej, A., Fischer-Kern, M., Doering, S., Hörz-Sagstetter, S., Rentrop, M., & Buchheim, A. (2021). Borderline patients before and after one year of transference-focused psychotherapy (TFP): A detailed analysis of change of attachment representations. *Psychoanalytic Psychology, 38*, 12–21.

Tomlinson, J. M., Feeney, B. C., & Peters, B. J. (2020). Growing into retirement: Longitudinal evidence for the importance of partner support for self-expansion. *Psychology and Aging, 35*, 1041–1049.

Tomlinson, J. M., Feeney, B. C., & Van Vleet, M. (2016). A longitudinal investigation of relational catalyst support of goal strivings. *Journal of Positive Psychology, 11*, 246–257.

Tosone, C., Bettmann, J. E., Minami, T., & Jasperson, R. A. (2010). New York City social workers after 9/11: Their attachment, resiliency, and compassion fatigue. *International Journal of Emergency Mental Health, 12*, 103–116.

Toth, S. L., & Gravener, J. (2012). Bridging research and practice: Relational interventions for maltreated children. *Child and Adolescent Mental Health, 17*, 131–138.

Toth, S. L., Maughan, A., Manly, J. T., Spagnola, M., & Cicchetti, D. (2002). The relative efficacy of two interventions in altering maltreated preschool children's representational models: Implications for attachment theory. *Development and Psychopathology, 14*, 877–908.

Toth, S. L., Michl-Petzing, L., Guild, D., & Lieberman, A. F. (2018). Child–parent psychotherapy: Theoretical bases, clinical applications, and empirical support. In H. Steele & M. Steele (Eds.), *Handbook of attachment-based interventions* (pp. 296–317). Guilford Press.

Toth, S. L., Rogosch, F. A., Manly, J. T., & Cicchetti, D. (2006). The efficacy of toddler–parent psychotherapy to reorganize attachment in the young offspring of mothers with major depressive disorder: A randomized preventive trial. *Journal of Consulting and Clinical Psychology, 74*, 1006–1016.

Toumbelekis, M., Liddell, B. J., & Bryant, R. A. (2018). Thinking of attachment figures blocks differential fear conditioning. *Social Cognitive and Affective Neuroscience, 13*, 989–994.

Toumbelekis, M., Liddell, B. J., & Bryant, R. A. (2021a). Secure attachment primes reduce fear consolidation. *Depression and Anxiety, 38*, 1078–1086.

Toumbelekis, M., Liddell, B. J., & Bryant, R. A.

(2021b). Secure attachment priming protects against relapse of fear in young adults. *Translational Psychiatry, 11*, Article 584.
Tracy, J. L., Shaver, P. R., Albino, A. W., & Cooper, M. L. (2003). Attachment styles and adolescent sexuality. In P. Florsheim (Ed.), *Adolescent romance and sexual behavior: Theory, research, and practical implications* (pp. 137–159). Erlbaum.
Tracy, R. E., Wilson, J. P., Slepian, M. L., & Young, S. G. (2020). Facial trustworthiness predicts ingroup inclusion decisions. *Journal of Experimental Social Psychology, 91*, Article 104047.
Tran, S., & Simpson, J. A. (2009). Pro-relationship maintenance behaviors: The joint roles of attachment and commitment. *Journal of Personality and Social Psychology, 97*, 685–698.
Travis, L. A., Bliwise, N. G., Binder, J. L., & Horne-Moyer, H. (2001). Changes in clients' attachment styles over the course of time-limited dynamic psychotherapy. *Psychotherapy, 38*, 149–159.
Trevino, K. M., Pargament, K. I., Krause, N., Ironson, G., & Hill, P. (2019). Stressful events and religious/spiritual struggle: Moderating effects of the general orienting system. *Psychology of Religion and Spirituality, 11*, 214–224.
Trief, P., Sandberg, J. G., Ploutz-Snyder, R., Brittain, R., Cibula, D., Scales, K., & Weinstock, R. S. (2011). Promoting couples collaboration in type 2 diabetes: The diabetes support project pilot data. *Families, Systems and Health, 29*, 253–261.
Tropp, L. R. (2021). Crossing to safety: Attachment processes in intergroup contact. *Journal of Social Issues, 77*, 86–104.
Troxel, W. M., Cyranowski, J. M., Hall, M., Frank, E., & Buysee, D. J. (2007). Attachment anxiety, relationship context, and sleep in women with recurrent major depression. *Psychosomatic Medicine, 69*, 692–699.
Troxel, W. M., & Germain, A. (2011). Insecure attachment is an independent correlate of objective sleep disturbances in military veterans. *Sleep Medicine, 12*, 860–865.
Troyer, D., & Greitemeyer, T. (2018). The impact of attachment orientations on empathy in adults: Considering the mediating role of emotion regulation strategies and negative affectivity. *Personality and Individual Differences, 122*, 198–205.
Tsvieli, N., & Diamond, G. M. (2018). Therapist interventions and emotional processing in attachment-based family therapy for unresolved anger. *Psychotherapy, 55*, 289–297.
Tsvieli, N., Lifshitz, C., & Diamond, G. M. (2022). Corrective attachment episodes in attachment-based family therapy: The power of enactment. *Psychotherapy Research, 32*, 209–222.
Tsvieli, N., Nir-Gottlieb, O., Lifshitz, C., Diamond, G. S., Kobak, R., & Diamond, G. M. (2020). Therapist interventions associated with productive emotional processing in the context of attachment-based family therapy for depressed and suicidal adolescents. *Family Process, 59*, 428–444.
Tuck, N. L., & Consedine, N. S. (2015). Breast cancer screening: The role of attachment. *Psychology, Health and Medicine, 20*, 400–409.
Tuckman, B. W. (1965). Developmental sequence in small groups. *Psychological Bulletin, 63*, 384–399.
Tuckman, B. W., & Jensen, M. A. (1977). Stages of small-group development revisited. *Group and Organization Studies, 2*, 419–427.
Tulloch, H., Greenman, P. S., Demidenko, N., & Johnson, S. M. (2017). *Healing Hearts Together: A cardiac couple in conversation with Dr. Sue Johnson* [DVD]. University of Ottawa Heart Institute.
Tulloch, H., Johnson, S. M., Demidenko, N., Clyde, M., Bouchard, K., & Greenman, P. S. (2021). An attachment-based intervention for patients with cardiovascular disease and their partners: A proof-of-concept study. *Health Psychology, 40*, 909–919.
Tung, E. S., Ruffing, E. G., Paine, D. R., Jankowski, P. J., & Sandage, S. J. (2018). Attachment to God as mediator of the relationship between God representations and mental health. *Journal of Spirituality in Mental Health, 20*, 95–113.
Twemlow, S. W., Fonagy, P., Campbell, C., & Sacco, F. C. (2018). Creating a peaceful school learning environment: Attachment and mentalization efforts to promote creative learning in kindergarten through fifthgrade elementary school students with broad extension to all grades and some organizations. In H. Steele & M. Steele (Eds.), *Handbook of attachment-based interventions* (pp. 360–374). Guilford Press.
Twemlow, S. W., Fonagy, P., Sacco, F. C., Gies, M. L., Evans, R., & Ewbank, R. (2001). Creating a peaceful school learning environment: A controlled study of an elementary school intervention to reduce violence. *American Journal of Psychiatry, 158*, 808–810.
Twemlow, S. W., & Sacco, F. C. (2012). *Preventing bullying and school violence*. American Psychiatric Publishing.
Tyrrell, C. L., Dozier, M., Teague, G. B., & Fallot, R. D. (1999). Effective treatment relationships for persons with serious psychiatric disorders: The importance of attachment states of mind. *Journal of Consulting and Clinical Psychology, 67*, 725–733.
Uchino, B. N., Cacioppo, J. T., & Kiecolt-Glaser, J. K. (1996). The relationship between social support and physiological processes: A review with emphasis on underlying mechanisms and implications for health. *Psychological Bulletin, 119*, 488–531.
Uhl, I., Klackl, J., Hansen, N., & Jonas, E. (2018). Undesirable effects of threatening climate change information: A cross-cultural study. *Group Processes and Intergroup Relations, 21*, 513–529.
Vail, K. E., III, Arndt, J., & Abdollahi, A. (2012). Exploring the existential function of religion and supernatural agent beliefs among Christians,

Muslims, Atheists, and Agnostics. *Personality and Social Psychology Bulletin, 38*, 1288–1300.

Valadez, E. A., Tottenham, N., Tabachnick, A. R., & Dozier, M. (2020). Early parenting intervention effects on brain responses to maternal cues among high-risk children. *American Journal of Psychiatry, 177*, 818–826.

Van der Asdonk, S., de Haan, W. D., van Berkel, S. R., van IJzendoorn, M. H., Rippe, R. C. A., Kuiper, C., . . . Alink, L. R. A. (2020). Effectiveness of an attachment-based intervention for the assessment of parenting capacities in maltreating families: A randomized controlled trial. *Infant Mental Health Journal, 41*, 821–835.

van der Mark, I. L., van IJzendoorn, M. H., & Bakermans-Kranenburg, M. J. (2002). Development of empathy in girls during the second year of life: Associations with parenting, attachment, and temperament. *Social Development, 11*, 451–468.

van der Vorst, H., Engels, R. C. M. E., Meeus, W., & Deković, M. (2006). Parental attachment, parental control, and early development of alcohol use: A longitudinal study. *Psychology of Addictive Behaviors, 20*, 107–116.

van IJzendoorn, M. H. (1995). Adult attachment representations, parental responsiveness, and infant attachment: A meta-analysis on the predictive validity of the Adult Attachment Interview. *Psychological Bulletin, 117*, 387–403.

van IJzendoorn, M. H., & de Wolff, M. S. (1997). In search of the absent father—meta-analysis of infant–father attachment: A rejoinder to our discussants. *Child Development, 68*, 604–609.

Van IJzendoorn, M. H., Sagi, A., & Lambermon, M. W. E. (1992). The multiple caretaker paradox: Data from Holland and Israel. In R. C. Pianta (Ed.), *Beyond the parent: The role of other adults in children's lives* (pp. 5–24). Jossey-Bass.

Van IJzendoorn, M. H., Schuengel, C., Wang, Q., & Bakermans-Kranenburg, M. J. (2022, January 17). Improving parenting, child attachment, and externalizing behaviors: Meta-analysis of the first 25 randomized controlled trials on the effects of video-feedback intervention to promote positive parenting and sensitive discipline. *Development and Psychopathology*. [Epub ahead of print].

Van Ryzin, M. J., Carlson, E. A., & Sroufe, L. A. (2011). Attachment discontinuity in a high-risk sample. *Attachment and Human Development, 13*, 381–401.

Van Vleet, M., & Helgeson, V. S. (2019). I am a rock; I am an island: Implications of avoidant attachment for communal coping in adults with type 2 diabetes. *Journal of Social and Personal Relationships, 36*, 3711–3732.

Van Zeijl, J., Mesman, J., van IJzendoorn, M. H., Bakermans-Kranenburg, M. J., Juffer, F., Stolk, M. N., . . . Alink, L. R. (2006). Attachment-based intervention for enhancing sensitive discipline in mothers of one- to three-year-old children at risk for externalizing behavior problems. *Journal of Consulting and Clinical Psychology, 74*, 994–1005.

Vancraeyveldt, C., Verschueren, K., Wouters, S., Craeyevelt, S., Noortgate, W., & Colpin, H. (2015). Improving teacher–child relationship quality and teacher-rated behavioral adjustment amongst externalizing preschoolers: Effects of a two-component intervention. *Journal of Abnormal Child Psychology, 43*, 243–257.

Vandenbroucke, L., Spilt, J., Verschueren, K., & Baeyens, D. (2017). Keeping the spirits up: The effect of teachers' and parents' emotional support on children's working memory performance. *Frontiers in Psychology, 8*, Article 512.

Vasconcellos, D., Parker, P. D., Hilland, T., Cinelli, R., Owen, K. B., Kapsal, N., . . . Lonsdale, C. (2020). Self-determination theory applied to physical education: A systematic review and meta-analysis. *Journal of Educational Psychology, 112*, 1444–1469.

Vasquez, A. C., Patall, E. A., Fong, C. J., Corrigan, A. S., & Pine, L. (2016). Parent autonomy support, academic achievement, and psychosocial functioning: A meta-analysis of research. *Educational Psychology Review, 28*, 605–644.

Vaughn, B. E., & Bost, K. K. (2016). Attachment and temperament as intersecting developmental products and interactive developmental contexts throughout infancy and childhood. In J. Cassidy & P. R. Shaver (Eds.), *Handbook of attachment: Theory, research, and clinical applications* (3rd ed., pp. 202–222). Guilford Press.

Venkataramani, V., Labianca, G., & Grosser, T. (2013). Positive and negative workplace relationships, social satisfaction, and organizational attachment. *Journal of Applied Psychology, 98*, 1028–1039.

Venta, A., & Sharp, C. (2015). Mentalizing mediates the relation between attachment and peer problems among inpatient adolescents. *Journal of Infant, Child and Adolescent Psychotherapy, 14*, 323–340.

Verhage, M. L., Fearon, R. M. P., Schuengel, C., van IJzendoorn, M. H., Bakermans-Kranenburg, M. J., Madigan, S., . . . Brisch, K.-H. (2018). Examining ecological constraints on the intergenerational transmission of attachment via individual participant data meta-analysis. *Child Development, 89*, 2023–2037.

Verhage, M. L., Schuengel, C., Madigan, S., Fearon, R. M. P., Oosterman, M., Cassibba, R., . . . van IJzendoorn, M. H. (2016). Narrowing the transmission gap: A synthesis of three decades of research on intergenerational transmission of attachment. *Psychological Bulletin, 142*, 337–366.

Verhees, M. W. F. T., Ceulemans, E., & Bosmans, G. (2019). Strengthening attachment-based therapies: A case for cognitive bias modification? *Journal of the American Academy of Child and Adolescent Psychiatry, 58*, 732–733.

Verschueren, K., & Koomen, H. M. Y. (2012). Teacher–child relationships from an attachment perspective. *Attachment and Human Development, 14,* 205-211.

Vicary, A. M., & Fraley, R. C. (2007). Choose your own adventure: Attachment dynamics in a simulated relationship. *Personality and Social Psychology Bulletin, 33,* 1279-1291.

Vilchinsky, N., Dekel, R., Asher, Z., Leibowitz, M., & Mosseri, M. (2013). The role of illness perceptions in the attachment-related process of affect regulation. *Anxiety, Stress and Coping, 26,* 314-329.

Vilchinsky, N., Dekel, R., Revenson, T. A., Liberman, G., & Mosseri, M. (2015). Caregivers' burden and depressive symptoms: The moderational role of attachment orientations. *Health Psychology, 34,* 262-269.

Vrijhof, C. I., Euser, S., Bakermans-Kranenburg, M. J., van den Bulk, B. G., Bosdriesz, J. R., Linting, M., . . . van IJzendoorn, M. H. (2020). Effects of parental sensitivity in different contexts on children's hot and cool effortful control. *Journal of Family Psychology, 34,* 459-468.

Waddington, C. H. (1957). *The strategy of the genes.* Allen & Unwin.

Walker, J. G., Johnson, S., Manion, I., & Cloutier, P. (1996). Emotionally focused marital intervention for couples with chronically ill children. *Journal of Consulting and Clinical Psychology, 64,* 1029-1036.

Wallin, D. J. (2007). *Attachment in psychotherapy.* Guilford Press.

Waraan, L., Rognli, E. W., Czajkowski, N. O., Aalberg, M., & Mehlum. L. (2021). Effectiveness of attachment-based family therapy compared to treatment as usual for depressed adolescents in community mental health clinics. *Child and Adolescent Psychiatry and Mental Health, 15,* Article PMC7881666.

Waslin, S. M., Kochendorfer, L. B., Blier, B., Brumariu, L. E., & Kerns, K. A. (2022, April 7). Parental emotion socialization: Relations with adjustment, security, and maternal depression in early adolescence. *Emotion.* [Epub ahead of print].

Waters, E., & Deane, K. E. (1985). Defining and assessing individual differences in attachment relationships: Q-methodology and the organization of behavior in infancy and early childhood. *Monographs of the Society for Research in Child Development, 50,* 41-65.

Waters, H. S., & Waters, E. (2006). The attachment working models concept: Among other things, we build script-like representations of secure base experiences. *Attachment and Human Development, 8,* 185-198.

Waters, T. E. A., Magro, S. W., Alhajeri, J., Yang, R., Groh, A., Haltigan, J. T., . . . Roisman, G. I. (2021). Early child care experiences and attachment representations at age 18 years: Evidence from the NICHD study of Early Child Care and Youth Development. *Developmental Psychology, 57,* 548-556.

Waters, T. E. A., Raby, K. L., Ruiz, S. K., Martin, J., & Roisman, G. I. (2018). Adult attachment representations and the quality of romantic and parent-child relationships: An examination of the contributions of coherence of discourse and secure base script knowledge. *Developmental Psychology, 54,* 2371-2381.

Waters, T. E. A., Ruiz, S. K., & Roisman, G. I. (2017). Origins of secure base script knowledge and the developmental construction of attachment representations. *Child Development, 88,* 198-209.

Watson, J. C., Steckley, P. L., & McMullen, E. J. (2014). The role of empathy in promoting change. *Psychotherapy Research, 24,* 286-298.

Weber, C., & Federico, C. M. (2007). Interpersonal attachment and patterns of ideological belief. *Political Psychology, 28,* 389-416.

Webster-Stratton, C. (2005). The Incredible Years: A training series for the prevention and treatment of conduct problems in young children. In E. D. Hibbs & P. S. Jensen (Eds.), *Psychosocial treatments for child and adolescent disorders: Empirically based strategies for clinical practice* (pp. 507-555). American Psychological Association.

Wegner, R., Roy, A. R. K., Gorman, K. R., & Ferguson, K. (2018). Attachment, relationship communication style and the use of jealousy induction techniques in romantic relationships. *Personality and Individual Differences, 129,* 6-11.

Weiss, R. S. (1973). *Loneliness: The experience of emotional and social isolation.* MIT Press.

Weiss, R. S. (1993). Loss and recovery. In M. S. Stroebe, W. Stroebe, & R. O. Hansson (Eds.), *Handbook of bereavement* (pp. 271-284). New York: Cambridge University Press.

Weissman, M. M., Klerman, G. L., Prusoff, B. A., Sholomskas, D., & Padian, N. (1981). Depressed outpatients: Results one year after treatment with drugs and/or interpersonal psychotherapy. *Archives of General Psychiatry, 38,* 51-55.

Weissman, M. M., Markowitz, J. C., & Klerman, G. L. (2000). *Comprehensive guide to interpersonal psychotherapy.* Basic Books.

Weissman, M. M., Markowitz, J. C., & Klerman, G. L. (2007). *Clinician's quick guide to interpersonal psychotherapy.* Oxford University Press.

Weissman, M. M., Markowitz, J. C., & Klerman, G. L. (2018). *The guide to interpersonal psychotherapy* (updated and expanded ed.). Oxford University Press.

Weissman, N., Batten, S. V., Rheem, K. D., Wiebe, S. A., Pasillas, R. M., Potts, W., . . . Dixon, L. B. (2018). The effectiveness of emotionally focused couples therapy with veterans with PTSD: A pilot study. *Journal of Couple and Relationship Therapy, 17,* 25-41.

Wenegrat, B. (1989). *The divine archetype: The sociobiology and psychology of religion.* Lexington Books.

Wentzel, K. R. (1998). Social relationships and motivation in middle school: The role of parents, teachers, and peers. *Journal of Educational Psychology, 90*, 202–209.

Wentzel, K. R., & Asher, S. R. (1995). The academic lives of neglected, rejected, popular, and controversial children. *Child Development, 66*, 754–763.

Werner, C. D., Vermeer, H. J., Linting, M., & van Ijzendoorn, M. H. (2018). Video-feedback intervention in center-based child care: A randomized controlled trial. *Early Childhood Research Quarterly, 42*, 93–104.

Westmaas, J., & Silver, R. C. (2001). The role of attachment in responses to victims of life crises. *Journal of Personality and Social Psychology, 80*, 425–438.

Wheeler, L., & Reis, H. T. (1991). Self-recording of everyday life events: Origins, types, and uses. *Journal of Personality, 59*, 339–354.

Wheeler, S. C., & DeMarree, K. G. (2009). Multiple mechanisms of prime-to-behavior effects. *Social and Personality Psychology Compass, 3*, 566–581.

Whipple, N., Bernier, A., & Mageau, G. A. (2011). A dimensional approach to maternal attachment state of mind: Relations to maternal sensitivity and maternal autonomy support. *Developmental Psychology, 47*, 396–403.

White, J. R., & Freeman, A. S. (Eds.). (2000). *Cognitive-behavioral group therapy: For specific problems and populations*. American Psychological Association.

Wickham, R. E., Reed, D. E., & Williamson, R. E. (2015). Establishing the psychometric properties of the self and perceived-partner Authenticity in Relationships Scale-Short Form (AIRS-SF): Measurement invariance, reliability, and incremental validity. *Personality and Individual Differences, 77*, 62–67.

Wiebe, S. A., Elliott, C., Johnson, S. M., Moser, M. B., Dalgleish, T. L., Lafontaine, M.-F., & Tasca, G. A. (2019). Attachment change in emotionally focused couple therapy and sexual satisfaction outcomes in a two-year follow-up study. *Journal of Couple and Relationship Therapy, 18*, 1–21.

Wiebe, S. A., & Johnson, S. M. (2016). A review of the research in emotionally focused therapy for couples. *Family Process, 55*, 390–407.

Wiebe, S. A., Johnson, S. M., Burgess Moser, M., Dalgleish, T. L., & Tasca, G. A. (2017). Predicting follow-up outcomes in emotionally focused couple therapy: The role of change in trust, relationship-specific attachment, and emotional engagement. *Journal of Marital and Family Therapy, 43*, 213–226.

Wiebe, S. A., Johnson, S. M., Lafontaine, M.-F., Burgess Moser, M., Dalgleish, T. L., & Tasca, G. A. (2017). Two-year follow-up outcomes in emotionally focused couple therapy: An investigation of relationship satisfaction and attachment trajectories. *Journal of Marital and Family Therapy, 43*, 227–244.

Wieselquist, J., Rusbult, C. E., Foster, C. A., & Agnew, C. R. (1999). Commitment, pro-relationship behavior, and trust in close relationships. *Journal of Personality and Social Psychology, 77*, 942–966.

Wilkinson, L. L., Rowe, A. C., & Heath, G. H. (2013). Eating me up inside: Priming attachment security and anxiety, and their effects on snacking. *Journal of Social and Personal Relationships, 30*, 795–804.

Williford, A. P., Carter, L. M., Pianta, R. C. (2016). Attachment and school readiness. In J. Cassidy & P. R. Shaver (Eds.), *Handbook of attachment: Theory, research, and clinical applications* (3rd ed., pp. 966–982). Guilford Press.

Williford, A. P., LoCasale-Crouch, J., Whittaker, J. V., DeCoster, J., Hartz, K. A., Carter, L. M., . . . Hatfield, B. (2017). Changing teacher–child dyadic interactions to improve preschool children's externalizing behaviors. *Child Development, 88*, 1544–1553.

Wilson, C. L., & Ruben, M. A. (2011). A pain in her arm: Romantic attachment orientations and the tourniquet task. *Personal Relationships, 18*, 242–265.

Wilson, C. L., & Simpson, J. A. (2016). Childbirth pain, attachment orientations, and romantic partner Support during labor and delivery. *Personal Relationships, 23*, 622–644.

Winkielman, P., & Gogolushko, Y. (2018). Influence of sub-optimally and optimally presented affective pictures and words on consumption-related behavior. *Frontiers in Psychology, 8*, Article 2261.

Wiseman, H. (2017). The quest for connection in interpersonal and therapeutic relationships. *Psychotherapy Research, 27*, 469–487.

Wiseman, H., & Tishby, O. (2014). Client attachment, attachment to the therapist and client–therapist attachment match: How do they relate to change in psychodynamic psychotherapy? *Psychotherapy Research, 24*, 392–406.

Wittenborn, A. K., Liu, T., Ridenour, T. A., Lachmar, E. M., Mitchell, E. A., & Seedall, R. B. (2019). Randomized controlled trial of emotionally focused couple therapy compared to treatment as usual for depression: Outcomes and mechanisms of change. *Journal of Marital and Family Therapy, 45*, 395–409.

Wong, T.-Y., Greenman, P. S., & Beaudoin, V. (2018). "Hold Me Tight": The generalizability of an attachment-based group intervention to Chinese Canadian couples. *Journal of Couple and Relationship Therapy, 17*, 42–60.

Woodhead, J., Bland, K., & Baradon, T. (2006). Focusing the lens: The use of digital video in the practice and evaluation of parent-infant psychotherapy. *Infant Observation, 9*, 139–150.

Woodhouse, S. S., & Gelso, C. J. (2008). Volunteer client adult attachment, memory for in-session emotion, and mood awareness: An affect regulation perspective. *Journal of Counseling Psychology, 55*, 197–208.

Woodhouse, S. S., Powell, B., Cooper, G., Hoffman, K., & Cassidy, J. (2018). The circle of security intervention: Design, research, and implementation. In H. Steele & M. Steele (Eds.), *Handbook of attachment-based interventions* (pp. 50–78). Guilford Press.

Woodhouse, S. S., Scott, J. R., Hepworth, A. D., & Cassidy, J. (2020). Secure base provision: A new approach to examining links between maternal caregiving and infant attachment. *Child Development, 91*, e249–e265.

Woolley, H., Hertzmann, L., & Stein, A. (2008). Video-feedback intervention with mothers with postnatal eating disorders and their infants. In F. Juffer, M. J. Bakermans-Kranenburg, & M. H. van IJzendoorn (Eds.), *Promoting positive parenting: An attachment-based intervention* (pp. 111–138). Taylor & Francis.

World Health Organization. (2018). *International classification of diseases for mortality and morbidity statistics* (11th rev.). Author.

Wu, C.-H., & Parker, S. K. (2017). The role of leader support in facilitating proactive work behavior: A perspective from attachment theory. *Journal of Management, 43*, 1025–1049.

Wu, L., Gu, R., Shi, X., Wang, B., & Zhang, J. (2020). Boosting attachment security to cope with threats: Behavioral and ERPs findings. *International Journal of Psychophysiology, 149*, 8–14.

Wysocki, T., Harris, M. A., Buckloh, L. M., Mertlich, D., Lochrie, A. S., Taylor, A., . . . White, N. H. (2008). Randomized, controlled trial of behavioral family systems therapy for diabetes: Maintenance and generalization of effects on parent–adolescent communication. *Behavior Therapy, 39*, 33–46.

Yagmur, S., Mesman, J., Malda, M., Bakermans-Kranenburg, M. J., & Ekmekci, H. (2014). Video-feedback intervention increases sensitive parenting in ethnic minority mothers: A randomized control trial. *Attachment and Human Development, 16*, 371–386.

Yalom, I. D. (1995). *The theory and practice of group psychotherapy* (4th ed.). Basic Books.

Yalom, I. D., & Leszcz, M. (2005). *The theory and practice of group psychotherapy* (5th ed.). Basic Books.

Yarger, H. A., Bernard, K., Caron, E., Wallin, A., & Dozier, M. (2020). Enhancing parenting quality for young children adopted internationally: Results of a randomized controlled trial. *Journal of Clinical Child and Adolescent Psychology, 49*, 378–390.

Yarger, H. A., Hoye, J. R., & Dozier, M. (2016). Trajectories of change in attachment and biobehavioral catch-up among high-risk mothers: A randomized clinical trial. *Infant Mental Health Journal, 37*, 525–536.

Yip, J., Ehrhardt, K., Black, H., & Walker, D. O. (2018). Attachment theory at work: A review and directions for future research. *Journal of Organizational Behavior, 39*, 185–198.

Yotsidi, V., Stalikas, A., Pezirkianidis, C., & Pouloudi, M. (2019). The relationships between client resistance and attachment to therapist in psychotherapy. *Journal of Contemporary Psychotherapy, 49*, 99–109.

Young, J. Z. (1964). *A model for the brain*. Oxford University Press.

Yu, C., & Frenkel, S. J. (2013). Explaining task performance and creativity from perceived organizational support theory: Which mechanisms are more important? *Journal of Organizational Behavior, 34*, 1165–1181.

Zafra-Tanaka, J. H., Pacheco-Barrios, K., Tellez, W. A., & Taype-Rondan, A. (2019). Effects of dog-assisted therapy in adults with dementia: A systematic review and meta-analysis. *BMC Psychiatry, 19*, Article 41.

Zajac, K., & Kobak, R. (2006). Attachment. In G. G. Bear & K. M. Minke (Eds.), *Children's needs III: Development, prevention, and intervention* (pp. 379–389). National Association of School Psychologists.

Zajac, L., Raby, K. L., & Dozier, M. (2020). Sustained effects on attachment security in middle childhood: Results from a randomized clinical trial of the Attachment and Biobehavioral Catch-up (ABC) intervention. *Journal of Child Psychology and Psychiatry, 61*, 417–424.

Zajdel, M., Helgeson, V. S., Kelly, C. S., & Berg, C. A. (2021). Shared illness appraisal and self-efficacy among adults with type I diabetes. *Journal of Health Psychology, 26*, 390–400.

Zajdel, M., Helgeson, V. S., Seltman, H. J., Korytkowski, M. T., & Hausmann, L. R. M. (2018). Daily communal coping in couples with type 2 diabetes: Links to mood and self-care. *Annals of Behavioral Medicine, 52*, 228–238.

Zajonc, R. B. (1984). On the primacy of affect. *American Psychologist, 39*, 117–123.

Zaporowska-Stachowiak, I., Stachowiak, K., & Stachnik, K. (2019). Two is a perfect number: Patient–doctor relationship and patient attachment style in palliative care. *Journal of Health Psychology, 24*, 549–560.

Zayas, V., Mischel, W., Shoda, Y., & Aber, J. L. (2011). Roots of adult attachment: Maternal caregiving at 18 months predicts adult peer and partner attachment. *Social Psychological and Personality Science, 2*, 289–297.

Zayas, V., & Shoda, Y. (2005). Do automatic reactions elicited by thoughts of romantic partner, mother, and self relate to adult romantic attachment? *Personality and Social Psychology Bulletin, 31*, 1011–1025.

Zeegers, M. A. J., Colonnesi, C., Stams, G.-J. J. M., & Meins, E. (2017). Mind matters: A meta-analysis on parental mentalization and sensitivity as predictors of infant–parent attachment. *Psychological Bulletin, 143*, 1245–1272.

Zeegers, M. A. J., de Vente, W., Nikolić, M., Majdandžić, M., Bögels, S. M., & Colonnesi, C. (2018). Mothers' and fathers' mind-mindedness influences physiological emotion regulation of infants across the first year of life. *Developmental Science, 21*, 1–18.

Zeifman, D., & Hazan, C. (2016). Pair bonds as attachments: Mounting evidence in support of Bowlby's hypothesis. In J. Cassidy & P. R. Shaver (Eds.), *Handbook of Attachment: Theory, research, and clinical applications* (3rd ed., pp. 416–434). Guilford Press.

Zhou, T., Guan, R., & Sun, L. (2021). Perceived organizational support and PTSD symptoms of frontline healthcare workers in the outbreak of COVID-19 in Wuhan: The mediating effects of self-efficacy and coping strategies. *Applied Psychology: Health and Well-Being, 13*, 745–760.

Zhou, Y., Arend, J., Mufson, L., & Gunlicks-Stoessel, M. (2021). Change in dysfunctional attitudes and attachment in interpersonal psychotherapy for depressed adolescents. *Psychotherapy Research, 31*, 258–266.

Zilberstein, K. (2014). The use and limitations of attachment theory in child psychotherapy. *Psychotherapy, 51*, 93–103.

Zilcha-Mano, S., Mikulincer, M., & Shaver, P. R. (2011a). An attachment perspective on human–pet relationships: Conceptualization and assessment of pet attachment orientations. *Journal of Research in Personality, 45*, 345–357.

Zilcha-Mano, S., Mikulincer, M., & Shaver, P. R. (2011b). Pet in the therapy room: An attachment perspective on animal-assisted therapy. *Attachment and Human Development, 13*, 541–561.

Zilcha-Mano, S., Mikulincer, M., & Shaver, P. R. (2012). Pets as safe havens and secure bases: The moderating role of pet attachment orientations. *Journal of Research in Personality, 46*, 571–580.

Zimmer-Gembeck, M. J., Rudolph, J., Edwards, E.-J., Swan, K., Campbell, S. M., Hawes, T., & Webb, H. J. (2022). The circle of security parenting program (COS-P): A randomized controlled trial of a low intensity, individualized attachment-based program with at-risk caregivers. *Behavior Therapy, 53*, 208–223.

Zimmermann, P., Mohr, C., & Spangler, G. (2009). Genetic and attachment influences on adolescents' regulation of autonomy and aggressiveness. *Journal of Child Psychology and Psychiatry, 50*, 1339–1347.

Zisk, A., Abbott, C. H., Bounoua, N., Diamond, G. S., & Kobak, R. (2019). Parent–teen communication predicts treatment benefit for depressed and suicidal adolescents. *Journal of Consulting and Clinical Psychology, 87*, 1137–1148.

Zuroff, D. C., & Blatt, S. J. (2006). The therapeutic relationship in the brief treatment of depression: Contributions to clinical improvement and enhanced adaptive capacities. *Journal of Consulting and Clinical Psychology, 74*, 199–206.

Zuroff, D. C., Kelly, A. C., Leybman, M. J., Blatt, S. J., & Wampold, B. E. (2010). Between-therapist and within-therapist differences in the quality of the therapeutic relationship: Effects on maladjustment and self-critical perfectionism. *Journal of Clinical Psychology, 66*, 681–697.

Index

Note. *f* or *t* following a page number indicates a figure or a table.